FETAL
AND MATERNAL
MEDICINE

FETAL
AND MATERNAL
MEDICINE

Edited by

E. J. QUILLIGAN, M.D.

Professor of Obstetrics and Gynecology and Associate Vice-President
   of Health Affairs
University of Southern California School of Medicine
Women's Hospital
Los Angeles, California

NORMAN KRETCHMER, M.D., Ph.D.

Director
National Institute of Child Health and Human Development
Bethesda, Maryland

A WILEY MEDICAL PUBLICATION
JOHN WILEY & SONS
New York • Chichester • Brisbane • Toronto

Library of Congress Cataloging in Publication Data:

Main entry under title:

Fetal and maternal medicine.

  (A Wiley medical publication)
  Includes index.
  1. Pregnancy, Complications of. 2. Fetus—Diseases.
3. Infants (Newborn)—Diseases. 4. Pregnancy.
I. Quilligan, Edward J. II. Kretchmer, Norman,
1923–   [DNLM: 1. Fetal diseases. 2. Infant,
Newborn, Diseases. 3. Pregnancy complications.
WQ211 F419]
RG571.F47   618.3′2   79-4345
ISBN 0-471-50737-7

Printed in the United States of America

10 9 8 7 6 5 4 3 2 1

Contributors

Charles Alford, Jr., M.D.
Meyer Professor of Pediatric Research
University of Alabama School of Medicine
Birmingham, Alabama

Tom P. Barden, M.D.
Professor of Obstetrics and Gynecology
Department of Obstetrics and Gynecology
University of Cincinnati College of Medicine
Cincinnati, Ohio

Frederick C. Battaglia, M.D.
Professor and Chairman of Pediatrics
Department of Pediatrics
University of Colorado School of Medicine
Denver, Colorado

Joseph A. Bellanti, M.D.
Professor of Pediatrics and Microbiology
Director, International Center for Interdisciplinary Studies of Immunology
Georgetown University Hospital
Washington, D.C.

Ricardo Bernales, M.D.
Fellow, Immunology Center
Georgetown University Hospital
Washington, D.C.

Barbara K. Burton, M.D.
Assistant Professor of Pediatrics
Department of Pediatrics
The Bowman Gray School of Medicine of Wake Forest University
Winston-Salem, North Carolina

William H. Clewell, M.D.
Assistant Professor of Gynecology
Department of Obstetrics and Gynecology
University of Colorado School of Medicine
Denver, Colorado

Larry N. Cook, M.D.
Director, Division of Neonatal Medicine
Assistant Professor of Pediatrics and Obstetrics and Gynecology
University of Louisville School of Medicine
Louisville, Kentucky

Marvin Cornblath, M.D.
Professor of Pediatrics
University of Maryland Hospital
Special Assistant to the Scientific Director for Clinical Programs
Intramural Research Program
National Institute of Child Health and Human Development
Bethesda, Maryland

Frank Falkner, M.D., F.R.C.P.
Professor of Maternal and Child Health
School of Public Health
University of Michigan
Ann Arbor, Michigan

Philip M. Farrell, M.D., Ph.D.
Assistant Professor of Pediatrics
Center for Health Sciences
University of Wisconsin-Madison
Madison, Wisconsin

Delbert A. Fisher, M.D.
Professor of Pediatrics and Medicine
University of California
Los Angeles School of Medicine
Los Angeles, California
Director, Perinatal Research Laboratories
Harbor General Hospital
Torrance, California

Steven G. Gabbe, M.D.
Associate Professor
Department of Obstetrics and Gynecology
Hospital University of Pennsylvania
Philadelphia, Pennsylvania

Charles H. Hendricks, M.D.
Distinguished Robert A. Ross Professor and Chairman
Department of Obstetrics and Gynecology
University of North Carolina
Chapel Hill, North Carolina

L. Stanley James, M.D.
Professor of Pediatrics and Obstetrics and Gynecology
Director, Division of Perinatal Medicine
College of Physicians and Surgeons of Columbia University
New York, New York

John D. Johnson, M.D.
Associate Professor of Pediatrics
Department of Pediatrics
University of New Mexico
Albuquerque, New Mexico

G. Eric Knox, M.D.
Perinatologist
Abbott-Northwestern Hospital Corporation
Minneapolis, Minnesota

William J. Ledger, M.D.
Professor and Chairman
Department of Obstetrics and Gynecology
Cornell University Medical Center
New York, New York

Ronald J. Lemire, M.D.
Professor, Department of Pediatrics
University of Washington School of Medicine
Seattle, Washington

Chester Martin, M.D.
Professor of Obstetrics and Gynecology
Stollenbergweg 58
Berg en Dal, The Netherlands

Jorge H. Mestman, M.D.
Clinical Professor of Obstetrics and Gynecology
University of Southern California Medical Center
Los Angeles, California

Henry L. Nadler, M.D.
Professor and Chairman of Pediatrics
Division of Genetics, Children's Memorial Hospital
Department of Pediatrics
Northwestern University Medical School
Chicago, Illinois

Richard H. Paul, M.D.
Chief, Division of Maternal and Fetal Medicine
Associate Professor of Obstetrics and Gynecology
School of Medicine
University of Southern California
Los Angeles, California

Roy M. Pitkin, M.D.
Professor and Chairman
Department of Obstetrics and Gynecology
University of Iowa Hospitals and Clinics
Iowa City, Iowa

John T. Queenan, M.D.
Professor and Chairman
Department of Obstetrics and Gynecology
University of Louisville School of Medicine
Louisville, Kentucky

Edward O. Reiter, M.D.
Associate Professor
Department of Pediatrics
University of South Florida College of Medicine
Tampa, Florida
The All Children's Hospital
St. Petersburg, Florida

David W. Reynolds, M.D.
Associate Professor of Pediatrics
Department of Pediatrics
University of Alabama School of Medicine
Birmingham, Alabama

William van B. Robertson, Ph.D.
Professor of Pediatrics and Biochemistry
Department of Pediatrics
Stanford University School of Medicine
Stanford, California

Allen W. Root, M.D.
Professor, Department of Pediatrics
University of South Florida College of Medicine
Tampa, Florida
The All Children's Hospital
St. Petersburg, Florida

Herbert C. Schwartz, M.D.
Professor of Pediatrics
Department of Pediatrics
Stanford University School of Medicine
Stanford, California

Robert Schwartz, M.D.
Professor of Pediatrics
Brown University Program in Medicine
Providence, Rhode Island

Daniel G. Seigel, S.D.
Deputy Chief
Office of Biometry and Epidemiology
National Eye Institute
Bethesda, Maryland

Thomas H. Shepard, M.D.
Professor of Pediatrics and Head
Central Laboratory for Human Embryology
University of Washington School of Medicine
Seattle, Washington

Fiona Stanley, M.D.
Fellow in Clinical Sciences
Unit of Clinical Epidemiology
University Department of Medicine
Perth Medical Centre
Shenton Park, Western Australia

Stanley J. Stys, M.D.
Assistant Professor of Obstetrics and Gynecology
University of Cincinnati
Cincinnati, Ohio

Philip Sunshine, M.D.
Professor of Pediatrics
Department of Pediatrics
Stanford University School of Medicine
Stanford, California

Evelyn B. Thoman, Ph.D.
Professor of Psychology
University of Connecticut
Storrs, Connecticut

Richard D. Zachman, M.D., Ph.D.
Associate Professor
Department of Pediatrics
University of Wisconsin-Madison
Madison, Wisconsin

Frederick P. Zuspan, M.D.
Professor and Chairman
Department of Obstetrics and Gynecology
College of Medicine
The Ohio State University
Columbus, Ohio

Preface

The objective of this book is to emphasize the field of perinatal medicine. This is a new field in terms of medical specialization, where current knowledge and latest advances in biomedical and behavioral science, pediatrics, and obstetrics can synergistically contribute to the benefit of the patients—mother, fetus, and family. The areas covered in this volume are those we have determined to be clinically current and significant to physicians, medical students, and nurses. Each section of the book presupposes knowledge of earlier sections.

This text, while not all-inclusive, is designed to encompass the most important aspects of perinatal medicine, focusing on those subject areas which have the greatest concern for the practitioner. In addition, the book is arranged so that each subject is discussed both by a pediatrician and an obstetrician, thus presenting to the reader an appraisal of the advances and approaches offered by each specialty. Fetal distress, infectious teratology, twinning, diabetes mellitus, endocrinology, and hematology are discussed with consideration of the interrelationship of the two patients and the various medical groups.

We know that the best care for our patients will derive from a coalition of all health personnel concerned with the mother and fetus. We hope that this volume will help to stimulate perinatal interests in our students, for we believe this is the field of the future where prevention of disease and disability should begin.

E. J. Quilligan, M.D.
Norman Kretchmer, M.D., Ph.D.

Contents

FETAL
AND MATERNAL
MEDICINE

Part 1

BASIC CONCEPTS IN PERINATAL MEDICINE

1

Statistics
on Perinatal
Morbidity
and Mortality

Daniel G. Seigel, S.D.
Fiona Stanley, M.D.

It is a common theme in biology that entry into the life stream is a perilous event. Rachel Carson's eloquent description of the journey of the mackerel from fertilized egg to free-living adult is not irrelevant to the human (1). The risk of death per unit of time is at its peak in early fetal life and does not reach its trough until early adolescence, when the protective human environment gives way to somewhat less sheltered living. The risk of death in the first year is finally attained again at age 60, when the challenges to life begin to come not only from the environment but from within the organism. Even so, the risk of death in the fetal period is never exceeded, at least in the age groupings provided to us by our computers.

Morbidity statistics for the several ages of life are not routinely collected and therefore are less conveniently compared than those on mortality. It is likely, though, that they would parallel the pattern just described. The illnesses that the newborn experiences have a long duration at a time when he is most susceptible to damage and thereby have a major impact on his own life and that of his society. This is manifestly clear for the serious chronic problems such as congenital malformations. Neonatal problems that appear to be acute, moreover, can often be demonstrated to lead to increased risk of disability at later ages.

The fact that the risk of illness is so high during the perinatal period and that the lifelong consequences can be so substantial offers to researchers and clinical practitioners potentially high rewards for their effort.

It is the purpose of this chapter to describe the basic statistics that are essential to all of us as a first step toward the realization of these rewards.

MORTALITY

Although the rate of spontaneous abortion during the first 5 months is not precisely known, it has been estimated that 10% of all pregnancies that reach the eighth week end in fetal death (2). Of all pregnancies reaching the 20th week, 2 in 80 do not survive

Table I. Proportion of Pregnancies Ending in Fetal Death Subsequent to Selected Gestational Ages, United States, 1972

Gestational age (weeks)	20	24	28	32	36	40
Fetal deaths thereafter per 1000 pregnancies	13	11	9	8	6	5

SOURCE: Reference 6.

beyond the first month of life, one dying before birth, i.e., a fetal death, and the other in the neonatal period (3). The risk that a pregnancy will thereafter result in fetal death declines as the pregnancy advances (Table I). At 40 weeks it is less than half that at 20 weeks.

Both fetal death ratios* (Table II) and infant and neonatal mortality rates (Table III) have continued to decrease in recent years. The considerably lower rates seen in some other countries (Table IV) suggest that further progress in the reduction of infant mortality in the U.S. is possible. Such comparisons with other countries should not divert attention from the great variation in infant mortality in the United States. The neonatal death rate in 1974 in the United States was 12.3 per 1000 live births, but ranged from 16.0 in Mississippi to 9.0 in Utah. Washington, D.C., the nation's capital, had a rate of 20.6, greater than that of any state (3).

Fetal Mortality

Fetal death ratios in the United States have fallen steadily over the last two decades (Table II). Although the rates for nonwhites have fallen more, proportionally they remain consistently higher. This difference is similar to those seen in populations with different socioeconomic and social class distributions. Both fetal and neonatal death ratios and the proportion of infants born who are of low birthweight are higher in lower social class populations. For all races, infants of multiple pregnancies are at higher risk of fetal death than those of singleton gestations (Table V). This follows from the fact that multiple pregnancies have an increased risk of complications—preeclampsia, hydramnios, and other maternal diseases (4); of complicated deliveries, e.g., breech

Table II. Fetal Death Ratios* in the United States by Race for Selected Years

Year	Total	White	All Other
1974	11.4	10.1	16.7
1972	12.7	11.2	19.5
1962	15.9	13.9	26.7
1952	18.3	16.1	32.2

SOURCE: National Center for Health Statistics.

* Ratios are fetal deaths equal to or greater than 20 weeks of gestational age per 1000 live births in the same year.

* For definitions of terms see tables in which data are presented.

Table III. Infant and Neonatal Mortality Rates* by Race for Selected Years, United States

Year	Infant Mortality			Neonatal Mortality		
	Total	White	All Other	Total	White	All Other
1974	16.7	14.8	24.9	12.3	11.1	17.2
1972	18.5	16.4	27.7	13.6	12.4	19.2
1962	25.3	22.3	41.4	18.3	16.9	26.1
1952	28.4	25.5	47.0	19.8	18.5	28.0

SOURCE: National Center for Health Statistics.

* Infant death rate defined by deaths occurring at less than 1 year of age per 1000 live births. Neonatal death rate defined by deaths occurring at less than 28 days of age per 1000 life births.

birth; and of a preterm or low birthweight outcome (4)—all of which are associated with a higher risk of fetal death (4).

Pregnancy in older women carries with it a greater risk of fetal death (Table VI), the risk in women over 40 years being three times that of women in their twenties, which seems to be the optimal age. Pregnancy at very low maternal ages also carries an increased risk of fetal death as compared with that in the optimal age group.

Table IV. Infant Mortality Rates,* Selected Countries, 1973

Rank	Country	Rate
1	Sweden	9.6
2	Finland	10.1†
3	Norway (1972)	11.3
4	Netherlands	11.6†
5	Japan (1972)	11.7
6	Switzerland	12.8†
7	Denmark (1971)	13.5
8	France (1972)	16.0
9	German Democratic Republic	16.0
10	New Zealand	16.2
11	Australia (1972)	16.7†
12	Canada	16.8
13	Belgium	17.0†
14	United Kingdom (1972)	17.5
15	United States	17.7
16	Ireland	17.8†
17	Federal Republic of Germany (1972)	20.4†
18	Singapore	20.4†
19	Czechoslovakia	21.2†
20	Israel	22.1

SOURCE: National Center for Health Statistics.

* Rates are deaths under 1 year of age per 1000 live births.

† Provisional.

Table V. Fetal Death Rates* by Plurality of Birth, United States, 1974

Single deliveries	10.8
Twin deliveries	40.2
Other plural deliveries	65.1
All births	11.4

SOURCE: National Center for Health Statistics.

* Fetal deaths are those occurring at gestational ages of 20 weeks or more.

Parity also exerts an effect independent of age on fetal mortality. At each age group, women of parity zero and parities over three have an increased risk of fetal mortality, and parities two and three seem optimal. Particularly at risk is the older woman having her first pregnancy (6).

Causes of fetal death are not routinely obtained in the United States. Pathological examination of a consecutive series of births in Great Britain (5) showed that, of those with anatomical lesions, 50% of deaths were due to intrauterine asphyxia and congenital malformations. The pattern was almost identical in the early neonatal deaths, suggesting that factors contributing to death in utero are similar to those contributing to early neonatal death.

Neonatal Mortality

A decline similar to that for fetal mortality is also seen for infant and neonatal mortality in the United States (Table III) as well as other industrial countries. However, rates for nonwhites lag approximately one generation behind whites. Proportionally more infants die in the first month than in all the first year, and the greatest portion of first month deaths occur in the first 24 hr (6).

Congenital malformations and conditions associated with low birthweight, such as respiratory distress syndrome, are now the major causes of neonatal death in the United States (Table VII). Certain complications of pregnancy and labor, including problems

Table VI. Fetal Death Ratios* by Age of Mother, United States, 1974

Age	Ratio
<15	21.8
15–19	12.8
20–24	10.0
25–29	9.9
30–34	14.0
35–39	22.5
40 and over	36.6

SOURCE: National Center for Health Statistics.

* Fetal deaths are those occurring at gestational ages of 20 weeks or more.

Table VII. Principal Causes of Death in Neonatal* Period, United States, 1974

Cause	Percentage of Deaths
Congenital anomalies	15
Immaturity (unqualified)	13
Asphyxia of newborn (unspecified)	12
Respiratory distress syndrome or hyaline membrane disease	21
Respiratory infection	2
Nonrespiratory infection	4
Complications of pregnancy and labor	19
Other	14

SOURCE: National Center for Health Statistics.

* Neonatal deaths occur at less than 28 days of age.

relating to the placenta and umbilical cord, as well as birth injury, are also important causes of neonatal mortality.

The probability of death in the first week climbs rapidly from being a rare event in babies over 3000 g birthweight to being highly likely in those less than 2000 g (Table VIII). Indeed, although babies less than 2500 g comprise less than 7% of all births, more than 70% of the neonatal deaths occur in this group (6). Furthermore, the risk of death during the first month is more than eight times greater than during the remainder of the first year for babies less than 2500 g; but in infants of normal birthweight, these two components of infant mortality are of the same magnitude (Table IX). Clearly, the distinction between the low birthweight baby and other neonates must be continually kept in mind in planning for neonatal health care.

Birthweight and gestational age are strongly correlated, and although birthweight is a better predictor of neonatal mortality, either could be used. For any birthweight group, babies with lower gestational age have a poorer prognosis for survival than do those with higher gestational age (7). Insofar as neonatal mortality is concerned, therefore, the concepts of "low birthweight for dates" and "appropriate for dates" are

Table VIII. Probability of Death in First Week by Birthweight

Birthweight (g)	Deaths in First Week per 1000 Births
1500 and less	575
1501–2000	140
2001–2500	32
2501–3000	6
3001–3500	3
Over 4000	2

SOURCE: Reference 5.

Table IX. Neonatal and Postneonatal Mortality Rates by Birthweight, United States, 1960

	Deaths per 1000	
Birthweight (g)	*Under 28 Days*	*28 Days–12 Months*
2500	171.6	22.6
Over 2500	5.5	5.8
Total	18.4	6.9

SOURCE: Reference 12.

misleading if used to imply that of two babies with identical weight the one who is "appropriate for date" will fare better. This is not to deny the implications of the "low-weight for dates" relationship as a signpost of intrauterine growth retardation and a possible predictor of poor infant development (8).

It is clear that preventive child health efforts that are directed toward decreasing mortality and morbidity in the neonate should be focused on the problem of low birthweight. As with mortality, whites have considerably smaller low birthweight rates than nonwhites. Unlike the mortality trends, however, the low birthweight rate has remained remarkably steady over the last 20 to 30 years in the United States (Table X) and other countries in which it has been recorded, even though dramatic changes in some factors normally associated with low birthweight, such as socioeconomic variables and maternal height, have occurred. Despite the strong association of mortality and low birthweight, apparently the decline in mortality has not been mediated through changes in the birthweight distribution.

MORBIDITY

Information on illness in the neonatal period is not routinely obtained for the United States. As a result we rely on an array of studies that are usually regional and cover a limited time period. Comparison among studies is hazardous because of variation in such factors as type of information obtained, medical coding practices, diagnostic groupings, and the special characteristics of the population under investigation. Reliable trends over time are particularly difficult to obtain. Recognition of these gaps in our knowledge led to the launching of two large studies of infants, one in the United States and the other in Great Britain, from which much of our current knowledge is obtained.

Table X. Proportion of Births That Are Less Than 2500 g, by Race for Selected Years, United States, All Registered Live Births

	1952	*1962*	*1972*	*1974*
Nonwhites	11.1	13.1	12.9	12.4
Whites	7.0	7.0	6.5	6.3
All Races	7.6	8.0	7.7	7.4

SOURCE: National Center for Health Statistics.

Table XI. Incidence of Major Malformations: Rates per 10,000 Live Births

Central nervous system:		Cardiorespiratory:	
Anencephaly	6	Pectus excavatum	21
Microcephaly	16	Hypoplasia or immaturity of lung	13
Hydrocephaly	14		
Abnormal separation of sutures	17	Cardiac enlargement	20
		Patent ductus arteriosus	8
Meningomyelocele; miningocele	7	Atrial septal defect	5
		Ventricular septal defect	11
Musculoskeletal:			
Fingers absent	5	Gastrointestinal:	
Toes absent	5	Pyloric stenosis	19
Torticollis	13	Inguinal hernia	130
Vertebral abnormality	10	Umbilical hernia	12
Contracture or tightness of hip	20		
Dysplasia of hip	23	Genitourinary:	
Talipes equinovarus	35	Hypospadias	40
Metatarsus adductus	200	Undescended testicles, bilateral	18
Talipes calcaneovalgus	34		
Scoliosis; lordosis; kyphosis	7	Urethral meatal stenosis	14
		Hydroureter; megaloureter	8
		Cystic kidney	6
Head:			
Cataract	9		
Cleft palate	11	Other:	
Cleft lip	11	Cavernous hemangioma	70
Micrognathia	8	Down syndrome	11

SOURCE: Reference 10.

Table XII. Conditions Seen During First Week of Life—Singleton Survivors

Conditions	Percentage of Babies
Congenital abnormalities	4
Temperature 94° or less	1
Jaundice	19
Blood sugar 19 mg or less	0.2
Breathing difficulties	2
Cyanotic attacks	2
Fits or convulsions	0.3
Conditions requiring surgery	0.4
Cerebral signs	2

SOURCE: Reference 5.

Table XIII. Incidence of Selected Neonatal Conditions and Relative Risks of Neonatal Mortality and Neurologic Abnormality for Those With and Without Condition, by Birthweight

Condition	No./1000 Live Births		Relative Risk* of Neonatal Death		Relative Risk* of Neurologic Abnormality	
	Under 2501 g	Over 2500 g	Under 2501 g	Over 2500 g	Under 2501 g	Over 2500 g
Condition at birth:						
Resuscitation						
In first 5 min	140	50	58	22	2.2	2.0
After 5 min	106	21	98	63	2.2	1.8
Apgar less than 7						
1 min	350	184	12	6	1.4	1.8
5 min	170	34	18	21	2.2	2.3
Bilirubin over 12	210	54			1.8	1.7
Bilirubin over 15	110	24			2.2	2.0
Neurological signs:						
Brain abnormalities	37	6	12	115	8.5	26.4
Seizures	8	2	7	120		19.0
Myeclonus	4	2	2			7.5

Hypertonia	12	6	1	28		7.5
Hypotonia	80	13	8	44	6.3	13.0
Hypoactivity	51	7	9	63	4.5	10.2
Lethargy	29	5	9	52	3.2	6.6
Abnormal Moro reflex	47	9	7	45	7.0	8.9
Abnormal cry	43	7	8	60	5.1	11.9
Abnormal suck	31	4	8	90	4.4	17.8
Neonatal conditions:						
Cephalohematoma	7	11	7			
Intracranial hemorrhage	18	1	19	330		
Hyaline membrane disease	35	1	125	322		
Primary atelectasis	36	1	175	290		
Pneumonia	25	2	110	230		
Primary apnea	47	11	100	46		

* Relative risks in each column are ratios of risks of neonatal death, or neurologic abnormality, for those with and those without conditions specified, for infants with given birthweight.

NOTE: Where sample sizes are too small or no data are available, no rates appear.

The United States Collaborative Perinatal Study (9) summarized the experience of over 50,000 pregnancies in 12 university centers in the years 1959 to 1966. Data collected include illnesses in the neonatal period, results of an examination at one year, and follow-up through early childhood. Comparison of the numbers of congenital malformations diagnosed at birth and those diagnosed at one year indicates that only one-third of malformations are detected at birth. The incidence of the more common major malformations (10) among live births in the Collaborative Perinatal Study observed at any time during infancy is shown in Table XI. The diagnoses vary considerably in frequency and the extent to which they are associated with either mortality or morbidity. The sum of rates of malformations that are serious enough to cause severe, lifelong handicap is roughly 50% greater than the infant mortality rate with congenital malformations as the underlying cause; that is to say, for every two neonatal deaths from congenital malformations, three infants with serious malformations survive. Furthermore, in terms of emotional and financial cost to the family and society, the morbidity from congenital malformations is more devastating than the traumatic but brief impact of early mortality. Decreasing the incidence of congenital malformations in the newborn is clearly a high priority in medical care, whether achieved by identifying and removing responsible teratogens or by offering prenatal diagnosis and selective abortion to the mothers of affected fetuses.

The British study (5) traced all births of more than 24 weeks' gestation occurring in 1 week in Great Britain in 1970. Data were collected on 17,196 births, and detailed questionnaires were completed by physicians on the neonatal experience of the surviving infants. Follow-up studies are planned, but published data cover only the first week of life. Of the 16,432 singletons, nearly one-third developed one or more adverse conditions during the first week (5), and, as the authors note, there was probably under-reporting of certain of these which were less severe. Some conditions recorded in those infants who survived the first week of life are summarized in Table XII. One is impressed with the quantity and variety of morbidity seen in this brief episode of life.

This morbidity in the neonatal period may have consequences that extend into infancy and beyond. The Collaborative Perinatal Study permits some assessment of the impact of certain neonatal conditions on the risk of neonatal death or neurologic abnormalities at 1 year of age. Table XIII shows the incidence of selected neonatal conditions and the relative risk of neonatal death or neurologic abnormalities at 1 year of age by birthweight group. The "relative risk" figures presented are the ratios of neonatal mortality rates, or neurologic abnormality rates, in those with the neonatal condition and those without. The relative risk of 7, for example, implies that babies with low birthweight who have seizures have a risk of neonatal death seven times greater than babies with low birthweight who do not experience seizures. By way of definition, it is also important to note that neurologic abnormality at 1 year in Table XIII includes children for whom "the examiner is able to make a diagnosis of a recognized syndrome, those who he feels are definitely neurologically abnormal but who do not fit into any specific diagnostic category, and those with conditions which may not be themselves neurological but which are often related to central nervous system disorders" (9).

The first striking observation is the association that these conditions have with low birthweight. With the exception of cephalohematoma, the rate of occurrence of each condition listed is higher in babies weighing 2500 g or less at birth than in those with higher birthweights. The second major feature is the extent to which the presence of these conditions is associated with increases in the risk of death or neurologic abnormality. The presence of primary apnea, for example, increases the risk of death 100-fold in the low birthweight infant and 50-fold in the baby with normal birthweight. A 5-min Apgar of less than 7 predicts a doubling in the rate of neurologic abnormality observed 12 months later. A bilirubin of greater than 15 results in a doubling in the risk of neurologic abnormality at 1 year.

The relative risks in Table XIII for normal-weight babies are impressive and generally exceed those of the low birthweight infants. This probably is explained in two ways. First, the rates of neonatal mortality are higher in low birthweight infants, and there is less opportunity for multifold increases. Second, some of these conditions may only signify prematurity when appearing in the low birthweight infant but may convey a more sinister indication of severe pathology in the normal-weight baby.

CONCLUSION

Marshaling the statistics that describe the morbidity and mortality of the perinatal period makes one more keenly aware of data that are still needed.

For mortality, we have tended to use what is available in our vital statistics, which were designed, not for research, but for the legal requirements associated with the registration of vital events. As a result, in the United States we cannot tabulate the causes of infant mortality against the characteristics of the mother or even of the infant at birth. Such data are not on the death certificate, and linkage of infant deaths and birth certificates is done only at the level of some states. Of greater interest but of greater difficulty to obtain are data on several pregnancies in the same women. For example, data on the risk of prematurity in women who previously had premature births are not easily assembled.

For morbidity, data are really inadequate. We are highly dependent on studies that begin to grow outdated or come from other countries. Only recently have routine data become available on the incidence of congenital malformations. Even so, they are obtained in the neonatal period and consequently underestimate the true values (13).

Longitudinal data on the sequelae in later life to infant problems such as respiratory distress syndrome, prematurity, obesity, and jaundice are extremely difficult to obtain. Nor can we readily evaluate the long-term consequences of treatment strategies, such as intensive care or fetal monitoring.

The ease with which such data can be obtained is often not taken into consideration in planning our health care systems. Until we are able to obtain from our medical practice those statistics required for etiological research, evaluation of medical care, and assessing our health needs, perinatal medicine will be less successful than it needs to be.

ACKNOWLEDGMENT

Discussions with Dr. Stephen Lamm were particularly helpful in the preparation of this chapter.

REFERENCES

1. Carlson, R.: *Under the Sea Wind,* Oxford University Press, 1941.
2. Taylor, W. F.: The probability of fetal death. *Congenital Malformations: Proceedings of the Third International Conference,* Excerpta Medica, International Congress Series No. 204, 1970, pp. 307–320.
3. National Center for Health Statistics, Division of Vital Statistics, unpublished statistics.

4. The Editorial Team: The multiple births, in Butler, N. R., and Alberman, E. D. (eds.): *Perinatal Problems*. E. & S. Livingstone, 1969, pp. 122–140.

5. *British Births 1970*. A survey under the joint auspices of the National Birthday Trust Fund and the Royal College of Obstetricians and Gynaecologists. Vol. 1, *The First Week of Life*. Heinemann, London, 1975.

6. *Vital Statistics of the United States*. Vol. 2, Part A, *Mortality*, U.S. Government Printing Office, Washington, D.C.

7. Armstrong, R. J.: A study of infant mortality from linked records: By birth weight, period of gestation, and other variables. *Vital Health Stat.*, Ser. 20, No. 12, DHEW, HSMHA, NCHS, 1972.

8. Clinics in Developmental Medicine, No. 19. M. Dawkins and W. MacGregor (eds.): *Gestational Age, Size and Maturity*. The Spastics Society Medical Education and Information Unit in Association with Heinemann, London.

9. The Collaborative Perinatal Study of the National Institute of Neurological Diseases and Stroke. K. R. Niswander and M. Gordon (eds.): *The Women and Their Pregnancies*. DHEW, PHS, NIH, U.S. Government Printing Office, Washington, D.C., 1972.

10. Myrianthopoulos, N. C., and Chung, C. S.: *Congenital Malformations in Singletons: Epidemiologic Survey*. Report from the Collaborative Perinatal Project; Stratton Intercontinental Medical Book Corporation, 1974.

11. Hardy, J. B., Drage, J. S., and Jackson, E. C.: *The First Year of Life*. In preparation, via personal communication from Dr. Drage, NIH.

12. Chase, H.: Infant mortality and weight at birth: 1960 United States birth cohort. *Am. J. Public Health*, 59, September 1969.

13. Birth Defects Monitoring Program. *Congenital Malformations Surveillance Report*, July 1974–June 1975, issued December 1975. DHEW, PHS, CDC, Atlanta, Ga.

2

Human Perinatal Endocrinology

Allen W. Root, M.D.
Edward O. Reiter, M.D.

To a large extent the endocrine system of the fetus functions independently of the mother. Although maternal and placental steroid hormones enter the fetal circulation, the peptide and thyronine hormones do not cross the placental barrier. Therefore, the fetus is dependent on endogenous secretion of these hormones for satisfaction of its requirements for growth and maturation.

The majority of the fetal endocrine glands are organized and morphologically distinguishable within the first 6 weeks after conception. These structures become functional between 6 and 10 weeks, and by 12 weeks the hormonal products of the endocrine system can be demonstrated in the fetal circulation. Each gland has its unique temporal pattern of function during gestation, but the significance and importance of each component of the endocrine system for the growth, maturation, and development of the fetus are still not completely understood. By term the endocrine system has, for the most part, matured to the stage at which it is able to function immediately in the postpartum period.

HYPOTHALAMIC–PITUITARY AXIS

The hypothalamic-pituitary axis functions as an integrated unit. The hypothalamus produces small peptides that stimulate or inhibit the synthesis and secretion of anterior pituitary hormones. The hypothalamic hormones are stored and to some extent synthesized in the median eminence, the area of the hypothalamus immediately above the pituitary stalk. They are also synthesized in other areas of the hypothalamus and central nervous system. These hypothalamic products reach the pituitary gland through the pituitary portal vascular system.

Embryology

In man the anterior pituitary gland develops from the ectodermal roof of the stomodeum (1–4). This stomodeal pocket, or Rathke pouch, which appears in the 2.5-mm embryo

*Supported by National Foundation–March of Dimes Grants 1-323
and C-199 and Basil O'Connor Starter Grant 5-71.*

(5 to 6 weeks), is located anterior to the stomodeal-pharyngeal membrane and is adherent to a tubular projection from the floor of the neural tube (forebrain) that is immediately adjacent to the membrane. The tubular projection eventually becomes the infundibulum, which further differentiates into the neural (posterior) lobe of the pituitary and the pituitary stalk. By the 3-mm stage (7 weeks) the connection of the Rathke pouch with the oral epithelium has become merely a stalk of cells, and all connection is severed by 8 weeks' gestation as the pituitary becomes encased in the developing sphenoid bone. The cells at the pharyngeal end of this cell column may persist postnatally as the pharyngeal pituitary. Also at the 3-mm stage the anterior wall of the Rathke pouch thickens, and this eventually differentiates into the anterior pituitary gland. Cells from the posterior wall persist as the intermediate zone of the pituitary in adults. By 10 to 11 weeks of gestation, acidophilic and basophilic cells are histochemically distinguishable. The use of immunocytochemical techniques has permitted identification of hormone-containing cells in the pituitary glands of much younger fetuses. The number and size of acidophiles increase greatly between 16 and 21 weeks of gestation. Fetal pituitary weight increases from 3 mg between 10 and 14 weeks to 12 mg between 20 and 24 weeks and to 99 mg at term (one-fifth the weight of the adult pituitary).

Capillary formation in the region of the developing adenohypophysis and adjacent neural tissue is present by the tenth week of gestation, and the primary plexus of the hypothalamic-pituitary portal vascular system is present by 14 to 15 weeks (2). By 20 weeks of gestation the neurosecretory nerves and the primary portal plexus of capillaries are juxtaposed and the hypothalamic-pituitary portal vascular system is morphologically intact (3,5). There is concurrent development of the hypothalamic nuclei and other neural structures during this period. The neurochemical monoamine transmitters—dopamine, norepinephrine, serotonin—have been identified in the human fetal hypothalamus and median eminence by 10 to 13 weeks of gestation (6).

Very early in gestation the hypothalamic and pituitary hormones appear to be secreted independently. With advancing gestational age, there is increasing stimulation of pituitary hormone secretion secondary to uninhibited secretion of the hypothalamic hormones. In the last trimester of pregnancy and extending into early infancy, inhibitory neural influences over hypothalamic-pituitary activity become apparent (3). These developmental phases correlate with neurophysiological, histological, and electrical maturation of the central nervous system.

Hypothalamic Hormones

The chemical identity of three hypothalamic hormones has been established: thyrotropin releasing hormone (TRH); gonadotropin releasing hormone (Gn-RH), also termed luteinizing hormone–releasing hormone (LH-RH, LRF); and somatotropin release-inhibiting factor (SRIF, somatostatin). Development of radioimmunoassays for each of these hormones has permitted their quantitation in human fetal neural and extraneural tissue.

Thyrotropin Releasing Hormone (TRH)
TRH is the tripeptide

$$(Pyro)Glu-His-Pro-NH_2$$

Its structure is similar in all species from which it has been isolated. TRH stimulates the secretion of thyroid stimulating hormone (TSH, thyrotropin) and prolactin. However, the physiologic importance of the latter effect is not yet apparent. TRH has been identified in the hypothalamus, thalamus, pituitary, midbrain, cerebellum, brain stem, cerebral cortex, spinal cord, and pineal gland of the rat and other species (3,4,7). In the human fetus, TRH has been identified by radioimmunoassay in hypothalami between 10 and 22 weeks' gestation, in which concentrations range between 0.32 and 218 pg/mg, with content varying from 0.46 to 260 ng per hypothalamus (3,8). TRH has been detected in a whole brain extract from a human fetus of 4.5 weeks' gestational age. The tripeptide has also been identified in human fetal cerebrum and cerebellum. In the cerebral cortex of the human fetus between 10 and 22 weeks gestation, the TRH concentration varies between 0.28 and 93 pg/mg of tissue.

In monolayer cultures of human fetal pituitary tissue (10 to 14 weeks' gestation), TRH stimulates a two- to fivefold increase in TSH release over control levels; the increased secretion persists for 24 to 48 hr following removal of TRH from the incubation medium (9). TRH does not provoke prolactin secretion from these tissues, perhaps because prolactin secretion is already great. TRH does not consistently affect the production of growth hormone (GH), luteinizing hormone (LH), or follicle stimulating hormone (FSH) in these cell cultures.

Gonadotropin Releasing Hormone (Gn-RH)
Gn-RH is the decapeptide

$$\text{(Pyro)Glu-His-Trp-Ser-Tyr-Gly-Leu-Arg-Pro-Gly-NH}_2$$

Gn-RH stimulates the secretion of both LH and FSH. The bulk of Gn-RH is localized in the hypothalamus, principally in the median eminence and arcuate nucleus. In rodents it has also been demonstrated in the pituitary, midbrain, cerebral cortex, cerebellum, brain stem, and pineal gland (7). Gn-RH is present in human fetal hypothalami but is only occasionally detectable in human fetal cortex (10). In the human fetus Gn-RH was identified immunochemically in the extract of a whole brain from a 4.5-week fetus. In one study hypothalamic concentration of Gn-RH between 8 and 24 weeks' gestation ranged between 4 and 65 pg/mg (10). Kaplan et al. (3,8) measured Gn-RH in 35 fetal hypothalami between 10 and 22 weeks' gestation. Gn-RH concentration varied between 0.27 and 6.5 pg/mg of wet tissue, and Gn-RH content varied between 0.18 and 5.2 ng per hypothalamus. There was no relation between Gn-RH concentration or content and gestational age or sex in this study. These investigators (3,8) also detected Gn-RH in low concentrations in the cerebral cortex. Reyes et al. (11) recorded increased hypothalamic Gn-RH content (0.45 to 6 ng) in 10 human fetal hypothalamic extracts obtained between 8 and 18 weeks' gestation.

Exposure of human fetal pituitary tissue in culture between 13 and 19 weeks' gestation to Gn-RH for 4 hr increases LH and FSH secretion two- to fourfold (9). Increased secretion of the gonadotropins persists for 24 hr after removal of Gn-RH. This decapeptide has no consistent effect on secretion of GH, TSH, or prolactin in this system.

Somatotropin Release Inhibiting Factor (SRIF)
SRIF is the tetradecapeptide

$$\text{H-Ala-Gly-Cys-Lys-Asn-Phe-Phe-Trp-Lys-Thr-Phe-Thr-Ser-Cys-OH}$$

SRIF inhibits the secretion of growth hormone, ACTH, and TSH as well as many extrapituitary hormones (Table I). This tetradecapeptide is widely distributed throughout the central nervous system, the gastrointestinal tract, pancreas, and thyroid. The concentration of SRIF in human fetal (10 to 22 weeks) hypothalamic extracts increases and correlates with advancing gestational age (3,8). At 10 weeks the hypothalamic concentration of SRIF is 7.3 pg/mg of wet tissue, increasing to 10.2 pg/mg between 11 and 15 weeks and to 28.5 pg/mg by 20 weeks. Hypothalamic content of SRIF increases from 7.8 ng in early gestation to 36.6 ng at midgestation. SRIF is also detectable in extracts of human fetal cerebral cortex at concentrations one-fourth those in hypothalamic extracts and in pancreatic islets after 10 weeks of gestation (12).

SRIF inhibits secretion of GH from human fetal (10 to 18 weeks' gestation) pituitary monolayer cultures and explants in both the short term (within 4 hr) and during longer exposure (12 to 24 hr) (9). Following removal of SRIF from the culture medium, there is an immediate rebound increase in GH release. SRIF does not consistently affect the secretion of LH, FSH, TSH, or prolactin from human fetal pituitaries in vitro.

Pituitary Hormones

Growth Hormone (GH)

Human growth hormone (GH) is a peptide with 191 amino acids and a molecular weight of 21,500 with significant protein anabolic, lipolytic, and diabetogenic effects (13). The anabolic effects of GH are mediated by somatomedins, a family of serum peptides (molecular weight 4000 to 8000) which stimulate incorporation of radiolabeled sulfate into cartilage mucopolysaccharides in vitro and which are under the direct control of GH (14). Four somatomedins are known: somatomedin A, somatomedin C, nonsuppressible insulin-like activity, and multiplication stimulating activity. These bioactive materials circulate in plasma carried by a specific binding protein. In infants, children, and adolescents GH is essential for appropriate linear growth as well as for several homeostatic metabolic functions. However, the biologic role of GH in the human fetus is unclear.

Maternal Growth Hormone. Concentrations of GH in maternal serum and plasma are low (approximately 3 ng/ml) during pregnancy and do not change significantly with advancing gestation (15,16). GH levels increase in pregnant women after insulin-induced hypoglycemia but to a lesser extent than in nonpregnant females (16). Impaired maternal GH secretion persists postpartum, the result, perhaps, of hypothalamic-pituitary suppression by human chorionic somatomammotropin (17). Several studies suggest that maternal GH does not influence the fetus. GH does not cross the placental barrier either at 14 to 16 weeks of gestation or at term (18,19). Hypophysectomy of a woman with metastatic breast cancer at 26 weeks' gestation did not impair the growth of her fetus who was delivered at 35 weeks' gestation with a birthweight of 2300 g (20). Infants of normal birthweight have been delivered to women with isolated deficiency of GH or with hypersecretion of GH and acromegaly (21). The peak level of GH achieved in the mother during insulin-induced hypoglycemia in the postpartum period does not correlate with the infant's birthweight (22).

Fetal and Neonatal Growth Hormone. The human fetal anterior pituitary gland has the capacity to secrete GH within 5 weeks after conception. Siler-Khodr et al. (23)

Table I. Inhibitory Effects of Somatotropin Release Inhibiting Factor (SRIF)

Hormonal
  Pituitary hormones
    Growth hormone
    Thyrotropin
    Adrenocorticotropin
    Prolactin
  Pancreatic hormones
    Insulin
    Glucagon
  Gut hormones
    Gastrin
    Secretin
    Vasoactive intestinal polypeptide
    Motilin
    Gut glucagon
    Cholecystokinin-pancreozymin
  Renal products
    Renin

Nonhormonal
  Gastric emptying
  Gastric acid and pepsin secretion
  Pancreatic enzyme and electrolyte secretion
  Xylose absorption
  Gallbladder contraction
  Splanchnic blood flow
  Acetylcholine release from nerve endings
  Central nervous system neuron electrical activity

measured the synthesis and secretion of pituitary hormones by anterior pituitary glands of 44 human fetuses between 5 and 40 weeks' postconception maintained in tissue culture. All pituitaries, including that from the youngest fetus, synthesized and released GH for about 2 to 3 weeks irrespective of the gestational age of the donor, although the quantity of GH released increased with age and size of the fetus and pituitary. A similar study was conducted by Goodyer et al. (9), who reported maximal release of GH from the fetal pituitary in the first week of culture with decline in secretion over the next several weeks. The daily secretion rate of GH in the first week of culture increases with the gestational age of the pituitary between 10 and 19 weeks. GH release in vitro is not affected by exposure to TRH or Gn-RH but is suppressed by SRIF and stimulated by the addition of dibutyryl cyclic AMP to the culture medium. Other investigators using a variety of techniques, including tissue culture, immunofluorescence, immunoelectrophoresis, and bio- and radioimmunoassay, have detected GH in the pituitary glands of fetuses between 7 and 15 weeks of gestation (24–27). Discrepant observations between investigators probably reflect the variable sensitivity of the methods used and the number and quality of the specimens with which the investigators worked.

Kaplan et al. (3,28–30) studied the pituitary and serum GH patterns in a large number of aborted fetuses. They detected immunoreactive GH in the pituitary of the youngest fetus (7 weeks) studied in their series. The mean pituitary content of GH increased from 0.44 mg per pituitary at 10 to 14 weeks to 577.6 mg per pituitary at 30 to 34 weeks with no substantial further increase during the last 6 weeks of gestation (Fig. 1). Bioassayable pituitary GH is present by 18 weeks' gestation and increases several-fold by term. Fetal pituitary GH is heterogeneous; extracts of fetal pituitaries contain the monomeric "little" GH (85%), the dimer "big" GH (10%), and small amounts of the heaviest material "big, big" GH (3,31).

Kaplan et al. detected GH in the serum of a fetus studied at 10 weeks' postconception (3). Serum concentrations of GH increased gradually from 65.2 ng/ml at 10 to 14 weeks to maximal levels at 20 to 24 weeks (131.9 ng/ml) and declined thereafter to values approaching those in umbilical venous blood (33.5 ng/ml) by 30 to 34 weeks of gestation (Fig. 2). The GH concentration in umbilical cord serum of preterm infants is significantly greater than in term infants (50 versus 31.5 ng/ml) (31). The rather high umbilical cord levels of GH do not relate to duration of labor, maternal toxemia, perinatal distress, Apgar score, mode of delivery, body weight, body length, or blood

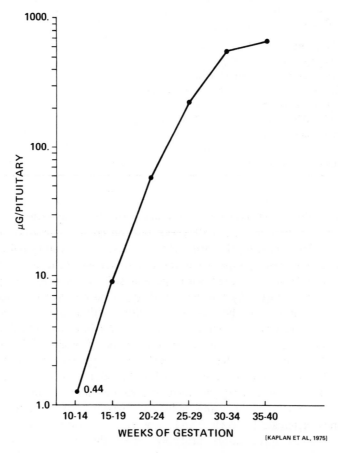

Figure 1. Pituitary content of immunoreactive growth hormone in human fetus. The ordinate is a log scale. Adapted from data of Kaplan et al. (3); reprinted from (198) with permission of publisher.

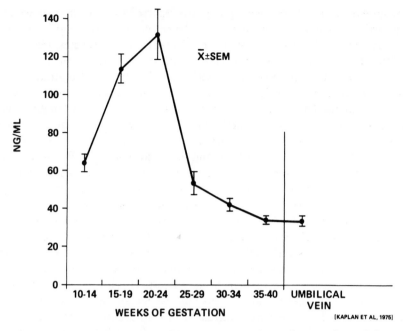

Figure 2. Serum concentration of growth hormone in human fetus. Adapted from data of Kaplan et al. (3); reprinted from (198) with permission of publisher.

glucose concentration (32). It has been suggested that early in gestation the secretion of GH occurs in an unrestrained and perhaps unregulated fashion (3). At midgestation there is augmented GH release due to stimulation by a theoretical hypothalamic GH-releasing factor. Later in development increasing inhibition, possibly by SRIF, of GH release is manifested by declining serum levels of GH as the organization of the central nervous system–hypothalamic-anterior pituitary axis matures.

In full-term infants GH levels remain unchanged for the first hours after birth (24 to 32 ng/ml), after declining slightly from cord values (42 ng/ml) (33). In premature infants GH levels increase immediately after birth (34). In the early neonatal period serum concentrations of GH are elevated in both full-term and prematurely born infants. In the former, GH levels gradually decline by 14 days of age, and in premature infants serum GH values may remain elevated for more than 56 days (35). Hypoglycemia, hyperglycemia, glucagon, and arginine evoke GH release in full-term and premature infants in the first postpartum week (36–38). In anencephalic newborn infants, levels of GH in cord blood are quite low. Postnatally there is variable growth hormone secretion in response to a variety of stimuli, including hypoglycemia and arginine infusion (3). Pituitary content of GH may also be low in such infants.

Role of Growth Hormone in the Fetus. The endogenous hormones that regulate fetal growth are not known with certainty. Fetal insulin is thought to be of prime importance, but the significance of growth hormone and other anterior pituitary products remains speculative. It has been suggested from clinical observations and experimental studies that endogenous growth hormone has no effect on fetal growth (28). Thus infants born with congenital aplasia of the pituitary, familial isolated deficiency of growth hormone, or anencephaly are reported to be of normal weight and length at birth, excluding the contribution of the cranial vault to weight and length in anencephalic infants. However, in a study of 147 anencephalic neonates, Honnebier and Swaab (39) reported that birthweights were significantly decreased relative to the control group of newborns even after compensating for the absence of brain tissue. Laron (40) commented that the birth length of neonates with isolated deficiency of GH was decreased, as was the birth length of infants with the syndrome of familial dwarfism with high plasma levels of immunoreactive GH (41). In the latter syndrome, a defect in somatomedin generation may be a primary abnormality. Naeye and Blanc (42) quantitatively analyzed the morphology of body and organ structures in 59 newborn anencephalic infants, 37 of whom were born prematurely (29 to 38 weeks' gestation) and 22 of whom were born at term or beyond (40 to 50 weeks). In the prematurely born group, total body weight, after compensation for the absent cranial vault, and the weights of the heart, liver, spleen, kidneys, adrenal, and lungs were below values anticipated for gestational age. In the full-term anencephalic infants the weight of the heart, adrenals, kidneys, and lungs was significantly less than control values. Cytologic examination revealed decreased cell numbers in both premature and full-term anencephalic infants in the heart, spleen, kidneys, and permanent adrenocortical cells. Liver cell number was decreased in premature anencephalic infants but was not affected in full-term neonates. Thymic epithelial cell numbers were increased in both groups of anencephalics. (The latter observation is difficult to interpret. In contrast, in Snell-Bagg mice with congenital deficiency of GH and in hypophysectomized rats, decreased thymic size increases following the administration of GH (43). The effects of GH on thymic size and function in man have not been defined as yet.) As GH exerts a major effect on growth by regulating the rate of cell division (44), Naeye and Blanc (42) suggest that deficiency of this hormone may be responsible for the deficient growth of anencephalic infants. In infants with fetal pituitary dysplasia, renal morphology is similar to that observed in anencephalic neonates; that is, there is a subnormal number of nephrons and decreased cytoplasmic mass in renal tubular cells (45).

Decapitation of the fetal rabbit or hamster does not impair growth, but decapitation or encephalectomy of the fetal rat and mouse and hypophysectomy of the fetal sheep lead to depressed growth (46–49). Administration of GH to the decapitated rat fetus in utero leads to increased body size (47). Destruction of the pituitary in the fetal monkey in the last third of pregnancy does not affect in utero growth in surviving animals, nor does destruction of the maternal pituitary adversely affect fetal growth in this species (50); but decapitation of the rhesus monkey fetus at midgestation significantly inhibits subsequent growth (51).

Somatomedin. Somatomedin activity has been measured in cord and neonatal sera by bioassay—incorporation of radiolabeled sulfate into cartilage—and more recently by radioreceptorassay (RRA) using placental membranes as receptors, and radioimmunoassay using specific antisera to and labeled tracer of somatomedin C. (Somatomedin C stimulates radiolabeled sulfate uptake into cartilage from hypophysectomized rats.) Bioactive somatomedin is present in cord serum, and the level increases with gestational age, correlating with birthweight, length, and head circumference independently of gestational age (52). Cord somatomedin levels do not correlate with placental weight or umbilical cord serum levels of GH. There may be a negative correlation between cord somatomedin values and serum concentrations of insulin (52). Cord somatomedin levels measured by both radioreceptorassay and radioimmunoassay are low relative to adult values and increase over the first several years of life to adult values (53,54). Cord values of radioreceptor somatomedin C have been reported to be less in infants with intrauterine growth retardation and in postmature infants than in full-term and preterm infants of appropriate size for gestational age (55).

Somatomedin A stimulates radiolabeled sulfate incorporation into chick cartilage. Measurements of somatomedin A by radioreceptor assay reveals mixed umbilical cord blood values at term of 0.21 to 1.00 U/ml (mean 0.50) with no consistent change over the first 4 days of life (56). In women at delivery the mean somatomedin A (RRA) level is 0.54 U/ml, a value significantly below that of nonpregnant women (0.91 U/ml). The somatomedin A level in women delivered by cesarean section is lower than that of vaginally delivered subjects (0.39 versus 0.70 U/ml). The mean cord level of somatomedin B, measured by radioimmunoassay, is 7.5 µg/ml and does not change over the first 4 days of life. Maternal somatomedin B values are higher in women delivered vaginally than in those who undergo cesarean sections (92.3 versus 35.4 µg/ml). There is no correlation between somatomedin levels in umbilical cord and maternal serum. Differential measurement of somatomedin in umbilical artery and vein has not been reported.

Somatomedin bioactivity has been demonstrated in amniotic fluid at full term at values approximately one-fourteenth (0.07 U/ml) those present in normal adult sera and one-fourth those recorded in pregnant women at term (57). Amniotic fluid levels of somatomedin C measured by radioreceptor assay apparently peak at 17 to 20 weeks (190 µg/ml) and then decline to term (5 µg/ml) (58). However, there is a specific amniotic fluid binding substance for somatomedin that seems to differ from the plasma somatomedin binding protein (59). It reacts in the somatomedin radioceptor assay but has no bioactivity. Measurement of somatomedin A in amniotic fluid by radioreceptor assay has revealed a mean level of 15.3 U/ml (range 2.7 to 73.3 U/ml) between 16 to 23 weeks' gestation and 6.8 (range 2.1 to 16.7) U/ml between 32 and 40 weeks (60); low values (1.4 and 1.5 U/ml) were present in the amniotic fluids of an anencephalic fetus and an infant with severe damage to the central nervous system. The quantitative discrepancy in amniotic fluid somatomedin values between the bioassay and the radioreceptor assay may relate to the carrier protein for somatomedin in amniotic fluid that cross-reacts in the radioreceptor assay but has no bioactivity (59).

The role of somatomedin in fetal growth is unknown. In fetal pigs receptors for somatomedin have been demonstrated in the liver, kidney, heart, lungs, and placenta (55). The low levels of somatomedin in the fetus suggest that this factor may be of little importance or that fetal cells are extremely sensitive to small amounts of this material. Alternatively, since somatomedin circulates in serum bound to a carrier protein, it is possible that the measured cord levels of somatomedin may not reflect the biologically active material in vivo if the carrier protein is low in fetal blood.

Prolactin

Prolactin has been identified as a distinct hormone in the pituitary glands of humans and higher primates (61). Structural and physicochemical characteristics of human prolactin are quite similar to those of GH. The secretion of prolactin is regulated by uncharacterized hypothalamic prolactin release-inhibiting and releasing activities (4). The tripeptide, thyrotropin releasing hormone (TRH), also stimulates prolactin secretion (4). McNeilly and coworkers (62) demonstrated that hypothalamic extracts from human fetuses less than 16 weeks of gestation either had no effect on prolactin secretion or had prolactin release-inhibiting effects, as tested in vivo in the ovariectomized, estrogen-progesterone treated rat. After 16 weeks of gestation all fetal hypothalamic extracts demonstrated prolactin release-inhibiting activity. No correlation between bioactivity and the hypothalamic content of immunoreactive TRH could be demonstrated in this study.

Maternal Prolactin. Maternal concentrations of serum prolactin begin to increase approximately 30 days after the midmenstrual cycle peak of luteinizing hormone that immediately precedes the ovulation leading to conception. Serum prolactin levels continue to rise as the levels of estradiol increase (63). Serum prolactin concentrations achieve peak levels at term (64,65). If the woman does not breast-feed, serum prolactin concentrations decline rapidly after parturition. In the woman who breast-feeds, levels of prolactin increase sharply with each feeding period; after several months of breast feeding there is decreased prolactin secretion during suckling (66,67). In the pregnant rhesus monkey serum prolactin concentrations do not increase until the last week of gestation, coinciding with but perhaps independent of rising maternal values of estradiol and estrone (68).

The role of maternal prolactin in the maintenance of human pregnancy is uncertain. In rats prolactin is necessary for maintenance of pregnancy during the first 6 days of gestation but is unnecessary thereafter (69,70). In humans, prolactin, acting synergistically with other hormones, is important for the mammary growth of pregnancy. In humans, monkeys, and hamsters maternal prolactin may cross the placenta and enter the fetal circulation in small amounts (71,72).

Prolactin may be found in amniotic fluid at concentrations that are 100-fold higher than maternal or fetal levels of prolactin (73). Although the source of amniotic fluid prolactin is unknown, recent data suggest that it may be derived primarily from the fetus (74). During the first 20 weeks of gestation amniotic fluid levels of immunoreactive prolactin range from 1.2 to 7.0 μg/ml, falling to 0.35 μg/ml at term (73).

Fetal and Neonatal Prolactin. Siler-Khodr et al. (23) reported that the pituitary gland of a human fetus of 5 weeks' gestation maintained in tissue culture released immunoreactive prolactin, as did pituitaries of older and larger fetuses. The quantity of prolactin secreted increased with gestational age and pituitary size. In this study prolactin secretion continued in vitro for as long as 200 days, whereas release of GH ceased after 17 to 18 days in culture, suggesting that the release of prolactin, but not that of GH, might be independent of hypothalamic stimulation in the human fetus. These findings were confirmed by Goodyer et al. (9), who observed increasing secretion of prolactin into culture medium from fetal pituitary tissue over a period of several weeks. The amount of prolactin released increased with the gestational age of the fetal pituitary. In this system the secretion of prolactin was not affected by exposure to TRH, Gn-RH, or SRIF but was increased by the addition of dibutyryl cyclic AMP to the incubation medium after 15 weeks' gestation (9). Prolactin has been identified in the human fetal pituitary gland by histochemical and bioassay techniques as early as 18 weeks' gestation (27). Using antisera to bovine prolactin, Baker and Jaffe (27) found immunoreactive prolactin-containing cells in the pituitary of a fetus of 16.5 weeks.

Aubert and coworkers (3,75) measured the pituitary content and serum concentration of prolactin in a large number of human fetuses. Immunoreactive prolactin was detectable in the alkaline (pH 8.2) extract of a pituitary from a fetus of 10 weeks' gestation, but, between 10 and 16.5 weeks, prolactin was below limits of detection (<2 ng) in 25 of 33 specimens. Thereafter pituitary prolactin content increased steadily until term (2000 ng per pituitary), correlating with gestational age but not with fetal sex (Fig. 3). Fetal pituitary contents of GH and prolactin are positively correlated, but the content of GH is 125- to 290-fold higher than that of prolactin. In the same study (75) prolactin was measurable in the plasma of a fetus of 12.5 weeks' gestation. Between this age and 29 weeks, serum prolactin concentrations remained relatively constant, with a mean of 20 ng/ml. After 30 weeks there was a rapid increment in prolactin levels to term, when the mean was 268 ng/ml followed by a decline to 168 ng/ml in umbilical vein blood (Fig. 4). Winters et al. (76) reported a similar pattern of intrauterine plasma prolactin levels. The late gestational rise in circulating fetal prolactin levels correlates with a rise in fetal estradiol values, and it has been suggested that the increase in estrogen levels is, in part, responsible for the prolactin secretory surge (3). There is a weak but positive correlation between maternal and fetal levels of prolactin (75). At term maternal prolactin concentrations are slightly lower (112 ng/ml) than in umbilical vein blood (75). In the neonate there is a brief increase in prolactin levels within 30 min after delivery, paralleling the rise in TSH values at this time (33). Postpartum prolactin levels in the neonate decline to stationary values by 6 weeks of age (77). Prolactin concentrations are higher in preterm than in term infants during this period.

McNeilly et al. measured human fetal prolactin levels in acidic (pH 4.5) extracts of

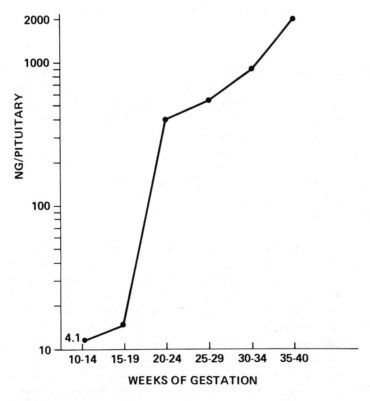

Figure 3. Pituitary content of prolactin in human fetus. The ordinate is a log scale. Adapted from data of Kaplan et al. (3); reprinted from (198) with permission of publisher.

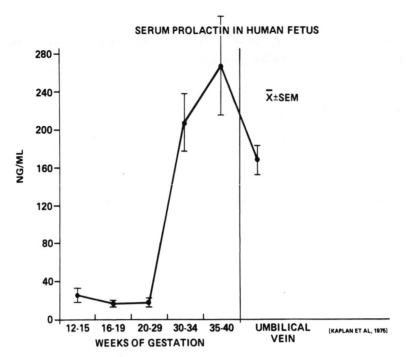

Figure 4. Serum concentration of prolactin in human fetus. Adapted from data of Kaplan et al. (3); reprinted from (198) with permission of publisher.

the pituitary and reported values of 26 to 40 ng per pituitary before 12 weeks' gestation, increasing to 45 to 200 ng at 13 to 17 weeks (196). The discrepancy between these data and those of Aubert et al. (75) may be related to the pH of the medium used to extract prolactin from the pituitary. McNeilly et al. (62) were also able to detect prolactin in the serum of a fetus of 10 weeks' gestation.

In anencephalic infants the concentration of serum prolactin is at least comparable to that of intact neonates and increases appropriately following administration of TRH (3). These and other observations (9,23,62) suggest that after the fourth month of gestation the fetal hypothalamus exerts primarily an inhibitory influence on pituitary synthesis and secretion of prolactin.

Role of Prolactin in Fetal Life. Prolactin has more than 20 known actions in mammals and additional effects in submammalian species (78). These actions may be classified in five categories: (1) reproductive, including lactation; (2) osmoregulatory; (3) growth promoting; (4) synergistic action with other hormones, particularly steroids; and (5) effects on ectodermal structures. In addition to its effects on mammary gland growth and lactation, prolactin has several biologic activities that are similar to growth hormone. In hypopituitary human subjects ovine prolactin induces nitrogen retention, hypercalciuria, and skeletal growth and impairs carbohydrate tolerance. In other species the hormone affects salt and water metabolism, function of the corpus luteum, and behavior (79). It stimulates somatomedin generation in rat livers (80). Nevertheless the basic biologic role of prolactin in the child and the adult male is poorly understood, and there are few data that define its role in the fetus.

Winters et al. (76) suggest that prolactin is essential for the growth of the human fetal adrenal gland in concert with adrenocorticotropin and estrogen. Skutch (81,82) hypothesizes that maternal prolactin may be responsible for the suppression of the maternal immune response to the fetus. It is known that there is decreased fetal and maternal lymphocyte mitotic responsivity to phytohemagglutinin due to a circulating inhibitory material (83,84) and that ovine prolactin suppresses the immune response of adult rats (85). Nevertheless, the exact circulating component in maternal and fetal serum that suppresses the immune responses, be it corticosteroids, progesterone, estrogens, chorionic gonadotropin, or prolactin, is unknown at present. It has been reported recently that in rabbit fetuses prolactin enhances the pulmonary synthesis of phospholipid and lecithin, important components of surfactant (86). Prolactin is also important for testicular function. Prolactin enhances the binding of luteinizing hormone to interstitial cells of the testes (87). However, in anencephalic male infants with normal levels of prolactin the external genitalia are often hypoplastic; this has been attributed to depressed secretion of gonadotropins by the fetal pituitary of such infants (3).

Posterior Pituitary Hormones

Arginine vasopressin and the nonapeptide, vasotocin, have been identified in the posterior pituitary gland of the human fetus, and arginine vasotocin has also been found in the human fetal pineal gland. Between 12 and 19 weeks of gestation the mean pituitary concentration of immunoreactive arginine vasopressin is 0.8 U/mg and that of arginine vasotocin 1.2 U/mg (88,89). The percentage of arginine vasopressin relative to the total content of this peptide plus the nonapeptide increases significantly with advancing gestational age over this interval. By bioassay vasotocin is detectable in the human fetal neurohypophysis by 8 to 9 weeks of gestation (90). The human fetal pineal contains both bioassayable and immunoassayable vasotocin and also synthesizes vasotocin in vitro by 14 weeks of gestation (91).

Oxytocin is demonstrable in umbilical cord plasma at values between 15 and 100 μU/ml (92).

PITUITARY-GONADAL AXIS

Embryology

Gonadal Differentiation

Primordial germ cells located in the dorsal endoderm of the yolk sac have been identified in the first week of gestation (93,94). These cells migrate under unknown influence to the urogenital ridge by the fifth and sixth weeks of life and are the sole sources of gonocytes. The undifferentiated structure that develops in the urogenital ridge must then differentiate into either a testis or ovary.

Testicular differentiation (93,94), chromosomally controlled by loci on the short arm of the Y chromosome (95), proceeds with development of Leydig cells from interstitial fibroblasts that demonstrate active steroidogenesis by 60 days of gestation. Leydig cell proliferation reaches its peak by 14 weeks of gestation, when this cell type accounts for more than half of the gonadal volume. Simultaneously, the seminiferous tubules elongate, thicken, and coil. Primitive spermatogonia and Sertoli cells develop, but no further intrauterine differentiation of the germinal epithelium occurs. The Leydig cells gradually decrease in number during the middle trimester and are almost absent at birth. In the last third of intrauterine life, the lumenized seminiferous tubules are separated by small amounts of interstitial tissue and scattered Leydig cells. The testis is surrounded by a thick tunica albuginea and gradually occupies a more caudal position in the peritoneal cavity with ultimate progression of the testis into the scrotum with closure of the inguinal canal.

Ovarian differentiation (93,94,96) determined by multiple loci on both X chromosomes (93,97) proceeds somewhat differently, as there is not only active steroidogenesis but also considerable follicular and oocytic differentiation. The primordial germ cells undergo proliferation and then differentiate into oogonia and finally oocytes, which remain in the diplotene phase of the first meiotic division. Primitive ovarian granulosa cells organize around the oocytes to form primordial and then primary follicles by the sixth month of intrauterine life. Later in gestation, granulosa cell proliferation and development of small antral follicles parallel the growth of the ovary. Steroidogenic epithelioid cells surround the several granulosa cell layers of the growing follicles by the end of the midtrimester of gestation. As further evidence of the capacity for considerable intrauterine maturation of ovarian function, follicular atresia, or germ cell degeneration, is seen by the end of the first trimester and is present until term. Antral follicles develop late in the second trimester and are seen until term.

Genital Duct Development
By the seventh week of fetal development, the anlage of the internal genital duct systems are present. The Wolffian, or mesonephric, ducts develop into the male epididymis, vas deferens, seminal vesicles, and the ejaculatory ducts; the Mullerian, or paramesonephric, ducts develop into the female uterus, fallopian tubes, and upper third of the vagina. Under the local influence of the fetal testis (see below) the Wolffian ducts differentiate and grow, and the Mullerian ducts involute; the absence of the testis, but not necessarily the presence of the ovary, leads to the development of Mullerian derivatives with resorption of Wolffian elements (98).

Differentiation of the External Genitalia
After 2 months of intrauterine life, the sexual dimorphism of the external genitalia has not yet become evident, but by 10 weeks the two sexes may be distinguished. The urogenital slit has an anterior genital tubercle, with glans and cavernous tissue, and is bounded laterally by urethral folds and, further laterally, by the labial-scrotal swellings. These basic structures develop respectively into the male penis, corpus spongiosum, and scrotum and into the female clitoris, labia minora, and labia majora. Again, as in the case of the internal ducts, the fetal testis and its secretions are necessary for the masculinization of the external genitalia. In the absence of the testis, feminization occurs. Normal testicular function during the first 12 weeks of intrauterine life is needed for complete differentiation of the male external genitalia.

Gonadotropins

Luteinizing Hormone (LH)
The glycoprotein hormones—LH, FSH, TSH, HCG—are made up of two noncovalently bound subunits, α and β chains (99). The α subunit is species-specific but similar in each of the human glycoprotein hormones; the β subunit confers biologic and immunologic specificity. The generation of subunit-specific antisera has permitted sensi-

tive and highly specific quantitation of both hLH and also hCG during intrauterine life (3,100,101). Such specificity of measurement had not been possible with the anti-hLH or anti-hCG sera previously available, as the degree of cross-reactivity was often complete.

Fetal. In vitro production of both LH and FSH by cultured fetal anterior pituitaries has been demonstrated by 5 weeks of intrauterine life (23). From 17 to 28 weeks, total pituitary release of LH is greater in females than in males. Kaplan and Grumbach demonstrated the presence of immunoreactive LH in the human fetal pituitary gland by 68 days of life (3,99,100). Mean LH content in both male and female pituitaries rises between 10 and 14 weeks of gestation and 30 and 40 weeks. Levels in females are higher than in males from 10 to 29 weeks of gestation (100). Serum LH levels are in the castrate range in many female fetuses prior to 20 weeks and then fall to undetectable levels by term (100,101). Serum concentrations are greater in female than in male fetuses between 12 and 20 weeks (101). Amniotic fluid levels of gonadotropins presumably reflect fetal urinary excretion. (In postnatal life, the urinary excretion of LH and FSH reflects the integrated value of pituitary production of these hormones and the mean serum levels.) Clements and coworkers (101) found that amniotic fluid levels of LH are quite low prior to 12 weeks and then rise to a peak at 16 weeks, with levels in amniotic fluid from female fetuses being significantly greater than in male. Amniotic fluid concentrations then fall into the undetectable range after 32 weeks. The LH concentrations in pituitary glands, sera, and amniotic fluid correlate closely in midgestation and demonstrate that LH production is increasing at a time that chorionic gonadotropin levels are falling (Figs. 5 and 6). Additionally, serum LH levels fall while pituitary LH content increases. This inverse relationship suggests that the pituitary

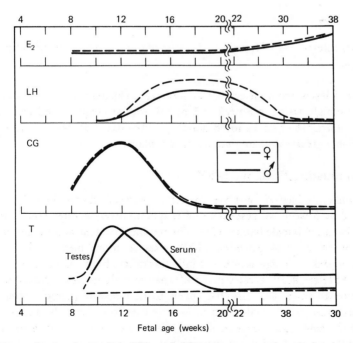

Figure 5. Serum levels of estradiol, LH, and CG and serum and testicular concentrations of testosterone in the fetus. Reprinted from (11) with permission of authors and publisher.

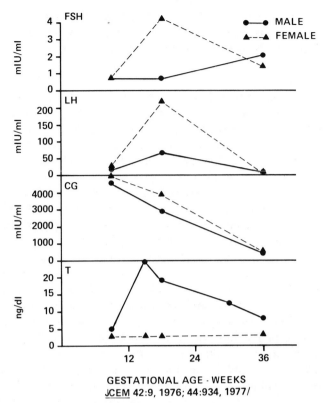

Figure 6. Amniotic fluid concentrations of gonadotropins in human fetus. Adapted from (101,200).

gonadotropes release less LH, perhaps because of diminished stimulation by Gn-RH, in late gestation.

Neonatal. LH levels are undetectable in cord sera. During the first week of life serum LH levels are high, rising to a peak at 1 month with subsequent decline to low prepubertal levels during the first 12 to 18 months of life (102,103). Serum concentrations of LH are variably greater in male than in female infants.

Follicle-Stimulating Hormone (FSH)

Fetal. In vitro production of FSH by fetal pituitary glands in culture has been demonstrated by 5 weeks of gestation and is quantitatively greater and of longer duration in pituitaries of female fetuses (23). The pituitary content of immunoreactive FSH, detectable by 68 days of gestation (100), rises to term; mean FSH concentration increases to a peak in midgestation and falls thereafter. Both content and concentration of pituitary FSH are much greater in female than in male fetuses. Immunoreactive FSH has been detected in fetal serum (101) prior to 12 weeks of gestation, with distinctly greater concentrations in female than in male fetuses from 12 to 20 weeks. FSH levels are often in the adult castrate range during this period (100,101). In many serum samples from male fetuses FSH is not detectable during this period. After 20 weeks serum

FSH levels fall into the low or undetectable range and remain so in cord sera. Umbilical cord FSH levels are greater in female than in male neonates (104,105). Amniotic fluid concentrations of FSH remain undetectable or very low in males but rise considerably in females with mean levels in females significantly greater throughout the midtrimester (Fig. 6). Amniotic fluid FSH values decrease to term and exhibit no sex-related difference in the last trimester (101). Maternal serum FSH levels during pregnancy have been generally extremely low or undetectable (106). This is presumably secondary to suppression by the high levels of serum estrogens.

Neonatal. FSH levels rise from birth to the second or third month of life and then gradually decrease into the prepubertal range by 2 years of life. FSH concentrations have generally been greater in female than in male infants (103,105).

Chorionic Gonadotropin (CG)

Maternal. Maternal serum levels of CG are often greater than 60 IU/ml during the first trimester, declining to a mean of less than 10 IU/ml by midterm. CG concentrations then rise significantly with advancing gestation in bearers of female children, but not in those of male children. At term, CG levels are greater in mothers with female infants; cord sera concentrations of CG generally exhibit no sex-related difference (107) other than in the studies of Penny et al., who found higher levels in male fetuses (104).

Fetal. During the period from 12 to 20 weeks, there is a decline in fetal serum levels of CG that parallels that seen in the mother and is not influenced by sex (101). The maternal-to-fetal ratio of serum CG during this period is about 30:1. Amniotic fluid levels of CG reflect those in sera, with a peak at 11 to 14 weeks and a marked decline to term (Figure 6). CG is present in amniotic fluid in high concentrations by 8 weeks of gestation and probably earlier. CG is undetectable in most fetal pituitary specimens and, when reported, appears to be accounted for by minor antigenic similarities leading to cross-reactivity of pituitary LH with the anti-hCG serum used in the radioassay.

The role of CG in fetal sexual differentiation is discussed below, but the peak at 11 to 14 weeks suggests that this hormone is the primary agent stimulating fetal Leydig cells. Clements et al. (101) also note that despite the considerable fall in CG concentration during the midtrimester of gestation, levels are still 3 to 50 times greater than those of LH (Fig. 5). Further radioreceptor and in vitro bioassay data (108,109) suggest a two- to sixfold greater potency-weight of CG than LH. This suggests an important role for CG in fetal Leydig cell function to at least 20 weeks of gestation and possibly longer.

Subunits of Glycoprotein Hormones

As noted above, the glycoprotein hormones are comprised of a β subunit, conferring biologic and immunologic specificity, and an α subunit. The α subunits are immunologically indistinguishable among the four glycoprotein hormones, although the amino acid sequences are not identical (99). Kaplan and coworkers demonstrated the presence of an α subunit from 17 weeks of gestation in both pituitary homogenates and serum, although β subunit is barely detectable (110). The α subunit is the predominant glycoprotein hormone in both the pituitary and serum and is present in greater concentration than is intact LH or FSH. No sex-related differences in subunit levels are recorded (110).

Sex Steroids

Testosterone

Fetal. Histochemical, in vitro synthetic, and gas-liquid chromatographic techniques have documented the capacity of fetal testes to produce androgens. Testosterone is the major androgen found in fetal testicular extracts (11,111,112). Fetal testicular concentrations of testosterone are greatest between 12 and 15 weeks of gestation and decrease thereafter. Ovaries contain negligible quantities of testosterone. Serum concentrations of testosterone are higher in males than in females from 9 to 25 weeks (113). The pattern of serum testosterone levels in males mirrors that in the testes, with highest amounts in the 11- to 17-week period, often in the adult male range (as high as 580 ng/dl). After 17 weeks of gestation, testosterone values decline to less than 100 ng/dl. Levels in female fetuses do not exceed 130 ng/dl and do not change during midgestation. Amniotic fluid levels of testosterone reflect gonadal and serum patterns and clearly demonstrate the sex-related difference (114). The pattern of testosterone production (Fig. 7) correlates well with Leydig cell proliferation and ultrastructural differentiation as well as with the in vitro production of testosterone (115). The importance of fetal testosterone production in sexual differentiation is discussed below.

At birth, the levels of free testosterone, i.e., not bound to the sex-hormone binding globulin, are three-fold greater than in adults (116). The greater capacity of the placenta to aromatize testosterone to estrogens, as well as the "protective role" of high concentrations of estradiol (E_2), may impede the manifestations of excessive androgen bioactivity in the normal infant. A protective situation is also evident in females born of mothers with androgen-producing neoplasms (117) in whom the degree of clitoral enlargement is quite small relative to the high testosterone exposure.

Postnatal. Testicular androgen production is present at birth, and there is a striking increase in postnatal androgen synthesis (116) (Fig. 8). In cord samples, testosterone levels are slightly greater in male than in female fetuses (34.2 ± 1.0 versus 25.8 ± 1.0

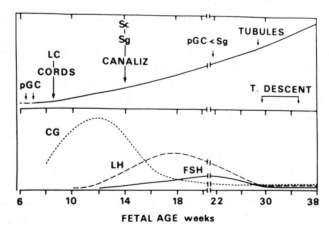

Figure 7. Levels of serum gonadotropins as correlated with changes of testicular histology (pGC = primordial germ cells; LC = Leydig cells; cords = germinal cords; Sc = Sertoli cells; Sg = spermatogonia; canaliz = canalization). Reprinted from (11) with permission of authors and publisher.

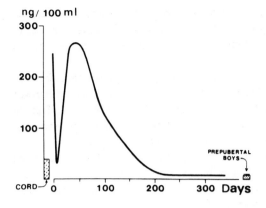

Figure 8. Changing levels of plasma testosterone in males during the first year. Reprinted from (116) by permission of author and publisher.

ng/dl), reflecting the placental aromatizing capacity. Within the first few hours of life serum concentrations of testosterone are substantially higher in male 242 ± 100 ng/dl) than in female neonates (28.6 ± 14 ng/dl). There is then a sharp decrement in testosterone levels in both male and female infants until the end of the first week of life, with a subsequent rise in males to a peak at 1 to 2 months. By 7 months of age, testosterone values fall to the prepubertal range. In female infants serum testosterone concentrations decline to the prepubertal range by 2 weeks of age.

As noted above, a lower percentage of testosterone is bound to sex-hormone binding globulin (SHBG) at birth than in adulthood. SHBG levels rise abruptly after birth with consequent change in the quantity of bound testosterone. Nonetheless, during the first 30 to 60 days of age, free (biologically active) testosterone (116) concentrations are 40-fold greater in males than in females and are in the midpubertal range.

Estradiol

Maternal estradiol (E_2) levels gradually increase throughout gestation and do not differ with the sex of the fetus. Fetal and maternal serum levels of E_2 are similar in midpregnancy and are 2 to 30 times greater than in the nonpregnant state. In the fetus gonadal and adrenal E_2 is generally undetectable (111). Serum E_2 levels are slightly higher in female than in male fetuses from 10 to 18 weeks, but considerable overlap exists. Payne and Jaffe (118) were unable to demonstrate in vitro aromatization of androgens by ovarian tissue, confirming earlier studies suggesting that most of fetal E_2 is of placental origin (119). Nonetheless, Pinkerton et al. (120) did demonstrate histochemical differences between fetal and prepubertal ovaries, suggesting active thecal steroidogenesis. Ross (96) has noted that the slope of the line relating the growth of the fetal uterus to gestational age is coincident with epithelioid transformation of the theca interna, again suggesting fetal ovarian estrogen production and response to intense gonadotropin stimulation.

Sex-Hormone Secretion and Sexual Differentiation (121)

Female

Embryologic studies by Jost (98) have demonstrated that sexual differentiation of the female fetus is a passive process. In the absence of a functional testis, internal (Mullerian) ducts become fallopian tubes and uterus, and Wolffian ducts involute; the external genitalia feminize. In the human syndrome of ovarian dysgenesis, internal and external genital development is feminine. Exposure to androgens prior to 12 weeks of gestation causes fusion of the labia minora, clitoral hypertrophy, and virilization of the external genitalia.

The absence of a distinct sex-related difference of serum E_2 suggests that the fetal ovary is not the primary source of this hormone, despite indirect evidence of estrogen synthesis by the ovary. The distinct elevations of endogenous fetal FSH and LH in the female and the considerable degree of ovarian follicular differentiation and growth indicate that the hypothalamic-pituitary-ovarian axis may be functional in the female fetus in utero (Fig. 9). Ross has deduced from data in anencephalic female infants and fetuses that fetal pituitary gonadotropin production may be necessary for appropriate follicular maturation, as ovaries of anencephalic fetuses weigh less and have diminished interstitial tissue and arrested follicular development (96).

In the immediate postpartum period and during the first 3 to 6 months of life, a slight rise in serum E_2 levels occurs (122). The reason for this subtle increment is unknown. Concentrations then fall into the undetectable range of less than 5 pg/ml.

Male

The importance of the fetal testes in sexual differentiation has been well established (98). The needs for local androgen to stimulate male internal (Wolffian) duct growth, for systemic androgens in the differentiation of the external genitalia, and for a nonsteroidal locally acting macromolecule to cause Mullerian duct involution (123) have been documented. In adults, the cellular effects of androgen are mediated largely by dihydrotestosterone (DHT); this 5α-reduced metabolite of testosterone is largely

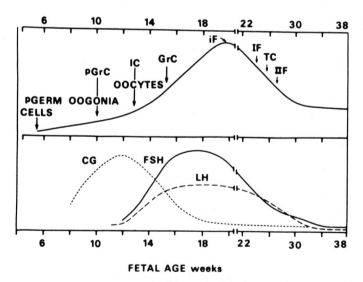

FETAL AGE weeks

Figure 9. Levels of serum gonadotropins as correlated with changes of ovarian histology (p germ cells; Gre = primordial germ cells; Gre = pregranulosa cells; IC = interstitial cells; GrC = granulosa cells; iF = primordial follicles; IF = primary follicles; TC = theca cells; IIF = secondary follicles). Reprinted from (11) by permission of authors and publisher.

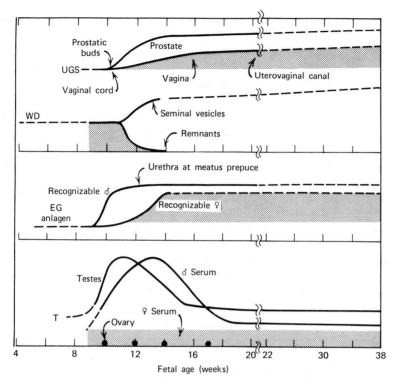

Figure 10. Pattern of sexual differentiation as related to serum and gonadal testerone levels. Reprinted from (11) by permission of authors and publisher.

produced intracellularly by target tissues and is then transported to the nuclear chromatin by the highly specific DHT-receptor protein (124). In the male fetus the urogenital sinus, labioscrotal swellings and folds, and the genital tubercle have the capacity to reduce testosterone to DHT, suggesting that masculine external genital differentiation is initiated by DHT (115). In contrast, the Wolffian ducts do not have 5α reductase, and the capacity for reduction of testosterone to DHT is not present during this critical period (124). Testosterone is the androgen responsible for the differentiation of the Wolffian ducts into the seminal vesicles, vas deferens, and epididymis (Fig. 10). In patients with deficiency of 5α reductase (pseudovaginal peroneal hypospadias syndrome), the anatomical defect is limited to the external genitalia, as there is development of the vas deferens, epididymis, and seminal vesicles (125).

The role of fetal and placental gonadotropin regulation of testicular function has been examined. Peak fetal serum levels of CG are present at 11 to 14 weeks, but they are already high by 8 weeks, during the period of gonadal, especially Leydig cell, and genital sex differentiation. The rise in serum testosterone in the male fetus parallels the levels of CG and occurs before the increment in fetal LH production (Fig. 5). The greater concentration of immunoreactive CG and its higher biopotency than LH suggest that CG is the gonadotropin responsible for fetal Leydig cell function during the early critical period of differentiation of the internal and external genitalia. During mid- to late gestation, immunoreactive fetal LH is secreted, but testosterone levels fall. The biopotency of endogenous LH has not been evaluated, however, and it may not be so bioactive as its immunoreactive levels suggest. Kaplan and coworkers suggest that rising levels of fetal serum prolactin may impair gonadal responsivity to LH and decrease testosterone synthesis and release (3,30,75). Nevertheless, late gestational pituitary LH-mediated secretion of testosterone is important for the normal growth of the male external genitalia in the last trimester. Male children with hypogonadotropic hypogonadism or anencephaly have normal anatomic sexual differentiation but may have diminished growth of the external genitalia (3,96). Despite the normal fall in testosterone levels in the second half of gestation, it is apparent that basal production of testosterone is necessary for normal genital growth and that the Leydig cells require fetal pituitary gonadotropic stimulation. Patients with abnormalities of testosterone biosynthesis have variably ambiguous development of the external genitalia (121).

Differentiation of the Mullerian ducts occurs in the absence of a fetal testis or ovary. Josso and her coworkers (123) have demonstrated that fetal Sertoli cells produce a nonsteroidal polypeptide that causes involution of the Mullerian ducts, i.e., an "anti-Mullerian hormone." Josso has also demonstrated that cultured human fetal testes but not postnatal testes inhibit Mullerian duct growth (123,126).

Between the second and twenty-eighth weeks of life, serum concentrations of testosterone are greater than in cord sera in the mid- to late-pubertal range (116). A similar increment in E_2 values is not seen in female infants. Despite extensive psychological studies, the role of the normal androgen increment, or of abnormal androgen levels such as may occur in females with congenital adrenal hyperplasia, in later development is unclear. The available data suggest that the hypothalamic-pituitary axis may be normal even following excessive androgen exposure in the neonatal period (127).

Maturation of Intrauterine Negative Feedback

Immunoreactive and bioactive Gn-RH have been found in human fetal hypothalami (8,11). Levina (128) demonstrated that hypothalamic fragments from third trimester fetuses stimulate less release of pituitary gonadotropins in vitro than do hypothalamic fragments from younger fetuses. The pituitary of midtrimester fetuses is capable of secreting LH and FSH in vitro in response to Gn-RH (129). In vivo Gn-RH administration during hysterotomies for abortions between the fifteenth and twenty-second weeks of gestation did not evoke pituitary release of gonadotropin (130), though specific immunoreactive LH was not quantitated. The failure of Gn-RH to release LH despite large amounts of pituitary LH during this period of gestation suggests either that the high levels of circulating estrogen and progesterone impair the responsivity of the gonadotropes or that more specific radioimmunologic techniques are required to assess the dynamic release of LH at this period.

Between 12 and 20 weeks of gestation, serum levels of LH and FSH in the female fetus are frequently in the castrate range despite very high levels of E_2. Deficiency of hypothalamic E_2 receptors has been suggested to explain this observation (101). Later in gestation, levels of gonadotropins fall to low or undetectable values in both sexes. Kaplan and coworkers (3) suggest that these data reflect maturational progress of hypothalamic regulation of pituitary gonadotropin secretion. The hypothalamic gonadostat becomes increasingly sensitive to sex steroid inhibitory feedback, leading to decreased Gn-RH release and consequent decline in secretion of LH and FSH (Fig. 11).

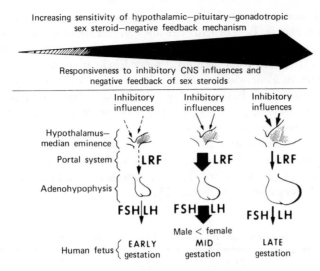

Figure 11. Development of the regulatory system for control of FSH and LH production in the fetus. Reprinted from (3) by permission of authors and publisher.

PITUITARY–THYROID AXIS

Embryology

The major part of the human thyroid gland is derived from the floor of the primitive buccal cavity and is first visible 16 to 17 days after conception, when the fetus is in the 3- to 4-mm stage. The lateral aspects of the thyroid gland are derived from the fourth pharyngeal pouches, the same embryological structures that give rise to the calcitonin-secreting parafollicular cells of the thyroid gland. By the fifth week of gestation the thyroid gland is a bilobed structure, and by 7 weeks it is situated in its accustomed midcervical site. The fetal thyroid gland is able to concentrate iodine by 10 weeks of gestation. Thyroxine (T_4) is present in the fetal thyroid by 12 weeks of gestation, but serum levels of T_4 remain low until midgestation. By the twelfth week of gestation the pituitary gland contains thyrotropin (TSH) secreting cells (131).

Thyrotropin (TSH)

Fetal pituitary TSH content is low before 18 weeks' gestation and increases thereafter. Fetal serum levels of TSH are low until 18 weeks' gestation, when there is an abrupt increase to approximately 9 μU/ml by 22 weeks (132,133). Thereafter the serum levels of TSH remain relatively constant until term. Hypothalamic thyrotropin releasing hormone (TRH) is detectable by 10 weeks of gestation and increases to 5 to 10 pg/mg of tissue by midgestation (8). Initially function of the fetal thyroid gland is probably independent of hypothalamic-pituitary control, but by midgestation it is likely that some regulation is exerted.

Thyroid Hormones

The midtrimester increase in serum levels of TSH is followed by a rise in serum concentrations of T_4 (132,133). Thyroxine-binding-globulin (TBG) concentrations also increase at this time, as do levels of free T_4, suggesting that there is increase in the absolute secretion rate of T_4. The fetus has low concentrations of triiodothyronine (T_3), and levels of reverse T_3 (rT_3) are high. Since the majority of the circulating triiodothyronine is derived from peripheral monodeiodination of T_4, the fetus must be relatively deficient in 5′ deiodinase activity. Reverse T_3 is biologically inactive in the human adult, but its role in fetal physiology is unknown. Total and free T_3 values and turnover of T_3 are low and the T_4/T_3 ratio high in the fetus. It is likely that T_4 is the major bioactive thyroid hormone of the fetus.

Fetal serum T_4 levels increase steadily throughout the last trimester of pregnancy. There is an increase in cord T_4 concentrations with increasing gestational age and birthweight (134) (Table II). Cord T_4 levels are low in infants who subsequently develop the respiratory distress syndrome (135).

Table II. Serum Concentrations of Pituitary and Thyroid Hormones in Relation to Age

	TSH ($\mu U/ml$)	T_4 ($\mu g/dl$)	T_3 (ng/dl)	Reverse T_3 (ng/dl)
Fetus	ND–20	4–16	15–126	
Amniotic fluid	1.5	0.54	30	82
	(ND–3.7)	(ND–1.75)	(25–35)	(ND–232)
Cord	9.5	12	50	315
	(1–20)	(6–17)	(10–90)	(175–455)
30 weeks		9.4		
		(5.7–15.6)		
35 weeks	14	10.1		
		(6.6–16.8)		
40 weeks		10.9		
		(6.6–18.1)		
45 weeks	8	11.7		
		(7.1–19.4)		
24 hr	20	21	300	150
		(16–26)	(220–400)	(100–200)
48 hr	18	18	180	125
		(12–20)	(130–230)	(100–150)
3–5 days	6	15	130	60
	(ND–20)	(9–20)	(50–210)	(30–100)
2 weeks–2 months	4	11	160	40
	(ND–10)	(7–15)	(160–240)	(10–60)
1 year	1.9	11.0	176	31
	(0.6–6.3)			
1–5 years	1.9	10.5	168	33
	(0.6–6.3)	(7.3–15.0)	(105–269)	(15–71)
5–10 years	1.9	9.3	150	36
	(0.6–6.3)	(6.4–13.3)	(94–241)	(17–79)
10–15 years	1.9	8.1	133	41
	(0.6–6.3)	(5.6–11.7)	(83–213)	(19–88)
15 years	1.9	7.6	125	43
	(0.6–6.3)			
Adults	ND–10	5–13	60–220	36–84

ND indicates nondetectable.

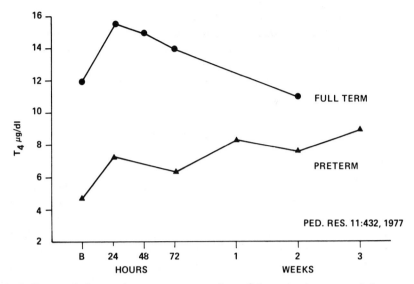

Figure 12. Postnatal changes in serum concentrations of thyroxine in preterm infants compared with full-term infants. Data adapted from Uhrmann et al. (139).

The fetal thyroid axis is independent of the mother, as TSH, T_4, and T_3 do not cross the placental barrier in either direction in significant amounts (133). The physiologic role of thyroid hormone in fetal growth and development is incompletely known, but it is important for the development of the fetal central nervous system, particularly the cerebral and cerebellar cortices.

Postnatal Changes

In the full-term neonate immediately after birth there is a surge in TSH concentration that peaks within 0.5 hr and returns to base line values by 48 to 72 hr (132,133,136). The rise in TSH is triggered by delivery of the infant into a cool environment; the rise is blunted if the neonate's temperature is not permitted to fall. No other major changes in TSH levels occur throughout childhood. Shortly after delivery T_4 and free T_4 values increase, probably in response to the antecedent rise in TSH secretion. Mean peak levels of T_4 (16 μg/dl) and free T_4 (7 ng/dl) are reached by 24 to 48 hr and decline slowly thereafter; values remain elevated and reach base line values only after several weeks. T_4 values continue to decline steadily throughout childhood to reach adult values by 15 years (137).

Values of T_3 and free T_3 increase after birth from low cord levels (50 ng/dl; 146 pg/dl) to hypertriiodothyroninemic concentrations (419 ng/dl; 1260 pg/dl) by 24 hr of life; values return to basal levels over the next several days. The surge in T_3 values reflects not only the antecedent increase in T_4 secretion but also the neurogenic effects of the cutting of the umbilical cord, as delay in cord cutting delays the rise in T_3 levels. The mean serum levels of T_3 decline throughout infancy and childhood (137).

The levels of rT_3 present in cord blood remain high for several days, declining to adult values by 10 to 14 days. The role of thyroid hormone in the immediate postpartum period relates to its effects on substrate mobilization and thermogenesis.

Data are incomplete concerning the changes in thyroid function that occur in the preterm infant following delivery. Available data suggest that serum thyroid hormone levels are low in such children and do not increase as in the full-term infant (138,139) (Fig. 12). Thyroid hormone concentrations may also be low in sick infants. Thus when assessing thyroid function in the neonate, it is important to know the gestational age, birthweight, postpartum age, and clinical status of the individual infant. Normal ranges for each of the thyroid hormones should be established, depending on these parameters.

THE FETAL PITUITARY–ADRENOCORTICAL AXIS

Embryology

The human fetal adrenal cortex is derived from the dorsal coelomic mesothelium beginning in the fourth week of gestation (140). It is composed of two histologically distinct zones. The inner fetal zone is predominant during fetal life, accounting for 85% of the weight of the fetal adrenal cortex. It is composed of large, eosinophilic cells. The outer zone, or neocortex, is composed of undifferentiated, probably nonfunctional cells. After birth the cells of the neocortex enlarge and proliferate, and the inner zone begins to deteriorate by the fourth postpartum day. The combined weight of the two fetal adrenal glands is approximately 2.5 g at the end of the fourth gestational month, 5.3 g in the eighth month, and 9.3 g by term. There is a 50% decline in combined fetal weight within the first postnatal month, which continues to a nadir of 3.3 g per pair at 18 months. Thereafter there is a slow increase in adrenal weight to the adult value of 10 g per pair by adolescence.

The human, the chimpanzee, and to some extent the rhesus monkey are the only species to have a distinct fetal adrenal cortical zone (141). The significance of the fetal cortical zone to the embryological development, growth, and well-being of the fetus is poorly understood. That the growth of the fetal zone in the second half of pregnancy is under fetal pituitary ACTH regulations is indicated by the observation that adrenocortical growth is imparied in fetuses with decreased secretion of ACTH, i.e., in infants with anencephaly, aplasia, or hypoplasia of the pituitary and in those whose mothers received large amounts of glucocorticoids during the pregnancy. However, the early development of the fetal adrenal is independent of ACTH because the adrenals of anencephalic fetuses grow normally in the first half of gestation (140,141). Fetal adrenal growth also coincides with increased concentrations of prolactin in fetal serum, and it has been postulated that prolactin may also be a corticotropic agent in utero (76). The fetal zone of the adrenal gland is deficient in the enzyme 3β-hydroxysteroid dehydrogenase (3βHSD), and as a consequence large amounts of Δ^5-19-carbon and Δ^5-21-carbon steroids are produced by and circulate in the fetus. The fetal cortex is able to produce Δ^4-3-keto-21-carbon steroids such as cortisol, using placental progesterone as substrate (142,143).

Fetal Adrenocorticotrophin (ACTH)

ACTH is a straight-chain, 39-amino-acid peptide, the biological activity of which resides in the 24-amino-acid sequence beginning at the amino-terminal end of the molecule. This sequence is identical in all species studied. ACTH is synthesized by specific basophiles of the pituitary as a larger molecule, "big" ACTH, which may be the precursor for both ACTH and β-lipotrophin (144). In addition, "big" ACTH may be the precursor for the two ACTH fragments-α-melanocyte-stimulating hormone (αMSH), a molecule composed of the first 13 amino acids from the amino terminus of ACTH, and corticotrophin-like intermediate lobe peptide (CLIP), both of which are found only in human fetal pituitary glands. Between 12 weeks and term the human fetal pituitary contains large quantities of these small ACTH fragments relative to the intact molecule, but at birth the proportion changes rapidly, and the major pituitary corticotropin fraction consists of authentic ACTH thereafter (144). The significance of the ACTH fragments, αMSH and CLIP, during fetal life is unknown, but it has been postulated that these peptides may specifically stimulate growth of the inner fetal zone of the adrenal cortex and that intact ACTH is responsible for stimulation of the growth of the neocortex and development of the adult adrenal zone at term.

Immunoreactive ACTH is detectable in the fetal pituitary by 7 weeks of gestation and bioassayable ACTH by 9 weeks (3). The mean immunoreactive ACTH content of the fetal pituitary at midterm is 16 ng per pituitary (range 3.6 to 38.8); the mean concentration is 2.01 ng/mg (range 0.44 to 5.71); the amount of pituitary ACTH increases in late gestation. In one anencephalic infant pituitary ACTH content was 76 ng (145). Siler-Khodr et al. (23) reported that in vitro culture of fetal pituitary tissue resulted in release of immunoreactive ACTH. Secretion was detected in a pituitary from a 5-week fetus and increased significantly in pituitaries obtained from fetuses between 15 and 20 weeks' gestation and term. ACTH release continued for approximately 17 days in culture and then declined to low levels. Bioassayable ACTH is released from fetal pituitaries in vitro by 11 weeks' gestation (9). The mean fetal serum concentration of ACTH has been reported to be 250 pg/ml at 12 to 19 weeks, decreasing thereafter to 143 pg/ml by 35 to 40 weeks of gestation (146). Allen et al. (145) and Kaupila et al. (147) reported a mean mixed umbilical cord serum ACTH value of 226 pg/ml (range, 53 to 570) in both full-term and premature infants.

Arai et al. (148) demonstrated higher levels of ACTH in umbilical arterial blood (602 pg/ml) than in umbilical vein blood (262 pg/ml) in full-term infants delivered vaginally. These data are consistent with endogenous fetal secretion and lack of transplacental passage of ACTH. In infants delivered by cesarean section without prior labor, ACTH values are similar in umbilical vein (333 pg/ml) and artery (385 pg/ml) specimens. Serial fetal sampling during labor reveals a significant increase in fetal ACTH levels as labor progresses. These observations indicate that fetal ACTH secretion increases during vaginal delivery, perhaps as a response to the stress of uterine contraction, trauma, or hypoxia. Maternal levels of ACTH at delivery are approximately 200 pg/ml (147).

Amniotic fluid also contains immunoreactive ACTH (149). The mean ACTH concentration is 209 pg/ml between 10 and 18 weeks, increases to 430 pg/ml between 26 and 30 weeks, and thereafter decreases to 173 pg/ml until term. The source of amniotic ACTH is unknown, but it is presumably of fetal origin. In the first voiding of the neonatal period urine contains 160 pg/ml of immunoreactive ACTH. In one pregnancy in a patient with Nelson's syndrome (ACTH-producing pituitary adenoma) in whom serum ACTH levels were 5000 to 23,000 pg/ml, amniotic fluid values for ACTH ranged between 20 and 221 pg/ml (126), suggesting that maternal levels did not influence amniotic fluid content. Amniotic fluid concentrations of ACTH in anencephalic infants are low at term (20 pg/ml).

The placenta secretes an ACTH-like peptide that has been identified in both placental extracts and tissue cultures (150). Its physiologic role is uncertain.

Fetal Adrenocortical Function

The fetal adrenal cortex and the placenta function as a unit during pregnancy, the biochemical function of each component complementing the other (141–143). The adrenal cortex of the fetus is relatively deficient in 3βHSD and Δ^5-isomerase activities and thus secretes a number of Δ^5-3βOH steroids, the principal ones of which are dehydroepiandrosterone (DHA) and its sulfoconjugate. The fetal adrenal cortex has marked 16α-hydroxylase activity. The 16α-OH-DHA serves as the precursor for estriol after it has been aromatized by the placenta. The placenta secretes progesterone, which the fetal adrenal cortex converts to cortisol. There is also transplacental passage of both progesterone and cortisol from the maternal to the fetal circulation. However, the bulk of maternal cortisol is metabolized to cortisone by the placenta and thus inactivated (151). The hydroxylating enzymes necessary for cortisol synthesis are demonstrable in the fetal adrenal cortex by the eighth gestational week, when these glands are capable of cortisol synthesis using progesterone as substrate (142). There is increasing production of cortisol by the fetal adrenal in vitro as gestation advances. However, since the plasma cortisol level of cord blood of the anencephalic infant with an atrophic adrenal gland has been reported to be similar to that of the normal newborn, it had been thought that the majority of circulating cortisol in the fetus was of maternal origin (152). This observation has been challenged by the report of low umbilical arterial concentrations of cortisol in such infants (153). Although there is approximately four times more cortisol in maternal than in fetal circulation, this is due in large part to the higher levels of transcortin, the cortisol binding protein, in maternal (8 to 9 mg/dl) than in fetal (1.5 to 2.0 mg/dl) serum (143). Other data imply also that the bulk of circulating cortisol in the fetus is of endogenous origin. There is cortisol in the umbilical cord blood of infants born to women with hypoadrenocorticism. Studies involving infusion of radiolabeled cortisol and cortisone into pregnant women at term indicate that approximately 75% of fetal circulating cortisol is secreted by the fetus, with the mother contributing 25% of this level (154). In infants with congenital adrenal hyperplasia due to an inborn error of cortisol biosynthesis with attendant hyperandrogenism, maternal cortisol is unable to prevent the fetal pituitary-adrenal hypersecretory response to deficient fetal cortisol secretion (155).

Cortisone, corticosterone, desoxycorticosterone, and aldosterone are also present in fetal blood (141–143). Cortisone, which is biologically inactive in the fetus, is derived from maternal cortisol after placental degradation (151). It is present in the fetal circulation in larger amounts than is cortisol, a pattern that persists throughout the first postnatal month. The serum concentration of aldosterone (20 to 80 ng/dl) at delivery is 2 to 21 times that of the mother's level and varies inversely with the quantity of sodium ingested by the mother (156).

Murphy (157) reports that the human fetus secretes cortisol as early as 10 to 18 weeks of gestation. She notes that the umbilical arterial concentration of cortisol is higher than that in the umbilical vein (0.8 verses 0.4 μg/ml), and the reverse is observed for cortisone and progesterone values. There is an increase in fetal cortisol levels as gestation progresses. In mixed arterial-venous umbilical cord samples, the mean cortisol level between 12 and 18 weeks' gestation is 0.7 μg/dl. The level of cortisol rises to 2.3 μg/dl between 36 and 41 weeks' gestation (158). The cortisol concentration in umbilical cord blood at delivery reflects to a large extent the mode of delivery. Thus, in spontaneous vaginal deliveries of term infants, the umbilical artery concentration of cortisol is significantly increased when compared with umbilical vein levels (7.9 verses 6.2 μg/dl), a difference not observed in induced labor—umbilical artery, 5.8; umbilical vein, 5.1 μg/dl (159). Maternal cortisol levels also rise impressively during labor, but since umbilical arterial cortisol concentrations are higher than umbilical venous values, the elevated fetal cortisol levels do not primarily reflect changes in maternal adrenocortical function but probably reflect the change in endogenous adrenocortical secretory activity during labor. Whether the increased umbilical cord levels of cortisol precede or coincide with labor is uncertain. Ohrlander et al. (160) measured fetal scalp blood cortisol levels serially during labor and observed a significant rise in values during both induced and spontaneous labor, although initial concentrations were similar in the two groups. These investigators concluded that the elevated cord levels of cortisol recorded in vaginally delivered infants were a consequence of the stress of labor. In a similar experiment Arai and Yanachara (161) were unable to demonstrate any significant changes in scalp plasma cortisol values between initiation and completion of spontaneous labor in primiparous mothers but did observe significant increase in concentrations of pregnenolone, progesterone, dehydroepiandrosterone, 16α-hydroxy-DHA, and estriol during labor. They concluded that there was increase in fetal adrenal secretory activity during labor. Some of the confusion in this area may stem from the nature of the specimen obtained. Thus mixed cord blood may be expected to contain primarily umbilical venous blood, because the umbilical artery may constrict and thus restrict flow. It is important to measure umbilical arterial blood in order to estimate endogenous fetal production of a substance.

Amniotic fluid free cortisol reaches detectable levels by 8 weeks' gestation (5 ng/ml), increases at 10 to 25 weeks' gestation (10 ng/ml), and remains constant until abruptly increasing between 38 and 40 weeks (15 to 20 ng/ml) (162). In other studies the sharp rise in amniotic fluid cortisol levels at term is not clearly evident. There is no increase in amniotic fluid cortisol levels during labor at term (163). There is a significant correlation between amniotic fluid and umbilical cord concentrations of cortisol; the latter is approximately twofold higher than amniotic fluid values. Amniotic fluid levels of cortisol are low in anencephalic infants and infants of diabetic pregnancies and high in stressed infants of toxemic mothers, those with Rh incompatibility and postmaturity, and during premature labor (162,163). Since there is wide variation in amniotic fluid cortisol levels, in part because of dilutional effects, individual values do not necessarily reflect fetal gestational age, weight, or pulmonary maturation and therefore are not useful alone as reliable indicators of fetal maturity or well-being (164–166). The cortisol/cortisone ratio of amniotic fluid increases as the fetus ages and correlates with fetal lung maturation more significantly than do cortisol or cortisone levels alone (167). Although much of amniotic fluid free cortisol is of fetal origin, the amniotic membrane converts cortisone to cortisol between 17 weeks gestation and term. This conversion probably contributes significantly to the rising amniotic fluid cortisol levels and cortisol/cortisone ratio observed in the last half of pregnancy (168,169). The amniotic membrane–produced cortisol may account for reasonably normal lung development observed in anencephalic infants.

Role of the Fetal Adrenal Cortex

The roles of the fetal adrenal cortex and placenta are complementary (141). The placenta provides the fetus with a precursor (progesterone) that permits fetal synthesis of the glucocorticoids—cortisol and 6β-hydroxycortisol—and the fetal adrenal provides the substrates—DHA, DHA sulfate, and 16α-hydroxy DHA—for placental production of estrogens, particularly estriol. The placenta synthesizes progesterone from cholesterol with a small part derived from pregnenolone supplied by the fetal adrenal cortex. The placentae of man and of the chimpanzee differ from those of other species in the large quantity of progesterone that they contain. In addition these species are the only ones in which there are high circulating levels of progesterone in both mother and fetus. Eberlein (141) has suggested that the relative deficiency of 3βHSD activity in the human fetal adrenal cortex may be due to substrate inhibition of this enzymatic activity by progesterone. Inability to produce cortisol would then provoke an increase in ACTH secretion from the fetal pituitary, causing hyperplasia of the fetal adrenal zone. Following delivery, progesterone levels fall, leading to decreased enzyme inhibition, increased cortisol secretion, decreased ACTH release, and degeneration of the fetal adrenal cortex. Whatever advantage, if any, may accrue to the fetus by this sequence of events remains enigmatic.

It has been suggested that a rise in endogenous fetal cortisol levels is important in the initiation of labor, but the role of this hormone in human parturition remains uncertain (158). There may be a surge of cortisol secretion immediately prior to the onset of human labor, which occurs in the sheep, as suggested by the rise in amniotic fluid cortisol levels near term and the increase in umbilical artery concentrations of cortisol following spontaneous labor and vaginal delivery. These phenomena could be secondary to the stress of labor or other factors. Clinically it is observed that the duration of pregnancies with defective fetal adrenal function—anencephaly, congenital adrenal hypoplasia—is prolonged. Labor has been induced in prolonged human pregnancies by intraamniotic administration of dexamethasone and cortisol, but it is uncertain whether this reflects mechanical trauma or a pharmacologic effect (163).

It is clearly established that cortisol is important for fetal lung maturation and production of surfactant (170,171). The human fetal lung has glucocorticoid receptors, and these hormones activate enzymes required for surfactant synthesis (172). Umbilical cord and amniotic fluid cortisol levels are lower in neonates who develop respiratory distress than in those who do not (166,167,170). Nevertheless, amniotic fluid cortisol values do not correlate well with lecithin/sphingomyelin (L/S) ratios, which indicate the degree of fetal lung maturation (164–166). Prenatal administration of glucocorticoids to the mother enhances fetal lung maturation and increases L/S ratios in amniotic fluid (173–174). Hydrocortisone, prednisolone, betamethasone, and especially dexamethasone have been reported to be useful in this regard (175,176). Premature rupture of membranes 16 to 24 hr before birth accelerates lung maturation, presumably because of increased endogenous fetal cortisol secretion. Other factors such as thyroid hormone (135), prolactin (86), and insulin (177) are also important for fetal lung maturation.

Postnatal Changes in Pituitary-Adrenal Function

The serum concentration of ACTH in the neonate declines after delivery from a mean cord level of 226 pg/ml to 49 pg/ml at 12 hr of life, increasing slightly by 24 hr to 193 pg/ml (145–148,178). In the first week of life the serum ACTH concentrations range between 35 and 120 pg/ml. Prenatal administration of dexamethasone does not signifi-cantly affect cord levels of ACTH (147), but infusion of hydrocortisone immediately prior to cesarean section may depress ACTH concentration. Mixed umbilical cord serum concentrations of ACTH are relatively independent of gestational age and birth-weight (148).

Although antenatal administration of betamethasone may depress cord levels of cortisol, the total radioreceptor-measurable glucocorticoid levels remain in the stress-associated range (179,180). There is a spontaneous rapid rebound in cortisol values in the first day of life following prenatal treatment. Cortisol responsiveness to exogenous ACTH is also not impaired under these conditions (181).

The mean serum corticoid level in full-term infants between 1 and 13 days of age is 4.6 µg/dl (range, 1.0 to 20.4). In infants with the respiratory distress syndrome, corticoid values are often several fold higher than in well infants (182).

The adrenal androgen, dehydroepiandrosterone sulfate (DHAS) is nearly fourhold higher in "sick" full-term infants than in normal term infants (183). Ill premature infants have even greater concentrations of serum DHAS than normal prematures, but there is considerable variability (Fig. 13). The higher levels of DHAS in infancy, greater in the premature than in the full-term, are consistent with a relatively decreased activity of the 3βhydroxysteroid dehydrogenase-Δ4.5-isomerase enzyme complex in the fetus and neonate. The further elevated DHAS concentration in the "sick" infants may reflect either a stress-induced adrenal response or a greater diminution of the enzymatic conversion of Δ5 to Δ4 compounds in such infants.

Maternal Hypercortisolism

Under usual conditions endogenous or exogenous maternal hypercortisolism has no dele-terious effects on fetal or neonatal adrenal function. Rarely transient adrenal hypofunc-tion may be observed in the offspring of such women (141).

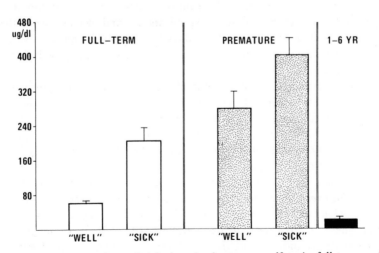

Figure 13. Serum concentrations of dehydroepiandrosterone sulfate in full-term and preterm infants. Reprinted from (183) with permission of publisher.

CALCIOSTATIC HORMONES

Maternal total calcium concentrations decline steadily throughout pregnancy as a consequence of both a decrease in serum albumin levels and a slight decrease in ionized calcium values. Maternal concentrations of PTH increase throughout gestation, reflecting the decline in ionized calcium values and the fetal drain on the maternal stores of calcium. Total calcium concentrations are higher in the fetus than in the mother throughout gestation, ranging between 11 and 13 mg/dl. The difference reflects the active transport of this cation from maternal to fetal circulation against a concentration gradient (184). During the last trimester 140 to 280 mg of calcium is transferred from the mother to the fetus daily. Immediately after birth there is a rapid decline in serum total and ionized calcium values in the neonate. The nadir in calcium levels is achieved at 48 hr wth subsequent stabilization and return to normal values by 5 to 10 days.

The parathyroid glands are derived from the third and fourth pharyngeal pouches, which differentiate by the fifth or sixth week of gestation (185). The derivatives of the third pouches become the inferior and the derivatives of the fourth pouches become the superior parathyroid glands. The parathyroids are capable of secreting parathyroid hormone (PTH) as early as 12 to 13 weeks of gestation in the human fetus. Both high and low concentrations of PTH in the serum of prematurely born infants have been reported (186,187). The discrepancy may be due in part to a difference in specificity between the anti-PTH sera used in different studies. In full-term infants PTH values are quite low in cord blood and remain suppressed for 48 to 72 hr after birth even in infants with significant hypocalcemia (188). Hillman et al. (189) reported that PTH concentrations, undetectable in umbilical cord sera in both full-term and premature infants, increase at 48 hr and remain elevated at 7 days of age. Levels of PTH are somewhat higher in premature than in term infants at this age. Thereafter PTH levels decline into the normal adult range and do not fluctuate appreciably.

Fetal and maternal concentrations of calcitonin, a hypocalcemic product of the thyroid parafollicular cells (neural crest cells that migrate into the lateral margins of the last pharyngeal pouch) are quite high and decline only slowly postpartum (190). Hillman et al. (189) reported that umbilical cord serum concentrations of calcitonin are higher in premature (146 pg/ml) than in term (91 pg/ml) infants and increase two to threefold 48 hr later. Levels decline only slowly by 7 days to values still considerably above cord levels. Hypercalcitonemia has been suggested as one of the pathogenetic factors of neonatal hypocalcemia.

Recently data concerning the metabolism of vitamin D in the pregnant woman, fetus, and neonate have been reported. Vitamin D is first hydroxylated in the liver at the carbon-25 position to produce 25-OHD. Another hydroxylation occurs in the kidney at the carbon-1 position to produce $1,25(OH)_2D$, the most potent biological form of vitamin D (184). The renal tubules and also chondrocytes synthesize $24,25(OH)_2D$, a material whose action is suspected to be primarily on bone. There is transplacental transport of both 25-OHD and $1,25(OH)_2D$. Serum concentrations of 25-OHD and $24,25(OH)_2D$ in pregnant women at term are significantly lower than in nonpregnant females (191) (Fig. 14, 15). Umbilical cord levels of 25-OHD and $24,25(OH)_2D$ are lower than, and correlated with, maternal values (191,192). In serum the majority of 25-OHD circulates bound to a specific α-globulin, D binding protein (DBP). The mean concentration of DBP is significantly lower in cord serum than in maternal serum (26.8 versus 57.4 mg/dl respectively) (193). Although the 25-OHD level is also lower in cord

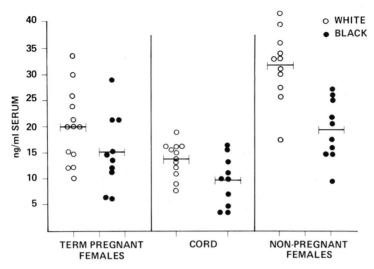

Figure 14. Concentrations of 25-hydroxyvitamin D in maternal and cord serum and in non-pregnant women.

serum, the calculated "free 25-OHD" values in cord and maternal specimens are quite similar. Serum values of 25-OHD remain relatively constant in the first week of life in full-term infants but decline in some premature infants during this period (192). Serum concentrations of $24,25(OH)_2D$ are lower in neonates than in older children (194) (Fig. 16). It has been recently reported that mean maternal concentrations of $1,25(OH)_2D$ at term are twofold higher than in nonpregnant adults (63 versus 29 pg/ml) and significantly higher than in placental vein blood (18 pg/ml) (195). In the full-term neonate serum levels of this metabolite increase to 31 pg/ml by 24 hr of life as the concentration of ionized calcium declines.

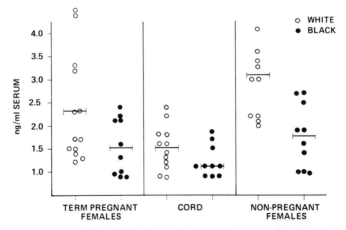

Figure 15. Concentrations of 24,25-dihydroxyvitamin D in maternal and cord serum and in non-pregnant women.

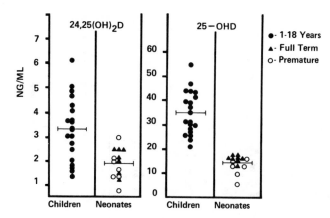

Figure 16. Serum concentrations of 24,25-dihydroxyvitamin D and 25-hydroxyvitamin D in neonates and older children. Reprinted from (194) with permission of publisher.

CONCLUSIONS

The hormonal environment of the fetus is the result of a complex interaction among the endocrine organs of the fetus, the mother, and the placenta. Each component contributes essential elements for normal fetal growth and development; there are also significant postnatal effects of the in utero hormonal environment. The growth, reproductive function, behavior, and psychosocial orientation of patients with congenital adrenal hyperplasia may be permanently altered, presumably as a consequence of in utero and postnatal exposure to high levels of androgens (196). Other functional and anatomic disorders have also been attributed to fetal exposure to an abnormal hormonal milieu (197). Future studies of the endocrinologically active fetus will provide data that may ultimately be of major therapeutic significance.

ACKNOWLEDGMENT

The competent, conscientious, and concerned assistance of Mrs. Virginia Hofmann in the preparation of this manuscript is acknowledged with great appreciation.

ABBREVIATIONS

ACTH	Adrenocorticotrophin
AF	Amniotic fluid
CG	Chorionic gonadotropin
CLIP	Corticotropin-like intermediate peptide
DBP	D binding protein
DHA	Dehydroepiandrosterone
DHAS	Dehydroepiandrosterone sulfate
DHT	Dihydrotestosterone
E_2	Estradiol

FSH	Follicle-stimulating hormone
GH	Growth hormone
Gn-RH	Gonadotropin releasing hormone
3βHSD	3β-Hydroxysteroid dehydrogenase
LH	Luteinizing hormone
MSH	Melanocyte-stimulating hormone
PRL	Prolactin
PTH	Parathyroid hormone
RRA	Radioreceptor assay
SHBG	Sex-hormone binding globulin
SRIF	Somatotropin release inhibiting factor (somatostatin)
T	Testosterone
T_3	Triiodothyronine
T_4	Thyroxine
rT_3	Reverse T_3
TBG	Thyroid binding globulin
TRH	Thyrotropin releasing hormone
TSH	Thyroid-stimulating hormone (thyrotropin)
25-OHD	25-Hydroxyvitamin D
24,25(OH)$_2$D	24,25-Dihydroxyvitamin D
1,25(OH)$_2$D	1,25-Dihydroxyvitamin D

REFERENCES

1. Arey, L. B.: *Developmental Anatomy,* 7th ed. W. B. Saunders Co., Philadelphia, 1974, pp. 230–232.
2. Kirgis, H. O., and Locke, W.: Anatomy and Embryology, in Locke, W., and Schally, A. V. (eds.): *The Hypothalamus and Pituitary in Health and Disease.* Charles C Thomas, Springfield, 1972, pp. 3–65.
3. Kaplan, S. L., Grumbach, M. M., and Aubert, M. L.: The ontogenesis of pituitary hormones and hypothalamic factors in the human fetus: Maturation of central nervous system regulation of anterior pituitary function. *Rec. Prog. Horm. Res.* 32:161, 1976.
4. Root, A. W., Reiter, E. O., and Weisman, Y.: Current status and clinical application of the hypothalamic hormones. *Adv. Pediat.* 23:151, 1976.
5. Monroe, B. G., and Paull, W. K.: Ultrastructural changes in the hypothalamus during development and hypothalamic activity: The median eminence. *Prog. Brain. Res.* 41:185, 1974.
6. Hyyppa, M.: Hypothalamic monoamines in human fetuses. *Neuroendocrinology* 9:257, 1972.
7. Wilber, J. F., Montoya, E., Plotnikoff, N. P., White, W. F., Gendrich, R., Renaud, L., and Martin, J. B.: Gonadotropin-releasing hormone and thyrotropin-releasing hormone: Distribution and effects in the central nervous system. *Rec. Prog. Horm. Res.* 32:117, 1976.
8. Aubert, M. L., Grumbach, M. M., and Kaplan, S. L.: The ontogenesis of human fetal hormones: IV. Somatostatin, luteinizing hormone releasing factor, and thyrotropin releasing factor in hypothalamus and cerebral cortex of human fetuses 10–22 weeks of age. *J. Clin. Endocrinol. Metab.* 74:1130, 1977.
9. Goodyer, C. G., Hall, C. S., Guyda, H., Robert, F., and Giroud, C. J. P.: Human fetal pituitary in culture: Hormone secretion and response to somatostatin, luteinizing hormone releasing factor, thyrotropin releasing factor and dibutyryl cyclic AMP. *J. Clin. Endocrinol. Metab.* 45:73, 1977.
10. Mortimer, C. H., McNeilly, A. S., Rees, L. W., Lowry, P. J., Gilmore, D., and Dobbie, H. G.: Radioimmunoassay and chromatographic similarity of circulating endogenous gonadotropin releasing hormone and hypothalamic extracts in man. *J. Clin. Endocrinol. Metab.* 43:882, 1976.

11. Reyes, F. I., Winter, J. S. D., and Faiman, C.: Gonadotropin-gonadal interrelationships in the fetus, in New, M. I., and Fiser, R. H., Jr. (eds.): *Diabetes and Other Endocrine Disorders During Pregnancy and in the Newborn.* Alan R. Liss, Inc., New York, 1976, pp. 83–106.

12. Dubois, P. M., Paulin, C., Assan, R., and Dubois, M. P.: Evidence for immunoreactive somatostatin in the endocrine cells of human fetal pancreas. *Nature* 256:731, 1975.

13. Raiti, S. (ed.): *Advances in Human Growth Hormone Research.* DHEW publication No. (NIH) 74-612, 1974, pp. 1–963.

14. Van Wyk, J. J., Underwood, L. E., Hintz, R. L., Clemmons, D. R., Voina, S. J., and Weaver, R. P.: The somatomedins: A family of insulin-like hormones under growth hormone control. *Rec. Prog. Horm. Res.* 30:259, 1974.

15. Kaplan, S. L., and Grumbach, M. M.: Serum chorionic "growth hormone–prolactin" and serum pituitary growth hormone in mother and fetus at term. *J. Clin. Endocrinol. Metab.* 25:1370, 1965.

16. Yen, S. S. C., Samaan, N., and Pearson, O. H.: Growth hormone levels in pregnancy. *J. Clin. Endocrinol. Metab.* 27:1341, 1967.

17. Katz, H. P., Grumbach, M. M., and Kaplan, S. L.: Diminished growth hormone response to arginine in the puerperium. *J. Clin. Endocrinol. Metab.* 29:1414, 1969.

18. King, K. C., Adam, P. A. J., Schwartz, R., and Teramo, K.: Human placental transfer of human growth hormone I^{125}. *Pediatrics* 48:534, 1971.

19. Gitlin, D., Kumate, J., and Morales, C.: Metabolism and maternofetal transfer of human growth hormone in the pregnant woman at term. *J. Clin. Endocrinol. Metab.* 25:1599, 1965.

20. Little, B., Smith, O. W., Jessiman, A. G., Selenkow, H. A., Van't Hoff, W., Eglin, J. M., and Moore, F. D.: Hypophysectomy during pregnancy in a patient with cancer of the breast: Case report with hormone studies. *J. Clin. Endocrinol. Metab.* 18:425, 1958.

21. Rimoin, D. L., Holzman, G. B., Merimee, T. J., Rabinowitz, D., Barnes, A. C., Tyson, J. E. A., and McKusick, V. A.: Lactation in the absence of human growth hormone. *J. Clin. Endocrinol. Metab.* 28:1183, 1968.

22. Parekh, M. C., Benjamin, F., and Castillo, N.: The influence of maternal growth hormone secretion on the weight of the newborn infant. *Am. J. Obstet. Gynecol.* 115:197, 1973.

23. Siler-Khodr, T. M., Morgenstern, L. L., and Greenwood, F. C.: Hormone synthesis and release from human fetal adenohypophyses *in vitro. J. Clin. Endocrinol. Metab.* 39:891, 1974.

24. Pavlova, E. B., Pronino, T. S., and Skebelskaya, Y. B.: Histostructure of adenohypophysis of human fetuses and contents of somatotropic and adrenocorticotropic hormones. *Gen. Comp. Endocrinol.* 10:269, 1968.

25. Matsuzaki, F., Irie, M., and Shizume, K.: Growth hormone in human fetal pituitary glands and cord blood. *J. Clin. Endocrinol. Metab.* 33:908, 1971.

26. Pierson, M., Malaprade, D., Grignon, G., Hartemann, P., Belleville, F., Lemoine, I., and Nabet, P.: Etude de la secretion hypophysaire du foetus humain: Correlations entre morphologie et activite secretoire. *Ann. Endocrinol.* 34:418, 1973.

27. Baker, B. L., and Jaffe, R. B.: The genesis of cell types in the adenohypophysis of the human fetus as observed with immunocytochemistry. *Am. J. Anat.* 143:137, 1975.

28. Kaplan, S. L., Grumbach, M. M., and Shepard, T. H.: The ontogenesis of human fetal hormones: I. Growth hormone and insulin. *J. Clin. Invest.* 51:3080, 1972.

29. Grumbach, M. M., and Kaplan, S. L.: Fetal pituitary hormones and the maturation of central nervous system regulation of anterior pituitary function, in Gluck, L. (ed.): *Modern Perinatal Medicine.* Year Book Medical Publishers, Chicago, 1974, pp. 247–271.

30. Grumbach, M. M., and Kaplan, S. L.: Ontogenesis of growth hormone, insulin, prolactin and gonadotropin secretion in the human fetus, in *Foetal and Neonatal Physiology.* Cambridge University Press, Cambridge, 1973, pp. 462–487.

31. Eshet, R., Assa, S., and Laron, Z.: Heterogeneity of pituitary and endogenous plasma human growth hormone from fetuses, premature and full-term newborns. *Biol. Neonate* 29:354, 1976.

32. Von Muhlendahl, K. E., Pachaly, J., and Schmidt-Gollwitzer, M.: Lack of correlation between clinical data and growth hormone concentrations in cord blood. *Biol. Neonate* 29:281, 1976.

33. Sack, J., Fisher, D. A., and Wang, C. C.: Serum thyrotropin, prolactin, and growth hormone levels during the early neonatal period in the human infant. *J. Pediat.* 89:298, 1976.

34. Turner, R. C., Schneeloch, B., and Paterson, P.: Changes in plasma growth hormone and insulin of the human foetus following hysterotomy. *Acta Endocrinol.* 66:577, 1971.

35. Cornblath, M., Parker, M. L., Reisner, S. H., Forbes, A. E., and Daughaday, W. H.: Secretion and metabolism of growth hormone in premature and full-term infants. *J. Clin. Endocrinol. Metab.* 25:209,1965.

36. Van der Schueren-Lodeweyckx, M., Eggermont, E., and Eeckels, R.: The role of growth hormone during foetal and neonatal life. *Acta Paediatr. Belg.* 26:241, 1972.

37. Ponte, C., Gaudier, B., Deconinck, B., and Fourlinnie, J. C.: Blood glucose, serum insulin, and growth hormone response to intravenous administration of arginine in premature infants. *Biol. Neonate* 20:262, 1972.

38. Turner, R. C., Oakley, N. W., and Beard, R. W.: Human fetal plasma growth hormone prior to onset of labour: Effects of stress, glucose, arginine and maternal diabetes. *Biol. Neonate* 22:169, 1973.

39. Honnebier, W. J., and Swaab, D. F.: The influence of anencephaly upon intrauterine growth of fetus and placenta and upon gestation length. *J. Obstet, Gynaecol. Br. Commonw.* 80:577, 1973.

40. Laron, Z.: The role of growth hormone on fetal development *in utero. Adv. Exp. Med. Biol.* 27:391, 1972.

41. Laron, Z., Karp, M., Pertzelan, A., Kauli, R., Keret, R., and Doron, M.: The syndrome of familial dwarfism and high plasma immunoreactive human growth hormone (IR-HGH), in Pecile, A., and Muller, E. E. (eds.): *Growth and Growth Hormone.* Excerpta Medica, Amsterdam, 1972, pp. 458–482.

42. Naeye, R. L., and Blanc, W. A.: Organ and body growth in anencephaly: A quantitative, morphological study. *Arch. Pathol.* 91:140, 1971.

43. Talwar, G. P., Pandian, M. R., Kumar, N., Hanson, S. N. S., Saxena, R. K., Krishnaraj, R., and Gupta, S. L.: Mechanism of action of pituitary growth hormone. *Rec. Prog. Horm. Res.* 31:141, 1975.

44. Cheek, D. B., and Hill, D. E.: Muscle and liver cell growth: Role of hormones and nutritional factors. *Fed. Proc.* 29:1503, 1970.

45. Naeye, R. L., Blanc, W. A., Milic, A. M. B.: Renal development in dysplasia of the fetal pituitary, *Pediatr. Res.* 4:257, 1970.

46. Jost, A., DuPovy, J.-P., and Rieutort, M.: The ontogenetic development of hypothalamo-hypophyseal relations. *Prog. Brain Res.* 43:209, 1974.

47. Jost, A.: Anterior pituitary function in foetal life, in Harris, G. W., and Donovan, B. T. (eds.): *The Pituitary Gland,* vol. 2. University of California Press, Berkeley, 1966, pp. 299–323.

48. Swaab, D. F., and Honnebier, W. J.: The influence of removal of the fetal brain upon intrauterine growth of the fetus and the placenta and on gestation length. *J. Obstet. Gynaecol. Br. Commonw.* 80:589, 1973.

49. Turner, R. C., and Cohen, N. M.: The role of insulin and growth hormone in fetal growth. *Dev. Med. Child. Neurol.* 16:371, 1974.

50. Chez, R. A., Hutchinson, D. L., Salazar, H., and Mintz, D. H.: Some effects of fetal and maternal hypophysectomy in pregnancy. *Am. J. Obstet. Gynecol.* 108:643, 1970.

51. Novy, M. J., Walsh, S. W., and Kittinger, G. W.: Experimental fetal anencephaly in the rhesus monkey: Effect on gestational length and fetal and maternal plasma steroids. *J. Clin. Endocrinol. Metab.* 45:1031, 1977.

52. Gluckman, P. D., and Brinsmead, M. W.: Somatomedin in cord blood: Relationship to gestational age and birth size. *J. Clin. Endocrinol. Metab.* 43:1378, 1976.

53. D'Ercole, A. J., Underwood, L. E., and Van Wyk, J. J.: Serum somatomedin-C in hypopituitarism and in disorders of growth. *J. Pediat.* 90:375, 1977.

54. Furlanetto, R. W., Underwood, L. E., Van Wyk, J. J., and D'Ercole, A. J.: Estimation of somatomedin C levels in normal patients and patients with pituitary disease by radioimmunoassay. *J. Clin. Invest.* 60:648, 1977.

55. D'Ercole, A. J., Foushee, D. B., and Underwood, L. E.: Somatomedin-C receptor ontogeny and levels in porcine fetal and human cord serum. *J. Clin. Endocrinol. Metab.* 43:1069, 1976.

56. Svan, H., Hall, K., Ritzen, M., Takano, K., and Skottner, A.: Somatomedin A and B in serum from neonates, their mothers and cord blood. *Acta Endocrinol.* 85:636, 1977.

57. Bala, R. M., and Smith, G. R.: Partial characterization of somatomedin bioactivity in term human amniotic fluid. *J. Clin. Endocrinol. Metab.* 43:907, 1976.

58. Chochinov, R. H., Ketupanya, A., Mariz, I. K., Underwood, L. E., and Daughaday, W. H.: Amniotic fluid reactivity detected by somatomedin C radioreceptor assay: Correlation with growth hormone, prolactin, and fetal renal maturation. *J. Clin. Endocrinol. Metab.* 42:983, 1976.

59. Chochinov, R. H., Mariz, I., K., Hajek, A. S., and Daughaday, W. H.: Characterization of a protein in mid-term human amniotic fluid which reacts in the somatomedin-C radioreceptor assay. *J. Clin. Endocrinol. Metab.* 44:902, 1977.

60. Moberg, P. J., Efendic, S., Hall, K., and Fryklund, L.: Amniotic fluid somatomedin A and fetal CNS damage. *Lancet* 1:1016, 1976.

61. Niall, H. D., Hogen, M. C., Tregear, G. W., Segre, G. V., Hwang, P., and Friesen, H.: The chemistry of growth hormone and the lactogenic hormones. *Rec. Prog. Horm. Res.* 29:387, 1973.

62. McNeilly, A. S., Gilmore, D., Dobbie, G., and Chard, T.: Prolactin releasing activity in the early human foetal hypothalamus. *J. Endocr.* 73:533, 1977.

63. Barberia, J. M., Abu-Fadil, S., Kletzky, O. A., Nakamura, R. M., and Mishell, D. R., Jr.: Serum prolactin patterns in early human gestation. *Am. J. Obstet. Gynecol.* 121:1107, 1975.

64. Tyson, J. E., Hwang, P., Guyda, H., and Friesen, H. G.: Studies of prolactin secretion in human pregnancy. *Am. J. Obstet. Gynecol.* 113:14, 1972.

65. Jacobs, L. S., and Daughaday, W. H.: Physiologic regulation of prolactin secretion in man, in Josimovich, J. B., Reynolds, M., and Cobo, E. (eds.): *Lactogenic Hormones, Fetal Nutrition, and Lactation.* John Wiley, New York, 1974, pp. 351–377.

66. Hwang, P., Guyda, H., and Friesen, H.: A radioimmunoassay for human prolactin. *Proc. Nat. Acad. Sci. (USA)* 68:1902, 1971.

67. Frantz, A. G., Kleinberg, D. L., and Noel, G. L.: Studies on prolactin in man. *Rec. Prog. Horm. Res.* 28:527, 1972.

68. Weiss, G., Butler, W. R., Hotchkiss, S., Dierschke, D. J., and Knobil, E.: Peri-parturitional serum concentrations of prolactin, the gonadotropins, and the gonadal hormones in the rhesus monkey. *Proc. Soc. Exp. Biol. Med.* 151:113, 1976.

69. Yang, W. H., Sairam, M. R., and Li, C. H.: The effect of ICSH-B and its combination with prolactin on the maintenance of pregnancy in the rat. *Acta Endocrinol.* 72:173, 1973.

70. Dohler, K. D., and Wuttke, W.: Total blockade of phasic pituitary prolactin release in rats: Effect on serum LH and progesterone during the estrous cycle and pregnancy. *Endocrinology* 94:1595, 1974.

71. Josimovich, J. B., Weiss, G., and Hutchinson, D. L.: Sources and disposition of pituitary prolactin in maternal circulation, amniotic fluid, fetus and placenta in the pregnant rhesus monkey. *Endocrinology* 94:1364, 1974.

72. Thompson, S. A., and Terranova, P. F.: Serum prolactin levels in fetal and neonatal hamsters and the relationship to maternal levels. *Proc. Soc. Exp. Biol. Med.* 150:461, 1975.

73. Friesen, H. G.: Structure and function of human prolactin, in *The Endocrine Milieu of Pregnancy, Puerperium and Childhood.* Third Ross Conference on Obstetric Research, Columbus, Ohio, 1974, pp. 111–114.

74. Fang, V. S., and Kim, M. H.: Study on maternal, fetal, and amniotic human prolactin at term. *J. Clin. Endocrinol. Metab.* 41:1030, 1975.

75. Aubert, M. L., Grumbach, M. M., and Kaplan, S. L.: The ontogenesis of human fetal hormones: III. Prolactin. *J. Clin. Invest.* 56:155, 1975.

76. Winters, A. J., Colston, C., MacDonald, P. C., and Porter, J. C.: Fetal plasma prolactin levels. *J. Clin. Endocrinol. Metab.* 41:626, 1975.

77. Guyda, H. J., and Friesen, H. G.: Serum prolactin levels in humans from birth to adult life. *Pediat. Res.* 7:534, 1973.

78. Cowle, A. T.: Physiological actions of prolactin. *Proc. R. Soc. Med.* 66:861, 1973.

79. Daughaday, W. H.: The adenohypophysis, in Williams, R. H. (ed.): *Textbook of Endocrinology*, 5th ed. W. B. Saunders, Philadelphia, 1974. pp. 46–50.

80. Francis, M. J. O., and Hill, D. J.: Prolactin-stimulated production of somatomedin by rat liver. *Nature* 255:167, 1975.

81. Skutch, G. M: Reserpine, prolactin, allergy and breast cancer. *Lancet* 2:967, 1974.

82. Skutch, G. M.: Prolactin and maternal immune reaction against fetus. *Lancet* 1:585, 1975.

83. Purtilo, D. T., Hallgren, H. M., and Yunis, E. J.: Depressed maternal lymphocyte response to phytohaemagglutinin in human pregnancy. *Lancet* 1:769, 1972.

84. Yu, V. Y. H., Waller, C. A., MacLennan, I. C. M., and Baum, J. D.: Lymphocyte reactivity in pregnant women and newborn infants. *Br. Med. J.* 1:428, 1975.

85. Kelly, J. D., and Dineen, J. K.: The supression of rejection of *Nippostrongylus brasiliensis* in Lewis strain rats treated with ovine prolactin: The site of the immunological defect. *Immunology* 24:551, 1973.

86. Hamosh, M., and Hamosh, P.: The effect of prolactin on the lecithin content of fetal rabbit lung. *J. Clin. Invest.* 59:1002, 1977.

87. Bohnet, H. G., Aragona, C., and Friesen, H. G.: Effect of changes in serum prolactin on prolactin and gonadotropin binding to Leydig cells and tubules of the rat testes. *Clin. Res.* 23:613A, 1975.

88. Skowsky, W. R., and Fisher, D. A.: Fetal neurohypophyseal arginine vasopressin and arginine vasotocin in man and sheep. *Pediat. Res.* 11:627, 1977.

89. LeGros, J. J., Louis, F., Demoulin, A., and Franchimont, P.: Immunoreactive neurophysins and vasotocin in human foetal pineal glands. *J. Endocr.* 69:289, 1976.

90. Pavel, S., Dumitru, I., Klepsh, I., and Dorcescu, M.: A gonadotropin inhibiting principle in the pineal of human fetuses. *Neuroendocrinology* 13:41, 1973.

91. Pavel, S., Dorcescu, M., Petrescu-Holban, R., and Ghinea, E.: Biosynthesis of a vasotocin-like peptide from pineal glands of human fetuses. *Science* 181:1252, 1973.

92. Piron-Bossuyt, C., Bossuyt, A., Brauman, H., and Van Den Driessche, R.: Development of a radioimmunoassay for oxytocin. *Ann. d'Endocrinol.* (Paris) 27:389, 1976.

93. Jirasek, J.: Principles of reproductive embryology, in Simpson, J. L. (ed.): *Disorders of Sexual Differentiation.* Academic Press, New York, 1976, pp. 51–110.

94. Jirasek, J. E.: Morphogenesis of the genital system in the human, in Blandau, R. J., and Bergsma, D. (eds.): *Morphogenesis and Malformation of the Genital System.* Birth Defects: Original Series, Vol. XIII, Alan R. Liss, Inc., New York, 1977, pp. 13–40.

95. Simpson, J. L.: The nature of sex determination, in Simpson, J. L. (ed.): *Disorders of Sexual Differentiation.* Academic Press, New York, 1977, pp. 141–155.

96. Ross, G. T.: Gonadotropins and preantral follicular maturation in women. *Fertility Sterility* 25:522, 1974.

97. Lyon, M. F.: Mechanism and evolutionary origins of variable X-chromosome activity in mammals. *Proc. Roy. Soc. Lond.* (Biol.) B187:243, 1974.

98. Jost, A.: Problems of fetal endocrinology: The gonadal and hypophyseal hormones. *Rec. Prog. Horm. Res.* 8:379, 1953.

99. Pierce, J. G., Liao, T-H., Howard, S. M., Shome, B., and Cornell, J. S.: Studies on the structure of thyrotropin: Its relationship to luteinizing hormone. *Rec. Prog. Horm. Res.* 27:165, 1971.

100. Kaplan, S. L., and Grumbach, M. M.: The ontogenesis of human fetal hormones: II. Luteinizing hormone (LH) and follicle stimulating hormone (FSH). *Acta Endocrinol.* 81:808, 1976.

101. Clements, J. A., Reyes, F. I., Winter, J. S. D., and Faiman, C.: Studies on human sexual development: III. Fetal pituitary and serum, and amniotic fluid concentrations of LH, CG, and FSH. *J. Clin. Endocrinol. Metab.* 42:9, 1976.

102. Faiman, C., and Winter, J. S. D.: Gonadotropin and sex hormone pattern in puberty: Clinical data, in Grumbach, M. M., Grave, G. D., and Mayer, F. E. (eds.): *The Control of the Onset of Puberty.* John Wiley., New York, 1974, pp. 32–55.

103. Forest, M. G., Sizonenko, P. C., Cathiard, A. M., and Bertrand, J.: Hypophysogonadal function in humans during the first year of life: I. Evidence for testicular activity in early infancy. *J. Clin. Invest.* 53:819, 1974.

104. Penny, R., Olambiwonnu, N. O., and Frasier, S. D.: Follicle stimulating hormone (FSH) and luteiniz-

ing hormone–human chorionic gonadotropin (LH-HCG) concentrations in paired maternal and cord sera. *Pediatrics* 53:41, 1974.

105. Winter, J. S. D., Faiman, C., Hobson, W. C., Prasad, A. V., and Reyes, F. I.: Pituitary-gonadal relation in infancy: I. Pattern of serum gonadotropin concentration from birth to four years of age in man and chimpanzees. *J. Clin. Endocrinol. Metab.* 40:545, 1975.

106. Jaffe, R. B., Lee, P. A., and Midgley, A. R.: Serum gonadotropin before, at the inception of, and following human pregnancy. *J. Clin. Endocrinol. Metab.* 29:1281, 1969.

107. Boroditsky, R. S., Reyes, F. I., Winter, J. S. D., and Faiman, C.: Serum human chorionic gonadotropin and progesterone pattern in the last trimester of pregnancy: Relationship to fetal sex. *Am. J. Obstet. Gynecol.* 121:238, 1975.

108. Lee, C. Y., and Ryan, R. J.: Interaction of ovarian receptors with human luteinizing hormone and human chorionic gonadotropin. *Biochem.* 12:4609, 1973.

109. Dufau, M. L., Catt, K. J., and Tsuruhara, T.: A sensitive gonadotropin responsive system: Radioimmunoassay of testosterone production by the rat testes *in vitro. Endocrinology* 90:1032, 1972.

110. Kaplan, S. L., Grumbach, M. M., and Aubert, M. L.: α and β glycoprotein subunits (hLH, hFSH, hCG) in the serum and pituitary of the human fetus. *J. Clin. Endocrinol. Metab.* 42:995, 1976.

111. Reyes, F. I., Winter, J. S. D., and Faiman, C.: Studies in human sexual development: I. Fetal gonadal and adrenal sex steroids. *J. Clin. Endocrinol. Metab.* 37:74, 1973.

112. Winter, J. S. D., Faiman, C., and Reyes, F. I.: Sex steroid production by the human fetus: Its role in morphogenesis and control by gonadotropins, in Blandau, R. J., and Bergsma, D. (eds.): *Morphogenesis and Malformation of the Genital System.* Birth Defects: Original Article Series, Vol. XIII, Alan R. Liss, New York, 1977, pp. 41–58.

113. Reyes, F. I., Boroditsky, R. S., Winter, J. S. D., and Faiman, C.: Studies on human sexual development: II. Fetal and maternal serum gonadotropin and sex steroid concentrations. *J. Clin. Endocrinol.* 38:612, 1974.

114. Judd, H. L., Robinson, J. D., Young, P. E., and Jones, O. W.: Amniotic fluid testosterone levels in midpregnancy. *Obstet. Gynecol.* 48:690, 1976.

115. Siiteri, P. K., and Wilson, J. D.: Testosterone formation and metabolism during male sexual differentiation in the human embryo. *J. Clin. Endocrinol. Metab.* 38:113, 1974.

116. Forest, M. G.: Differentiation and development of the male. *Clin. Endocrinol. Metab.* 4:569, 1975.

117. Verkauf, B. S., Reiter, E. O., Hernandez, L., and Burns, S. A.: Virilization of mother and fetus associated with luteoma of pregnancy: A case report with endocrinologic studies. *Am. J. Obstet. Gynecol.* 129:274, 1977.

118. Payne, A. H., and Jaffe, R. B.: Androgen formation from pregnenolone sulfate by the human fetal ovary. *J. Clin. Endocrinal. Metab.* 39:300, 1974.

119. Diczfalusy, E., and Troen, P.: Endocrine function of human placenta. *Vit. Horm.* 19:229, 1961.

120. Pinkerton, J. H. M., McKay, D. G., Adams, E. C., and Hertig, A. T.: Development of the human ovary: Study using histochemical techniques. *Obstet. Gynecol.* 18:152, 1961.

121. Grumbach, M. M., and Van Wyk, J. J.: Disorders of sexual maturation, in Williams, R. H. (ed.): *Textbook of Endocrinology,* 5th ed. W. B. Saunders, Philadelphia, 1974, pp. 423–501.

122. Winter, J. S. D., Hughes, I. A., Reyes, F. I., and Faiman, C.: Pituitary-gonadal relations in infancy: 2. Pattern of serum gonadal steroid concentration in man from birth to two years of age. *J. Clin. Endocrinol. Metab.* 42:679, 1976.

123. Josso, N., Picard, J.-Y., and Tran, D.: The antimullerian hormone. *Rec. Prog. Horm. Res.* 33:117, 1977.

124. Lipsett, M. B., and Sherins, R. J.: The testes, in Bondy, P. K., and Rosenberg, L. E. (eds.): *Diseases of Metabolism.* W. B. Saunders, Philadelphia, 1974, pp. 1553–1584.

125. Peterson, R. E., Imperato-McGinley, J., Gautier, T., and Sturla, E.: Male pseudohermaphroditism due to steroid 5α-reductase deficiency. *Am. J. Med.* 62:170, 1977.

126. Josso, N., Picard, J.-Y., and Tran, D.: The anti-mullerian hormone, in Blandau, R. J., and Bergsma, D. (eds.): *Morphogenesis and Malformation of the Genital System.* Birth Defects: Original Series, Vol. XIII, Alan R. Liss, Inc., New York, 1977, pp. 59–84.

127. Reiter, E. O., Grumbach, M. M., Kaplan, S. L., and Conte, F. A.: The response of pituitary

gonadotropes to synthetic LRF in children with glucocorticoid-treated congenital adrenal hyperplasia: Lack of effect of intrauterine and neonatal androgen excess. *J. Clin. Endocrinol. Metab.* 40:318, 1975.

128. Levina, S. E.: Reguliatsilia sekretsii giporizarnykh gonadotropinov v embiolgenze cheloveka. *Probl. Endokrinol.* 16:353, 1970.

129. Groom, G. U., and Boyns, A. R.: Effect of hypothalamic releasing factors and steroids on release of gonadotropin by organ cultures of human fetal pituitaries. *J. Endocr.* 59:511, 1973.

130. Gennser, G., Liedholm, P., and Thorell, J.: Pituitary hormone levels in plasma of the human fetus after administration of LRH. *J. Clin. Endocrinol. Metab.* 43:470, 1976.

131. Shepard, T. H.: Development of the thyroid gland, in Gardner, L. I. (ed.): *Endocrine and Genetic Diseases of Childhood and Adolescence*, 2nd ed. W. B. Saunders Co., Philadelphia, 1975, pp. 220–226.

132. Fisher, D. A.: Thyroid physiology in the fetus and newborn: Current concepts and approaches to perinatal thyroid disease, in New, M. I., and Fiser, R. H., Jr. (eds.): *Diabetes and Other Endocrine Disorders During Pregnancy and in the Newborn*. Alan R. Liss, Inc., New York, 1976, pp. 221–233.

133. Fisher, D. A., Dussault, J., Sack, J., and Chopra, I. J.: Ontogenesis of hypothalamic-pituitary-thyroid function in man, sheep and rat. *Rec. Prog. Horm. Res.* 33:59, 1977.

134. Bernard, B., Oddie, T. H., and Fisher, D. A.: Correlation between gestational age, weight, or ponderosity and serum thyroxine at birth. *J. Pediat.* 91:199, 1977.

135. Cuestas, R. A., Lindall, A., and Engel, R. R.: Low thyroid hormones and respiratory distress syndrome of the newborn, studies on cord blood. *New Engl. J. Med.* 295:297, 1976.

136. Fisher, D. A., and Burrow, G. N. (eds.): *Perinatal Thyroid Physiology and Disease*. Raven Press, New York, 1975, pp. 1–277.

137. Fisher, D. A., Sack, J., Oddie, T. H., Pekary, A. E., Hershman, J. M., Lam, R. W., and Parslow, M. E.: Serum T_4, TBG, T_3 uptake, reverse T_3 and TSH concentrations in children 1 to 15 years of age. *J. Clin. Endocrinol. Metab.* 45:191, 1977.

138. Abassi, V., Merchant, K., and Abramson, D.: Postnatal triiodothyronine concentration in healthy preterm infants and in infants with respiratory distress syndrome. *Pediat. Res.* 11:802, 1977.

139. Uhrmann, S., Marks, K. H., Maisels, H. J., Freedman, Z., Murray, F., Kulin, H., Kaplan, M., and Utiger, R.: Thyroid function in infants admitted to a neonatal intensive care unit (NICU): A longitudinal assessment. *Pediat. Res.* 11:432A, 1977.

140. Gardner, L. I.: Development of the normal fetal and neonatal adrenal, in Gardner, L. I. (ed.): *Endocrine and Genetic Diseases of Childhood and Adolescence*, 2nd ed. W. B. Saunders Co., Philadelphia, 1975, pp. 460–476.

141. Eberlein, W. R.: The fetal adrenal cortex, in Christy, N. P. (ed.): *The Human Adrenal Cortex*. Harper & Row, New York, 1971, pp. 317–327.

142. Peterson, R. E.: Metabolism of adrenal cortical steroids, in Christy, N. P. (ed.): *The Human Adrenal Cortex*. Harper & Row, New York, 1971. pp. 87–189.

143. Peterson, R. E., and Imperato-McGinley, J.: Cortisol metabolism in the perinatal period, in New, M. I., and Fiser, R. H., Jr. (eds.): *Diabetes and Other Endocrine Disorders During Pregnancy and in the Newborn*. Alan R. Liss, Inc., New York, 1976, pp. 141–172.

144. Rees, L. H.: ACTH, lipotrophin and MSH in health and disease. *Clin. Endocrinol. Metab.* 6:137, 1977.

145. Allen, J. P., Cook, D. M., Kendall, J. W., and McGilvra, R.: Maternal-fetal ACTH relationship in man. *J. Clin. Endocrinol. Metab.* 37:230, 1973.

146. Winters, A. J., Oliver, C., Colston, C., MacDonald, P. C., and Porter, J. C.: Plasma ACTH levels in the human fetus and neonate as related to age and parturition. *J. Clin. Endocrinol. Metab.* 39:269, 1974.

147. Kauppila, A., Simila, S., Ylikorkala, O., Koivisto, M., Makela, P., and Haapalahti, J.: ACTH levels in maternal, fetal and neonatal plasma after short-term prenatal dexamethasone therapy. *Brit. J. Obstet. Gynec.* 84:124, 1977.

148. Arai, K., Yanaihora, T., and Okinaga, S.: Adrenocorticotropic hormone in human fetal blood at delivery. *Am. J. Obstet. Gynecol.* 125:1136, 1976.

149. Tuimala, R., Kauppila, A., and Haapalahti, J.: ACTH levels in amniotic fluid during pregnancy. *Brit. J. Obstet. Gynec.* 83:853, 1976.

150. Liotta, A., Osathanondh, R., Ryan, K. J., and Krieger, D. T.: Presence of corticotropin in human placenta: Demonstration of *in vitro* synthesis. *Endocrinology* 101:1552, 1977.

151. Murphy, B. E. P., Clark, S. J., Donald, I. R., Pinsky, M., and Vedady, D.: Conversion of maternal cortisol to cortisone during placental transfer to the human fetus. *Am. J. Obstet. Gynecol.* 118:538, 1974.

152. Sybulski, S., and Maughan, G. B.: Cortisol levels in umbilical cord plasma in relation to labor and delivery. *Am. J. Obstet. Gynecol.* 125:236, 1976.

153. Fencl, M. de M., Osathanondh, R., and Tulchinsky, D.: Plasma cortisol and cortisone in pregnancies with normal and anencephalic fetuses *J. Clin. Endocrinol. Metab.* 43:80, 1976.

154. Beitins, I. Z., Bayard, F., Ances, I. G., Kowarski, A., and Migeon, C. J.: The metabolic clearance rate, blood production, interconversion and transplacental passage of cortisol in pregnancy near term. *Pediat. Res.* 7:509, 1973.

155. Root, A. W., Bongiovanni, A. M., and Eberlein, W. R.: The adrenogenital syndrome, in Christy, N. P. (ed.): *The Human Adrenal Cortex.* Harper and Row, New York, 1971, pp. 427–474.

156. Beitins, I. Z., Bayard, F., Levitsky, L., Ances, I. G., Kowarski, A., and Migeon, C. J.: Plasma aldosterone concentration at delivery and during the newborn period. *J. Clin. Invest.* 51:386, 1972.

157. Murphy, B. E. P.: Steroid arteriovenous differences in umbilical cord plasma: Evidence of cortisol production by the human fetus in early gestation. *J. Clin. Endocrinol. Metab.* 36:1037, 1973.

158. Murphy, B. E. P.: Does the human fetal adrenal play a role in parturition? *Am. J. Obstet. Gynecol.* 115:521, 1973.

159. Leong, M. K. H., and Murphy, B. E. P.: Cortisol levels in maternal venous and umbilical cord arterial and venous serum at vaginal delivery. *Am. J. Obstet. Gynecol.* 124:471, 1976.

160. Ohrlander, S., Gennser, G., and Eneroth, P.: Plasma cortisol levels in human fetus during parturition. *Obstet. Gynec.* 48:381, 1976.

161. Arai, K., and Yanaihara, T.: Steroid hormone changes in fetal blood during labor. *Am. J. Obstet. Gynecol.* 127:879, 1977.

162. Murphy, B. E. P., Patrick, J., and Denton, R. L.: Cortisol in amniotic fluid during human gestation. *J. Clin. Endocrinol. Metab.* 40:164, 1975.

163. Nwosu, U. C., Bolognese, R. J., Wallach, E. E., and Bongiovanni, A. M.: Amniotic fluid cortisol concentrations in normal labor, premature labor and postmature pregnancy. *Obstet. Gynec.* 49:715, 1977.

164. Sharp-Cageorge, S. M., Blicher, B. M., Gordon, E. R., and Murphy, B. E. P.: Amniotic-fluid cortisol and human fetal lung maturation. *New Engl. J. Med.* 296:89, 1977.

165. Gewolb, I. H., Hobbins, J. C., and Tan, S. Y.: Amniotic fluid cortisol as an index of fetal lung maturity. *Obstet. Gynec.* 49:462, 1977.

166. Gewolb, I. H., Hobbins, J. C., and Tan, S. Y.: Amniotic fluid cortisol in high-risk human pregnancies. *Obstet. Gynec.* 49:466, 1977.

167. Smith, B. T., Worthington, D., and Maloney, A. H. A.: Fetal lung maturation: III. The amniotic fluid cortisol-cortisone ratio in preterm human delivery and the risk of respiratory distress syndrome. *Obstet. Gynec.* 49:527, 1977.

168. Murphy, B. E. P.: Chorionic membrane as an extra-adrenal source of foetal cortisol in human amniotic fluid. *Nature* 266:179, 1977.

169. Tanswell, A. K., Worthington, D., and Smith, B. T.: Human amniotic membrane corticosteroid 11-oxidoreductase activity. *J. Clin. Endocrinol. Metab.* 45:721, 1977.

170. Murphy, B. E. P.: Evidence of cortisol deficiency at birth in infants with the respiratory distress syndrome. *J. Clin. Endocrinol. Metab.* 38:158, 1974.

171. Murphy, B. E. P.: Cortisol and cortisone levels in the cord blood at delivery of infants with and without the respiratory distress syndrome. *Am. J. Obstet. Gynecol.* 119:1112, 1974.

172. Ballard, P. L., and Ballard, R. A.: Cytoplasmic receptor for glucocorticoids in lung of the human fetus and neonate. *J. Clin. Invest.* 53:477, 1974.

173. Liggins, C. C., and Howie, R. N.: A controlled trial of antepartum glucocorticoid treatment for prevention of the respiratory distress syndrome in premature infants. *Pediatrics* 50:515, 1972.

174. Zuspan, F. P., Cordero, L., and Semchyshyn, S.: Effects of hydrocortisone on lecithin-sphingomyelin ratio. *Am. J. Obstet. Gynecol.* 128:571, 1977.

175. Szabo, I., Csaba, I., Novak, P., and Drozgyck, I.: Single dose glucocorticoid for prevention of respiratory distress syndrome. *Lancet* 2:243, 1977.

176. Ballard, R. A., and Ballard, P. L.: Use of prenatal glucocorticoid therapy to prevent respiratory distress syndrome. *Am. J. Dis. Child.* 130:982, 1976.

177. Smith, B. T., Giroud, C. J. P., Robert, M., and Avery, M. E.: Insulin antagonism of cortisol action on lecithin synthesis by cultured fetal lung cells. *J. Pediat.* 87:953, 1975.

178. Cacciari, E., Cicognani, A., Pirazoli, P., Dallacasa, P., Mazzarachio, M. A., Tassoni, P., Bernardi, F., Salardi, S., and Zappulla, F.: GH, ACTH, LH and FSH behaviour in the first seven days of life. *Acta Paediatr. Scand.* 65:337, 1976.

179. Sybulski, S.: Effect of antepartum betamethasone treatment on cortisol levels in cord plasma, amniotic fluid, and the neonate. *Am. J. Obstet. Gynecol.* 127:871, 1977.

180. Ballard, P. L., Granberg, P., and Ballard, R. A.: Glucocorticoid levels in maternal and cord serum after neonatal betamethasone therapy to prevent respiratory distress syndrome. *J. Clin. Invest.* 56:1548, 1975.

181. Ohrlander, S., Gennser, G., Nilsson, K. O., and Eneroth, P.: ACTH test to neonates after administration of corticosteroids during gestation. *Obstet. Gynec.* 49:691, 1977.

182. Bacon, G. E., George, R., Koeff, S. T., and Howatt, W. F.: Plasma corticoids in the respiratory distress syndrome and in normal infants. *Pediatrics* 55:500, 1975.

183. Reiter, E. O., Fuldauer, V. G., and Root, A. W.: Secretion of the adrenal androgen dehydroepiandrosterone sulfate, during normal infancy, childhood, and adolescence, in sick infants, and in children with endocrinologic abnormalities. *J. Pediat.* 90:766, 1977.

184. Root, A. W., and Harrison, H. E.: Recent advances in calcium metabolism: I. Mechanisms of calcium homeostasis. *J. Pediat.* 88:1, 1976.

185. Anast, C.: Development of the normal embryonic, fetal and neonatal parathyroid, in Gardner, L. I. (ed.): *Endocrine and Genetic Diseases of Childhood and Adolescence*, 2nd ed. W. B. Saunders Co., Philadelphia, 1975, pp. 355–358.

186. Dirksen, H. C., and Anast, C. S.: Elevated circulating immunoreactive parathyroid hormone (iPTH) in premature infants. *Pediat. Res.* 11:319A, 1977.

187. Tsang, R. C., Chen, I-W., Friedman, M. A., and Chan, I.: Neonatal parathyroid function: Role of gestational age and postnatal age. *J. Pediat.* 83:728, 1973.

188. David, L., and Anast, C. S.: Calcium metabolism in newborn infants: The interrelationship of parathyroid function and calcium, magnesium and phosphorus metabolism in normal, "sick" and hypocalcemic newborns. *J. Clin. Invest.* 54:287, 1974.

189. Hillman, L. S., Rojanasathit, S., Slatopolsky, E., and Haddad, J. G.: Serial measurements of serum calcium, magnesium, parathyroid hormone, calcitonin, and 25-hydroxy-vitamin D in premature and term infants during the first week of life. *Pediat. Res.* 11:739, 1977.

190. Samaan, N. A., Anderson, G. D., and Adam-Mayne, M. E.: Immunoreactive calcitonin in the mother, neonate, child and adult. *Am. J. Obstet. Gynecol.* 121:622, 1975.

191. Weisman, Y., Occhipinti, M., Knox, G., Reiter, E., and Root, A.: Concentrations of 24,25-dihydroxyvitamin D and 25-hydroxyvitamin D in paired maternal-cord sera. *Am. J. Obstet. Gynecol.* 130:704, 1978.

192. Hillman, L. S., and Haddad, J. G.: Human perinatal vitamin D metabolism: I. 25-hydroxyvitamin D in maternal and cord blood. *J. Pediat.* 84:742, 1974.

193. Bouillon, R., Van Baelen, H., and deMoor, P.: 25-Hydroxyvitamin D and its binding protein in maternal cord serum. *J. Clin. Endocrinol. Metab.* 45:679, 1977.

194. Weisman, Y., Reiter, E., and Root, A.: Measurement of 24,25-dihydroxyvitamin D in sera of neonates and children. *J. Pediat.* 91:904, 1977.

195. Steichen, J. J., Gratton, T. L., Tsang, R. C., and DeLuca, H. F.: Perinatal vitamin D homeostasis: 1,25(OH)$_2$D in maternal, cord and neonatal blood. *Clin. Res.* 25:567A, 1977.

196. Lee, P. A., Plotnick, L. P., Kowarski, A. A., and Migeon, C. J. (eds.): *Congenital Adrenal Hyperplasia*, University Park Press, Baltimore, 1977, pp. 3–532.

197. Herbst, A. L., Scully, R. E., Robboy, S. J., and Welch, W. R.: Complications of prenatal therapy with diethyl-stilbestrol. *Pediatrics* 62(suppl.):1151, 1978.

198. Root, A. W.: Growth hormone and prolactin in the fetus, in New, M. I., and Fiser, R. H., Jr. (eds.): *Diabetes and Other Endocrine Disorders During Pregnancy and in the Newborn.* Alan R. Liss, Inc., New York, 1976, pp. 107–126.

199. Gerich, J. E.: Somatostatin: Its possible role in carbohydrate homeostatis and the treatment of diabetes mellitus. *Arch. Int. Med.* 137:659, 1977.

200. Warne, G. L., Faiman, C., Reyes, F. I., and Winter, J. S. D.: Studies on human sexual development: V. Concentrations of testosterone, 17-hydroxyprogesterone and progesterone in human amniotic fluid throughout gestation. *J. Clin. Endocrinol. Metab.* 44:934, 1977.

3
Genetics

Henry L. Nadler, M.D.
Barbara K. Burton, M.D.

There is no doubt that genetic disorders may have a profound impact on the perinatal patient from long before conception to the neonatal period and beyond. Genetic disorders in either parent may affect fertility and, in the mother, may significantly influence the course of a pregnancy and the well-being of the infant. Genetic disease in the fetus may result in spontaneous abortion, premature birth, or subtle or overt disease in the neonate. It is the obstetrician and the pediatrician who are initially called on to recognize and manage such disorders. They also are in a position to provide the most meaningful and effective genetic counseling to families affected by genetic disorders or birth defects.

It is unreasonable to assume that the physician involved in perinatal medicine could be familiar with the diagnosis and management of all genetic disorders occurring in man, many of which are very rare. It is reasonable, however, to expect a physician to have an understanding of the principles of medical genetics so that once a diagnosis has been made, by himself or by a consultant, he can help the family to understand its implications. The physician should be acutely aware of the importance of making an accurate diagnosis before offering genetic counseling. The obstetrician must be aware of the availability of prenatal diagnosis for many genetic disorders and of his obligation to make this information available to the patient.

Neonatologists and other physicians dealing with the newborn should recognize those common congenital malformations and chromosomal abnormalities which are obvious in the neonatal period. They must also be cognizant of the fact that a number of inborn errors of metabolism may present as acute, life-threatening illnesses requiring immediate intervention in the newborn period. They must be prepared to answer the question, "Will this happen again?" in dealing with the parents of affected infants. The pediatrician must be familiar with any newborn screening procedures directed toward the detection of genetic disorders. Both the obstetrician and pediatrician must know where to turn for help in diagnosis and management of the patient with a rare familial disorder.

In this chapter, an attempt is made to discuss the basic principles of inheritance and their implications for genetic counseling and to touch on those genetic disorders which most often affect the well-being of the fetus or the newborn infant. For more detailed discussion of any of these topics, additional references are provided.

PATTERNS OF INHERITANCE IN MAN

Single Gene Defects

All the genetic material in an individual is contained in the nucleus of each cell. There all the genes that determine the characteristics of the individual are packaged into structures called chromosomes, which occur in pairs. The cells of every normal individual contain 46 chromosomes or 23 pairs; 22 of these pairs are the same in the two sexes and are referred to as the autosomes. The other pair, the pair of sex chromosomes, consists of two X chromosomes in the female and an X and a Y chromosome in the male. One chromosome of each pair is derived from the mother and the other from the father. When eggs and sperm are formed by the process of meiosis, the chromosomes segregate so that one from each pair is in the egg or sperm, giving a total number of 23.

Thousands of genes are located on each chromosome, and, in the case of the autosomes, each gene is matched by a corresponding gene for the same characteristic on the other chromosome of the pair. Thus, genes as well as chromosomes "come in pairs." The X chromosomes contain a full complement of genes, but no corresponding genes are present on the Y chromosomes. Clearly, some genes are present on the Y, particularly those dealing with the development of male sexual characteristics, but these have no corresponding match on the X chromosomes. In the female, therefore, those genes carried on the X chromosome are present in pairs, and in males they are not. This difference between the sexes has important implications with regard to those disorders coded for by genes on the X chromosome. This is discussed in more detail under the topic of X-linked inheritance.

Over 2000 disorders in man have now been attributed to single mutant genes. These are the disorders that follow the classical Mendelian patterns of inheritance. In many cases, the specific gene product is unknown or cannot be measured, but pedigree studies are clearly indicative of a specific inheritance pattern.

Those disorders which have been reported to occur on the basis of a single gene defect have been cataloged by McKusick in the volume *Mendelian Inheritance in Man*. Discussions of the four basic Mendelian patterns of inheritance are included here.

Autosomal Dominant Inheritance

The typical pedigree of a family with an autosomal dominant disorder is illustrated in Figure 1a. The gene for such disorders is located on one of the 22 autosomes, and the term *dominant* implies that the mutant gene is dominant over its normal counterpart. Thus, only one of the two genes in a pair need be abnormal for the individual to be affected with a particular disease. Autosomal dominant disorders are transmitted from generation to generation by affected individuals of both sexes, and males and females are equally affected. On the average, one-half of the offspring of an affected individual are also affected. In any pregnancy, the risk to an affected individual of having an affected child is 1 out of 2. Except in an unusual circumstance, where an autosomal dominant gene exhibits incomplete penetrance, unaffected family members have essentially no risk of passing the disorder on to their offspring. This is diagramed in Figure 1b.

In some circumstances, the manifestations and severity of an autosomal dominant disorder may vary considerably among affected individuals in the same family. This is referred to as variable expressivity. Usually an individual who has the gene for an autosomal dominant disease has that disease, and one who is completely free of the

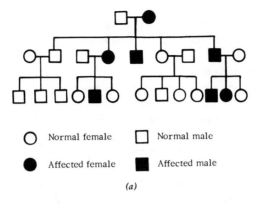

(a)

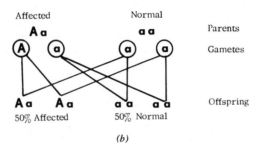

(b)

Figure 1. (a) Autosomal dominant inheritance; (b) offspring of a couple in whom one has an autosomal dominant disorder. A = mutant dominant gene; a = normal gene.

disorder can be assumed not to be a carrier of the gene. In unusual circumstances, however, an individual may carry the gene for an autosomal dominant disorder presumably without any manifestations of that disorder. This is referred to as incomplete penetrance. A dominant gene with complete penetrance always results in some clinical manifestations, although they may vary in degree.

Occasionally, a child who clearly has an autosomal dominant disorder is born to two parents who are normal and have no family history of other affected family members. When false paternity is excluded, this can be assumed to reflect the new mutation of a normal gene to the mutant form in one of the germ cells or in the zygote. Parents of a child with an autosomal dominant disorder secondary to a new mutation have essentially the same risk as the general population of having an affected child on a subsequent pregnancy. The affected individual, on the other hand, naturally faces a risk of 1 in 2 of passing the mutant gene on to each of his offspring. One factor that has been related to an increased incidence of autosomal dominant disorders related to new mutations is advanced paternal age. One note of caution should be entered here. Before any autosomal dominant disorder is assumed to represent a new mutation, both parents, siblings, and, occasionally, other family members must be carefully examined. It is well known that the manifestations of many autosomal dominant disorders are quite variable and may be so subtle as to be overlooked unless carefully sought.

Examples of autosomal dominant disorders include achondroplasia (the most common form of short-limbed dwarfism), Huntington's chorea, neurofibromatosis, adult polycystic kidney disease, and the common form of osteogenesis imperfecta.

Autosomal Recessive Inheritance

Autosomal recessive genes are located on the autosomes but, in contrast to autosomal dominant genes, do not exert an overt effect if a normal gene of the same pair is present. Thus, for an autosomal recessive disorder to be manifested clinically, both members of the gene pair must be abnormal. This implies that one of the mutant genes must be donated by each of the parents who, if normal, are by definition carriers of the disorder. Carriers, who have one normal gene and one gene for the disease, are usually normal, since the mutant gene "recedes" behind the normal one. The pedigree of a family with an autosomal recessive disorder is illustrated in Figure 2a. Such disorders occur with equal frequency in males and females and often occur in multiple siblings born to normal parents. Other affected family members are usually not found. Two carriers of an autosomal recessive disorder face a risk of 1 in 4 on each pregnancy of having an affected child. Of the normal siblings, two-thirds are carriers like the parents and one-third are not carriers. This is illustrated in Figure 2b. It is important for such parents to recognize that each pregnancy represents a new event and the outcome is not altered

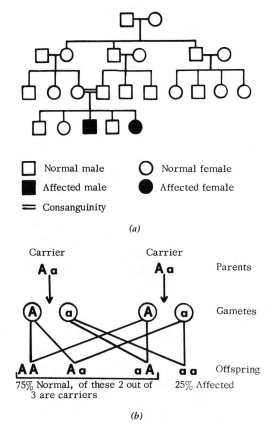

Figure 2. (a) Autosomal recessive inheritance; (b) offspring of a couple who are both carriers of an autosomal recessive disorder. A = normal gene; a = mutant recessive gene.

by the outcome of previous pregnancies. For example, if the first pregnancy results in an affected child, this does not imply that the next three will be normal.

Siblings of individuals with an autosomal recessive disorder often request genetic counseling regarding their risks of having children with the same disorder. Although such individuals have a two-thirds chance of being a carrier of the disorder, their risk of having affected children is usually quite low, essentially always less than 1 percent, since it is dependent on their mating with someone else who is also a carrier. The precise risk is dependent on the frequency of carriers for the disorder in the general population, but even the most common autosomal recessive genes have a carrier frequency of 1 in 20 or less.

Examples of autosomal recessive disorders include cystic fibrosis, sickle cell anemia, beta-thalassemia, and Tay-Sachs disease. It is generally accepted that every individual is the carrier of at least four or five deleterious autosomal recessive genes. Because these genes are individually quite rare, it is unusual for two individuals carrying the same gene to marry and have children. The birth of an affected child is usually the first indication to either parent that he or she is a carrier of a specific gene. In certain circumstances, this event is more likely to occur than in the general population. Individuals in the same family are likely to be carriers of some of the same genes, since these are transmitted through common ancestors. Thus, autosomal recessive disorders may occur with an increased frequency among children of consanguineous parents, as in first-cousin marriages.

Certain autosomal recessive disorders occur almost exclusively in certain racial or ethnic groups. Tay-Sachs disease, for example, occurs most commonly in the Ashkenazi Jewish population and sickle cell anemia in the black population. All disorders can occur in any population, but, at times, the common occurrence in one specific group can increase the index of suspicion for a given disorder. Screening methods are available for the detection of carriers of some of these disorders and, when desired by the individual, can be of benefit to the population at risk. Many individuals of Ashkenazi Jewish descent request screening for Tay-Sachs disease. In this way, carriers at risk can occasionally be identified prior to the birth of an affected child. Since prenatal diagnosis is available for this disorder, very precise genetic counseling can then be offered. Individuals with sickle cell trait who are carriers of sickle cell anemia can also be identified by simple screening methods. Prenatal diagnosis of this disorder has also recently become possible, although the procedure, to date, has had limited application.

X-Linked Recessive Inheritance
Genes that code for X-linked disorders are located on the X chromosome. An X-linked recessive gene is not manifested as long as it is balanced by a normal gene on the other X chromosome. Thus, females who have a mutant gene on one X chromosome and a normal gene on the other are usually normal. Males, on the other hand, have no genes on the Y chromosome to match those on the X. Thus, all the genes on the X chromosome of the male, whether dominant or recessive, are "exposed" and exert their full effect.

The pedigree of a family with an X-linked recessive disorder is illustrated in Figure 3a. It should be clear that such disorders occur almost exclusively in males and are transmitted through the family by carrier females, who themselves are usually normal. A female carrier of such a disorder faces a risk of 1 in 4 on any pregnancy of having an affected child, but this risk is 1 in 2 if the child is a male and essentially zero if it is a

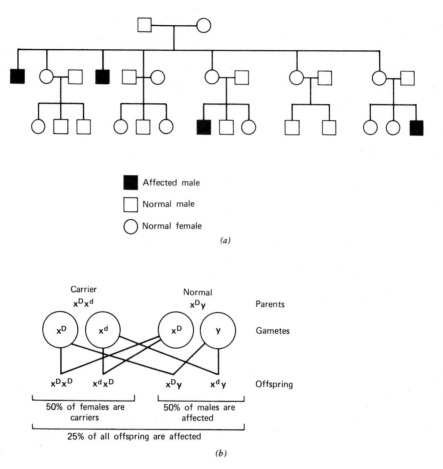

Figure 3. (a) X-Linked recessive inheritance; (b) offspring of a couple in whom the mother is the carrier of an X-linked recessive disorder. D = normal gene; d = mutant recessive gene.

female; 1 out of 2 daughters will be a carrier, however, like the mother. This is illustrated in Figure 3b. This risk figure is not affected by a carrier's choice of mates unless one happens to be affected by the X-linked recessive disorder in question.

The normal sisters of males with an X-linked recessive disorder, in general, have a risk of 1 in 2 of being a carrier. Their risk on any pregnancy of having an affected child is thus $\frac{1}{2} \times \frac{1}{4} = \frac{1}{8}$; or $\frac{1}{4}$ if the child is a male and essentially zero if it is a female, although some of their daughters might also be carriers. The only exception to this is in the family with only one affected male in whom, in some cases, this has occurred as the result of a new mutation. In such an instance, other family members may not be at increased risk of having affected children. It can never be automatically assumed, however, that an isolated case actually represents a new mutation.

Occasionally, an X-linked recessive disorder is observed in a female. This may occur by one of any number of different mechanisms. A female with Turner's syndrome (45,XO), for example, exhibits all the traits coded for by genes on her one X chromosome in the same way that this occurs in the male. Alternatively, if a male with an X-linked recessive disorder mates with a female who is a carrier of the same disorder, they may have a daughter with the recessive gene on both of her X chromosomes. This is an extraordinarily rare event unless the parents are blood relatives. Finally, an occasional carrier of an X-linked recessive disorder may exhibit some clinical manifestations of the disorder, although usually not with the same degree of severity observed in the male. This is thought to be explained by the phenomenon of X chromosome inactivation. In each cell of the female, early in fetal life, one of the two X chromosomes becomes condensed and functionally inactive. From this time on, all the cells derived from each parent cell have the same X chromosome inactivated. Therefore, each normal female is actually a mosaic with respect to the genes on the X chromosome. This can be thought of as nature's way of equalizing the amount of functionally active chromosome material in male and female cells. In some of the cells, only one X chromosome is active, and, in the others, only the other X chromosome is active. The phenomenon of X chromosome inactivation, sometimes referred to as the Lyon hypothesis, is presumably random, and most females have either X chromosome active in about 50 percent of the cells. Occasionally, however, a single X chromosome is active in substantially more than half of the cells. If this is an X with a recessive gene, clinical manifestations of the recessive disorder may be observed in the carrier female.

Examples of X-linked recessive disorders include hemophilia A and B, Duchenne muscular dystrophy, hemolytic anemia related to glucose-6-phosphate dehydrogenase deficiency, and deutan color blindness. Screening methods are now available for the detection of carriers of some of these disorders in families at risk.

X-Linked Dominant Inheritance

X-Linked dominant genes exert their effects in both males and females, since only a single dose of the mutant gene need be present for the disorder to be manifested. The feature that distinguishes X-linked dominant inheritance from autosomal dominant inheritance is the absence of male-to-male transmission. An affected father obviously cannot pass the gene on to his sons, since he gives his sons the Y chromosome instead of the X. An affected female has a risk of 1 in 2 on any pregnancy of having an affected child, and the risk is the same if the child is a male or a female. An affected male, on the other hand, always passes the disorder on to his daughters, since they all receive his X chromosome, and never to his sons. As a result, X-linked dominant disorders are twice as common in females as in males. This is illustrated in Figures 4a and b.

Examples of X-linked dominant disorders, which are actually quite rare, include familial hypophosphatemic vitamin D–resistant rickets, pseudohypoparathyroidism, ornithine transcarbamylase deficiency (a urea cycle defect), and incontinentia pigmenti. Some of these disorders are much more severe in the male than in the female or may actually be lethal in the male. Males with ornithine transcarbamylase deficiency usually die in the neonatal period, and affected females frequently survive. Incontinentia pigmenti is virtually never seen in the male and presumably results in the loss of male fetuses early in gestation.

Multifactorial Inheritance

There are a number of familial disorders, including some of the most common isolated congenital malformations, that cannot be attributed to the effect of a single mutant gene but are attributable to the additive effects of several mutant genes and environmental factors. Such disorders are said to exhibit multifactorial inheritance. Congenital malformations in this group include neural tube defects, cleft lip and palate, clubfoot, congenital hip dislocation, and some types of congenital heart disease. The principles of multifactorial inheritance and recurrence risks for individual disorders are primarily derived from statistical studies of large numbers of affected families. The number of genes involved in the determination of a given disorder is unknown, as is the nature of the environmental influences that may exert any additive effect.

Several basic principles separate disorders with multifactorial inheritance from single gene defects. First degree relatives of an affected individual, including parents, siblings, and offspring, are all equally likely to be affected. For example, a couple who has had a child with cleft lip and palate face a risk of about 4 percent that the next child will also be affected. Similarly, if one parent has cleft lip and palate, the risk is about 4 percent that the first child will be affected. Recurrence rates for malformations with multifactorial inheritance tend to cluster in the range of 3 to 7 percent. The risk of recurrence is increased if there are multiple affected family members.

Many multifactorial disorders are more common in one sex than in the other, implying that more mutant genes may be required for the malformation to be manifested in the less commonly affected sex. As expected in such circumstances, the individual of the less commonly affected sex is more likely to have affected offspring. This presumably is a reflection of his or her increased pool of mutant genes. The severity of the defect in an

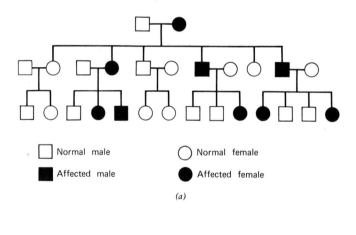

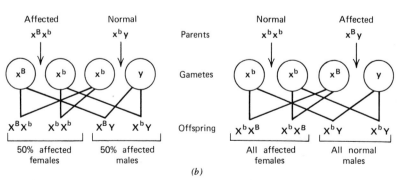

Figure 4. (a) X-Linked dominant inheritance; (b) offspring of a couple in whom one has an X-linked dominant disorder. B = dominant mutant gene; b = normal gene.

Table I. Recurrence Risks for Common Congenital Malformations

Malformation	Percentage of Risk for Each Subsequent Child
Cleft lip with or without cleft palate*	
One affected child	4
Two affected children	9
One affected parent	4
One affected parent and one affected child	17
Cleft palate only	
One affected child	2
Two affected children	10
One affected parent	6
One affected parent and one affected child	15
Neural tube defects (anencephaly, myelomeningocele, encephalocele)	
One affected child	4–5
Two affected children	12–15
Congenital heart disease	
Ventricular septal defect	5
Atrial septal defect	3
Patent ductus arteriosus	4
Pulmonic stenosis	3
Aortic stenosis	2
Tetralogy of Fallot	3
Transposition of great vessels	2
Coarctation of aorta	2
Clubfoot	3
Congenital hip dislocation	4–5
Pyloric stenosis	
One affected child	3
Mother affected	16
Father affected	5

SOURCE: Data compiled from multiple sources.

* All the risk figures are somewhat increased if affected individual is female or if cleft is severe.

affected individual also influences the recurrence risk in his relatives, presumably on a similar basis. The more severely affected individual may carry more mutant genes than his less severely affected counterpart. In Table I, the specific recurrence risks for some common congenital malformations with multifactorial inheritance are outlined.

GENETIC DISORDERS AND FERTILITY

A variety of genetic disorders have been related to infertility in both the male and female. Leading the list are the sex chromosome abnormalities, including Turner syndrome in the female (XO gonadal dysgenesis) and Klinefelter syndrome in the male (47, XXY). Individuals with true Turner syndrome, unless they are mosaics, have streak ovaries and primary amenorrhea and are invariably sterile. Such individuals are usually diagnosed prior to attempts at conception because of their associated short stature or other somatic stigmata or during the course of the evaluation of primary amenorrhea. In addition to the XO chromosomal complement, individuals with structural abnormalities of the X chromosome may exhibit many of the stigmata of Turner syndrome, including infertility. Infertile females with XY or XX gonadal dysgenesis are also occasionally encountered. Females with a 47, XXX karyotype, many of whom are normal, may exhibit an increased incidence of infertility. Phenotypic females with testicular feminization (XY genotype) are, by definition, infertile.

Males with the Klinefelter syndrome are invariably sterile. This diagnosis is usually suspected on the basis of the unusual body habitus and small testes, although other anomalies may be present as well. More complex sex chromosomal abnormalities in the male (48, XXXY; 49, XXXXY; etc.) are also associated with infertility but usually include mental retardation and multiple somatic anomalies as well. Studies of infertile couples have indicated that about 2 percent of males with oligospermia have a recognizable chromosomal abnormality. Thus, chromosome analysis may occasionally be indicated in the evaluation of such couples.

A number of Mendelian disorders have also been associated with infertility in individuals with normal chromosomal complements. Myotonic dystrophy, an autosomal dominant disorder with manifestations in many organ systems besides the neuromuscular system, is associated with decreased fertility in both sexes. Cystic fibrosis, an autosomal recessive disorder that was once almost uniformly fatal in childhood, is now compatible with survival into early adult life, and some affected individuals marry. Affected males are almost uniformly sterile, regardless of the severity of their disease. Many other examples could be cited of generalized disorders with impact on the reproductive system.

GENETIC DISORDERS IN THE MOTHER AND THEIR IMPACT ON THE DEVELOPING FETUS

A number of genetic disorders are known to alter the normal course of pregnancy and thereby influence the well-being of the developing fetus. One of the most outstanding examples is that of maternal hyperphenylalaninemia, with or without phenylketonuria, which has been shown to be associated with the almost invariable occurrence of mental retardation in the offspring. About one-half of all cases of hyperphenylalaninemia actually represent classical phenylketonuria. In the past, most of these individuals were severely retarded and did not reproduce. With the advent of neonatal screening and dietary therapy, however, affected individuals are now reaching child-bearing age with normal intelligence. Dietary therapy in phenylketonuria is usually discontinued in the early school years. In addition to those individuals with classical phenylketonuria about an equal number of individuals have hyperphenylalaninemia without mental retardation or any other manifestations. Although such individuals are now also identified by neonatal screening, there would have been, in the past, no way of clinically recognizing such an individual. It has been suggested that dietary restriction of phenylalanine during pregnancy in women with hyperphenylalaninemia may avert damage to the fetus. Adequate clinical studies in this population of pregnant women have not yet been reported. Because of the high risk of recurrence of mental retardation, a blood phenylalanine determination is indicated in any woman who has given birth to one or more children with undiagnosed mental retardation. One might also suggest that blood phenylalanine levels be determined in all women during early pregnancy.

Although hyperphenylalaninemia is the outstanding example, there is no reason to believe that other metabolic derangements in the mother might not have similar adverse effects on fetal development. The effects of maternal diabetes mellitus on the fetus are well known and are extensively discussed in Chapter 24.

Genetic disorders other than the inborn errors of metabolism may also affect the outcome of pregnancy and the well-being of the fetus. Many of the genetically determined skeletal dysplasias such as classical achondroplasia, the most common form of short-limbed dwarfism, alter the anatomy of the pelvis to such an extent that delivery by cesarean section is necessary. Certain inherited disorders of connective tissue, including some forms of the Ehlers-Danlos syndrome, are associated with an increased incidence of prematurity. Many other examples could be cited of genetic disorders in the mother affecting fetal well-being.

THE PROBLEM OF RECURRENT SPONTANEOUS ABORTION AND ITS IMPLICATIONS FOR GENETIC COUNSELING

It is well known that spontaneous abortion in the first trimester of pregnancy is often a reflection of fetal abnormalities. Indeed, a number of studies have documented the presence of chromosomal abnormalities in approximately 50 percent of first trimester abortuses. It is clear that accidents in meiosis resulting in an abnormal chromosomal complement in the egg or sperm are common events. Because many chromosomal abnormalities are incompatible with fetal survival and are never seen in liveborn infants, many such accidents result in miscarriage. Other chromosomal abnormalities that are seen in living children, such as Turner syndrome (45, XO), exhibit a high rate of spontaneous abortion as well.

Miscarriage is, in itself, a common event, occurring in 15 to 20 percent of all pregnancies. Therefore, a history of one or two spontaneous abortions in a couple is rarely a cause for excessive concern. When three or more miscarriages occur, however, the situation is somewhat different. With the knowledge that first trimester abortion is often associated with chromosomal abnormalities in the fetus, chromosome analysis has been performed on a number of couples with a history of recurrent miscarriages. Such cytogenetic studies, when performed with newer banding techniques, indicate that in about 10 percent of such couples a balanced chromosomal rearrangement (translocation) can be found in one of the parents. The carrier of such a translocation is himself normal, since the correct amount of chromosomal material is present. The repackaging of this material by means of a translocation, however, interferes with the normal segregation of chromosomes at meiosis and may lead to the production of gametes with too much or too little chromosomal material. If the resulting unbalanced chromosomal abnormality in the fetus is incompatible with survival, miscarriage results. This is illustrated in Figure 5.

The advantages of detecting this type of chromosomal rearrangement in one member of a couple are numerous. Simply understanding the underlying basis for recurrent abortion is reassuring to some individuals. In certain situations, estimates can be made of the risk of miscarriage on subsequent pregnancies. A very rare individual is found to

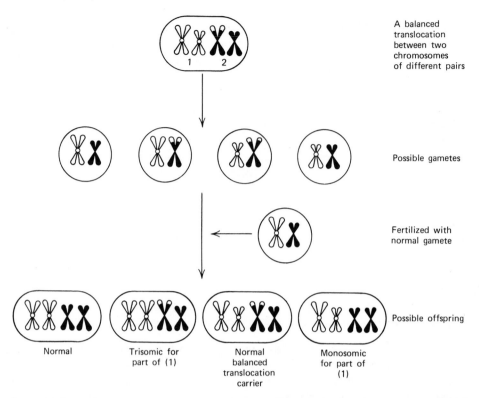

A balanced
translocation
between two
chromosomes
of different pairs

Possible gametes

Fertilized with
normal gamete

Possible offspring

Normal   Trisomic for   Normal   Monosomic
                part of (1)   balanced   for part of
                                    translocation   (1)
                                    carrier

Figure 5. Diagrammatic representation of the possible outcome of a pregnancy in an individual with a balanced chromosomal translocation. Some of the unbalanced zygotes formed might be inviable, and others might result in the birth of children with anomalies.

be the carrier of a type of translocation that never allows the production of normal gametes. For example, an occasional individual is detected in whom the two chromosomes of a given pair are joined to form a single larger chromosome. When meiosis occurs in such an individual, the gamete receives either two "doses" or no "dose" of that particular chromosome. When fertilization occurs, the resulting zygote is either trisomic or monosomic for that chromosome. If neither of these states is compatible with fetal survival, the outcome of every pregnancy is abortion. If either state is compatible with survival, the individual is at risk for having children with a chromosomal abnormality as well.

Fortunately, most balanced translocations do not preclude the production of normal offspring. However, in addition to the risk of additional miscarriages, the carrier of a balanced translocation may also be at risk for having children with an unbalanced chromosomal translocation that is compatible with fetal survival. Thus, depending on the type of translocation, amniocentesis for prenatal diagnosis may be indicated in pregnancies continuing beyond the first trimester. When a translocation is found in one individual, other family members are often anxious to have chromosome analysis, since many such translocations are familial.

With techniques of chromosome banding now becoming widely available, it would seem prudent to perform chromosome analysis on all couples with a history of three or more unexplained first trimester abortions.

GENETIC DISORDERS MANIFESTED IN THE NEWBORN

Chromosomal Abnormalities

Alterations in the normal number or structure of chromosomes are not rare in the newborn infant. Numerous cytogenetic studies of consecutive newborn infants have documented an incidence of gross chromosomal abnormalities of about 1 in 150. Most of these studies were performed using conventional techniques of chromosome analysis. With the development of more sophisticated banding techniques, more subtle chromosomal aberrations can now be identified, and it is possible that the true incidence of significant chromosomal abnormalities may actually be somewhat higher.

The normal human karyotype is illustrated in Figure 6. The banding techniques developed in recent years have made it possible to identify individually each of the 23 pairs of chromosomes, which originally were grouped and numbered on the basis of size and position of the centromere. Karyotypes are ordinarily derived from actively dividing cells during the part of meiosis referred to as metaphase, when the chromosomes are most dense and line up in the center of the cell in preparation for cell division. The tissues most commonly used for chromosome analysis are peripheral lymphocytes and cultivated skin fibroblasts.

A brief explanation of nomenclature applicable to chromosomal abnormalities is included here. The normal number of chromosomes, which in man is 46, is referred to as the diploid number. The haploid number is 23, that is, the number present in the gametes. The presence of additional complete sets of chromosomes in a cell is referred to as polyploidy. Triploidy refers to the presence of 69 chromosomes; tetraploid cells contain 92. Aneuploidy refers to an abnormality in chromosome number resulting from the presence or absence of a single chromosome or several chromosomes. The most common examples of this are trisomy, in which three chromosomes of a given pair are

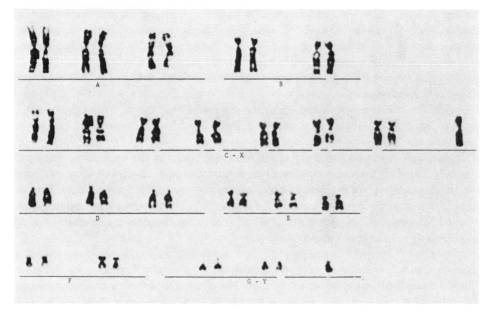

Figure 6. Normal male karyotype, 46, XY.

present, and monosomy, in which only one member of the pair is present. Occasionally one encounters, in a given individual, two or more populations of cells, each containing a different chromosomal complement. This is referred to as mosaicism and presumably results from an accident in cell division, or mitosis, occurring in the zygote following fertilization.

Structural anomalies of the chromosomes are being recognized with increased frequency since the development of banding techniques. The most commonly encountered structural abnormality is a translocation, in which part or all of a particular chromosome is attached to another chromosome. This is referred to as balanced if the appropriate amount of chromosomal material is present, although rearranged, and unbalanced if part of a chromosome is missing or extra. In reality, there is probably no such thing as a completely balanced translocation, since translocations are the result of chromosome breakage followed by recombination. The amount of material lost can apparently be so small as to be insignificant. Breakage of a chromosome with complete loss of the broken segment gives rise to a deletion. A ring chromosome is the result of breakage of both ends of a chromosome with subsequent fusion. More complex structural abnormalities such as inversions and duplications also occur but to date have been of limited clinical significance.

It should be pointed out that the possibilities for different structural and numerical abnormalities of the chromosomes are infinite. As previously mentioned, many types of chromosomal abnormalities are incompatible with fetal survival and are never seen in the infant. Of those abnormalities observed in the infant or child, clinically recognizable syndromes are associated with the more common ones. This is particularly true of the abnormalities of number, i.e., the trisomic states. Although some deletion syndromes have also been delineated, the clinical features associated with structural anomalies tend to be more variable. Clearly, the amount of missing chromatin can itself be variable and the specific genes left "unopposed" on the homologous (matching) chromosome may contribute to the clinical picture.

Chromosome analysis is clearly indicated when a specific chromosomal abnormality such as Down syndrome is suspected. It is also indicated in infants with multiple congenital anomalies of unknown etiology and in infants who have neurologic abnormalities in combination with physical anomalies that may be subtle.

Autosomal Abnormalities

The most common autosomal abnormalities observed in the neonate are trisomies 21, 18, and 13. Patients have been reported who are trisomic for one of the other autosomes, but most other autosomal trisomies are incompatible with fetal survival. It is unreasonable to expect the physician to recognize clinically the unusual patient with another trisomic state such as trisomy 8. Such patients will be diagnosed cytogenetically if the basic guidelines for performing chromosome analysis in infants, i.e., multiple malformations in an unrecognized pattern, are followed. With the possible exception of two reported patients, monosomy for an autosome is also incompatible with survival and is not observed in the liveborn infant.

Down Syndrome. Down syndrome, or mongolism, is by far the most common and most widely known abnormality of the autosomes. The clinical syndrome was recognized and well delineated long before its cytogenetic basis could be established. It is now known that the clinical features of this syndrome are related to the presence of an extra "dose" of chromosome 21 in the cells of the affected individual.

The major features of Down syndrome are listed in Table II with the frequency in which they occur. Most affected individuals are readily recognizable on the basis of the characteristic facial features, as illustrated in Figure 7. Clinical recognition may be somewhat more difficult in the neonatal period, since overall appearance at this age is not always typical. One very helpful clinical finding in the neonate is that of hypotonia, observed in over 95 percent of newborns with Down syndrome. This may alert the clinician to search for more subtle features of the disorder.

The most significant problem associated with Down syndrome is undoubtedly mental retardation, which is invariably present, although some variation in IQ's within the retarded range may be observed. The average individual with Down syndrome is ultimately able to walk, dress himself, say some words, and learn other simple tasks but is never able to become self-sufficient. More severely retarded individuals are not uncommon.

In addition to the characteristic physical features of the disorder, several life-threatening anomalies occur with an increased incidence in Down syndrome. It has been calculated that 40 to 60 percent of affected individuals have congenital heart disease, the most commonly encountered lesions being endocardial cushion defect and ventricular septal defect. Duodenal atresia and Hirschsprung disease both occur with increased frequency in the neonate with Down syndrome, and there appears to be an increased incidence of leukemia of a variety of types in children with Down syndrome.

In the absence of serious physical anomalies, the life span of the individual with

Table II. Major Clinical Features of Down Syndrome (%)

Mental retardation	100
Hypotonia (neonatal period)	95
Flat facial features	90
Slanted palpebral fissures	80
Flat occiput	78
Short, broad hands with short fingers	70
High-arched palate	70
Dysplastic pelvis on X-ray	67
Open mouth with protruding tongue	65
Short fifth middle phalanx	62
Brushfield spots in iris	50
Abnormal ears	50
Clinodactyly	50
Congenital heart disease	40–60
Simian crease	48
Increased space between first and second toes	45
Epicanthal folds	40
Single flexion crease, fifth finger	20
Strabismus	20
Duodenal atresia	8

SOURCE: Adapted from *Birth Defects Atlas and Compendium,* D. Bergsma (Ed.), Williams and Wilkins, Baltimore, 1973.

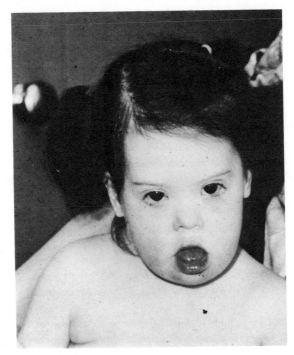

Figure 7. Child with Down syndrome.

Down syndrome may be normal or comparable with that of other retarded individuals, many of whom are institutionalized in adulthood if not before. Approximately 25 percent of infants with Down syndrome do not survive beyond the first year of life, however, and another 25 percent die by the age of 8 to 10 years. Most of these deaths are related to the complications of congenital heart disease.

As previously mentioned, the underlying defect in Down syndrome is the presence of an extra dose of chromosome number 21. In about 95 percent of patients with Down syndrome, chromosome analysis reveals the presence of 47 chromosomes in each cell, the extra one being a number 21. This is illustrated in Figure 8. This finding gives rise to the descriptive term for the disorder, trisomy 21. The occurrence of this disorder, and of other trisomic states, is thought to be the result of an accident in meiosis during the formation of the egg or the sperm. When the two members of a chromosome pair fail to segregate appropriately during meiosis, an event referred to as nondisjunction, both may be included in the gamete. When this combines with the normal gamete, a zygote trisomic for the chromosome pair results.

All the factors responsible for the occurrence of nondisjunction are not well understood. It is certainly a very common event, as evidenced by the common observation of numerical chromosomal abnormalities in spontaneous abortuses and by the relatively high incidence of Down syndrome and other chromosomal abnormalities in the general population. One factor that has definitely been associated with an increased incidence of chromosomal abnormalities and thus, presumably, of nondisjunctional events is that of advanced maternal age. This is best illustrated with reference to Down syndrome, which occurs with an incidence of approximately 1 in 700 live births in the general population. The incidence exhibits a marked increase with advancing maternal age. At

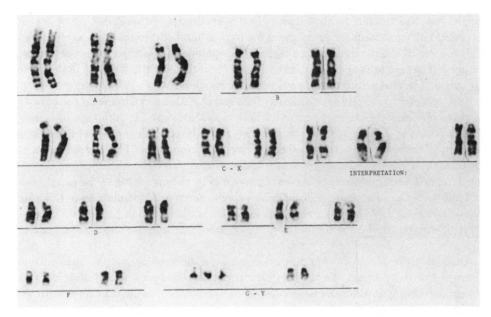

Figure 8. Karyotype of a female with trisomic Down syndrome, 47, XX, +21.

the age of 25, the incidence is about 1 in 2000; by 35, it is 1 in 250 to 300; by 40, it is 1 in 100; and by 45, it is 1 in 40. The same phenomenon applies to essentially all chromosomal abnormalities, and the overall incidence of chromosomal abnormalities as a function of maternal age is illustrated in Figure 9.

A second factor that appears to increase the likelihood of a nondisjunctional event occurring in a given individual is its previous occurrence in the same individual. Once a

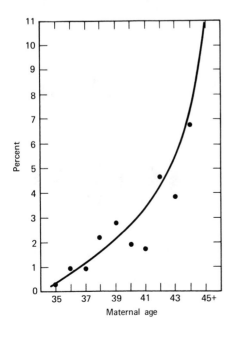

Figure 9. Graph of the incidence of all chromosomal abnormalities versus maternal age.

couple has had a child with trisomic Down syndrome, for example, they are at increased risk in subsequent pregnancies for having another affected child as compared with couples of comparable age in the general population. The exact risk is dependent on age but generally is three- to sixfold higher than that of other couples in the same age group. The reasons for this phenomenon are not clear.

Approximately 5 percent of individuals with classical Down syndrome do not have 47 chromosomes and thus cannot be said to have typical trisomy 21. Although such individuals are found to have 46 chromosomes, they have the equivalent of 47 with the extra number 21 chromosome being attached to another chromosome. This is referred to as the translocation type of Down syndrome and is clinically indistinguishable from the trisomic type. The only difference between the two is in the packaging of the extra chromosome material. The extra chromosome is most commonly attached to a D group chromosome in a D/G or D/21 translocation. This is illustrated in Figure 10. Alternatively, it may be attached to another G group chromosome, either number 21 or number 22.

Although there are no clinical differences between the trisomic and the translocation forms of Down syndrome, the finding of a translocation has great significance in terms of genetic counseling. When a child is diagnosed to have the translocation form of Down syndrome, chromosome analyses must be performed on both of the parents. In about one-third of the cases, one of the parents is found to have 45 chromosomes with a balanced translocation between a number 21 and one of the D or G group chromosomes. The karyotype of an individual who is a carrier of a D/G translocation is illustrated in Figure 11. The importance of this finding is that it gives the carrier a

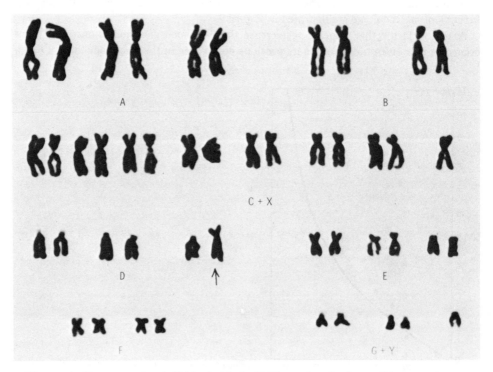

Figure 10. Karyotype of an individual with the D/G translocation form of Down syndrome.

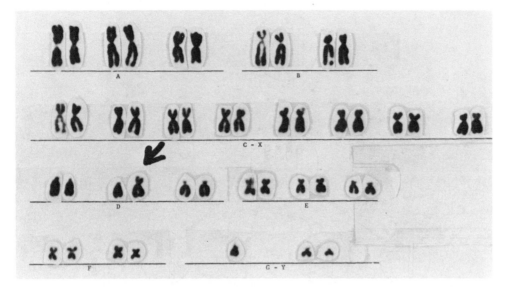

Figure 11. Karyotype of a D/G translocation carrier, mother of child with Down syndrome.

substantial risk of having additional children with Down syndrome, since the attached chromosomes cannot segregate normally at meiosis. The theoretical risk to a D/G translocation carrier of having a child with Down syndrome is 1 in 3 on any pregnancy. This is illustrated in Figure 12. In practice, the risk is substantially lower than this and is dependent on whether the male or the female is a carrier of the translocation. Female carriers of a D/G translocation have a risk of about 10 to 15 percent on any pregnancy of having a child with Down syndrome. For male carriers, the risk is about 2 to 3 percent. The reasons for the discrepancy between theoretical and actual risk values are not clear but may include decreased viability of embryos with unbalanced chromosomal complements and decreased fitness of sperm with abnormal complements.

The recurrence risk for other types of translocations varies as well. One remarkable and fortunately rare circumstance is that of the individual who is a carrier of a 21/21 translocation. Such an individual can produce only two types of gametes, those with two doses of the number 21 chromosome and those with no number 21 chromosome. With fertilization, the former results in the production of a child with Down syndrome and the latter results in a zygote monosomic for chromosome 21 that is spontaneously aborted. Thus, such an individual can only have children with Down syndrome.

It should be obvious that once a translocation is found in a family, other family members should be studied as well, since some of them may well be carriers of the same translocation.

Trisomy 18. Trisomy 18, or E trisomy, is the second most common autosomal abnormality, occurring with an incidence of about 1 in 3500 live births. Females are affected three times more commonly than males. This is a disorder that is readily recognizable in the neonatal period on the basis of the multiple malformation pattern observed. Recognition at this time is of utmost significance because of the prognositic implications. Fifty percent of affected infants die by 2 months of age and 90 percent by 1 year of age. The survivors are uniformly severely retarded. Therefore, the physician should take

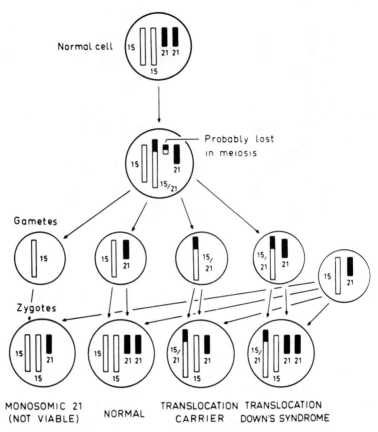

Figure 12. Theoretical scheme of the formation of a 15/21 (D/G) translocation and subsequent meiosis. The products after fertilization by normal gametes (sperm) will give rise to four types of zygotes. One will be inviable. Of the three possible viable zygotes, one will result in the birth of a child with Down syndrome. From Saxen, L., and Rapola, J. *Congenital Defects,* New York, Holt, Rinehart and Winston, Inc., 1969, p. 68.

these facts into consideration before instituting extraordinary measures for prolongation of life.

The major features of trisomy 18 are summarized in Table III. A wide variety of other abnormalities can also occasionally be observed. Some of the characteristic clinical features are seen in infants pictured in Figure 13. The exact cause of death in affected infants is often not known. Apneic episodes are common in the neonatal period, and poor sucking commonly leads to severe feeding problems.

The etiology of trisomy 18 is presumably meiotic nondisjunction in the majority of cases. An increasing incidence is observed with advanced maternal age. As with Down syndrome, a number of cases are related to a chromosomal translocation, some of which may be familial. When one patient is the carrier of a balanced translocation, the recurrence risk is high in subsequent pregnancies. Parents of trisomic cases probably also face a somewhat increased risk on subsequent pregnancies.

Trisomy 13. Trisomy 13, or D_1 trisomy, is the third major autosomal abnormality observed in the neonatal period. It occurs with an incidence of about 1 in 5000 births.

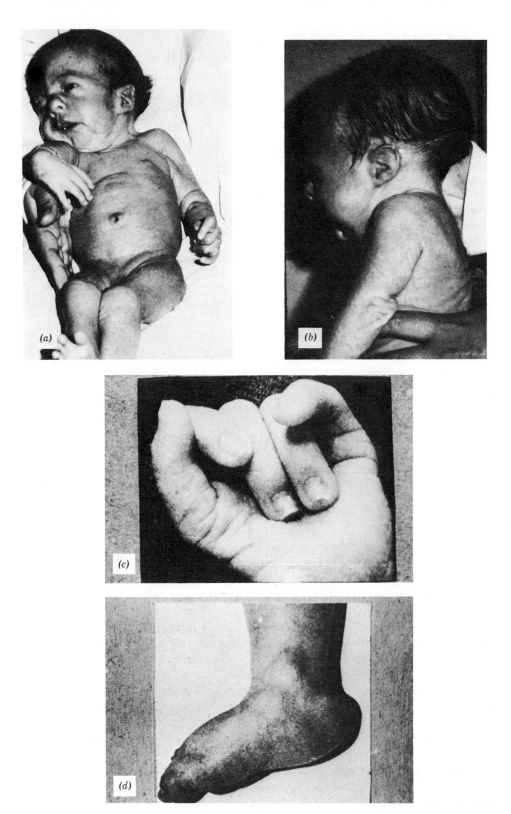

Figure 13. (*a*) Infant with trisomy 18, illustrating (*b*) the prominent occiput, (*c*) overlapping fingers, and (*d*) rocker bottom feet.

Table III. Major Clinical Features of Trisomy 18 (%)

Developmental and mental retardation	100
Failure to thrive	100
Cryptorchidism (males)	>95
Congenital heart disease (VSD, PDA)	>95
Abnormal ears	>80
Prominent occiput	>80
High-arched palate	>80
Micrognathia	>80
Short sternum	>80
Single umbilical artery	>80
Overlapping fingers	>80
Simple arches on six or more digits	>80
Small pelvis	>80
Limited hip abduction	>80
Umbilical or inguinal hernia	50–80
Rocker bottom feet	50–80
Renal malformations	50–80
Clubfoot	40–60
Microphthalmus	10–50
Abnormal flexion creases	10–50
Partial syndactyly	10–50
Hypoplastic nails	10–50
Omphalocele	10–20
Myelomeningocele	10–20
Cleft lip or palate	10–20
Tracheoesophageal fistula	<10

SOURCE: Adapted from *Birth Defects Atlas and Compendium,* D. Bergsma (Ed.), Williams and Wilkins, Baltimore, 1973.

As with trisomy 18, this disorder is usually recognizable clinically on the basis of the malformation pattern observed. The major clinical features of this disorder are listed in Table IV. Again, variability is the rule, and many other abnormalities may be observed. Some of the outstanding clinical features are depicted in Figure 14.

Anomalies of the midface, eye, and forebrain are characteristic of the trisomy 13 syndrome. The presence of holoprosencephaly, varying in severity from cyclopia or cebocephaly to less severe forms, in combination with the extracephalic anomalies should suggest this diagnosis. In other infants, the triad of microphthalmia, cleft lip and palate, and polydactyly should bring the diagnosis to mind.

The prognosis for this disorder is extremely poor; 44 percent of affected infants die within the first month of life and 80 percent within the first year. The survivors have severe mental retardation and failure to thrive. Once again, the physician should consider these facts before initiating extraordinary methods of life support in the neonatal period.

As with other trisomic states, advanced maternal age has been associated with the occurrence of trisomy 13. Parents of trisomic cases probably have an increased risk of recurrence on subsequent pregnancies as compared with couples of comparable age in the general population, but this risk remains low, probably less than 1 percent. Occasionally, this syndrome is related to a translocation, which is usually of the D/D type. In such instances, chromosome analysis of the parents is indicated. If one is the carrier of such a translocation, the recurrence risk might be quite high.

Autosomal Deletion Syndromes. A number of clinical syndromes have been associated with a deletion of chromosome material from one of the autosomes. With the widespread use of banding techniques, there is no doubt that additional deletion syndromes will be described. It is beyond the scope of this chapter to describe in detail the features of the specific syndromes recognized to date. Again, variability is the rule in

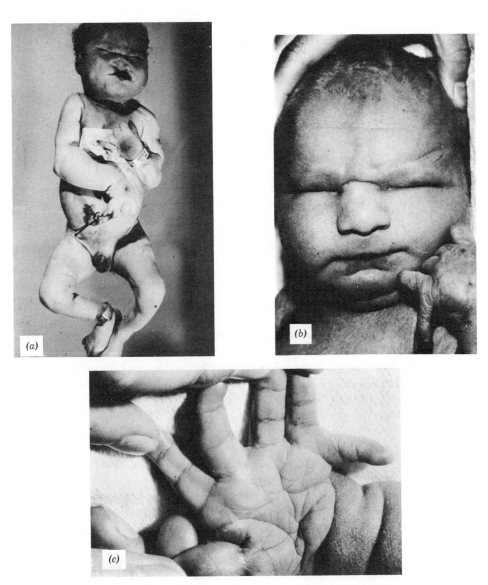

Figure 14. Two infants with trisomy 13, illustrating (*a*) cleft lip and palate, (*a* and *b*) microphthalmia, and (*c*) polydactyly.

Table IV. Major Clinical Features of Trisomy 13 (%)

Developmental and mental retardation	100
Cryptorchidism (males)	100
Elevated fetal hemoglobin during infancy	100
Hypertelorism	>80
Abnormal ears	>80
Congenital heart disease (VSD, PDA, ASD)	>80
Renal anomalies	>80
Brain anomalies	70–80
Apneic spells	50–80
Microcephaly	50–80
Microphthalmia	50–80
Cleft lip or palate	50–80
Polydactyly	50–80
Epicanthal folds	50–80
Micrognathia	50–80
Hyperconvex nails	50–80
Simian crease	50–80
Seizures	20–30
Scalp defects	10–50
Iris colobomata	10–50
Inguinal or umbilical hernia	10–50
Single umbilical artery	10–50
Omphalocele	10–20
Limited hip abduction	10–20

SOURCE: Adapted from *Birth Defects Atlas and Compendium,* D. Bergsma (Ed.), Williams and Wilkins, Baltimore, 1973.

these disorders. Instead, an example is given of one of the more commonly encountered deletion syndromes.

The cri-du-chat syndrome is a clinically recognizable disorder associated with a deletion of the short arm of chromosome 5. A representative karyotype is illustrated in Figure 15. Some of the typical features of the disorder can be seen in Figure 16. Affected infants are typically small for gestational age, grow poorly, and have a peculiar catlike cry in infancy. Most are hypotonic and exhibit microcephaly, hypertelorism, epicanthal folds, downslanting palpebral fissures, and simian creases. About 30 percent have congenital heart disease, variable in type. A variety of other anomalies are occasionally noted. Although most infants with this disorder survive the neonatal period, the prognosis is for severe mental retardation, the average IQ being in the 20 to 30 range.

The deletion of the short arm of chromosome 5 is a sporadic occurrence in most cases of the cri-du-chat syndrome. The etiologic factors related to its occurrence are unknown. In 10 to 15 percent of cases, however, a balanced chromosomal translocation is found in one of the parents, with the deleted material from the short arm of chromosome 5 being attached to another chromosome. When this is the case, the recurrence risk for this syndrome is quite high. Such individuals obviously might also have an increased risk of having offspring with other unbalanced chromosomal abnormalities, depending on the nature of the translocation.

Chromosome analysis is indicated in the parents of any child who is found to have a chromosomal deletion or translocation, since the possible occurrence of a familial translocation has great implications for genetic counseling.

Sex Chromosome Abnormalities

Abnormalities of the sex chromosomes are relatively common findings in liveborn infants, occurring with an incidence of about 1 in 400 births. They are twice as common in phenotypic males as in phenotypic females. In general, most children with sex chromosome abnormalities are not recognized in the neonatal period. Multiple major anomalies are not the rule in such disorders. The major stigmata of sex chromosomal abnormalities tend to revolve around body habitus and ultimate stature and sexual development. Mental retardation and other somatic abnormalities are seen with an increased frequency in some of these disorders but not to the same extent as in the autosomal abnormalities. Abnormalities of this chromosome pair, in general, seem to have less widespread implications than the abnormalities of the autosomes. Both numerical and structural anomalies of the sex chromosomes may be observed.

Turner Syndrome. Turner syndrome (45, XO), also referred to as XO gonadal dysgenesis, is the only monosomic chromosomal abnormality seen with any frequency in man. It occurs with an incidence of about 1 in 3000 newborn females and is the most common significant sex chromosomal abnormality in females. The incidence of the XO karyotype in the newborn does not begin to reflect the true occurrence of this condition in the zygote, since the vast majority of XO fetuses are spontaneously aborted. This observation suggests that the presence of a second sex chromosome (X or Y) may be far more critical in early fetal life than it is in postnatal life.

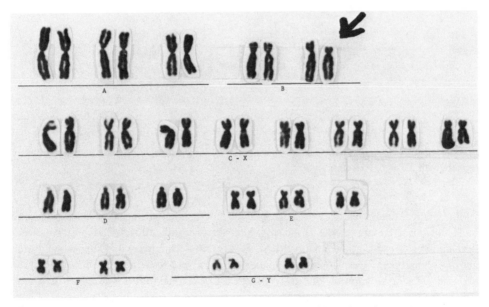

Figure 15. Karyotype of an infant with cri-du-chat syndrome. Note the deletion of the short arm of chromosome 5.

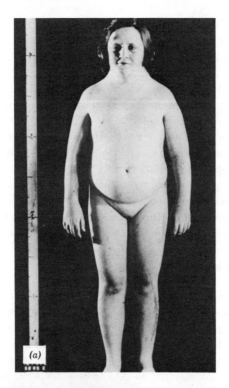

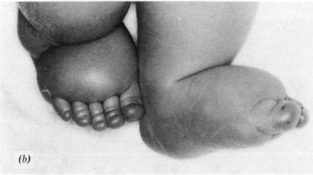

Figure 16. (*a*) Older child with Turner syndrome; (*b*) lymphedema of the dorsum of the feet in a neonate with Turner syndrome.

The major clinical features of Turner syndrome are listed in Table V. Because the most obvious stigmata of the disorder, short stature and failure of secondary sexual development, are not apparent until later in life, many infants with Turner syndrome are not recognized. Occasionally, however, suggestive features may be noted in the neonate. The most common one is lymphedema of the dorsum of the hands and feet, illustrated in Figure 16b. Any female infant with this finding should be suspected of having this disorder. A rare patient also exhibits swelling of the nape of the neck. Webbing of the neck or coarctation of the aorta in a female infant may also alert the physician to this diagnosis.

When the diagnosis of Turner syndrome is suspected, a buccal smear may be of value as a simple preliminary screening test. A negative buccal smear (absence of Barr bodies) in a phenotypic female would be presumptive evidence for this diagnosis, although it should always be confirmed by chromosome analysis. A positive buccal smear does not, in any way, rule out a sex chromosome abnormality. XO/XX, XO/XY, and more complex forms of mosaicism exist that are detectable only by further evaluation. In addition, a significant number of patients with the clinical stigmata of Turner syndrome have been reported who are 46, XX but have a structural abnormality of one of the X chromosomes. Such patients often have a normal percentage of Barr bodies on buccal smear. Thus, any patient suspected of having Turner syndrome or any other sex chromosomal abnormality must have a complete chromosome analysis.

The 45, XO karyotype is thought to result from the loss of a sex chromosome during the early meiotic divisions in the zygote following fertilization. It is presumably not a result of meiotic nondisjunction in either of the parents. Thus, parents of an affected child are not at substantially increased risk on subsequent pregnancies for having children with this or any other chromosomal abnormality.

Triple X Female (47, XXX). Trisomy for the X chromosome occurs with a frequency of about 1 in 1600 newborn females. Affected individuals are almost never recognized in the neonatal period, unless cytogenetic screening is performed. Indeed, the vast majority of 47, XXX females appear normal. A slight increase in the incidence of mental retardation and amenorrhea may be observed in this disorder, but the magnitude of the increase is as yet unknown. It is obvious that affected individuals with problems will be diagnosed much more commonly than asymptomatic individuals so that published data may be misleading as to the true incidence of abnormalities.

An interesting implication of this diagnosis relates to reproductive counseling. As many as one-sixth of the offspring of a fertile 47, XXX female may have a sex chro-

Table V. Major Clinical Features of Turner Syndrome (%)

Short stature	100
Ovarian dysgenesis	95
Congenital lymphedema of the hands and feet	80
Shield chest with widely spaced nipples	80
Low posterior hairline	80
Abnormal ears	80
Cubitus valgus	70
Narrow, hyperconvex nails	70
Renal anomalies, usually minor	60
Perceptive hearing loss	50
Excessive pigmented nevi	50
Webbed neck	50
Short fourth metacarpal or metatarsal	50
Epicanthal folds	40
Congenital heart disease (usually coarctation of aorta)	20
Ptosis	16
Mental retardation	10

SOURCE: Adapted from *Birth Defects Atlas and Compendium,* D. Bergsma (Ed.), Williams and Wilkins, Baltimore, 1973.

mosomal abnormality. Thus, a woman giving birth to two such infants should probably have a chromosome analysis.

Klinefelter Syndrome. The Klinefelter syndrome, or XXY syndrome, affecting 1 in 500 newborn males, is the single most common sex chromosome abnormality in man. Similar to the XXX syndrome, it is almost never suspected in the neonatal period, as most affected infants appear grossly normal. The most significant feature of the disorder is hypogonadism and infertility. Indeed, this represents the most common single cause of infertility in the adult male. Testes that are significantly smaller than normal are occasionally noted in the neonate. Without hormonal therapy, the penis and testes remain prepubertal, since testosterone production is almost invariably inadequate. An occasional affected individual exhibits cryptorchidism and hypospadius.

The second major feature of the Klinefelter syndrome is tall stature related to the pubertal hypogonadism, with a low upper-to-lower body segment ratio. The average IQ is reduced in this disorder, and 15 to 20 percent of patients are mentally retarded. Other features may include radioulnar synostosis and multiple minor anomalies such as dermatoglyphic abnormalities.

In most cases, the XXY syndrome is presumably the result of meiotic nondisjunction in one of the parents. A maternal age factor has been demonstrated. As with other nondisjunctional abnormalities, parents of an affected child are at increased risk on subsequent pregnancies. The magnitude of this increased risk is not currently known.

XYY Syndrome. The XYY karyotype is a sex chromosomal abnormality that has recently received a good deal of public attention because of a reported association with criminal behavior and psychiatric disorders. Newborn screening studies have demonstrated that this is a common abnormality, occurring with a frequency of about 1 in 800 newborn males. Although common, it is seldom diagnosed in the child or even in the adult, since many individuals with this karyotype are normal. It now appears clear, however, that there is an increased incidence of significant behavioral problems among individuals with this disorder. Aggressive behavior, occasionally accompanied by mild mental retardation, may result in juvenile delinquency or in overt criminal behavior. The XYY karyotype is 24 times more common among institutionalized juvenile delinquents than among the general male population.

The second major feature that may be associated with the XYY karyotype is that of accelerated growth, resulting in tall stature and long hands and feet. Severe acne is common in affected adolescents. Other abnormalities, including hypogonadism and poor fine motor coordination, may occasionally be observed.

In dealing with the parents of a child found to have the XYY karyotype, it is important to emphasize that affected individuals may develop normally. The public notoriety this disorder has achieved may create undue anxiety in the families of such individuals. The risk of recurrence in siblings of affected individuals has not yet been established. The offspring of affected individuals have also not yet been studied to see what percentage have sex chromosomal abnormalities.

Other Sex Chromosome Abnormalities. Phenotypic males and females with up to five X chromosomes have been reported. The incidence and severity of mental retardation observed appears to rise in direct relationship to the number of X chromosomes present beyond the normal one or two. Genital abnormalities and infertility are commonly seen in all these syndromes. The OY karyotype is incompatible with fetal survival.

Isolated Congenital Malformations

It has been estimated that as many as 4 percent of newborn infants have at least one congenital malformation. Although minor and insignificant malformations are often included in such estimates, major malformations are certainly not uncommon. Certain basic principles must be kept in mind in evaluating an infant who, at birth, is found to have a congenital anomaly. The first is that any infant who has one major malformation or a combination of minor malformations has an increased risk of having other malformations. Thus, once a single anomaly has been identified, others must be carefully sought. Children who have multiple malformations may have a chromosomal abnormality, some of which have been described, or a recognizable malformation complex. A number of excellent textbooks and atlases have been devoted to the problem of malformation syndromes. Some of these have been related to a single mutant gene, and, for others, a specific environmental or teratogenic cause has been identified. In other instances, the etiology has not been established, but the specific recurrence risks have been calculated and the natural history has been documented. In evaluating the infant with multiple malformations, every effort should be made to establish a specific diagnosis. This has obvious significance in terms of predicting the long-term prognosis for the affected infant and for providing precise genetic counseling.

In some instances, the presence of a specific anomaly prompts a search for specific disorders in which that anomaly is a common component. For example, it has been demonstrated that about 11 percent of infants born with an omphalocele have the Beckwith syndrome. The other common features of this disorder, including large size for gestational age, macroglossia, neonatal hypoglycemia, visceromegaly, and unusual ear creases may occasionally be overlooked or disregarded if the physician is unfamiliar with this syndrome. The implications of making this diagnosis are obvious. First, affected infants should have their blood sugar carefully monitored. Second, the recurrence risk for the Beckwith syndrome, an autosomal recessive disorder, is 1 in 4, and for an isolated omphalocele it is less than 1 percent.

A number of infants born with anencephaly or an encephalocele have other malformations compatible with the diagnosis of Meckel syndrome, another autosomal recessive disorder. Other significant abnormalities associated with this disorder include microphthalmia, cleft palate, polydactyly, and polycystic kidneys. Here again, the recurrence risk for this disorder is 1 in 4 as opposed to the recurrence risk of 4 to 5 percent for isolated neural tube defects.

Cleft lip and palate, occurring with an incidence of 1 to 2 per 1000 live births, is one of the most common congenital malformations in man. About 10 percent of individuals with this anomaly have a recognizable malformation syndrome, some of which are attributable to a single mutant gene. Genetic counseling is obviously different in these cases than in isolated cleft lip and palate.

Certain types of congenital malformations, although not part of a specific syndrome, are known to occur commonly together. The association of low-set or abnormally formed ears with renal anomalies is well known, and every infant with this type of finding should have an intravenous pyelogram. By the same token, an infant with one or more features of the Vater association should be carefully examined for the other anomalies in this group, which include vertebral anomalies, anal atresia, tracheoeso-phageal fistula, renal anomalies, radial dysplasia, and congenital heart lesions. Such associations, although not strictly malformation syndromes, represent the nonrandom association of specific anomalies in combination with one another. Many more examples of such associations could be cited.

In some circumstances, information from the prenatal history may prompt a search for specific types of malformations in the newborn. Chronic alcoholism, for example, has been associated with a high incidence of specific abnormalities in the neonate. These may include growth deficiency, short palpebral fissures, and microcephaly. Other teratogenic drugs, such as methotrexate, warfarin, and diphenylhydantoin, and terato-genic viruses, such as rubella, have been identified and are discussed elsewhere in this text.

It is a common assumption that infants with multiple malformations also inevitably exhibit mental retardation, and this is a concern invariably expressed by the parents of such infants. Indeed, many disorders associated with physical anomalies are also associated with mental retardation, and any infant with significant birth defects is at increased risk of also having abnormalities of the central nervous system. This, however, is by no means universally true. Many malformation complexes could be cited that are usually associated with normal intelligence. In such instances, the establishment of a specific diagnosis can be most reassuring to the parents and physician and can guide them toward vigorous rehabilitative efforts for the affected infant.

When a newborn has been carefully examined and a single isolated congenital malformation detected, genetic counseling can then be provided for that anomaly. The etiology of most of the more common isolated malformations in man is very poorly understood. Many of these exhibit multifactorial inheritance, as previously described. For these disorders, data and recurrence risks are tabulated from studies of large numbers of families with affected individuals. The recurrence risks for some common congenital malformations are listed in Table I. It is important, as always, that a careful family history be elicited before counseling is provided. Multiple affected family members may imply a higher risk of recurrence than in the isolated case. Examination of other family members, especially the parents and siblings, may be indicated. Certain types of isolated congenital heart lesions, for example, may occasionally be inherited in a dominant fashion, even though the majority of cases show multifactorial inheritance. Affected individuals may be unaware of the presence of a clinically insignificant lesion.

It is a good general rule in dealing with congenital malformations, as with other genetic disorders, to collect as much information as possible via all possible routes before providing genetic counseling. Precise and accurate counseling is always based on accurate diagnosis and knowledge of the disorder with which one is dealing.

Inborn Errors of Metabolism

Although many of the inborn errors of metabolism are individually quite rare, collectively, they are not rare. With new diagnostic methods and mass screening programs, a number of these disorders are being found to be significantly more common than previously believed. There is, in addition, no doubt that a significant number of children with these disorders still go undiagnosed. Manifestations of inherited metabolic disorders, whether overt and life-threatening or more subtle, are often present in the neonatal period. The significance of the precise diagnosis of metabolic disease, when possible, cannot be overemphasized. Increasing numbers of these once "hopeless" disorders are now lending themselves to medical management, and when treatment means the prevention of significant mental retardation or death, even when the numbers are small, it is clearly worth pursuing. The remarkably successful dietary therapy of phenylketonuria and galactosemia is but one example of this. More recently, coenzyme therapy such as the use of vitamin B_{12} in methylmalonic acidemia or pyridoxine in homocystinuria has been shown to be of dramatic benefit in selected cases. A variety of other treatment modalities have been tried in a large number of the inborn errors of metabolism with variable success. The success of most treatment regimens is contingent on the institution of early therapeutic maneuvers, stressing the importance of diagnosis in the newborn period.

For the majority of the inborn errors of metabolism, of course, there is still no effective treatment available. Diagnosis is of equal importance in these cases, however, for purposes of genetic counseling. Disorders in this group are essentially all inherited in either an autosomal recessive or sex-linked recessive fashion so that parents of an affected child face a significant risk of recurrence. Without a diagnosis, appropriate counseling can certainly never be given. For many of the inborn errors of metabolism for which the underlying biochemical defect, usually an enzyme deficiency, has been identified, prenatal diagnosis and selective abortion is now possible. Once a definitive diagnosis has been made in these cases, the parents can be offered this option.

A number of the known inborn errors of metabolism follow a fulminating course leading to death in the neonatal period, which again underlines the need for a prompt and accurate diagnosis. Everyone involved in genetic counseling is from time to time confronted by a couple who has had a child die in the neonatal period following a poorly defined and undiagnosed, or misdiagnosed, illness and who are concerned about the risk of recurrence. In most metabolic disorders, the autopsy findings are nonspecific and unrevealing unless special biochemical studies are done. The recurrence risks for such a couple may be essentially zero if the diagnosis was infection, asphyxia, or some other nonhereditary neonatal disorder or as high as 1 in 4 in the case of most inborn errors of metabolism. Even if a biochemical disorder is suspected, it is essentially impossible to make a diagnosis in retrospect and although carrier detection is possible for some disorders, it would never be feasible to screen parents for all disorders known to cause fulminating neonatal disease.

As with many devastating illnesses in the neonate, the clinical manifestations of the inborn errors of metabolism are protean and often nonspecific. For many of these disorders, the predominant clinical signs and symptoms are those of poor feeding, lethargy, and failure to gain weight—the same general features seen in neonatal sepsis, a much more common event in the newborn. For certain disorders, there are more specific findings that might provide a clue to the clinician, and it is important to be aware of these. In general, however, it is a constellation of findings, unexplained by the existence of other neonatal disorders (such as sepsis, respiratory distress syndrome, or asphyxia), that should alert the physician to the possibility of metabolic disease.

It is the purpose of this section to attempt to define that constellation of findings in the newborn which should alert the clinician to this possibility. Once the suspicion of an inborn error of metabolism has arisen, the physician has crossed the first major hurdle toward making an accurate diagnosis. We confine the discussion to those disorders for which manifestations have been observed in the neonatal period and do not discuss the many disorders that typically present in later infancy or childhood. A series of simple laboratory studies, available to all clinicians, can often confirm the suspicion of an inborn error of metabolism, and it is our feeling that all physicians dealing with newborn infants should be familiar with these. An additional goal of this discussion, then, is to provide an approach to the use of these simple laboratory tools in a selective fashion in infants suspected of having a metabolic disease.

Using the approach outlined here, many more infants will be screened for metabolic disease than will actually be shown to have these disorders. However, the importance of recognizing the individual infant with such a disorder is so critical that we feel such an approach will indeed be rewarding. It is certainly true that once the diagnosis of an inborn error of metabolism is made, the infant is best cared for in a center with experience in the treatment and diagnosis of such disorders. It is only by careful scrutiny on the part of the primary physician, however, that such infants will reach the appropriate facilities.

Major Clinical Manifestations Associated with the Inborn Errors of Metabolism in the Neonatal Period

An outline of those inborn errors of metabolism which have been described clinically in the newborn infant is found in Table VI. This summary can by no means be considered to be complete in that it includes only those disorders for which neonatal manifestations have been documented in the literature. It is likely that disorders typically occurring later in childhood may occasionally present in the first month of life. In addition, new

Table VI. Inborn Errors of Metabolism Which May Present In The Neonatal Period

Disorders of carbohydrate metabolism
1. Galactosemia (galactose-1-phosphate uridyl transferase deficiency)
2. Hereditary fructose intolerance (fructose-1-phosphate aldolase deficiency)
3. Fructose-1,6-diphosphatase deficiency
4. Glycogen storage disease, type I (von Gierke disease, glucose-6-phosphatase deficiency)
5. Glycogen storage disease, type II (Pompe disease, α-1,4-glucosidase deficiency)
6. Glycogen storage disease, type III (limit dextrinosis, debrancher deficiency)
7. Glycogen storage disease, type IV (amylopectinosis, brancher deficiency)

Disorders of lipid metabolism
8. GM_1 gangliosidosis, type I (generalized gangliosidosis, β-galactosidase deficiency)
9. GM_3 gangliosidosis
10. Wolman disease (acid lipase deficiency)
11. Niemann-Pick disease, types A and B (sphingomyelinase, deficiency)

Disorders of mucopolysaccharide metabolism
12. Hurler syndrome (mucopolysaccharidosis I, α-L-iduronidase deficiency)
13. Hunter syndrome (mucopolysaccharidosis II, iduronic acid sulfatase deficiency)
14. β-Glucuronidase deficiency

Urea cycle defects
15. Carbamyl phosphate synthetase deficiency (hyperammonemia type I)
16. Ornithine transcarbamylase deficiency (hyperammonemia type II)
17. Citrullinemia
18. Argininosuccinic aciduria
19. Arginase deficiency

Table VI. (Continued)

Disorders of amino acid metabolism or transport
  20.   Maple syrup urine disease
  21.   Hypervalinemia
  22.   Hyperlysinemia
  23.   Hyper-β-alaninemia
  24.   Nonketotic hyperglycinemia
  25.   Phenylketonuria
  26.   Oasthouse syndrome (methionine malabsorption)
  27.   Tyrosinemia (tyrosinosis)
  28.   Hypermethioninemia
  29.   Homocystinuria
  30.   Hartnup disease
  31.   Hypersarcosinemia

Disorders of organic acid metabolism
  32.   Methylmalonic acidemia
  33.   Propionic acidemia (ketotic hyperglycinemia)
  34.   Isovaleric acidemia
  35.   Butyric and hexanoic acidemia (green acyl dehydrogenase deficiency)
  36. β-Methyl crotonyl CoA carboxylase deficiency

Miscellaneous disorders
  37.   Adrenogenital syndrome
  38.   Lysosomal acid phosphatase deficiency
  39.   Renal tubular acidosis
  40.   Nephrogenic diabetes insipidus
  41.   Menke kinky hair syndrome
  42.   Orotic aciduria
  43.   Congenital lactic acidosis
  44.   Cystic fibrosis
  45.   Hypophosphatasia
  46.   Fucosidosis
  47.   Crigler-Najjar syndrome
  48. α_1-Antitrypsin deficiency
  49.   I-Cell disease (mucolipidosis II)
  50.   Albinism
  51.   Lesch-Nyhan syndrome

disorders causing neonatal disease will undoubtedly continue to be described. For general reference, however, this should serve as a useful guide.

Table VII includes a summary of the major clinical findings seen in neonates with the inborn errors of metabolism and the disorders with which they have been associated. Table VIII serves as a guideline for abnormal laboratory findings seen in these disorders.

Failure to Thrive, Lethargy, and Poor Feeding. As mentioned previously, these findings may be associated with essentially all the inborn errors of metabolism presenting in the neonatal period and indeed may be seen in any sick infant, regardless of the nature of the illness. Certainly sepsis and asphyxia, among others, are more common causes of such problems. In the absence of evidence of any of these and particularly when other

Table VII. Major Clinical Manifestations of the Inborn Errors of Metabolism in the Neonatal Period

Clinical Finding	Associated Disorders (numbers refer to those listed in Table VI)
1. Failure to thrive, poor feeding	Essentially all
2. Lethargy	8,9,15–24,28,32–34,41,43
3. Vomiting	1–4,10,15–22,25,27,31–34,37–41,51
4. Diarrhea	1,10,27,30,44
5. Jaundice	1,2,7,10,11,15,47,48
6. Hypotonicity or hypertonicity	1,3–5,8,9,15–20,24,26,31–33,36, 41,43,46,51
7. Seizures	1,2,4,6,9,15–20,22–24,26,32,33,37–41, 43,45
8. Hepatomegaly	1–14,16,18,27,28,31,32,37,46,48,49
9. Dehydration	15–19,33,37,40
10. Coarse facial features	8,9,12–14,49
11. Abnormal urinary odor	20,25–28,34–36
12. Abnormal hair	18,25,29,41,50
13. Respiratory distress	5,9,16,18,43
14. Gingival hyperplasia	8,9,49
15. Macroglossia	5,8,9

supportive clinical or laboratory features are present, metabolic disease must be considered. It is important to recognize that many infants with metabolic disorders may be debilitated, and it is not uncommon for them to have, in fact, sepsis also.

Vomiting. Persistent vomiting is a distinctly unusual finding in the neonate and usually signals significant underlying disease. It is a prominent feature of a number of the inborn errors of metabolism, particularly those associated with protein intolerance. In virtually every instance, the vomiting associated with inherited metabolic disorders begins only after feedings have been instituted. In the infant who begins vomiting after

Table VIII. Laboratory Findings Associated with the Inborn Errors of Metabolism in the Neonatal Period

Laboratory Finding	Associated Disorders (numbers refer to those listed in Table VI)
1. Metabolic acidosis	2–4,6,15,32–35,39,43
2. Hypoglycemia	2–4,6,20,27,28,32,38,43,48
3. Reducing substances in the urine	1,2,27
4. Ferric chloride test (Phenistix) positive on urine	20,25–27
5. Hyperammonemia	15–19,22
6. Neutropenia	15,27,32–35,42
7. Thrombocytopenia	27,32–36
8. Vacuolated lymphocytes on peripheral smear	4,8,10–13,46

this time and in whom no evidence of a gastrointestinal anomaly is found, these disorders must be strongly considered.

Neonatal vomiting has been described in phenylketonuria, a disorder whose other major clinical manifestations, severe mental retardation and seizures, do not become obvious until later in infancy. Although some retrospective studies of infants with phenylketonuria have revealed that neonatal vomiting occurs in approximately 50 percent, it is probably significantly less common than this figure would indicate. In most states, screening of newborn infants for phenylketonuria is routinely performed by measurements of blood phenylalanine levels in a central laboratory. If the diagnosis is suspected, however, it can be substantiated before these results are available by the immediate quantitation of urine and blood phenylalanine or occasionally by a positive ferric chloride test on the urine or a positive dipstick for phenylketones (Phenistix, Ames Co.). It is important to note that elevated blood phenylalanine can be documented before phenylketones are present in the urine and that an infant must be taking protein feedings for at least 24 hr or more before any biochemical abnormality can be documented.

Perhaps the group of disorders most notably associated with persistent vomiting is the group of urea cycle defects, those disorders characterized by hyperammonemia secondary to a deficiency of one of the five enzymes of the urea cycle, the major known pathway for ammonia detoxification in man. Affected infants exhibit marked protein intolerance characterized clinically by postprandial vomiting, lethargy, and occasional changes in muscle tone. The obvious diagnostic clue here is the plasma ammonia level, most reliably elevated following a protein feeding. Infants on intravenous fluids only, often necessitated by their poor condition, may or may not show the expected elevation of ammonia.

A number of other metabolic disorders may be associated with protein intolerance and recurrent vomiting. Among the most prominent are the disorders of organic acid metabolism, including methylmalonic acidemia, propionic acidemia, and isovaleric acidemia. A major feature of these disorders is a profound metabolic acidosis, easily demonstrable by arterial or capillary blood gases. Neutropenia and thrombocytopenia may also be noted.

When a metabolic disorder associated with protein intolerance is suspected, it is essential that protein feedings be immediately discontinued. Samples should be obtained immediately for blood ammonia and blood gases, as mentioned previously, and for blood and urine amino acids. Infants with these disorders frequently die in the neonatal period if treatment is not rapidly instituted. In selected cases, vigorous attempts to reverse the hyperammonemia or acidosis by exchange transfusion or peritoneal dialysis may be indicated.

Other metabolic disorders associated with neonatal vomiting are listed in Table VII.

Diarrhea. Diarrhea is described in relatively few of the inborn errors of metabolism in contrast to vomiting, which is seen in so many. Notable exceptions to this are galactosemia, certain cases of cystic fibrosis, and less familiar disorders such as intestinal disaccharide deficiency, Wolman disease (acid lipase deficiency), and tyrosinemia.

Jaundice. Neonatal jaundice that is unusual or prolonged and not explained by hemolytic disease, congenital infection, or other obvious etiologic factors might be related to the presence of an inborn error of metabolism.

For most of the inborn errors of metabolism associated with jaundice, the elevated serum bilirubin is of the direct-reacting type, speaking for liver disease rather than hemolysis. This generalization, of course, does not include those inborn errors of red blood cell metabolism such as glucose-6-phosphate dehydrogenase deficiency or pyruvate kinase deficiency which are occasionally responsible for hemolytic disease in the newborn. The best-known metabolic disease associated with jaundice is galactosemia, in which the deficiency of the enzyme galactose-1-phosphate uridyl transferase results in an accumulation of galactose-1-phosphate and other metabolites such as galactitol that are thought to have a direct toxic effect on the liver and other organs. The jaundice in this disease is progressive and usually appears during the second week of life along with hepatomegaly, vomiting, diarrhea, poor weight gain, and cataract formation, provided the infant is receiving a galactose-containing formula. When galactosemia is suspected, the urine should be tested simultaneously with Benedict's reagent (Clinitest tablets, Ames Co.) and with a glucose oxidase method (Clinistix, Ames Co.). The glucose oxidase method is specific for glucose, whereas Benedict's reagent detects any reducing substance, so that a negative dipstick for glucose with a positive Benedict's reaction means that a nonglucose reducing substance is present. With appropriate clinical findings, this is most likely to be galactose. Paper chromatography can be used to identify the reducing substance positively. Similar to the situation with disorders of protein intolerance, the urine may be negative if the child is not receiving galactose in the diet.

If the diagnosis of galactosemia is suspected, whether or not reducing substances are present in the urine, galactose feedings should immediately be replaced by lactose-free feedings, pending the results of appropriate enzyme assays on red blood cells to confirm the diagnosis. Untreated galactosemics, if they survive the neonatal period, will have persistent liver disease, cataracts, and severe mental retardation. Treatment of this disorder by simple dietary restriction of galactose results in complete reversal of essentially all the physical manifestations and enables affected individuals to develop normal or near normal intelligence.

Another inborn error of metabolism that occasionally presents in the newborn period with jaundice, hepatomegaly, and the presence of reducing substances in the urine is hereditary fructose intolerance, which is also characterized by episodes of profound hypoglycemia, vomiting, and metabolic acidosis. This disorder is uncommonly seen in the neonate, however, because most newborns are not immediately exposed to a fructose-containing diet. In the uncommon event that an infant who has been receiving fructose should present with these findings, this diagnosis should be considered. Once again, analysis of the urine reveals the presence of a nonglucose reducing substance that on paper chromatography can be demonstrated to be fructose. Treatment of this disorder is by dietary restriction of fructose and results in a complete resolution of all clinical signs and symptoms. Confirmation of the diagnosis is by assay of the deficient enzyme, fructose-1-phosphate aldolase, in liver tissue.

An additional disorder that may be associated with neonatal jaundice is α_1-antitrypsin deficiency, a puzzling disorder that has recently been diagnosed in a number of individuals with neonatal hepatitis and cirrhosis. The clinical manifestations of this disorder may be identical with those of traditional neonatal or "giant-cell" hepatitis, and a determination of serum α_1-antitrypsin or a serum protein electrophoresis should be a part of the initial evaluation of all children presenting with this syndrome. α_1-

Antitrypsin is the major component of the α_1 fraction of serum globulins, so that this diagnosis is virtually ruled out by a normal electrophoretic pattern of serum proteins.

In contrast to the disorders previously mentioned in which there is an elevation of the direct-reacting bilirubin, a persistent elevation of indirect bilirubin beyond the limits of physiologic jaundice, without evidence of hemolysis, is suggestive of the diagnosis of the Crigler-Najjar syndrome. The hyperbilirubinemia in this disorder is related to a partial or complete deficiency of glucuronyl transferase, the liver enzyme responsible for the normal conjugation of bilirubin to bilirubin diglucuronide. There is no effective long-term therapy for some patients with this disorder, but the standard modalities of phototherapy and exchange transfusion may be of value in preventing the development of kernicterus in the neonatal period. Individuals with a partial deficiency of the enzyme may respond to phenobarbital therapy.

Hypotonicity or Hypertonicity. The nonspecific findings of hypotonicity or hyper-tonicity may be seen in a great variety of the inborn errors of metabolism, as seen in Table VII, as well as in sepsis, central nervous system disorders, Down syndrome, and other diseases. As an isolated finding, it is difficult to know how much significance to attach to either of these conditions. Once again, the overall clinical picture must be evaluated.

Seizures. Seizures are a very common and important manifestation of many inborn errors of metabolism in the neonatal period. Although seizures may be secondary to perinatal asphyxia, hypoxia, central nervous system anomalies, or hemorrhage, menin-gitis, or a variety of other causes, their occurrence should always alert the physician to the possibility of a metabolic derangement. A number of excellent reviews have been published on the subject of neonatal seizures, and, in most centers, the initial evaluation of a seizure disorder now routinely includes determination of serum glucose, calcium, and electrolytes. Hypoglycemia, hypocalcemia, or electrolyte imbalance may certainly occur as an isolated finding in otherwise normal newborns, especially in premature infants, but when the disturbance is not readily correctable, there are complicating fac-tors, or the etiology is not immediately apparent, the underlying cause of the disturb-ance must be investigated.

The salt-losing form of the adrenogenital syndrome leads to progressive salt wasting and potassium conservation with the development of hyponatremia and hyperkalemia, classically at the end of the first week of life. If unrecognized and untreated, infants with this disorder often die as a result of the profound fluid and electrolyte disturbances. In female infants one is usually aided in making this diagnosis by the presence of virilized external genitalia, and, of course, the adrenogenital syndrome is high on the list in the differential diagnosis of the infant with ambiguous genitalia and a positive buccal smear. In male infants, the genitalia are usually normal; so one is without this early diagnostic clue. Because of the difficulty in making the diagnosis in males and the substantial rate of death in unrecognized cases, it was thought for many years that the disorder was more common in female infants than in males. This, of course, is not the case, since all of the well-known forms of the adrenogenital syndrome are inherited as autosomal recessive disorders, but during this time the statistics were biased because of the death of significant numbers of male infants with this disorder.

A number of the other inborn errors of metabolism are occasionally associated with the development of dehydration and subsequent electrolyte imbalance and may be related to seizures through this mechanism. An example of these disorders is nephrogenic diabetes insipidus, in which the primary problem is excessive urinary loss of free water.

Those inborn errors of metabolism associated with hypoglycemia may, of course, be associated with seizures on that basis. Among the best-known disorders in this category are the glycogen storage diseases of which types I (von Gierke disease or glucose-6-phosphatase deficiency) and III (limit dextrinosis or debrancher deficiency) are the most likely to be associated with manifestations in the neonatal period. The hypoglycemia in these disorders is related to the inability of the liver to release glucose from glycogen; so it is most profound during periods of fasting. In addition to hypoglycemia, hepatomegaly, hypotonia, and metabolic acidosis are prominent features of these disorders. It should be noted here that hypoglycemia is not a feature of glycogen storage disease type II (Pompe disease or α-1,4-glucosidase deficiency), since cytoplasmic glycogen metabolism and release is normal in this disorder, in which glycogen accumulates in lysosomes as a result of the deficiency of the lysosomal enzyme, α-1,4-glucosidase. The clinical manifestations of this well-described disorder include macroglossia, hypotonia, cardiomegaly with congestive failure, and hepatomegaly. Of these, the cardiomegaly is most striking, and congestive failure is the cause of death in most cases.

A disorder that presents clinically with findings virtually indistinguishable from the hepatic glycogen storage diseases, types I and III, is fructose-1,6-diphosphatase deficiency, a newly described disorder of gluconeogenesis. The basic immediate treatment of all these disorders is frequent feedings, and the definitive diagnosis is made by liver biopsy and assay of appropriate hepatic enzymes.

Other disorders that may be associated with hypoglycemia and seizures include hereditary fructose intolerance, discussed previously, maple syrup urine disease, congenital lactic acidosis, and lysosomal acid phosphatase deficiency. Of these maple syrup urine disease, although rare, is perhaps the best described and is associated with a fulminating course of poor feeding, hypertonicity, and seizures, often leading to death in the neonatal period. This disorder is related to a deficiency of the enzyme, branched-chain ketoacid decarboxylase, and results in an accumulation of the branched-chain amino acids valine, leucine, and isoleucine and their derivatives, the branched-chain ketoacids, in plasma and urine. The hypoglycemia observed in this disease is thought to be related to the very high levels of leucine observed, which are known to provoke hypoglycemia even in normal individuals. The presence of the ketoacids in the urine results in a positive ferric chloride reaction, and a positive reaction with Phenistix, that is distinguishable from that seen in phenylketonuria on the basis of the color change observed. Treatment of maple syrup urine disease by dietary restriction of the branched-chain amino acids has been attempted in a number of cases with variable success.

Hypercalcemia, although not usually associated with seizures, is occasionally seen in infants with hypophosphatasia and may be accompanied by vomiting. Seizures do occasionally occur in infants with this disease as a result of increased intracranial pressure resulting from abnormalities of the skull.

Many other inborn errors of metabolism may be associated with neonatal seizures without abnormalities of serum glucose or electrolytes. When the etiology of the seizure disorder is unknown, these should always be considered. A determination of urine amino acids is a valuable part of the evaluation of neonatal seizures and should be performed in these cases. In addition, as mentioned previously, a number of these disorders are associated with a positive ferric chloride reaction in the urine, and since this test is one that is readily available to any physician, it is worthwhile in the immediate evaluation of such infants.

Hepatomegaly. Most of the inborn errors of metabolism associated with hepatomegaly in the neonatal period have already been mentioned in the discussions of jaundice and seizures. Those disorders associated with hepatomegaly fall into two general categories, the storage diseases on the one hand and those disorders associated with liver damage or cirrhosis on the other. Many of the well-known lipid storage diseases such as Gaucher disease do not typically present in the neonatal period. Among those which may be associated with hepatomegaly in the neonatal period, however, are GM_1 gangliosidosis, type I (generalized gangliosidosis), and Wolman disease, both of which are also associated with splenomegaly. The glycogen storage diseases that are associated with hepatomegaly in the newborn have previously been discussed and are listed in Table VII. Among the mucopolysaccharidoses, the only ones in which abnormalities such as hepatomegaly have been reported in the neonatal period are types I and II, the Hurler and Hunter syndromes. Even in these disorders, however, it is unusual to observe clinical abnormalities in the first month of life. Indeed, newborns who appear to have the typical features of these syndromes such as coarse facial features, hepatosplenomegaly, skeletal abnormalities, and hernias are more likely to have GM_1 gangliosidosis. β-Glucuronidase deficiency, which is probably appropriately classified as a mucopolysaccharidosis, may present in the neonatal period with features virtually indistinguishable clinically from those of the Hurler and Hunter syndromes. I-Cell disease or mucolipidosis type II also occasionally presents in the newborn period. A single infant with GM_3 gangliosidosis and a similar clinical presentation has also been reported.

When one of these disorders is suspected, a simple urine spot test for mucopolysaccharides may be performed. It will be positive in the Hurler and Hunter syndromes, slightly positive in GM_1 gangliosidosis and β-glucuronidase deficiency, and negative in I-cell disease. It should be noted that false positives on the spot test are not uncommon in neonates. The definitive diagnosis of these disorders of lipid or mucopolysaccharide metabolism is made by skin biopsy and appropriate biochemical studies on the cultivated fibroblasts.

Among the inborn errors of metabolism associated with actual liver disease and hepatomegaly on that basis are α_1-antitrypsin deficiency, galactosemia, hereditary fructose intolerance, and fructose-1,6-diphosphatase deficiency. Tyrosinemia is typically characterized by cirrhosis with hepatomegaly, vomiting, diarrhea, rickets, and failure to thrive. Other disorders in which hepatomegaly has been reported but is poorly understood include: methylmalonic acidemia, lysosomal acid phosphatase deficiency, and two of the urea cycle defects, ornithine transcarbamylase deficiency and argininosuccinic aciduria.

Dehydration. Already mentioned briefly in the section on seizures with electrolyte imbalance, those disorders which may be associated with dehydration in the neonatal period include nephrogenic diabetes insipidus, the adrenogenital syndrome, and the urea cycle defects.

Coarse Facial Features. Coarse facial features, a classical finding in older infants with mucopolysaccharidoses and certain lipid storage diseases, are observed occasionally in neonates with GM_1 gangliosidosis, the Hurley and Hunter syndromes, β-glucuronidase deficiency, I-cell disease, and GM_3 gangliosidosis.

Abnormal Urinary Odor. Abnormal urinary odor, most likely to be noted by nurses or mothers rather than physicians, is an important but often overlooked clue to the diagnosis of several of the inborn errors of metabolism and indeed may be the most specific clinical finding in such patients. This is best described for phenylketonuria for which the urine was noted to have a peculiar musty odor years before the biochemical basis of the disease was understood. In maple syrup urine disease, the urine has a distinctive sweet odor reminiscent of maple syrup or burnt sugar. Several of the less well-known inborn errors of metabolism are also associated with an abnormal urinary odor.

It is advisable for the clinician who suspects a metabolic disorder and intends to test the urine with ferric chloride or for reducing substances to take a moment to actually smell the urine himself. Here again, simple clinical tests are frequently the most rewarding.

Abnormal Hair. Abnormal hair, although frequently difficult to evaluate in the newborn, may be a clue to the diagnosis of argininosuccinic aciduria and Menke kinky hair syndrome.

Respiratory Distress. Respiratory distress without other obvious etiology such as hyaline membrane disease, pneumothorax, or pneumonia has been described in several of the urea cycle defects. Tachypnea, of course, may be a manifestation of the response to metabolic acidosis seen in glycogen storage disease, fructose-1,6-diphosphatase deficiency, organic acidemias, congenital lactic acidosis, and others.

Gingival Hyperplasia. This unusual clinical finding has occasionally been reported in newborn infants with GM_1 gangliosidosis, I-cell disease, and GM_3 gangliosidosis.

Macroglossia. Macroglossia is a typical finding in Pompe disease (glycogen storage disease, type II) as previously described. It has also been described in neonates with GM_1 and GM_3 gangliosidosis.

NEWBORN SCREENING FOR GENETIC DISORDERS

The emphasis on preventive medicine of recent years has led to a great deal of interest in screening for disease. Many of the screening programs developed have quite reasonably focused on the newborn, and most have related to the detection of familial metabolic disorders. The success of the phenylketonuria screening programs has provided great impetus to the movement to expand the realm of the screening process. At the same time, there is growing concern in the medical community and in society about the implications of widespread screening programs. In response to this concern, the National Academy of Sciences and the American Academy of Pediatrics have recently established guidelines for the formulation of genetic screening programs.

The major objective of any newborn screening program is presumably to identify individuals with unrecognized disease by the application of simple, rapidly accomplished procedures. The goals of such an undertaking may include one or more of the following:

1. To provide opportunities for medical intervention to prevent or minimize the effect of the disorder in question
2. To provide opportunities for genetic counseling to family members
3. To collect basic knowledge regarding the incidence and natural history of the disease and to allow identification of cases for early experimental therapy

Screening programs established for research purposes must be clearly distinguished from those in which a direct benefit may be derived by the screened individual or his family. Informed consent is important in all screening endeavors but, in the latter circumstance, is critical.

Before any proposed screening program is adopted on a large-scale basis, a number of important criteria must be met. Briefly, these include the following:

1. The disorder in question must be reasonably common so that a reasonable return can be expected from the investment of time, money, and facilities required by the screening endeavor. In other words, the cost/benefit ratio must be acceptable.
2. The screening method should be relatively simple, adaptable to widespread use, and reasonably inexpensive. It should be highly accurate, so that few false negative results occur. The degree of specificity of screening tests is somewhat variable, but the false positive rate should also be acceptable.
3. Except in special research programs, the benefits to the screened individual or his family must be clearly defined. This implies that the disorder should be one with some clinical significance. The detection of an asymptomatic biochemical disorder with no prognostic significance is of little relevance.
4. Adequate follow-up and treatment facilities should be available to ensure confirmation of diagnosis, good patient care, and family counseling. The regionalization of treatment centers may be the optimal way of achieving this goal.

The phenylketonuria screening programs currently underway in this country serve as a prototype for neonatal screening programs and illustrate the basic principles of such an undertaking. Although originally instituted before the effectiveness of treatment was thoroughly established, these screening programs have proved to be remarkably effective. Phenylketonuria is a common biochemical disorder, occurring with an incidence of about 1 in 15,000 live births. At one time, individuals with phenylketonuria were uniformly severely retarded and comprised about 1 percent of the severely retarded institutionalized population. When affected individuals are detected in the neonatal period and dietary therapy is initiated, ultimate intellectual development is essentially normal. The screening procedures used in this disorder are simple and reasonably inexpensive. A drop of blood from a heelstick is spotted on filter paper, and the blood phenylalanine is subsequently measured, usually in a central laboratory, When an elevated level is detected, the patient is referred to a regional treatment center for confirmation of the diagnosis and institution of therapy.

Despite the fact that phenylketonuria provides a prototype for metabolic screening, problems still exist in this disorder. It has been estimated that at least 5 percent of affected individuals may be missed by the screening procedures in operation in this country. Infants with phenylketonuria are born with normal blood phenylalanine levels and must be exposed to protein feedings for a certain period of time before elevated levels can be documented. The exact length of time required is dependent on the sex, protein intake, and a number of other factors. The current policy of early hospital discharge forces many infants to be screened at an earlier than optimal time. An additional problem in this country is the not infrequent delay in the institution of therapy for affected infants.

Perhaps the most dramatic extension of newborn screening is that currently in operation in Massachusetts. The Massachusetts Metabolic Disorders Screening Program, first initiated in 1968, includes screening for virtually all disorders of amino acid and organic acid metabolism, galactosemia, and a number of other disorders. The information derived from this widespread screening program has added to our knowledge of the incidence and natural history of a number of disorders and has provided a unique opportunity to initiate early experimental therapy for a number of others. For these purposes, this type of extensive screening program is certainly valuable, although it is by no means applicable to widespread use at the present time. At this point, it can be thought of as a useful information-gathering device that may provide us with data applicable to the rational development of widespread screening programs.

Of the specific disorders for which screening procedures are now being developed and tested, congenital hypothyroidism may be among the most promising. Estimates of the frequency of this disorder place the incidence at about 1 in 4000 live births, indicating that it is a relatively common disorder. Since affected infants often appear normal at birth, diagnosis may be delayed for as long as several months. Normal intellectual development is dependent on the early institution of thyroid replacement therapy. By the time overt clinical signs are apparent, irreparable brain damage may already have occurred. Relatively simple methods for screening newborn infants with blood T_4 or TSH determinations have now been developed and applied in selected populations. When the most effective screening method has been determined and subjected to adequate clinical trials, congenital hypothyroidism may well prove to be a disorder amenable to widespread screening and early therapeutic intervention.

Cystic fibrosis is an example of another disorder for which widespread screening has been extensively discussed in recent years. This is the most common fatal genetic disorder among Caucasians, occurring with an incidence of about 1 in 2000 live births. A simple dipstick for the detection of albumin in meconium has recently been developed that theoretically detects 85 percent of infants with this disorder. Infants with cystic fibrosis who do not have pancreatic insufficiency would be missed by this method. Proponents of this screening test have suggested that its use be extended to include all newborns. At the present time, this appears to be unjustified for a number of basic reasons. The first and most significant argument against mass screening for this disorder is that there is no really effective therapy for cystic fibrosis at the present time. There is no doubt that symptomatic treatment, including chest physiotherapy, antibiotics, and pancreatic enzyme replacement therapy, has prolonged the life of many individuals with this disorder. There is no evidence, however, to suggest that any additional benefit is derived from the initiation of therapy before symptoms occur. An additional argument against mass screening with the meconium dipstick is that the false positive rate is quite high. Infants with positive screening tests require follow-up sweat testing, and facilities are not currently available for such a massive undertaking.

Proponents of the meconium test have argued that the identification of affected infants may provide the parents with information that is useful in subsequent family planning. There is some merit to this argument, since multiple siblings with cystic fibrosis are often born before the diagnosis is made. Before this is used as a rationale for screening, however, adequate facilities for genetic counseling and family follow-up must be firmly established.

PRENATAL DIAGNOSIS OF GENETIC DISORDERS

One of the great contributions to the field of perinatal medicine in recent years has been the development of safe and accurate methods for the prenatal diagnosis of genetic disorders. The initial attempts at early intrauterine diagnosis were directed toward the determination of fetal sex in pregnancies at risk for X-linked recessive disorders and later toward the detection of chromosomal abnormalities in cultivated amniotic fluid cells. Subsequently, methods were developed for the biochemical diagnosis of a number of inborn errors of metabolism in utero. Exciting recent developments have opened the door to the diagnosis of a number of severe congenital malformations and of the hemoglobinopathies. There is little doubt that currently available methods will be refined and new methods developed to enable us to diagnose significantly more disorders antenatally. Since this subject has been extensively reviewed in numerous texts and scientific journals during the past few years, only an overview is presented below.

The disorders that can now be accurately detected prenatally are listed in Table IX. A number of other disorders, not included, may be diagnosable under certain circumstances. Therefore, attempts at prenatal diagnosis are not necessarily limited to those disorders listed.

The rationale for prenatal diagnosis for most of these disorders requires no explanation. Many of these disorders are associated with severe mental and physical disability and early death. Others are associated with severe mental retardation but do allow prolonged survival. For most of these, effective therapy is not available. The availability of prenatal diagnosis has greatly expanded the ability of the physician to help families at risk for having children with these disorders. Couples who were once afraid to attempt additional pregnancies can now be virtually assured of having normal children.

The major diagnostic tool used for prenatal diagnosis is amniocentesis, which is performed at about 16 weeks' gestation. Cells of fetal origin, suspended in amniotic fluid, can be cultivated and used for chromosome analysis or biochemical studies. Alternatively, the cell-free amniotic fluid can be used for a number of chemical determinations, including the measurement of α-fetoprotein levels, used in the prenatal diagnosis of neural tube defects.

A recent nationwide collaborative study has documented that the risk to the mother and fetus associated with midtrimester amniocentesis is really quite low. There does appear to be a low risk of spontaneous abortion following the procedure, but this probably occurs no more than 0.5 percent of the times the procedure is performed. Needle puncture marks have been observed in several newborn infants following midtrimester amniocentesis, but significant trauma has not been observed in infants surviving to term. It has been suggested that Rh isoimmunization may occur as a result of placental puncture during amniocentesis, but as yet this has not been documented.

Table IX. Disorders Which Are Detectable in the Midtrimester of Pregnancy

Chromosomal abnormalities
    Essentially all significant cytogenetic disorders

Sex-linked recessive disorders, by fetal sex determination

Neural tube defects
    Anencephaly
    Myelomeningocele
    Encephalocele

Inborn errors of metabolism
    Disorders of lipid metabolism
        Cholesterol ester storage disease
        Fabry disease
        Familial hypercholesterolemia
        Farber disease
        Gaucher disease, infantile and adult types
        GM_1 gangliosidosis, types I and II
        GM_2 gangliosidosis, type I (Tay-Sachs disease)
        GM_2 gangliosidosis, type II (Sandhoff disease)
        GM_2 gangliosidosis, type III
        GM_3 gangliosidosis
        Krabbe disease
        Metachromatic leukodystrophy
        Niemann-Pick disease, types A, B, and C
        Refsum disease
        Wolman disease

    Disorders of carbohydrate metabolism
        Fucosidosis
        Galactokinase deficiency
        Galactosemia
        Glucose-6-phosphate dehydrogenase deficiency
        Glycogen storage disease, types II, III, IV, VI, and IX
        Mannosidosis
        Pyruvate decarboxylase deficiency
        Pyruvate dehydrogenase deficiency

    Disorders of mucopolysaccharide (MPS) metabolism
        Hurler syndrome (MPS I)
        Scheie syndrome (MPS I)
        Hunter syndrome (MPS II A and B)
        Sanfilippo syndrome (MPS III A and B)
        Morquio syndrome (MPS IV)
        Maroteaux-Lamy syndrome (MPS VI A and B)
        Beta-glucuronidase deficiency (MPS VII)

    Disorders of amino acid and organic acid metabolism
        Arginase deficiency
        Argininosuccinic aciduria
        Aspartylglucosaminuria
        Citrullinemia
        Cystathioninuria
        Dihydropteridine reductase deficiency (PKU variant)
        Histidinemia

Table IX. (Continued)

Homocystinuria (cystathionine synthetase deficiency)
Hypervalinemia
Isovaleric acidemia
Maple syrup urine disease, severe and intermittent types
Methylenetetrahydrofolate reductase deficiency
Methylmalonic acidemia
Propionic acidemia (ketotic hyperglycinemia)
Miscellaneous disorders
Adenosine deaminase deficiency
Congenital erythropoietic porphyria
Congenital nephrotic syndrome
Cystinosis
Hypophosphatasia
I-Cell disease
Lesch-Nyhan syndrome
Lysosomal acid phosphatase deficiency
Lysyl-protocollagen hydroxylase deficiency
Menke kinky hair syndrome
Orotic aciduria
Xeroderma pigmentosum
Hemoglobinopathies
Sickle cell anemia
Thalassemia

The majority of amniocenteses performed in the past for prenatal diagnosis were done for chromosome analysis of the amniotic fluid cells. Indications for such cytogenetic studies include advanced maternal age or the previous birth of a child with Down syndrome or another chromosomal abnormality.

Chromosome analysis for fetal sex determination is performed in pregnancies at risk for X-linked recessive disorders. The magnitude of the risk in each of these situations is dependent on the individual circumstances and has been discussed elsewhere in this chapter. Cytogenetic studies of the amniotic fluid cells are at least 99 percent reliable in the detection of all major chromosomal abnormalities.

Amniocentesis for the detection of an inborn error of metabolism is usually performed only after the birth of one affected child. In unusual circumstances, carriers of a specific mutant gene, such as the gene for Tay-Sachs disease, may be identified in heterozygote screening programs before the birth of an affected child. In situations in which both parents are carriers, amniocentesis may be indicated.

Developments in the past several years have made amniocentesis a valuable tool in the prenatal diagnosis of neural tube defects, including anencephaly and myelomeningocele. Significant open neural tube defects are now detectable with 90 to 95 percent accuracy, using a combination of α-fetoprotein determination on the amniotic fluid and diagnostic ultrasound. Maternal serum α-fetoprotein levels are currently being studied as a potential tool for screening all pregnancies for neural tube defects.

In addition to its use in the detection of neural tube defects, ultrasound is of value when performed prior to any diagnostic amniocentesis for a number of reasons.

Measurements of biparietal diameter provide an accurate means of assessing gestational age in the midtrimester. Placental localization is also readily achieved. An important role of ultrasound is in the identification of twin pregnancies prior to amniocentesis, although multiple pregnancies may be missed even when this tool is used. When a twin pregnancy is suspected, the first amniocentesis may be followed by the injection of a water-soluble dye. If clear fluid is obtained on a second amniocentesis, it is assumed that the second amniotic sac has been entered. More sophisticated techniques of ultrasound using specialized equipment are currently being developed that may provide a means of diagnosing other structural anomalies in the fetus, including polycystic kidneys, omphalocele, hydrocephalus, and others.

In the past several years, a number of centers have been involved in the development of the fetoscope, an instrument that provides a means of direct visualization of the fetus and the placental blood vessels. With this instrument, small samples of fetal blood have been obtained from these placental vessels and used in the prenatal diagnosis of certain hemoglobinopathies, including sickle cell anemia and β-thalassemia. Direct placental aspiration has also been used for this purpose. Further refinements of these techniques will be necessary to minimize the associated risk and to make them available for more widespread application. Fetoscopy may one day also be of value in the diagnosis of specific structural anomalies in the fetus for which no cytogenetic or biochemical markers are available.

Fetal radiographs, obtained late in the second trimester of pregnancy, have been of value in selected cases for the diagnosis of specific disorders of the skeletal system. Such an approach may be applicable to the diagnosis of many of the chondrodystrophies, particularly those associated with severe manifestations in the neonate. It may also be applicable to the diagnosis of disorders associated with radial aplasia, such as Fanconi anemia, the thrombocytopenia-absent radius (TAR) syndrome, and others. Again, this approach is largely experimental, and the risk associated with fetal radiation exposure is as yet unknown.

Regardless of the approach used, it is essential that all intrauterine diagnosis be confirmed by appropriate studies on the fetus or the newborn infant. Only in this way can the procedures used be improved and expanded.

In summary, the generally accepted indications for midtrimester prenatal diagnosis now include the following:

1. Maternal age greater than 35 years
2. Previous birth of a child with trisomic Down syndrome or another chromosomal abnormality
3. Balanced chromosomal translocation in either parent, usually detected after the birth of a child with a chromosomal abnormality or through family studies
4. Mother a known or suspected carrier of an X-linked recessive disorder, identified by family history or carrier detection methods
5. Family history of a neural tube defect, i.e., previous child, either parent, or, at times, another family member
6. Previous birth of a child with an inborn error of metabolism known to be detectable in utero
7. Both parents identified as carriers of a disorder detectable in utero, i.e., Tay-Sachs disease

BIBLIOGRAPHY

Patterns of Inheritance in Man: Single Gene Defects

McKusick, V. A.: *Mendelian Inheritance in Man*. The Johns Hopkins Press, Baltimore, 1971.

Nora, J. J., and Fraser, F. C.: *Medical Genetics: Principles and Practice*. Lea & Febiger, Philadelphia, 1974.

Genetic Disorders and Fertility

Hammerton, J. L.: *Human Cytogenetics*. Academic Press, London, Vol. 2, 1971.

Dewhurst, C. J.: Sex chromosome abnormalities and the gynaecologist, *J. Obstet. Gynaecol. Brit. Commonwlth.* 78:1058–1076, 1971.

Taussig, L. M., Lobeck, C. C., di Sant'Agnese, P. A., Ackerman, D. R., and Kattwinkel, J.: Fertility in males with cystic fibrosis. *N. Engl. J. Med.* 287:586–589, 1972.

Reame, N. E., and Hafez, E. S. E.: Hereditary defects affecting fertility. *N. Engl. J. Med.* 292:675–681, 1975.

Genetic Disorders in the Mother and Their Impact on the Developing Fetus

Frankenburg, W. K., Duncan, B. R., Coffelt, R. W., Koch, R., Coldwell, J. G., and Son, C. D.: Maternal phenylketonuria: Implications for growth and development. *J. Pediat.* 73:560–570, 1968.

Perry, T. L., Hansen, S., Tischler, B., Richards, F. M., and Sokol, M.: Unrecognized adult phenylketonuria: Implications for obstetrics and psychiatry. *N. Engl. J. Med.* 289:395–398, 1973.

McKusick, V. A.: *Heritable Disorders of Connective Tissue*. C. V. Mosby Co., St. Louis, 1972.

The Problem of Recurrent Spontaneous Abortion and Its Implications for Genetic Counseling

Kim, H. J., Hsu, L. Y. F., Paciuc, S., Cristian, S., Quintana, A., and Hirschhorn, K.: Cytogenetics of fetal wastage. *N. Engl. J. Med.* 293:844–847, 1975.

Lucas, M., Wallace, I., and Hirschhorn, K.: Recurrent abortions and chromosome abnormalities. *J. Obstet. Gynaecol. Brit. Commonwlth.* 79:1119–1127, 1972.

Hsu, L. Y. F., Barcinski, M., Shapiro, L. R., Valderrama, E., Gertner, M., and Hirschhorn, K.: Parental chromosomal aberrations associated with multiple abortions and an abnormal infant. *Obstet. Gynecol.* 36:723–730, 1970.

Jacobson, C. B., and Barter, R. H.: Some cytogenetic aspects of habitual abortion. *Am. J. Obstet. Gynecol.* 97:666–680, 1967.

McConnell, H. D., and Carr, D. H.: Recent advances in the cytogenetic study of human spontaneous abortions. *Obstet. Gynecol.* 45:547–552, 1975.

Genetic Disorders Manifested in the Newborn: Chromosomal Abnormalities

Miller, O. J., and Breg, W. R.; Autosomal chromosome disorders and variations. *N. Engl. J. Med.* 294:596–598, 1976.

Gerald, P. S.: Sex chromosome disorders. *N. Engl. J. Med.* 294:706–708, 1976.

Day, R. W.; The epidemiology of chromosome aberrations. *Am. J. Human Genet.* 18:70–80, 1966.

Goad, W. B., Robinson, A., and Puck, T. T.: Incidence of aneuploidy in a human population. *Am. J. Human Genet.* 28:62–68, 1976.

Hamerton, J. L., Canning, N., Ray, M., and Smith, S.: A cytogenetic survey of 14,069 newborn infants: I. Incidence of chromosome abnormalities. *Clin. Genet.* 8:223–243, 1975.

Nielsen, J., and Sillesen, I.: Incidence of chromosome aberrations among 11,148 newborn children. *Humangenetik* 30:1–12, 1975.

Lewandowski, R. C., and Yunis, J. J.: New chromosomal syndromes. *Am. J. Dis. Child.* 129:515–529, 1975.

Genetic Disorders Manifested in the Newborn: Isolated Congenital Malformations

Smith, D. W.: *Recognizable Patterns of Human Malformation: Genetic, Embryologic, and Clinical Aspects.* W. B. Saunders Co., Philadelphia, 1970.

Warkany, J.: *Congenital Malformations.* Year Book Medical Publishers, Chicago, 1971.

Bergsma, D. (ed.): *Birth Defects Atlas and Compendium.* Williams and Wilkins Co., Baltimore, 1973.

Goodman, R. M., and Gorlin, R. J.: *The Face in Genetic Disorders.* C. V. Mosby Co., St. Louis, 1970.

Holmes, L. B.: Congenital malformations. *N. Engl. J. Med.* 295:204–207, 1976.

Fraser, F. C.: The genetics of cleft lip and cleft palate. *Am. J. Human Genet.* 22:336–352, 1970.

Nora, J. J., McGill, C. W., and McNamara, D. G.: Empiric recurrence risks in common and uncommon congenital heart lesions. *Teratology* 3:325–330, 1970.

Genetic Disorders Manifested in the Newborn: Inborn Errors of Metabolism

Stanbury, J. B., Wyngaarden, J. B., and Fredrickson, D. S. (eds.): *The Metabolic Basis of Inherited Disease.* McGraw-Hill Book Co., New York, 1972.

Nyhan, W. L. (ed.): *Heritable Disorders of Amino Acid Metabolism: Patterns of Clinical Expression and Genetic Variation.* John Wiley & Sons, New York, 1974.

O'Brien, D., and Goodman, S. I.: The critically ill child: Acute metabolic disease in infancy and early childhood. *Pediatrics* 46:620–626, 1970.

Frequency of inborn errors of metabolism, especially PKU, in some representative newborn screening centers around the world: A collaborative study. *Humangenetik* 30:273–286, 1975.

Newborn Screening for Genetic Disorders

The pediatrician and genetic screening, The Task Force on Genetic Screening of The American Academy of Pediatrics, 1976.

Genetic Screening: Programs, Principles, and Research. Committee for the Study of Inborn Errors of Metabolism, Division of Medical Science, Assembly of Life Sciences, NRC, Washington, D.C., National Academy of Sciences, 1975.

Komrower, G. M.: The philosophy and practice of screening for inherited diseases. *Pediatrics* 53:182–188, 1974.

Buist, N. R. M., and Jhaveri, B. M.: A guide to screening newborn infants for inborn errors of metabolism. *J. Pediat.* 82:511–522, 1973.

Levy, H. L., Madigan, P. M., and Shih, V. E.: Massachusetts Metabolic Disorders Screening Program: I. Technics and results of urine screening. *Pediatrics* 49:825–836, 1972.

Holtzman, N. A., Mellits, E. D., and Kallman, C. H.: Neonatal screening for phenylketonuria: II. Age dependence of initial phenylalanine in infants with PKU. *Pediatrics* 53:353–357, 1974.

Holtzman, N. A., Meek, A. G., Mellits, E. D., and Kallman, C. H.: Neonatal screening for phenylketonuria: III. Altered sex ratio; extent and possible causes. *J. Pediat.* 85:175–181, 1974.

Dontanville, V. K., and Cunningham, G. C.: Effect of feeding on screening for PKU in infants. *Pediatrics* 51:531–538, 1973.

Prenatal Diagnosis of Genetic Disorders

Nadler, H. L.: Prenatal detection of genetic defects, in I. Schulman (ed.): *Advances in Pediatrics.* Year Book Medical Publishers, Chicago, pp. 1–81, 1976.

Milunsky, A.: Prenatal diagnosis of genetic disorders. *N. Engl. J. Med.* 295:377–380, 1976.

Milunsky, A.: *The Prenatal Diagnosis of Hereditary Disorders.* Charles C Thomas, Springfield, 1973.

4

The Effects of Drugs on Uterine Contractility

Tom P. Barden, M.D.

In order to understand the actions of drugs on uterine activity, it is necessary to consider first the basic mechanisms of myometrial cell function and the mechanisms that control the onset of labor. Billions of myometrial cells combine to form the smooth muscle wall of the uterus. The contractile elements of myometrial cells are the intercellular myofibrils that contain the threadlike proteins, myosin and actin. During contractions, the two types of myofibrils slide on each other, and the protein threads combine. It is now well established that the actin-myosin interaction is calcium-sensitive. As early as 1909, Blair-Bell and Hick (1) reported that administration of calcium chloride to a pithed rabbit produced uterine contractions. Later, in 1939, Danforth and Ivy (2) reported increased uterine activity in dogs and rabbits after administration of calcium chloride. However, there has been no convincing evidence from human observations to indicate that blood calcium levels have a specific influence on uterine activity.

In a series of reports during recent years, Carsten has clarified the mechanism of action of certain oxytocic drugs, namely, oxytocin and prostaglandin (3–6). By working with tissue fractions largely derived from the sarcoplasmic reticulum, she demonstrated a release of calcium in the presence of prostaglandins E_2 and F_{2a}, or oxytocin. As illustrated in Figure 1, current evidence suggests that when relaxed, the cell functions in part by expending energy to pump calcium across the cell membrane or into intracellular storage areas that consist of mitochondria, sarcoplasmic reticulum, and cell membrane vesicles. During contraction, the cell permits calcium to enter from the storage sites or from the higher concentration of the extracellular space and then uses energy to contract.

In 1928, Bourne and Burn reported that the intravenous injection of epinephrine inhibited uterine contractions in humans (7). Twenty years later, in 1948, Ahlquist concluded that the action of sympathomimetic amines on smooth muscle is mediated through two sets of receptors, which he designated as "alpha" and "beta adrenergic receptors" (8). From this work it became evident that norepinephrine is the prototype of the alpha-receptor-active drugs, producing increased uterine activity, and isoproterenol is the prototype of the beta adrenergic drug, producing uterine relaxation. By 1960, the studies of Sutherland and his associates began to clarify the nature of the beta receptor

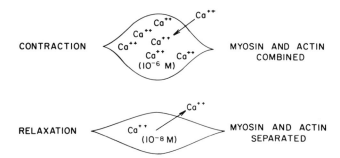

Figure 1. Calcium flux and calcium-sensitive actin-myosin interaction during contraction and relaxation of myometrial cells.

(9). First, messenger hormones, such as epinephrine, interact with the target cell membrane to release adenyl cyclase, which, as illustrated in Figure 2, catalyzes the intracellular metabolism of adenosine triphosphate to cyclic adenosine monophosphate, so-called cyclic AMP. Cyclic AMP in turn activates a class of enzymes, the protein kinases, that facilitate the transport of calcium to sequestration sites to facilitate relaxation of the cell. The nature of the alpha receptor is not well understood. Evidence suggests that it may function through the same basic mechanism as the beta receptor by enhancing the action of phosphodiesterase, the enzyme responsible for metabolism of cyclic AMP, or it may act through guanosine monophosphate, cyclic GMP, a counterpart nucleotide to cyclic AMP.

The action of drugs on myometrial cell function is logically extended to a consideration of the mechanism of labor onset. Maternal hypophyseal release of oxytocin has long been considered a primary element of this mechanism, for when administered in late pregnancy, it usually produces clinical labor. However, to date there has been no clear evidence that the onset of labor in humans is associated with a surge of oxytocin released by the maternal pituitary. Current evidence suggests that oxytocin is released in spurts, mainly in late labor. At delivery, levels of oxytocin are higher in fetal blood than in maternal blood (10,11). Also, there is evidence of fetal oxytocin release in meconium that may trigger labor and serve as an escape mechanism for the fetus exposed to intrauterine asphyxia (12).

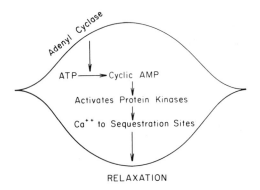

Figure 2. Intracellular events with beta-adrenergic receptor stimulation.

The relaxing influence of progesterone on the uterus has long been considered a plausible component of the control mechanism. Csapo introduced the concept that placental production of progesterone produces a local block of myometrial contractility that persists until shortly before the onset of labor (13). The hypothesis was supported when Kumar and associates found that the concentration of progesterone was higher in myometrium underlying the placenta than in that from other sites (14). Most human studies have failed to detect a measurable fall in blood levels of progesterone prior to the onset of labor. However, Turnbull and associates detected falling peripheral plasma progesterone levels, when measured serially, in a series of patients during late pregnancy (15). Schwarz and associates reported that levels of progesterone in human fetal membranes are significantly lower in those obtained after vaginal delivery than those obtained at cesarean section, prior to the onset of labor (16).

In agreement with the initial report of Siiteri and MacDonald (17), it is now well established that estrogen is produced during pregnancy by the placenta from fetal adrenal precursors. Caldeyro-Barcia and associates reported evidence that increasing levels of estrogen during pregnancy are responsible for increasing sensitivity of myometrium to oxytocin (18). Also, there is evidence from several animal species that alpha-adrenergic receptor responsiveness increases after administration of estrogen and beta-receptor sensitivity increases after progesterone (19). There is also evidence that estrogen and progesterone influence microsomal binding sites for calcium in myometrial cells (5,20). Although there is no clear relationship of maternal blood levels of estrogen to the onset of labor, Raja and associates (21) reported higher levels of plasma estradiol in patients who subsequently developed spontaneous premature labor than in patients who delivered at term. In contrast, Cousins and associates (22) found significantly lower levels of both serum progesterone and serum estradiol in a series of patients prior to premature labor than in controls of similar gestational age. However, they found no significant change in either progesterone or estradiol levels prior to normal-term labor.

The role of fetal cortisol in onset of labor was suggested from studies in sheep when Liggins and associates (23) observed prolongation of pregnancy following destruction of the fetal pituitary and Drost and Holm (24) found the same result after fetal adrenalectomy. Liggins (25) subsequently reported that injection of hypophysectomized fetal lambs with ACTH or adrenalectomized fetal lambs with cortisol or dexamethasone was followed by premature labor. Additional observations in sheep revealed an elevation of fetal cortisol starting about 10 days prior to labor, followed by a sudden rise in the level of estrogen and fall in the level of progesterone in uterine venous blood during the 24 hr prior to labor (26,27). Evidence suggests that cortisol induces a steroid 17α-hydroxylase in the placenta that serves to reduce progesterone and elevate estrogen production (28). In contrast to the results in sheep, Mueller-Heubach and associates (29) reported that fetal adrenalectomy in a series of rhesus monkeys had no significant influence on the timing of labor onset. Also in rhesus monkeys, Walsh and Novy (30) reported that fetal ACTH infusions resulted in significant increases of fetal and maternal plasma estrogen, principally estrone, increases of amniotic fluid prostaglandin E_1, but no changes of maternal plasma progesterone levels prior to onset of labor.

From observations in human pregnancy, there have been several reports of higher levels of cortisol in cord blood after spontaneous labor in contrast to labor induced by oxytocin or after delivery by cesarean section without labor (31–33). However, from other studies, the fetal cortisol levels were similar with and without previous labor

(34,35). The role of cortisol in the mechanism of labor onset in human pregnancy is further suggested by observations that intraamniotic injection of hydrocortisone in late pregnancy usually serves to induce labor (36,37) and that postmature infants have low plasma cortisol levels (38,39).

Prostaglandins are another likely component of the mechanism controlling onset of labor, as suggested by their oxytocic activity throughout pregnancy and their appearance in amniotic fluid and blood at the onset of labor (40–42). There is now considerable evidence that arachidonic acid, the obligatory precursor for prostaglandin, is stored in fetal membranes and uterine decidua in its esterified, inactive form as a glycerophospholipid. During pregnancy progesterone serves to stabilize lysosomal phospholipase A_2 and prevent the synthesis of prostaglandin. When progesterone production decreases, this enzyme is released from fetal membranes and decidua to catalyze the hydrolysis of phospholipids. The unesterified arachidonate that is then released serves as precursor of prostaglandin formation in the decidua (43–48). The oxytocic effects of prostaglandins are likely mediated through alterations of myometrial cell calcium flux. Carsten (3,4) observed that prostaglandin inhibits the ATP-dependent sequestration of calcium by sarcoplasmic reticulum, leading to an increase of intracellular free calcium.

Other evidence suggests the relationship of myometrial stretching and production of prostaglandin. Kloeck and Jung (49) reported that small quantities of prostaglandins E and F were released during spontaneous activity of myometrial strips in vitro; however, after subjecting the strips to stretching, there was an increase of prostaglandin E and a decrease of prostaglandin F. Thus, increasing uterine volume in late pregnancy may trigger production of prostaglandin, which in turn stimulates uterine contractions. Csapo and associates (50) reported that addition of only 150 ml of isotonic solution to the amniotic fluid of patients at term consistently produced increased uterine activity.

The onset of labor, as well as the action of many drugs on myometrium, is related to changes in uterine blood flow. Increased uterine activity is associated with clinical conditions that compromise effective uterine blood flow such as hypertensive vascular disease, toxemia, multiple pregnancy, and the supine position. Indeed, evidence suggests that labor begins when the nutritional needs of the uterus or fetus are no longer met. Brotanek, Hendricks, and Yoshida (51) reported evidence of decreased uterine blood flow after administration of oxytocin and preceding the increase of uterine activity. From a more recent study in nonpregnant ewes, Resnik and Brink (52) reported that prostaglandin E_1 is a potent uterine vasodilator, increasing uterine blood flow to maximal levels achieved by estradiol-17β, and that prostaglandin F_{2a} has marked vasopressor properties. Thus, prostaglandins may variously influence uterine blood flow.

Uterine activity tends to decrease when uterine blood flow is increased by bed rest or by vasodilation produced by beta adrenergic drugs or by ethanol. Brotanek and Hodr (53) presented evidence of increased uterine blood flow in women treated with infusions of isoxsuprine hydrochloride, a beta adrenergic agonist. However, from studies in ovine pregnancy, where uterine vessels are maximally dilated in late pregnancy, Ehrenkranz and associates (54,55) reported significant decreases of uterine blood flow during infusions of beta adrenergic drugs. The decline in uterine blood flow was noted to exceed the decline in maternal blood pressure, which suggests that the agents increase uterine vascular resistance. Thus, the relationship between some drugs and uterine blood flow may be quite complex and not entirely predictable.

To understand the effects of drugs on uterine contractility demands quantitation of uterine activity data. It may be expressed as simply average intensity, frequency, duration, and interval tonus. However, in this form the data may be very difficult to interpret in relationship to clinical events. One of the most widely used methods for quantitation was introduced in 1957, when Caldeyro-Barcia and associates (56) described the "Montevideo unit" as the product of the average intensity multiplied by the frequency of contractions in consecutive 10-min periods. Subsequently, the "Alexandria unit" was described as the product of intensity, frequency, and duration of contractions (57). By 1973 Hon and Paul (58) suggested that the integrated area under the pressure curve was the most inclusive measure of uterine activity. Other investigators have used sophisticated mathematical methodology to evaluate the characteristics of individual contractions (59,60) and the regularity of serial contractions (61,62). Several of these studies have revealed that spontaneous uterine activity is not so regular and individual contractions are not so abrupt in onset as that induced by oxytocic drugs (63). During labor there is a progressive increase of both frequency and intensity of contractions. Effer and associates (61) observed that the intrinsic pattern of irregularity of contractions persists despite the crescendo of activity. The term "uterine hypertonus" has been applied to many forms of uterine activity. Considering only the interval tonus, hypertonus has been variously defined as pressure exceeding 10, 12, 15, 20, or 25 mm Hg. Caldeyro-Barcia and Poseiro (64) considered contraction frequency of five or more in 10 min as a form of hypertonus. There have been few attempts to define the normal limits of contraction intensity and duration. On a basis of most of the proposed definitions, uterine hypertonus is often present to some degree in spontaneous labor. From a clinical perspective, inadequate uterine activity in labor is associated with failure of progress, and excessive uterine activity may be associated with evidence of fetal distress, maternal trauma, or fetal trauma. Even "normal" uterine activity may produce evidence of fetal distress if there is concomitant reduction of uterine blood flow, abnormal placental function, or preexisting fetal compromise. Thus, the inexact limits of normal uterine activity in labor, and the many variables that influence fetal response to labor, produce inherent difficulty in the evaluation of the effect of drugs on uterine activity.

Oxytocin is the foremost drug with oxytocic properties in clinical usage at present. It is well established that myometrial sensitivity to oxytocin increases throughout pregnancy and may be further enhanced by administration of estrogen or prostaglandin (65,66). At term, the effective dosage to induce labor is in the range of 0.5 to 10 milliunits per minute, intravenously. The uterine response to intravenous oxytocin requires approximately 20 min to stabilize. The uterine effects of oxytocin decreases rapidly after the infusion is discontinued (67,68). In contrast, when administered by intramuscular injection or absorption through nasal or oral mucosa, the uterine response is less predictable and persists for a considerable period of time after the last dose. The lack of control produced by these alternative routes places the fetus in considerable danger in the event of excessive stimulation. The complications of uterine hypertonus include not only fetal asphyxia but also the risk of premature separation of the placenta and uterine rupture. Several reports have indicated that the administration of oxytocin at doses as low as 40 milliunits per minute may produce antidiuresis (69–71). There are no apparent maternal or fetal cardiovascular effects from the dose of oxytocin necessary for induction of labor. From one study (72) there was evidence that the occurrence of mild hyperbilirubinemia of neonates is related to the total dose of oxytocin administered during labor.

The prostaglandins are a family of closely related lipids with oxytocic properties that are actively synthesized by the gravid uterus and its contents. As with oxytocin, there is increasing myometrial sensitivity to prostaglandins during pregnancy. From the evidence discussed above, the prostaglandins are strongly implicated in the mechanism of labor onset. The ability of prostaglandins to induce or enhance labor is the likely explanation for the practice of Eskimo women ingesting prostaglandin-rich fat from the paws of polar bears for promoting labor or the ingestion of seminal fluid by women of certain African tribes for the same purpose. The technique of intraamniotic injection of prostaglandin F_{2a} has become established as the method of choice for termination of pregnancy from about 14 to 22 weeks' gestation. Intravaginal prostaglandin E_2 is effective for termination of pregnancies complicated by missed abortion, hydatid mole, or fetal death. The use of prostaglandins for induction of labor in late pregnancy has remained somewhat controversial, for although it is clear that they have oxytocic properties comparable with synthetic oxytocin, uterine hypertonus has been observed somewhat more often during infusions of prostaglandins (73–76). Also, prostaglandins rather frequently produce annoying gastrointestinal side effects.

Ergot alkaloids are derived from a fungus that grows on rye and other grains. If consumed in significant quantities, ergot produces poisoning manifested by gangrene of extremities or convulsions. In obstetrics, ergot is universally condemned as an antepartum oxytocic agent, even in low doses, because of its propensity to produce uterine hypercontractility (77).

Sparteine sulfate is an alkaloid derived from plants of the lupine family. It enjoyed a brief popularity as an antepartum oxytocic agent in the United States starting in 1958 (78); however, there were soon numerous reports of its similarity to ergot in producing uterine hypertonus capable of damaging a living fetus (79–82). This drug is now considered unsafe for antepartum administration.

Other drugs with known oxytocic properties include norepinephrine (83), acetylcholine (84), and propranolol (85,86). These drugs, which act as neurotransmitters and adrenergic-receptor-active agents, lack the necessary specificity for myometrial activity to be clinically useful oxytocic agents.

Dimenhydrinate (Dramamine) is an antihistamine, closely related to diphenhydramine (Benadryl), which is widely used for prevention or treatment of motion sickness. Several studies have revealed a definite oxytocic action of this drug (87–89). Its effectiveness and safety have not been established for induction of labor.

The characteristics of drugs capable of inhibiting uterine activity are as heterogeneous as those of drugs having oxytocic activity. Among those of clinical interest, the largest group is the beta-adrenergic-receptor stimulators. These agents, described as betamimetics, are phenylethylamines that include epinephrine, isoproterenol, isoxsuprine, ritodrine, orciprenaline, salbutamol, terbualine, fenoterol, and buphrenine. As described earlier, they act via the beta adrenergic receptors on the myometrial cell, but they all have some effect on beta receptors of other structures. Also, they all have some effect on alpha receptors.

The nature of the beta-adrenergic mechanism, initially studied by Sutherland and associates (9), was further elucidated by Lands and associates (90), who described two populations of beta receptors. The $beta_1$ receptors are responsible for actions such as increase of heart rate and force of contraction, lipolysis, and relaxation of intestinal smooth muscle, and the $beta_2$ receptors mediate glycogenolysis and smooth muscle relaxation of arterioles, the bronchus, and the uterus. The clinical effects of beta mimetics are quite complex, for, in addition to uterine relaxation, they all produce an increase of maternal heart rate, plus some degree of peripheral vasodilation. The result is a variable effect on uteroplacental blood flow. In addition, beta mimetics tend to elevate maternal and fetal blood glucose levels and through their lipolytic effects produce fetal ketosis. Although it has not been discovered, the ideal beta mimetic for inhibition of uterine activity would stimulate only the beta$_2$ receptors of the myometrium.

Isoxsuprine hydrochloride has been the most widely used beta mimetic in the United States for inhibition of uterine activity. Unfortunately, up to 10% of patients who receive an intravenous infusion of isoxsuprine adequate to inhibit labor also develop significant hypotension, compromise of uterine blood flow, and evidence of fetal distress (91–93). Ritodrine hydrochloride was synthesized for its more specific uterine relaxing effects (94). From a collaborative study in Europe, it proved to be an effective inhibitor of premature labor with relatively few side effects (95). Ritodrine is currently undergoing clinical trials in the United States in order to achieve approval of the Food and Drug Administration.

Ethanol presumably inhibits uterine activity by blocking the release of oxytocin from the maternal or fetal pituitary. Investigative and clinical experience has established the efficacy and relative safety of intravenous ethanol for inhibition of premature labor (96–98). However, clinical acceptance is limited by the annoying side effects of nausea, vomiting, headache, restlessness, and diuretic effect. From animal studies there is evidence of decreased uterine blood flow and fetal asphyxia during intravenous infusions of ethanol (99–101). However, from the clinical experience with ethanol for inhibition of premature labor in human pregnancy, there is no evidence of adverse effects on the fetus or neonate.

Aspirin, indomethacin, and other nonsteroidal antiinflammatory drugs are capable of inhibiting uterine activity by interfering with the synthesis of prostaglandins. Among the agents that have been studied to data are aspirin, indomethacin, naproxen, ibuprofen, fenoprofen, mecloflenamic acid, flufenamic acid, and phenylbutazone. From several studies in various animals there was evidence that these drugs may produce a significant delay in the onset of labor (102–104). From Israel, Zuckerman and associates reported successful inhibition of premature labor in 40 out of 50 patients treated by large doses of indomethacin (105). Despite such promising results, further evidence has suggested potential danger from use of these drugs during pregnancy. There has been convincing evidence from observations in animals and humans that exposure to these drugs during pregnancy may trigger premature closure of the fetal ductus arteriosus (106–108). Thus, the clinical application of these drugs for prophylaxis or treatment of premature labor should be deferred pending the results of carefully designed and well-controlled studies.

Diazoxide, an antihypertensive benzothiadiazine, was developed as an antihypertensive but was also found to relax smooth muscle. Although it is capable of inhibiting human labor at term (109), concomitant vasodilatation and lowering of blood pressure limit the clinical application of diazoxide for inhibition of premature or otherwise unwanted labor.

Aminophyllin, a methylxanthine derivative, is capable of relaxing myometrium by inhibition of the metabolic degradation of intracellular cyclic adenosine-3′,5′-monophosphate. It is capable of decreasing uterine motility in nonpregnant human subjects (110), but it has not been evaluated in pregnancy.

Magnesium sulfate depresses uterine activity in human pregnancy when maternal serum magnesium levels reach 6 to 8 mEq per liter (111,112). From observations in sheep there was evidence that the infusion of magnesium sulfate produced slightly increased uteroplacental blood flow (113). Although controlled studies have not been reported, some clinicians recommend a continuous intravenous infusion of magnesium sulfate in management of premature labor.

The inhalation anesthetic agents, halothane and ether, are potent uterine relaxants. Most other gas anesthetics used in obstetrics have no effect on uterine activity.

The effects of certain other drugs on uterine activity are not always predictable. Although evidence suggests that myometrium becomes progressively more sensitive to oxytocin and prostaglandin during pregnancy through increased exposure to estrogen, there has been sparse evidence of a direct oxytocic action of estrogen. Pinto and associates reported an oxytocic effect of intravenous and intraamniotic administration of estradiol 17-β in late human pregnancy (114,115). No confirmatory studies have been reported to date. The administration of progesterone during pregnancy delays the onset of labor in several animal species. Bengtsson (116) reported that injection of medroxy-progesterone into the anterior wall of the uterus temporarily inhibited labor in 9 out of 10 patients in clinical premature labor; however, Brenner and Hendricks (117) found no evidence that medroxyprogesterone taken orally in late human pregnancy had any effect on the timing of labor onset. From other studies it may be generally concluded that the administration of large doses of progestogens in late human pregnancy may produce a partial suppression of uterine activity (118,119). Johnson and associates (120), from a series of patients at risk of premature labor, reported that weekly injections of 17α-hydroxyprogesterone caproate (Delalutin) successfully delayed onset of labor to term while many patients in a placebo group delivered prior to term.

The effect of local anesthetic agents on uterine activity is a confusing subject because of the multitude of variables that exist during labor and among the drugs. For example, the myometrial response to these drugs is influenced by the characteristics of the individual drugs, the addition of epinephrine to the agent, the dose and route of administration, and the patient's position, blood pressure, stage of labor, and endogenous catecholamines. From studies in pregnant ewes, Greiss and associates (122) reported decreased uteroplacental blood flow and increased uterine activity following the intravascular injection of a series of local anesthetic agents. Evidence suggested that the vascular effect was direct rather than mediated by adrenergic receptors. From several studies in human pregnancy at term, epidural administration of local anesthetic agents was observed to produce a slight decrease or no effect on uterine activity (123–125).

The administration of analgesic agents during labor has long been thought to reduce uterine activity modestly. However, several studies using quantitative techniques have revealed a significant increase of uterine activity following administration of meperidine (126–128).

In conclusion, the effect of drugs on uterine activity is mediated through complicated control mechanisms and affected by many clinical variables. Although certain of the drugs discussed above have relatively predictable effects on uterine contractility, there are many that are quite unpredictable. No drugs are known at present that act exclusively at the myometrial cell. The evaluation of drugs in pregnancy is further complicated by the frequent discrepancy between quantitatable uterine activity and the clinical progress of labor. In addition, the effect of drugs on uterine activity must be considered in relation to any direct or indirect effects of the agent on the fetus.

REFERENCES

1. Blair-Bell, W., and Hick, P.: Observations on the physiology of the female genital organs. *Br. Med. J.* 1:177, 1909.

2. Danforth, D. N., and Ivy, A. C.: The effect of calcium upon uterine contractions and upon uterine response to intravenously injected oxytocics. *Am. J. Obstet. Gynecol.* 37:194, 1939.

3. Carsten, M. E.: Prostaglandins and cellular calcium transport in the pregnant human uterus. *Am. J. Obstet. Gynecol.* 117:824, 1973.

4. Carsten, M. E.: Prostaglandins and oxytocin: Their effects on uterine smooth muscle. *Prostaglandins* 5:33, 1974.

5. Carsten, M. E.: Hormonal regulation of myometrial calcium transport. *Gynecol. Invest.* 5:269, 1974.

6. Carsten, M. E., and Miller, J. D.: Prostaglandins: Calcium ionophores? *Gynecol. Invest.* 8:54, 1977.

7. Bourne, A., and Burn, J. H.: The dosage and action of pituitary extract and of the ergot alkaloids on the uterus in labor, with a note on the action of adrenalin. *J. Obstet. Gynaecol. Brit. Emp.* 34:249, 1927.

8. Ahlquist, R. P.: A study of the adrenotropic receptors. *Am. J. Physiol.* 153:586, 1948.

9. Sutherland, E. W., and Rall, T. W.: The relation of adenosine-3',5'-phosphate and phosphorylase to the actions of catecholamines and other hormones. *Pharmacol. Rev.* 12:265, 1960.

10. Chard, T., Hudson, C. N., Edwards, C. R. W., and Boyd, N. R. H.: Release of oxytocin and vasopressin by the human foetus during labour. *Nature* 234:352, 1971.

11. Dawood, M. Y., Wang, C. F., Gupta, R., and Fuchs, F.: Fetal contribution of oxytocin in human parturition. *Gyncol. Invest.* 8:33, 1977.

12. Seppala, M., and Aho, I.: Physiological role of meconium during delivery. *Acta Obstet. Gynecol. Scand.* 54:209, 1975.

13. Csapo, A.: Defense mechanism of pregnancy, *Ciba Foundation Study Groups: Progesterone and the Defense Mechanism of Pregnancy.* Boston, Little Brown and Co., 1961.

14. Kumar, D., Goodno, J. A., and Barnes, A. C.: Isolation of progesterone from human pregnant myometrium. *Nature (Lond.)* 195:1204, 1962.

15. Turnbull, A. C., Patten, P. T., Flint, A. P. F., Jeremy, J. Y., Keirse, M. J. N. C., and Anderson, A. B. M.: Significant fall in progesterone and rise in oestradiol levels in human peripheral plasma before onset of labour. *Lancet* 1:101, 1974.

16. Schwarz, B. E., Heaton, C. L., Milewich, L., Athey, R., and MacDonald, P. C.: Progesterone deprivation in the chorioamnion from laboring women. *Gynecol. Invest.* 8:98, 1977.

17. Siiteri, P. K., and MacDonald, P. C.: Placental estrogen biosynthesis during human pregnancy. *J. Clin. Endocrin.* 26:751, 1966.

18. Caldeyro-Barcia, R., and Sereno, J. A.: The response of the human uterus to oxytocin throughout pregnancy, in *Oxytocin,* Caldeyro-Barcia, R., and Heller, H. (eds.). Pergamon, New York, 1961, p. 177.

19. Roberts, J. M., Insel, P. A., Goldfien, R., and Goldfien, A.: The effect of progesterone and/or estradiol on uterine contractility and β-adrenergic receptor number. *Gynecol. Inves.* 8:56, 1977.

20. Carsten, M. E.: How does calcium control uterine contraction? *Contemp. Ob. Gyn.* 8:61, 1976.

21. Raja, R. L., Anderson, A. B. M., and Turnbull, A. C.: Endocrine changes in premature labor. *Brit. Med. J.* 4:67, 1974.

22. Cousins, L. M., Hobel, C. J., Chang, R. J., Okada, D. M., and Marshall, J. R.: Serum progesterone and estradiol: 17 β levels in premature and term labor. *Am. J. Obstet. Gynecol.* 127:612, 1977.

23. Liggins, G. C., Kennedy, P. C., and Holm, L. W.: Failure of initiation of parturition after electrocoagulation of the pituitary of the fetal lamb. *Am. J. Obstet. Gynecol.* 98:1080, 1967.

24. Drost, M., and Holm, L. W.: Prolonged gestation in ewes after foetal adrenalectomy. *J. Endocrinol.* 40:293, 1968.

25. Liggins, G. C.: Premature delivery of foetal lambs infused with glucocorticoids. *J. Endocrinol.* 45:515, 1969.

26. Anderson, A. B., Pierrepoint, C. G., Griffiths, K., and Turnbull, A. C.: Steroid metabolism in the adrenals of fetal sheep in relation to natural and corticotrophin induced parturition. *J. Reprod. Fertil. (Suppl.)* 16:25, 1972.

27. Liggins, G. C., Fairclough, R. J., Grieves, S. A., Kendall, J. Z., and Knox, B. S.: The mechanism of initiation of parturition in the ewe. *Recent Prog. Horm. Res.* 29:111, 1973.

28. Anderson, A. B., Flint, A. P., and Turnbull, A. C.: Mechanism of action of glucocorticoids in induction of ovine parturition: Effect on placental steroid metabolism. *J. Endocrinol.* 66:61, 1975.

29. Mueller-Heubach, E., Myers, R. D., and Adamsons, K.: Effects of adrenalectomy on pregnancy length in the rhesus monkey. *Am. J. Obstet. Gynecol.* 112:221, 1972.

30. Walsh, S. W., and Novy, M. J.: Fetal ACTH stimulation of steroidogenesis and its implications for parturition in chronically prepared rhesus monkeys. *Gynecol. Invest.* 8:32, 1977.

31. Cawson, M. J., Anderson, A. B. M., Turnbull, A. C., and Lampe, L.: Cortisol, cortisone, and 11-deoxycortisol levels in human umbilical and maternal plasma in relation to the onset of labour. *J. Obstet. Gynaecol. Br. Comm.* 81:737, 1974.

32. Goldkraud, J. W., Schulte, R. L., and Messer, R. H.: Maternal and fetal plasma cortisol levels at parturition. *Obstet. Gynecol.* 47:41, 1976.

33. Murphy, B. E. P.: Does the human fetal adrenal play a role in parturition? *Am. J. Obstet. Gynecol.* 115:521, 1973.

34. Sybulski, S., and Maughan, G. B.: Cortisol levels in umbilical cord plasma in relation to labor and delivery. *Am. J. Obstet. Gynecol.* 125:236, 1976.

35. Tuimala, R. J., Kaupila, A. J. I., and Haapalahti, J.: Response of pituitary-adrenal axis on partal stress. *Obstet. Gynecol.* 46:275, 1975.

36. Nwosu, U. C., Wallach, E. E., and Bolognese, R. J.: Initiation of labor by intra-amniotic cortisol instillation in prolonged human pregnancy. *Obstet. Gynecol.* 47:137, 1976.

37. Mati, J. K. G., Horrobin, D. F., and Bramley, P. S.: Induction of labour in sheep and humans by single doses of corticosteroids. *Brit. Med. J.* 2:149, 1973.

38. Nwosu, U. C., Wallach, E. E., Boggs, T. R., and Bongiovanni, A. M.: Possible adrenocorticol insufficiency in postmature neonates. *Am. J. Obstet. Gynecol.* 112:969, 1975.

39. Nwosu, U. C., Wallach, E. E., Boggs, T. R., Nemiroff, R. L., and Bongiovanni, A. M.: Possible role of the fetal adrenal glands in the etiology of postmaturity. *Am. J. Obstet. Gynecol.* 121:366, 1975.

40. Karim, S. M. M.: Appearance of prostaglandin F_{2a} in human blood during labour. *Brit. Med. J.* 4:618, 1968.

41. Karim, S. M. M.: Identification of prostaglandins in human amniotic fluid. *J. Obstet. Gynaecol. Br. Comm.* 73:903, 1966.

42. Karim, S. M. M., and Devlin, J.: Prostaglandin content of amniotic fluid during pregnancy and labor. *J. Obstet. Gynaecol. Br. Comm.* 74:230, 1967.

43. Akesson, G., and Gustavii, B.: Occurrence of phospholipase A_1 and A_2 in human decidua. *Prostaglandin* 9:667, 1975.

44. Gustavvi, B.: Release of lysosomal acid phosphatase into the cytoplasm of decidual cells before the onset of labor in humans. *Brit. J. Obstet. Gynaecol.* 82:177, 1975.

45. Keirse, M. J. N. C., and Turnbull, A. C.: Metabolism of prostaglandins within the pregnant uterus. *Brit. J. Obstet. Gynaecol.* 82:887, 1975.

46. MacDonald, P. C., Schultz, F. M., Duenhoelter, J. H., Gant, N. F., Jimenez, J. M., Pritchard, J. A., Porter, J. C., and Johnston, J. M.: Initiation of human parturition: I. Mechanism of action of arachidonic acid. *Obstet. Gynecol.* 44:629, 1974.

47. Schultz, F. M., Schwarz, B. E., MacDonald, P. C., and Johnston, J. M.: Initiation of human parturition: II. Identification of phospholipase A_2 in fetal chorioamnion and uterine decidua. *Am. J. Obstet. Gynecol.* 123:650, 1975.

48. Schwarz, B. E., Schultz, F. M., MacDonald, P. C., and Johnston, J. M.: Initiation of human parturition: III. Fetal membrane content of prostaglandin E_2 and F_2 and precursor. *Obstet. Gynecol.* 46:564, 1975.

49. Kloeck, F. K., and Jung, H.: In vitro release of prostaglandins from the myometrium under the influence of stretching. *Am. J. Obstet. Gynecol.* 115:1066, 1973.

50. Csapo, A. I., Jaffin, H., Kerenyi, T., Lipman, J. I., and Wood, C.: Volume and activity of the pregnant human uterus. *Am. J. Obstet. Gynecol.* 85:819, 1963.

51. Brotanek, V., Hendricks, C. H., and Yoshida, T.: Changes in uterine blood flow during uterine contractions. *Am. J. Obstet. Gynecol.* 103:1108, 1969.

52. Resnik, R., and Brink, G. W.: Modulating effects of prostaglandins on the uterine vascular bed. *Gynecol. Invest.* 8:10, 1977.

53. Brotanik, V., and Hodr, J.: The effect of isoxsuprine on uteroplacental circulation: Intra-uterine dangers to the fetus. Excerpta Medica Foundation, 1967, pp. 424–427.

54. Ehrenkranz, R. A., Walker, A. M., Oakes, G. K., McLaughlin, M. K., and Chez, R. A.: Effect of ritodrine infusion on uterine and umbilical blood flow in pregnant sheep. *Am. J. Obstet. Gynecol.* 126:343, 1976.

55. Ehrenkranz, R. A., Hamilton, L. A., Brennan, S. C., Oakes, G. K., Walker, A. M., and Chez, R. A.: Effects of salbutamol and isoxsuprine on uterine and umbilical blood flow in pregnant sheep. *Am. J. Obstet. Gynecol.* 128:287, 1977.

56. Caldeyro-Barcia, R., Pose, S. V., and Alvarez, H.: Uterine contractility in polyhydramnios and the effects of the withdrawal of the excess of amniotic fluid. *Am. J. Obstet. Gynecol.* 73:1238, 1957.

57. El-Sahwi, S. Gaafar, A. A., and Toppozada, H. K.: A new unit for evaluation of uterine activity. *Am. J. Obstet. Gynecol.* 98:900, 1967.

58. Hon, E. H., and Paul, R. H.: Quantitation of uterine activity. *Obstet. Gynecol.* 42:368, 1973.

59. Csapo, A., and Sauvage, J.: The evolution of uterine activity during human pregnancy. *Acta Obstet. Gynecol. Scand.* 47:181, 1968.

60. Seitchik, J., and Chatkoff, M. L.: Oxytocin-induced uterine hypercontractility pressure wave forms. *Obstet. Gynecol.* 48:436, 1976.

61. Effer, S. B., Bertola, R. P., Vrettos, A., and Caldeyro-Barcia, R.: Quantitative study of the regularity of uterine contactile rhythm in labor. *Am. J. Obstet. Gynecol.* 105:909, 1969.

62. Schulman, H., and Romney, S. L.: Variability of uterine contractions in normal human parturition. *Obstet. Gynecol.* 36:215, 1970.

63. Cerevka, J., Scheffs, J. S., and Vasicka, A.: Shape of uterine contractions (intra-amniotic pressure) and corresponding fetal heart rate. *Obstet. Gynecol.* 35:695, 1970.

64. Caldeyro-Barcia, R., and Poseiro, J. J.: Physiology of the uterine contraction. *Clin. Obstet. Gynecol.* 3:386, 1960.

65. Caldeyro-Barcia, R., and Sereno, J. A.: The response of the human uterus to oxytocin throughout pregnancy, *Oxytocin,* R. Caldeyro-Barcia and H. Heller (eds). Pergamon, New York, 1961, p. 177.

66. Favier, J., and Helfferich, M.: The effects on the fetus of an abnormal contraction pattern in the induction of labor with oxytocin. *Am. J. Obstet. Gynecol.* 112:1107, 1972.

67. Sica-Blanco, Y., and Sala, N. L.: Uterine contractility at the beginning and end of the oxytocin infusion, in *Oxytocin,* R. Caldeyro-Barcia and H. Heller (eds.). Pergamon, New York, 1961, p. 127.

68. Gonzalez-Panizza, V. H., Sica-Blanco, Y., and Mendez-Bauer, C.: The fate of injected oxytocin in the pregnant women near term, in *Oxytocin,* R. Caldeyro-Barcia and H. Heller (eds.). Pergamon, New York, 1961, p. 347.

69. Giglio, F. A., and Stewart, J. P.: Metabolic-endocrine effects of oxytocin stimulation. *Am. J. Obstet. Gynecol.* 93:543, 1965.

70. Morgan, D. B., Kirwan, N. A., Hancock, K. W., Robinson, D., Howe, J. G., and Ahmad, S.: Water intoxication and oxytocin infusion. *Brit. J. Obstet. Gynaecol.* 84:6, 1977.

71. Abdul-Karim, R., and Assali, N.S.: Renal function in human pregnancy. *J. Lab. Clin. Med.* 57:522, 1961.

72. Beazley, J. M., and Alderman, B.: Neonatal hyperbilirubinaemia following the use of oxytocin in labour. *Brit. J. Obstet. Gynaecol.* 82:265, 1975.

73. Anderson, G., Cordero, L., Hobbins, J., and Speroff, L.: Clinical use of prostaglandins as oxytocic substances. *Ann. N.Y. Acad. Sci.* 180:499, 1971.

74. Beazley, J. M., and Gillespie, A.: A double-blind trial of prostaglandin E_2 and oxytocin in induction of labor. *Lancet* 1:152, 1971.

75. Brown, A. A., Hamlett, J. D., Hibbard, B. M., and Howe, P. D.: Induction of labour by amniotomy and intravenous infusion of oxytocic drugs: A comparison between prostaglandin and oxytocin. *J. Obstet. Gynecol. Brit. Com.* 80:111, 1973.

76. Spellacy, W. M., and Gall, S. A.: Prostaglandin F_{2a} and oxytocin for term labor induction. *J. Reprod. Med.* 9:300, 1972.

77. Bruns, P. D., Snow, R. H., and Drose, V. E.: Effect of dihydroergotamine on human uterine contractility. *Obstet. Gynecol.* 1:188, 1953.

78. Gray, N. J., and Plentl, A. A.: Sparteine: A review of its use in obstetrics. *Obstet. Gynecol.* 11:204, 1958.

79. Hendricks, C. H., Reid, D. W. J., Van Praagh, I., and Cibils, L. A.: Effect of sparteine sulfate upon uterine activity in human pregnancy. *Am. J. Obstet. Gynecol.* 91:1, 1965.

80. Stander, R. W., Thompson, J. F., and Stanley, J. R.: Continuous intrauterine pressure recordings in the evaluation of sparteine sulfate. *Am. J. Obstet. Gynecol.* 86:281, 1963.

81. Newton, B. W., Benson, R. C., and McCorriston, C. C.: Sparteine sulfate: A potent, capricious oxytocic. *Am. J. Obstet. Gynecol.* 94:234, 1966.

82. Cibils, L. A., and Hendricks, C. H.: Effect of ergot derivatives and sparteine sulfate upon the human uterus. *J. Reprod. Med.* 2:147, 1969.

83. Cibils, L. A., Pose, S. V., and Zuspan, F. P.: Effect of 1-norepinephrine infusion on uterine contractility and cardiovascular system. *Am. J. Obstet. Gynecol.* 84:307, 1962.

84. Sala, N. L., and Fisch, L.: Effect of acetylcholine and atropine upon uterine contractility in pregnant women. *Am. J. Obstet. Gynecol.* 91:1069, 1965.

85. Barden, T. P., and Stander, R. W.: Myometrial and cardiovascular effects of an adrenergic blocking drug in human pregnancy. *Am. J. Obstet. Gynecol.* 101:91, 1968.

86. Mitrani, A., Oettinger, M., Abinader, E. G., Sharf, M., and Klein, A.: Use of propranolol in dysfunctional labour. *Br. J. Obstet. Gynaecol.* 82:651, 1975.

87. Klieger, J. A., and Massart, J. J.: Clinical and laboratory survey into the oxytocic effects of dimenhydriante in labor. *Am. J. Obstet. Gynecol.* 92:1, 1965.

88. Shephard, B., Cruz, A., and Spellacy, W.: The acute effects of Dramamine on uterine contractility during labor. *J. Reprod. Med.* 16:27, 1976.

89. Rotter, C. W., Whitaker, J. L., and Yared, J.: The use of intravenous Dramamine to shorten the time of labor and potentiate analgesic. *Am. J. Obstet. Gynecol.* 75:1101, 1958.

90. Lands, A. M., Arnold, A., McAuliff, J., Luduena, F. P., and Brown, T. G.: Differentiation of receptor systems activated by sympathomimetic amines. *Nature* 214:597, 1967.

91. Hendricks, C. H., Cibils, L. A., Pose, S. V., and Eskes, T. K. A. B.: Pharmacologic control of excessive uterine activity with isoxsuprine. *Am. J. Obstet. Gynecol.* 76:969, 1958.

92. Karim, M.: Isoxsuprine and the human parturient uterus. *J. Obstet. Gynaecol. Br. Commonw.* 70:992, 1963.

93. Stander, R. W., Barden, T. P., Thompson, J. F., Pugh, W. R., and Werts, C. E.: Fetal cardiac effects of maternal isoxsuprine infusion. *Am. J. Obstet. Gynecol.* 89:792, 1964.

94. Gamissans, O., Esteban-Altirriba, J., and Maiques, V.: Inhibition of human myometrial activity by a new β-adrenergic drug (DU 21220). *J. Obstet. Gynaecol. Br. Commonw.* 76:656, 1969.

95. Wesselius-de Casparis, A., Thiery, M., Yo Le Sian, A., Baumgarten, K., Brosens, I., Gamissans, O., Stolk, J. G., and Vivier, W.: Results of double-blind, multicenter study with ritodrine in premature labor. *Br. Med. J.* 3:144, 1971.

96. Fuchs, F., Fuchs, A. R., Poblete, V. F., Jr., and Risk, A.: Effect of alcohol on threatened premature labor. *Am. J. Obstet. Gynecol.* 99:627, 1967.

97. Zlatnik, F. J., and Fuchs, F.: A controlled study of ethanol in threatened premature labor. *Am. J. Obstet. Gynecol.* 112:610, 1972.

98. Lauersen, N. H., Merkatz, I. R., Tejani, N., Wilson, K. H., Roberson, A., Mann, L. I., and Fuchs, F.: Inhibition of premature labor: A multicenter comparison of ritodrine and ethanol. *Am. J. Obstet. Gynecol.* 127:837, 1977.

99. Dilts, P. V.: Effect of ethanol on uterine and umbilical hemodynamics and oxygen transfer. *Am. J. Obstet. Gynecol.* 108:221, 1970.

100. Horiguchi, T., Suzuki, K., Comas-Urrutia, A. C., Mueller-Heubach, E., Boyer-Milic, A. M., Baratz,

R. A., Morishima, H. O., James, L. S., Adamsons, K.: Effect of ethanol upon uterine activity and fetal acid-base state of the rhesus monkey. *Am. J. Obstet. Gynecol.* 109:910, 1971.

101. Mann, L. I., Bhakthavathsalan, A., Liu, M., and Makowski, P.: Placental transport of alcohol and its effect on maternal and fetal acid-base balance. *Am. J. Obstet. Gynecol.* 122:837, 1975.

102. Aiken, J. W.: Aspirin and indomethacin prolong parturition in rats: Evidence that prostaglandins contribute to expulsion of fetus. *Nature* 240:21.

103. Csapo, A. I., Csapo, E. E., Fay, E., Henzl, M. R., and Salau, G.: Delay of spontaneous labor by naproxen in the rat model. *Prostaglandins* 3:827, 1973.

104. Novy, J. J., Cook, M. J., and Manaugh, L.: Indomethacin block of normal onset of parturition in primates. *Am. J. Obstet. Gynecol.* 118:412, 1974.

105. Zuckerman, H., Reiss, U., and Rubinstein, I.: Inhibition of human premature labor by indomethacin. *Obstet. Gynecol.* 44:787, 1974.

106. Coceani, F., and Olley, P. M.: The response of the ductus arteriosus to prostaglandins. *Can. J. Physiol. Pharmacol.* 51:220, 1973.

107. Heymann, M. A., and Rudolph, A. M.: Effects of acetylsalicylic acid on the ductus arteriosus and circulation in fetal lambs in utero. *Circ. Res.* 38:418, 1976.

108. Archilla, J. A., Thilenius, O. G., and Ranniger, K.: Congestive heart failure from suspected ductal closure in utero. *J. Pediatr.* 75:74, 1969.

109. Landesman, R., de Souza, F. A., Coutinho, E. M., Wilson, H. K., and deSousa, F., M. B.: The inhibitory effect of diazoxide in normal term labor. *Am. J. Obstet. Gynecol.* 103:430, 1969.

110. Coutinho, E. M., and Vieira-Lopes, A. C.: Inhibition of uterine motility by aminophylline. *Am. J. Obstet. Gynecol.* 110:726, 1971.

111. Harbert, G. M., Cornell, G. W., and Thornton, Jr., W. M.: Effect of toxemia therapy on uterine dynamics. *Am. J. Obstet. Gynecol.* 105:94, 1969.

112. Petrie, R. H., Wu, R., Miller, F. C., Sacks, D. A., Sugarman, R., Paul, R., and Hon, E. H.: The effect of drugs on uterine activity. *Obstet. Gynecol.* 48:431, 1976.

113. Dandavino, A., Woods, Jr., J. R., Murayama, K., Brinkman III, C. R., and Assali, N. S.: Circulatory effects of magnesium sulfate in normotensive and renal hypertensive pregnant sheep. *Am. J. Obstet. Gynecol.* 127:769, 1977.

114. Pinto, R. M., Votta, R. A., Montuori, E., and Baleiron, H.: Action of estradiol 17 β on the pregnant human uterus. *Am. J. Obstet. Gynecol.* 94:876, 1966.

115. Pinto, R. M., Lerner, U., Mazzocco, N., and Glauberman, M.: The oxytocic action of intra-amniotic estradiol-17β on the pregnant human uterus. *Am. J. Obstet. Gynecol.* 94:876, 1966.

116. Bengtsson, L. P.: Experiments on suppressive effect of a synthetic progestogen on activity of the pregnant human uterus. *Acta Obstet. Gynecol. Scand.* 41:124, 1962.

117. Brenner, W. E., and Hendricks, C. H.: Effect of medroxyprogesterone acetate upon duration and characteristics of human gestation and labor. *Am. J. Obstet. Gynecol.* 82:1094, 1962.

118. Wood, C., Elstein, M., and Pinkerton, J. H. M.: The effect of progestogens upon uterine activity. *J. Obstet. Gynaec. Br. Commonw.* 70:839, 1963.

119. Bieniarz, J. Burd, L., Motew, M., Scommegna, A., Lin, S., Wineman, C., and Seals, C.: Inhibition of uterine contractility in labor. *Am. J. Obstet. Gynecol.* 111:874, 1971.

120. Johnson, J. W., Austin, K. L., Jones, G. S., Davis, G. H., and King, T. M.: Efficacy of 17 α-hydroxy-progesterone caproate in the prevention of premature labor. *New Eng. J. Med.* 293:675, 1975.

121. Schellenberg, J. C.: Uterine activity during lumbar epidural analgesia with bupivacaine. *Am. J. Obstet. Gynecol.* 127:26, 1977.

122. Greiss, Jr., F. C., Still, J. G., and Anderson, S. G.: Effects of local anesthetic agents on the uterine vasculature and myometrium. *Am. J. Obstet. Gynecol.* 124:889, 1976.

123. Raabe, N., and Belfrage, P.: Epidural analgesia in labour: IV. Influence on uterine activity and fetal heart rate. *Acta Obstet. Gynecol. Scand.* 55:305, 1976.

124. Schellenberg, J. C.: Uterine activity during lumbar epidural analgesia with bupivacaine. *Am. J. Obstet. Gynecol.* 127:26, 1977.

125. Lowensohn, R. I., Paul, R. H., Fales, S., Yeh, Si-Y., and Hon, E. H.: Intrapartun epidural anesthesia: An evaluation of effects on uterine activity. *Obstet. Gynecol.* 44:388, 1974.

126. Riffel, H. D., Nochimson, D. J., Paul, R. H., and Hon, H. G.: Effects of meperidine and promethazine during labor. *Obstet. Gynecol.* 42:738, 1973.

127. Filler, Jr., W. W., Hall, W. C., and Filler, N. W.: Analgesia in obstetrics: The effect of analgesia on uterine contractility and fetal heart rate. *Am. J. Obstet. Gynecol.* 98:832, 1967.

128. DeVoe, S. J., DeVoe, K., Rigsby, W. C., and McDaniels, B. A.: Effect of meperidine on uterine contractility. *Am. J. Obstet. Gynecol.* 105:1004, 1969.

5

Maternal-Infant Nutrition

William van B. Robertson, Ph.D.

Their satisfaction [nutritional needs in pregnancy] must
begin with the antenatal lives of the mothers of our race.
It must continue during the period of their growth up to,
during and following the period when they find their
fulfillment in motherhood; a fulfillment for which
nutrition prepares and makes ready the way.

McCarrison (1)

Reproduction poses a fascinating nutritional situation. From the time that the ovum is released until the infant is able to forage, grasp, and supplement breast feeding with other foods, the nutrition of the conceptus is entirely dependent on the physiological processes of the mother. Knowledge of the specific and detailed nutritional needs of the developing human organism and of the placental and mammary mechanisms involved in supplying these needs at differing stages of development is scanty. As knowledge accumulates, we should be able to establish appropriate recommendations for the successful outcome of reproduction and should become more capable of dealing successfully with the mother-fetus-infant in pathologic situations.

Many genetic and environmental factors that impinge on the mother may affect either the placental nourishment of her fetus or the quantity and quality of her breast milk (Fig. 1). This chapter deals primarily with the effects of one of these factors, maternal nutrition.

In all cultures for which we have sufficient evidence, the feeding of mother and infant is given special consideration. Special foods are often prescribed during pregnancy or lactation in order to endow the offspring with certain favorable characteristics. More commonly, certain foods are forbidden, presumably to prevent an untoward outcome for mother or child. Although many of the taboos are nutritionally harmless, others are less innocuous. For example, some African tribes prohibit the pregnant or lactating woman from eating eggs or milk; this restriction removes one of the only good protein sources from an already protein-poor diet. Modern medicine is also not yet free of recommendations reflecting nonscientific biases. At one time or another in the last 25 years, physicians have proscribed red meat, salt, or an adequate caloric intake for the pregnant woman. Mothers have been urged to forsake breast feeding and to feed solid foods as early as possible.

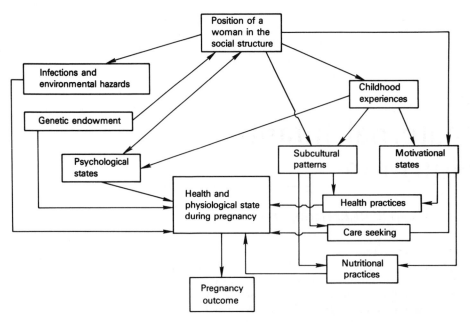

Figure 1. Theoretical model: Effect of social structure on women's physiological state and pregnancy outcome. Siegel and Morris (2). The model is equally applicable to lactation.

Although numerous studies have been undertaken during the last 50 years—for reviews of earlier literature see (3–6)—it has been difficult to obtain definitive scientific answers regarding many aspects of the role of maternal nutrition in the outcome of human reproduction. Several factors have contributed to the difficulty of obtaining reliable information. (1) The possibility that the offspring may be harmed by dietary manipulation, especially restriction of essential nutrients, erects an ethical barrier to carrying out this type of research in the healthy mother. (2) In most epidemiologic studies that take advantage of dietary variation resulting from underdevelopment, famine, or other catastrophe, as well as those variations in established populations, it has not been possible to separate the effects of maternal malnutrition from those of the socioeconomic environment. (3) Because it is far easier to organize research when a patient is confined to a hospital, studies have tended to be concentrated around the birth process and abnormal pregnancies. (4) Conclusions regarding nutritional status of mothers and infants have often been based on comparisons with healthy nonpregnant adults and have neglected the fact that some changes in physiologic parameters, e.g., blood hemoglobin concentration, are adaptive and not necessarily a result of poor nutrition. (5) Although animal experimentation has contributed significant information, the application to human reproductive processes is fraught with the possibility of error. No single physiologic activity exhibits such gross differences between mammalian species as does reproduction. Among these differences, all of which interact with nutrition, are estrus pattern, anatomy and function of the placenta, stage of development at birth, number of progeny per pregnancy, rate of growth of fetus and infant, composition of milk, and feeding pattern during lactation.

As a result, even authoritative recommendations for the nutrition of the pregnant woman and lactating mother have been based largely on uncontrolled empiric observations and have varied from time to time as one or another emphasis in nutrition becomes apparent. Thus, following Burke's Boston study (7) showing a high correlation of favorable outcome of pregnancy with good maternal nutrition, and influenced by the then current enthusiasm for vitamins and minerals in nutrition, it became commonplace to recommend major supplements during pregnancy and lactation. The apparent failure of supplemental nutrition to alter the incidence of prematurity, the documentation of experiences during the World War II famines in Leningrad, Holland, and postwar Germany showing no effect on pregnancy outcome other than a reduction of birthweight by a few hundred grams, the high birth rate in poor countries where mothers suffer from chronic malnutrition, and finally the careful study by Thomson of pregnancies in Aberdeen in which they could demonstrate no specific effect of maternal nutrition on birth outcome or maternal mortality (8) led scarcely two decades later to the concept that, except in extreme circumstances, maternal nutrition during pregnancy had little or no effect on the outcome of pregnancy. The fetus came to be regarded as an effective parasite that would thrive at the expense of the mother and irrespective of her nutrition. It was at this time common in the United States to limit weight gain during pregnancy severely by recommending extreme caloric and salt restriction.

In the past 5 to 10 years the pendulum of opinion has swung back, and eating a balanced diet during pregnancy is again regarded as important to the outcome. The American College of Obstetricians and Gynecologists has incorporated specific nutritional standards as part of its *Standards for Ambulatory Obstetric Care* (9) and called attention to special groups of women who are at risk of nutritional deficiency. Table I lists groups of women considered to be at nutritional risk. The Congress of the United States has authorized a program (WIC) that provides for nutritional supplementation of low-income pregnant and nursing mothers judged to be at nutritional risk. This change in viewpoint can be attributed to (1) careful epidemiologic and clinical studies demonstrating that maternal weight gain during pregnancy is a major factor influencing birthweight and perinatal health (11,12), (2) intervention studies demonstrating the effectiveness of nutritional supplements in reducing the incidence of low birthweight infants (13), and (3) demonstration of biochemical and cellular abnormalities in the reproductive tissues of malnourished pregnant women (14). It also reflects a renewed belief among both the lay public and professionals that good nutrition is important for the maintenance of health and prevention of disease.

In the present chapter, current information about the role of nutrition in reproduction

Table I. Pregnant Women at High Risk of Nutritional Deficiency

1. Adolescents, especially those who are not married
2. Women with low prepregnancy weights
3. Women with inadequate weight gain during pregnancy
4. Women with low income or for whom food purchase is an economic problem
5. Women with a history of frequent conceptions
6. Women with a history of infants having low birthweight
7. Women with diseases that influence nutritional status—diabetes, tuberculosis, anemia, drug addiction, alcoholism, or mental depression
8. Women known to be dietary faddists or with frank pica

SOURCE: Reference 10.

is examined with a view to establishing dietary regimens conducive to a successful out-come. Conception, followed by an uneventful, full-term pregnancy resulting in delivery of a healthy infant, who should then develop, fulfilling its genetic potential both physically and mentally, would be the primary considerations for a successful outcome. However, development should not occur in a nutritional environment that predisposes the future adult to disease or disability, e.g., obesity, cardiovascular disease, or cancer. A successful reproductive outcome should also consider the effects on the mother. She should have a reproductive episode free of somatic morbidity, she should enjoy emo-tional and mental well-being, and the episode should not affect her future health adversely.

Though not demonstrated with complete scientific rigor in all details, the general nutritional requirements for achieving some of the aspects of this goal, e.g., a healthy baby of adequate size and normal growth and development are well enough known to allow formulation of sound recommendations that should withstand the test of time. Requirements for specific nutrients during reproduction are less well established than for general nutrition. Conclusions are drawn from the results of experiments in animals, dietary histories of healthy populations, and comparison with established needs of non-pregnant, nonlactating adult women. For other aspects, such as the long-term conse-quences of nutrition on mother or child, the hard evidence is still scanty, and we must depend on the experience, perception, and judgment of expert groups for recommen-dations.

Both in the population at large and among professionals, size of the infant at birth is commonly used as a measure of success of a pregnancy. Although an individual baby may be small, healthy, and well developed, in all populations studied, low birthweight is associated with a high rate of perinatal mortality and morbidity. Figure 2 illustrates the relation of perinatal mortality to birthweight in full-term deliveries. The slope of the

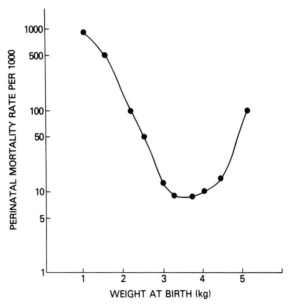

Figure 2. Perinatal motality related to birthweight. Adapted from Bergner and Susser (11) and others.

curve showing a decreased mortality as birthweight increases does not flatten out significantly until birthweight reaches about 2750 g. Minimum mortality is observed at about 3500 g, which is somewhat higher than the average mean birthweight at term. As birthweight increases excessively, an increased mortality is again observed. The curve relating perinatal death rate to birthweight for different populations or different durations of gestation would be displaced somewhat vertically but otherwise have the same general shape.

Although significant differences exist in the type of morbidity, management, and potential outcome associated with prematurity as opposed to intrauterine growth retardation, all small infants are at high risk for physical and intellectual impairment. It has been generally assumed that the excess risk was only significant for birthweights less than 2.5 kg. Laskey et al. (15), however, have reported that psychomotor performance at both birth and 6 months of age was significantly correlated with birthweights not only below 2.5 kg but in babies weighing 2.5 to 4.8 kg. This unexpected finding, if repeated in other studies, should influence birthweight goals.

Both genetic and environmental factors contribute to variation in birthweight. It has been estimated that in our society about 40% of the variation may be attributed to the former and 60% to the latter (16). The detailed mechanisms by which these factors, whether genetic or environmental, exert their effect are in most cases unknown, but it is probable that each of them somehow affects the capacity of the mother to nourish the fetus. This impact on the fetus could be mediated by effects on the size of the placenta or its perfusion and the capacity of the mother to mobilize nutrient stores as well as by specific nutrient deficits in the maternal diet.

The effect of maternal nutrition on reproduction may, for convenience, be considered during three major periods: prepregnancy, pregnancy, and lactation. Malnutrition at any stage leaves its imprint on the offspring, even though appropriate nutritional intervention at later stages may ameliorate some of the most damaging effects of poor nutrition at a previous stage.

Poor nutrition, when associated with low socioeconomic status, is often a woman's lot throughout her life span. When this condition exists for successive generations in families, it causes not only a high degree of reproductive wastage but adults who are smaller. The smallness, although it may appear hereditary and occur in successive generations, is not of genetic origin. Catch-up growth, sufficient for a people to express their full genetic potential, may require more than one reproductive cycle.

PREPREGNANT NUTRITION

The mother's prepregnant head circumference and height have each been found to correlate positively with birthweight (17). Variation of these two parameters in a population reflects early nutrition. Thus, inadequate nutrition while the mother was in her mother's womb and during the first 2 years of life results in smaller adult head circumference. Eventual height may be diminished by poor nutrition at any time through the age of 7 years (18). One can surmise that these prior events modify birthweight by limiting the ability of the placenta to deliver nutrients to the fetus. Specific nutrient deficiencies, such as vitamin D–deficiency rickets in early life, might lead to an unsuccessful pregnancy when they leave permanent residual anatomic or metabolic abnormalities.

Immediate prepregnant weight-for-height of the mother, to a large extent, a measure of recent nutrition, is correlated positively and independently of height and head circumference with birthweight (19). Thus the baby of the woman who enters pregnancy malnourished is already at greater risk than normal, even when adequate nutrition is supplied during pregnancy.

Severe prepregnant undernutrition, as observed in such famines as that during the seige of Leningrad, when average daily food intake was less than 500 kcal/day, or in patients with anorexia nervosa, is accompanied by decreased fertility as the incidence of amenorrhea and anovulation increases. In chronically undernourished populations, a delayed onset of menarche and regularization of ovulation is common. Although these phenomena seem to result from simple energy deprivation, the quality of the diets is poor, and a specific nutrient deficiency may be responsible. Frisch has postulated the existence of a threshold of adiposity necessary to allow ovulation (20). The mechanism of this relation, although unknown, is probably hormonally mediated. Wishik (21) believes it is more reasonable to postulate a complementary balance between maturation and body fat stores (available energy) as a determinant of ovulation; he cites the observation that even grossly undernourished women in developing countries are eventually fertile. In this regard, it is of interest that East Indian women reproduce regularly at levels of caloric intake that would cause anovulation in previously well-nourished Western women.

NUTRITION DURING PREGNANCY

In most major studies, the predominant positive correlate with birthweight of the infant has been weight gain of the mother during pregnancy (22). In general, this parameter is a good measure of the mother's dietary intake during this period. The average weight gains found in numerous studies of healthy mothers in different population groups who gave birth to healthy children has ranged between 10 and 12.5 kg. However, it should be emphasized that in every study individual variation was very large; healthy babies were born to mothers who gained less than 5 kg or to those who gained over 15 kg. Pitkin (23) points out that, although the range of 10 to 12.5 kg represents average rather than ideal weight gain, it coincides with the weight gain for best reproductive performance. The longer-term effect on the mother of either very little or excessive weight gain has not been systematically explored. However, the depletion of body stores in nutritionally deprived mothers, especially after multiple pregnancies, is presumed to contribute to premature aging and debility. It also seems probable that excessive deposition of fat during pregnancy might predispose to permanent obesity in women who do not nurse and live in a culture with abundant food. Good practice places less emphasis on maintaining total weight gain within narrow limits than on the pattern of accumulation (23).

As may be seen in Figure 3, the usual pattern of weight gain is not uniform throughout pregnancy. Very little weight is gained during the first 2 months, which comprises the embryonic stage of pregnancy. The weight then begins to increase slowly. From the tenth or twelfth week until near term the gain is linear; then it may slow slightly. Excessive and sudden deviations from linearity are probably not of nutritional origin and often herald reproductive pathology. Eighty percent of the increased weight of the second trimester is accounted for by maternal tissue and fluids, and in the third

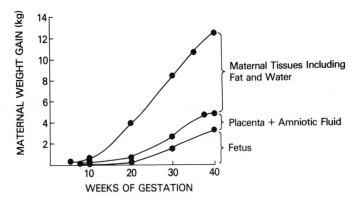

Figure 3. Weight gain of mother during pregnancy partitioned between maternal tissues and fetal tissues. Adapted from Hytten and Leitch (19).

trimester weight gain is distributed equally between mother and fetus. As might be expected, caloric deprivation during the third trimester results in a smaller baby than similar deprivation in earlier trimesters. Paradoxically, caloric supplementation of chronically undernourished women during the first trimester alone increases birth-weight as effectively as the same amount of supplementation during later periods (13). Early supplementation presumably permits laying down of fat stores that can be called on later. It would seem desirable to increase the nutrition of the underweight mother beginning as early in pregnancy as possible. Attempts to reduce the weight of the excessively obese mother during pregnancy are hazardous because of the danger of ketosis that often accompanies calorie-restricted diets and the nutritional inadequacies of such diets. Some control of weight gain by moderate limitation of energy intake using a well-balanced diet is feasible.

Although weight gain of mother and birthweight of infant are useful guides to caloric status, they are relatively crude indices of the satisfaction of total nutritional requirements of mother and fetus. In order to define these more precisely, knowledge is needed of the nutritional demands of the conceptus, of the manner in which nutrients are transferred from mother to fetus, and of changes in maternal requirements dictated by the altered metabolism of pregnancy and the growth of supporting tissues.

Nutrition for the ovum and blastocyst in the earliest stages of pregnancy is supplied directly from the maternal fluids bathing the cells. Beginning about the twentieth day after fertilization, the placenta begins to develop and gradually takes over the nutrition of the embryo while anatomic structures are being elaborated. The nutritional demands during this stage are quantitatively not large, for at 60 days the embryo weighs but 6 g. However, throughout this period, it is especially susceptible to nutritional and meta-bolic imbalances in the mother. For example, mild maternal deficiencies or excesses of vitamins or elevated blood levels of phenylalanine, having no consequences for the mothers, have caused malformations and abortions.

The next 7 months is a period of rapid growth for mother and fetus. The fetus has become almost entirely dependent on the placenta for its supply of oxygen and other nutrients and for the removal of waste products. The growth of the placenta, or more specifically the surface area on which transport of nutrients is dependent, parallels the growth of the fetus until shortly before term, when placental growth ceases (19).

Four basic mechanisms by which the placenta conveys nutrition to the fetus have been recognized.

1. *Simple diffusion.* Substances transferred by this pathway are at the same or slightly lower concentration in fetal blood than in maternal blood. The rate of transfer is limited by the permeability of the placenta to the substance in question. Sodium, potassium, pyridoxin, and the fat-soluble vitamins are among substances supplied by this mechanism. Relatively large amounts of certain nutrients whose transfer is slow, e.g., iron and other trace elements, may accumulate in the fetus if they are locked in by being changed to a form that cannot diffuse back into the maternal blood.

2. *Facilitated diffusion.* The concentration in fetal blood is about the same as in maternal blood, but the transfer may proceed at a much faster rate than would occur by simple diffusion. This mechanism is adapted to substances whose use by the fetus is rapid. Glucose, the primary fetal energy source, is supplied by this mechanism.

3. *Active transport.* The concentration of the nutrient is higher in fetal than in maternal blood. This mechanism provides for adequate supplies of essential nutrients for the fetus even though their concentration in maternal blood may be low. Amino acids, water-soluble vitamins, calcium, and magnesium are among substances supplied by this mechanism.

4. *Placental synthesis.* A few nutrients synthesized in the placenta, such as cholesterol and fatty acids, appear in fetal blood. The contribution of this mechanism to fetal nutrition is probably minor.

Although the normally functioning placenta has mechanisms for transferring nutrients effectively from mother to fetus, the fetus does not thrive in the face of maternal nutritional deprivation. Even in the case of amino acids that are actively concentrated by the placenta, dietary protein (amino acid) insufficiency in the mother results in fetal growth retardation (24,25). There is only limited validity to the view of the fetus as an effective parasite that can grow and develop successfully by draining nutrients from the mother and precipitating maternal nutritional deficiency. Indeed, the literature contains documented cases in which the fetus showed signs of a specific vitamin deficiency and the mother was spared. The low levels of some nutritional parameters in pregnant women that were once interpreted as supporting the concept of the infant as a parasite are now considered reflections of altered maternal physiology. Massive supplementation with vitamins or minerals may move these parameters toward values found in nonpregnant women, but this manipulation seems to have no beneficial effect on the outcome of pregnancy. Nor can we be certain that such massive supplementation is completely harmless.

The diet of a well-nourished pregnant woman should supply the additional nutrients necessary for normal growth of new tissues, both fetal and maternal, taking into account physiologic changes in maternal metabolism. When a woman presents evidence of malnutrition, either general or specific, this should be repaired, bearing in mind that the fetus may be harmed by either too vigorous supplementation or restriction.

Several approaches have been taken to determine nutrient requirements during pregnancy: (1) the factorial method, which sums the amounts of nutrient accumulated in new tissues and fluids and the amounts metabolized; the resultant value is then corrected for efficiency of the organism in using foods supplying the nutrients; (2) balance studies, which determine the amount of nutrient in a diet resulting in maximum positive balance (accumulation); (3) determination of the amount of a vitamin or mineral necessary to maintain serum concentrations or other biochemical parameters at what are considered to be normal levels; and (4) calculations of the dietary intakes of women who have had successful pregnancies yielding appropriately sized, healthy children. Not all approaches are applicable to all nutrients. Results obtained using one approach may differ widely from those obtained using another. Recommendations must finally be based on evaluation of the total data pool and may often reflect nonscientific biases. The Food and Nutrition Board of the National Academy of Sciences has established recommended daily allowances of 17 essential nutrients (26). These recommendations are under continuing review as new data become available and are revised about every 5 years. Table II gives the current recommendations. A diet supplying the recommended amounts of nutrients should assure adequate nutrition in almost every healthy woman. A woman's failure to meet these allowances does not mean that her diet is necessarily inadequate, and there may be an occasional woman who needs greater amounts of a particular nutrient. However, dietary recommendations that depart significantly from those given here are generally unnecessary and should only be made when clearly indicated in the individual case. The needs for essential nutrients, for which no recommendations are specified, are also met when a mixed diet is eaten.

A great variety of diets can fulfill nutritional recommendations. Table III outlines one of many adaptable meal patterns. Protein foods may be of plant or animal origin. Idiosyncrasies such as milk or gluten intolerance, specific allergies, or aversions can be accommodated in the same manner as before pregnancy. The significance of this sample meal pattern is to illustrate the similarity of a good diet for pregnancy to a good pre-pregnancy diet.

Additional comments may be pertinent concerning some of the recommended allowances. The estimated energy cost of pregnancy of 80,000 kcal is covered by the recommended allowance of an additional 300 kcal/day. This is an average daily value. It is apparently immaterial whether the increase is spread out evenly during the pregnancy or a smaller increase during the first trimester is balanced by a larger increase during the last two trimesters (28). Routinely limiting caloric intake to control weight gain increases the risk of fetal malnutrition by directly limiting available energy, by causing ketosis, or by diverting protein needed for new tissue to use as an energy source. The view that caloric intake leading to a large weight gain predisposes to preeclampsia is not supported by the evidence. The misconception probably arose because of failure to distinguish between calorie-produced weight gain or new adipose tissue and that caused by water retention associated with toxemia.

The recommended allowance for an additional 30 g of protein per day or 8 kg during gestation may seem excessive when compared with the approximately 1 kg of new maternal and fetal tissue protein. Although such a high protein intake cannot be justified by hard scientific evidence, among the factors leading to this recommendation were (1) the decreased efficiency of protein utilization during pregnancy; (2) the continuing increase in nitrogen retention, presumably reflecting synthesis of new tissue, in response to increasing levels of dietary protein; and a feeling that the new tissue may act as a source of protein during the last trimester of pregnancy and during lactation, when protein needs are greatest; and (3) the permanent deficit in the number of cells in the central nervous system of offspring when animals were fed a protein-deficient diet dur-

Table II. Food and Nutrition Board, National Academy of Sciences—National Research
Good Nutrition of Practically All Healthy People in the U.S.A.)

	Age	Weight		Height		Energy	Protein	Fat-Soluble Vitamins			
								Vita-min A Activity		Vita-min D	Vita-min E Activity[e]
	(years)	(kg)	(lbs)	(cm)	(in)	(kcal)[b]	(g)	(RE)[c]	(IU)	(IU)	(IU)
Infants	0.0–0.5	6	14	60	24	kg × 117	kg × 2.2	420[d]	1400	400	4
Females	11–14	44	97	155	62	2400	44	800	4000	400	12
	15–18	54	119	162	65	2100	48	800	4000	400	12
	19–22	58	128	162	65	2100	46	800	4000	400	12
	23–50	58	128	162	65	2000	46	800	4000		12
Pregnant						+300	+30	1000	5000	400	15
Lactating						+500	+20	1200	6000	400	15

[a] The allowances are intended to provide for individual variations among most normal persons as they live in the United States under usual environmental stresses. Diets should be based on a variety of common foods in order to provide other nutrients for which human requirements have been less well defined.

[b] Kilojoules (kJ) = 4.2 × kcal.

[c] Retinol equivalents.

[d] Assumed to be all as retinol in milk during the first six months of life. All subsequent intakes are assumed to be half as retinol and half as β-carotene when calculated from international units. As retinol equivalents, three fourths are as retinol and one fourth as β-carotene.

ing pregnancy. The significance of a similar finding in brains of protein-calorie malnourished children is not so clear, because of the inability to differentiate between the effects of protein and energy deficits (29).

Probably no nutritional recommendation has changed as radically during the past decade as that for sodium (salt). A low-salt diet used to be commonly advocated in the belief that a tendency to excessive salt retention was characteristic of pregnancy and that dietary salt restriction would be preventive against edema and preeclampsia. In order to maintain isotonicity and water balance in new fetal and maternal tissues and fluids, 1000 mEq of sodium must be retained during pregnancy. Because of increased glomerular filtration rates beginning early in pregnancy, the filtered sodium load increases as much as 10,000 mEq/day. Increased progesterone levels stimulate natruresis. Although increased activity of the renin-angiotensin-aldosterone system produces a compensatory renal tubular reabsorption of sodium, pregnancy tends to be a salt-wasting state. Decreased sodium levels caused by restriction of salt intake may lead to even higher and potentially harmful levels of angiotensin. Salt restriction seems antiphysiologic and therefore not to be recommended for the healthy pregnant woman. On the other hand, dietary salt intake in our culture is high enough to fulfill additional requirements without further supplementation.

No dietary recommendation provokes as much controversy as that for iron. Hemoglobin concentration in blood generally declines during pregnancy, anemia (hemoglobin < 12 g/dl) is not uncommon, and the incidence of anemia is higher during the second and subsequent pregnancies. One view regards the decline as indicative of iron depletion that should be prevented by giving supplemental iron to protect the mother's stores. The other view considers the lowered hemoglobin concentration during pregnancy a

Council Recommended Daily Dietary Allowances,[a] Revised 1974 (Designed for the Maintenance of

Water-Soluble Vitamins							Minerals					
Ascor-bic Acid (mg)	Fola-cin[f] (μg)	Nia-cin[g] (mg)	Ribo-flavin (mg)	Thia-min (mg)	Vita-min B_6 (mg)	Vita-min B_{12} (μg)	Cal-cium (mg)	Phos-phorus (mg)	Iodine (μg)	Iron (mg)	Mag-nesium (mg)	Zinc (mg)
35	50	5	0.4	0.3	0.3	0.3	360	240	35	10	60	3
45	400	16	1.3	1.2	1.6	3.0	1200	1200	115	18	300	15
45	400	14	1.4	1.1	2.0	3.0	1200	1200	115	18	300	15
45	400	14	1.4	1.1	2.0	3.0	800	800	100	18	300	15
45	400	13	1.2	1.2	2.0	3.0	800	800	100	18	300	15
60	800	+2	+0.3	+0.3	2.5	4.0	1200	1200	125	18+[h]	450	20
80	600	+4	+0.5	+0.3	2.5	4.0	1200	1200	150	18	450	25

[e] Total vitamin E activity, estimated to be 80 percent as α-tocopherol and 20 percent other tocopherols.

[f] The folacin allowances refer to dietary sources as determined by *Lactobacillus casei* assay. Pure forms of folacin may be effective in doses less than one fourth of the recommended dietary allowance.

[g] Although allowances are expressed as niacin, it is recognized that on the average 1 mg of niacin is derived from each 60 mg of dietary tryptophan.

[h] This increased requirement cannot be met by ordinary diets; therefore, the use of supplemental iron is recommended.

normal physiological adjustment that has not been shown to compromise mother or fetus and views increased erythrocyte mass following iron supplementation as a potentially harmful pharmacologic response.

The loss of iron from the mother at parturition has been estimated as between 350 and 500 mg, of which about two-thirds to three-fourths is in the fetus and placenta and the remainder is associated with blood loss. However, amenorrhea of pregnancy spares a loss of 100 to 150 mg of iron. Thus the net loss to the mother is between 250 and 400 mg. This amount must be absorbed from food in addition to usual requirements, if stores are to be maintained. Another 300 to 500 mg of iron is temporarily needed for the expansion of the maternal red cell pool, but this is returned to stores as the amount of circulating hemoglobin returns to normal following delivery. Thus, between 600 and 900 mg of iron must be absorbed from food or obtained from maternal stores, nearly all during the second half of pregnancy. If, as is sometimes claimed, most women have very small iron stores during the reproductive years and it is necessary to supply iron from the diet on a day-to-day basis, the amount needed would increase from about 1 mg/day at the beginning of pregnancy to over 8 mg/day near term, or an average of 3 to 4 mg/day throughout pregnancy. This is more than twice the estimated iron absorption by the nonpregnant woman from the usual American diet. Even though absorption from the gut is more efficient during pregnancy, this requirement might not be reached without the provision of supplemental iron. Routine iron supplementation is commonly prescribed but is probably not usually necessary. Women with low serum ferritin levels indicative of depleted iron stores are at risk for iron deficiency and should get 30 to 60 mg/day of elemental iron given orally as a ferrous salt to prevent hypochronic anemia.

Hypovitaminemia and biochemical test results that in the nonpregnant woman would be suggestive of actual or impending vitamin deficiency are common during pregnancy (30), even in women taking common multivitamin preparations (31). Pharmacologic dosages of vitamins are often required to bring plasma levels and functional tests to prepregnant levels. Extensive use of vitamin supplementation does not appear to have improved the outcome of pregnancy. Today, the prevailing opinion is that low vitamin levels are part of the metabolic adjustment to pregnancy; that a good dietary pattern, fulfilling daily allowances, should supply sufficient nutrients; and that additional supplementation is unnecessary and may be harmful. However, the vegetarian who eats neither eggs nor milk should probably receive vitamin B_{12}.

Although the need for including minute amounts of a number of trace elements in the diet has long been recognized, recent years have seen a resurgence of emphasis on their importance. This renewal of interest may be ascribed to (1) the results of animal experiments showing the essentiality of elements not previously recognized as being of nutritional value, e.g., chromium, selenium, and silicon; (2) identification of the metabolic functions of a number of trace elements; (3) improved analytical technology that permits routine, sensitive, and accurate assay of trace elements in body fluids and tissues; (4) recognition of the existence of trace element deficiency symptomatology in some human populations, e.g., hypogonadism and dwarfism as a result of zinc deficiency observed in the Middle East; and (5) evidence suggesting a marginal deficiency in some individuals in the United States of one or another trace element, possibly related to the increased

Table III. Adaptation of a Sample Dietary Pattern for Pregnant Women

Meal	Nonpregnant Woman	Pregnant Woman
Breakfast	1 serving of vitamin C–rich fruits and vegetables 1 serving of grain products 1 serving of milk and milk products	1 serving of vitamin C–rich fruits and vegetables 1 serving of grain products 1 serving of milk and milk products
Morning snack	Optional	Optional
Lunch	2 servings of grain products 1 serving of protein foods 1 serving of other fruits and vegetables 1 serving of milk and milk products	2 servings of grain products 1 serving of protein foods 1 serving of other fruits and vegetables 1 serving of milk and milk products
Afternoon snack	1 serving of protein foods ½ serving of milk and milk products	1 serving of protein foods ½ serving of milk and milk products
Dinner	1 serving of protein foods 2 servings of leafy green vegetables	2 servings of protein foods 2 servings of leafy green vegetables 1 serving of milk and milk products
Evening snack	½ serving of milk and milk products	½ serving of milk and milk products

SOURCE: Reference 27.

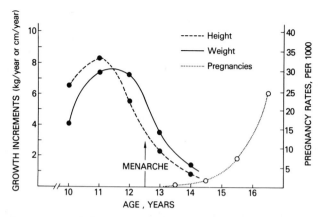

Figure 4. Growth rates around the mean age of menarche and incidence of pregnancies by age. Menarche is normalized at 12.5 years of age. The curves may be displaced horizontally for populations with different ages of menarche (32).

use of highly refined foods. However, except for iron, copper, iodine, and zinc, recommended dietary allowances have not been established. The evidence at this time not only does not warrant generalized trace element supplementation of the usual mixed diet but suggests that significant dietary increases of some trace elements are harmful.

The pregnant adolescent is at higher than average risk for morbidity and for delivery of a low birthweight baby. Inadequate nutrition, because of increased requirements to support the mother's growth, in addition to the needs associated with pregnancy, is often assumed to be a major factor contributing to the poor outcome.

Adolescence is often defined by age, but this is a physiologically unsatisfactory basis because of variations in the time of onset of menstruation. Although conception is possible at menarche, the probabilities are that most adolescent pregnancies do not occur until 2 or more years later, following physical maturation and regularization of ovulation. The pregnant adolescent is likely to be more mature physically than her nonpregnant contemporaries. Since rate of growth declines rapidly from a maximum reached about 1½ years prior to menarche, growth will usually have ceased by the onset of pregnancy, and the need for additional nutrients is likely to be negligible (see Fig. 4). The nutritional requirements of the pregnant adolescent are not significantly different from those of the older pregnant woman.

The incidence of adolescent pregnancy in the United States is highest among girls from groups of low economic status. Poor prepregnant nutrition is more common among this group than in the population at large. Eating patterns of adolescents in general are haphazard and not considered conducive to good nutrition. Thus, despite nutritional requirements that are not exceptional, pregnant adolescents as a group are at high nutritional risk. They are in need of intensive dietary counseling and the provision of appropriate foods.

POSTNATAL NUTRITION

The neonatal period is, from a nutritional standpoint, probably the most critical period in an individual's life. Following delivery, an infant's demands for energy increase rapidly to support maintenance of body temperature, muscle work associated with breathing, and increased activity. During the first 6 postnatal months, body weight doubles, and its composition changes as the proportion of lean muscle mass increases relative to fat and water. The food to supply the large amounts of essential nutrients needed for work, growth, and maturation must be metabolized, and waste products excreted, by a still underdeveloped organism whose tolerance to variation is limited.

Lactation has evolved as the final phase completing the reproductive cycle in mammals. Over many years of evolution, natural selection has functioned to adapt the nutrition of the newly born and its metabolism, so that a species has the best chance of survival. The result has been that the milk produced by various species differs widely in its composition (Table IV). The nursing interval in different species varies from once a day to almost continuous. The duration of lactation is less than the gestational period in some species and much longer in others. Infants of one species do not usually thrive when foster-nursed by mothers of another species.

Since the neolithic revolution 8000 years ago sociocultural evolution has outstripped biological evolution, and changes in our environment have perhaps reduced the adaptive value of human lactation. Modern technology has allowed the development of substitutes for human milk that appear to satisfy the nutritional needs of most infants. Nevertheless, complete breast feeding of the normal, full-term infant by a healthy, well-nourished mother is considered by most authorities to be the most satisfactory nutrition during the first 4 to 6 months of life. The Committee on Nutrition of the American Academy of Pediatrics recommends breast feeding for all full-term and vigorous preterm infants. Supplementation of breast-fed infants with iron, vitamin D, and fluoride is sometimes advocated, not because of demonstrated need, but because the concentrations

Table IV. Composition of Milk of Various Species (per 100 ml)

Species	Protein (g)	Fat (g)	Carbohydrate (g)	Energy (kcal)
Rat	9	9	3	129
Guinea pig	8	6	3	98
Rabbit	13	15	2	195
Cat	11	11	3	155
Dog	8	9	4	129
Sheep	6	8	4	128
Cow	3	4	5	68
Horse	2	2	6	50
Ass	2	2	6	50
Rhinoceros	2	0.5	6	37
Elephant	8	9	4	129
Pig	6	9	5	125
Hippopotamus	7	18	2	198
Man	1	4	7	68
Monkey	2	4	6	68
Seal	11	53	3	533
Whale	12	40	1	412

SOURCE: Reference 33.

in milk are low. Advocates of breast feeding also stress the antiinfective, immunologic, emotional, social, and economic benefits—all intimately related to nutritional health (34). There are also studies suggesting that in later life breast-fed infants may have a lower incidence of obesity, hypertension, and allergy than formula-fed infants.

The nutrients needed for milk production are derived from the maternal diet and from nutrients present in the mother's tissues, some of which, notably fat and protein, accumulated during pregnancy. Although stores of iron, other trace elements, and fat-soluble vitamins accumulated by the fetus during gestation contribute to the infant's nutrition, the volume of mother's milk available and its composition are major determinants of satisfaction of the infant's needs. The question then arises of what effect maternal nutrition has on these parameters. Jelliffe and Jelliffe (35), in a recent review, deplore the paucity of reliable data but feel the following generalization is warranted.

> The volume and composition of human milk in poorly nourished women is surprisingly good, possibly due to some metabolic adaptations but usually to their cumulative nutritional detriment ("maternal depletion"). However, it is often suboptimum in quantity and in quality with lower levels of fat (calories), water soluble vitamins, vitamin A and somewhat lower calcium and protein than in well nourished women.

The poorly nourished woman referred to is one who suffers the chronic malnutrition of the poor in the Third World, a degree of malnutrition not generally seen in developed countries. In the latter, most women following a normal pregnancy have enough nutrients available in their tissues to act as a buffer in maintaining the quality and quantity of milk, even in the face of moderate dietary deficiency. Compliance of lactating women with recommended dietary allowances (Table II) assures replacement of nutrients secreted in milk and prevents depletion of maternal tissues. This is not to say that milk is not affected by diet. For example, the composition of fat in milk reflects that of the maternal diet. Various amounts of almost anything ingested and absorbed appear in milk. Concentrations of drugs, including alcohol, may be sufficient to harm the nursing infant, and the necessity for drug use by the mother may warrant a recommendation against breast feeding. Steroidal contraceptives decrease the volume and modify the composition of milk. Considerable folklore exists about foods to eat and to avoid during lactation, but most beliefs, including a commonly held one that drinking lots of fluids increases milk yield, have no basis in fact.

The estimated amounts of milk consumed by healthy growing nursing infants and its composition form the basis for calculating nutrient requirements and for the development of recommended dietary allowances by the Food and Nutrition Board. Recent measurements of the volumes of milk consumed by the suckling infant and analyses by modern techniques have given results significantly different from those usually accepted. For example, daily milk output commonly ranged between 600 and 700 ml during the first 6 months instead of 800 to 1000 ml (35). A true protein value for human milk is $0.9 \pm 0.1\%$ instead of the previously quoted 1.2% that was based on determination of total nitrogen (36). The nonnutritionally based interpersonal variation, in both volume and composition, has proved to be far greater than formerly believed, and large variations between feedings in an individual and in composition during a feeding have been observed. Alfin-Slater and Jelliffe (37) review the potential impact of the newer data on dietary recommendations for infants and call for reassessment and possible revision.

Developers of surrogate human milk feeding for infants compose formulas that meet recommended nutrient allowances. The earlier formulas based on cow's milk deviated

Table V. Composition of Protein Nitrogen and Nonprotein Nitrogen in Human Milk and Cow's Milk

	Human Milk	Cow's Milk
Total nitrogen	1.93	5.31
Protein nitrogen	1.43 (8.9)	5.03 (31.4)
Casein nitrogen	0.40 (2.5)	4.37 (27.3)
Whey protein nitrogen	1.03 (6.4)	0.93 (5.8)
α-Lactalbumin	0.42 (2.6)	0.17 (1.1)
Lactoferrin	0.27 (1.7)	Traces
β-Lactoglobulin		0.57 (3.6)
Lysozyme	0.08 (0.5)	Traces
Serum albumin	0.08 (0.5)	0.07 (0.4)
Ig A	0.16 (1.0)	0.005 (0.03)
Ig G	0.005 (0.03)	0.096 (0.6)
Ig M	0.003 (0.02)	0.005 (0.03)
Nonprotein nitrogen	0.50	0.28
Urea nitrogen	0.25	0.13
Creatine nitrogen	0.037	0.009
Creatinine nitrogen	0.035	0.003
Uric acid nitrogen	0.005	0.008
Glucosamine	0.047	?
α-Amino nitrogen	0.13	0.048
Ammonia nitrogen	0.002	0.006
Nitrogen from other components	?	0.074

SOURCE: Reference 36.

Values refer to grams of nitrogen per liter.

Values in parentheses refer to grams of protein per liter.

from human milk even in proximate composition (calories, carbohydrate, protein, fat, and minerals). Gradually formulas have been modified so that, with respect to proximate principles, they resemble human milk. Vitamins and minerals have been added so that these meet recommended allowances. However, as may be seen in Table V, a comparison of bovine with human milk shows the presence of proteins in one that are not present in the other; the amino acid composition of the proteins is also significantly different, with larger amounts of phenylalanine, tyrosine, and methionine and smaller amounts of cystine and taurine in cow's milk. The fatty acid pattern of the two milks differ, with human milk containing more unsaturated fat. It is clear that bovine milk cannot be made similar to human milk by additions and dilutions. Attempts to "humanize" cow milk are now giving way to formulas built from selected proteins, vegetable oils, carbohydrates, vitamins, and minerals.

SUMMARY

Reproduction is so well adapted to variations in the nutritional environment that, except under conditions of severe malnutrition, it has been difficult to sort out nutritional effects from those caused by other environmental influences. It is, however, becoming increasingly evident that the well-being of the mother and the healthy growth and development of the offspring are fostered by satisfactory nutrition. Unless contraindicated in the specific situation, adequate nutrition for the healthy pregnant and lactating woman is achieved by simply increasing the amount of a well-balanced diet she should have been eating prior to pregnancy. Any routine supplementation or restriction of a nutrient is not necessary or desirable. If adequately nursed, her suckling child will also not need nutritional supplementation during the first 4 to 6 months.

The infant deprived of its hereditary right to complete breast feeding has available a variety of surrogates. Several of these seem reasonably satisfactory for many infants when used as directed, and efforts to develop the ideal substitute continue. However, as the knowledge of the constituents of milk and their interactions with metabolism of the developing organism increase, it appears unlikely that a completely equivalent nutritional substitute for human milk is technically feasible.

REFERENCES

1. McCarrison, R.: Nutritional needs in pregnancy. *Br. Med. J.* 2:256–257, 1937.

2. Siegel, E., and Morris, N.: *The Epidemiology of Human Reproductive Casualties with Emphasis on the Role of Nutrition: Maternal Nutrition and the Course of Pregnancy.* Committee on Maternal Nutrition, Food and Nutrition Board, National Research Council, National Academy of Sciences, Washington, 1970.

3. Garry, R. C., and Wood, H. O.: A review of recent work on dietary requirements in pregnancy and lactation with an attempt to assess human requirements. *Nutr. Abstract Rev.* 5:855–887, 1936.

4. Garry, R. C., and Wood, H. O.: Dietary requirements in human pregnancy and lactation: A review of recent work. *Nutr. Abstract Rev.* 15:591–621, 1946.

5. Food and Nutrition Board: *Maternal Nutrition and Child Health Bulletin 123.* National Research Council, National Academy of Sciences, Washington, 1951.

6. World Health Organization: *Nutrition in Pregnancy and Lactation.* WHO Tech. Rep. Ser. No. 302, Geneva, 1965.

7. Burke, B. S., Beal, V. A., Kirkwood, S. B., and Stuart, H. C.: Nutrition studies during pregnancy: I. Problem, methods of study and group studied; II. Relation of prenatal nutrition to condition of infant at birth and during first two weeks of life; III. Relation of prenatal nutrition to pregnancy, labor, delivery and postpartum period. *Am. J. Obstet. Gynecol.* 46:38–52. 1943.

8. Thomson, A. M.: Diet in pregnancy: 3. Diet in relation to the course and outcome of pregnancy. *Br. J. Nutr.* 13:509–525, 1959.

9. Committee on Obstetric Practice: *Standards for Ambulatory Obstetric Care.* The American College of Obstetricians and Gynecologists, Chicago, 1977.

10. Christaksis, G.: Maternal nutrition assessment. *Am. J. Public Health* 63 (Suppl.):57–63, 1973.

11. Bergner, L., and Susser, M. W.: Low birth weight and prenatal nutrition: An interpretative review. *Pediatrics* 46:946–966, 1970.

12. Niswander, K. R., and Gordon, M.: *The Women and Their Pregnancies: The Collaborative Perinatal Study.* National Institute of Neurological Diseases and Stroke. Saunders, Philadelphia, 1972.

13. Lechtig, A., Yarbrough, C., Delgado, H., Habicht, J. P., Martorell, R., and Klein, R. E.: Influence of maternal nutrition on birth weight. *Am. J. Clin. Nutr.* 28:1223–1233, 1975.

14. Minkowski, A., Roux, J. M., and Tordet-Caridroit, C.: Pathophysiologic changes in intrauterine malnutrition, Chap. 4, *Nutrition and Fetal Development,* Winick, M. (ed.), Current Concepts in Nutrition, Vol. 2. John Wiley & Sons, New York, 1974.

15. Lasky, R. E., Lechtig, A., Delgado, H., Klein, R. E., Engle, P., Yarbrough, C., and Martorell, R.: Birth weight and psychomotor performance in rural Guatemala. *Am. J. Dis. Child.* 129:566–569, 1975.

16. Lerner, I. M.: *Heredity, Evolution and Society.* Freeman, San Francisco, 1968, p. 148.

17. Hansman, C.: Anthropometry and selected data, *Human Growth and Development,* McCannon, R. W. (ed.). Charles C Thomas, Springfield, 1970.

18. Mönckeberg, F.: Effect of early marasmic malnutrition on subsequent physical and mental development, *Malnutrition Learning and Behavior,* Scrimshaw, N. S., and Gordon, J. E. (eds.). M.I.T. Press, Cambridge, 1968.

19. Hytten, F. E., and Leitch, I.: *The Physiology of Human Pregnancy,* 2nd ed. Blackwell, Oxford, 1971.

20. Frisch, R. E.: Critical weights: A critical body composition, menarche, and the maintenance of menstrual cycles, *Biosocial Interrelations in Population Adaptation,* Watts, E. S., Johnston, F. E., and Lasker, G. W. (eds.). Mouton, The Hague, 1975.

21. Wishik, S. M.: The implications of undernutrition during pubescence and adolescence on fertility, Chap. 3, *Nutritional Impacts on Women Throughout Life With Emphasis on Reproduction,* Moghissi, K. S., and Evans, T. N. (eds.). Harper and Row, Publishers, Hagerstown, Md., 1977, pp. 23–29.

22. Eastman, N. J., and Jackson, E.: Weight relationships in pregnancy: I. The bearing of maternal weight gain and pre-pregnancy weight on birth weight in full term pregnancies. *Obstet. Gynecol. Surv.* 23:1003–1025, 1968.

23. Pitkin, R. M.: Nutritional support in obstetrics and gynecology. *Clin. Obstet. Gynecol.* 19:489–513, 1976.

24. Metcoff, J. M., Mameesh, M., Jacobson, G., Costiloe, P., Crosby, W., Sandstead, H., and McClain, P.: Fetoplacental growth related to maternal nutritional status and leucocyte metabolism at mid-pregnancy. *Federation Proceedings* 35, 1–3 (1201):422, 1976.

25. Burke, B. S., Harding, V. V., and Stuart, H. C.: Nutrition studies during pregnancy: IV. Relation of protein content of mother's diet during pregnancy to birth length, birth weight and condition of infant at birth. *J. Pediatr.* 23:506–515, 1943.

26. Food and Nutrition Board, National Research Council: *Recommended Dietary Allowances,* 8th ed. National Academy of Sciences, Washington, 1974.

27. Jacobson, H. N.: Current concepts in nutrition: Diet in pregnancy. *N. Engl. J. Med.* 297:1051–1053, 1977.

28. Habicht, J. P., Yarbrough, C., Lechtig, A., and Klein, R. E.: Relation of maternal supplementary feeding during pregnancy to birth weight and other sociobiological factors, Chap. 7, *Nutrition and Fetal Development,* Winick, M. (ed.). John Wiley, New York, 1974.

29. Winick, M., and Rosso, P.: The effect of severe early malnutrition on cellular growth of human brain. *Pediat. Res.* 3:181–184, 1969.

30. Pitkin, R. M.: Vitamins and minerals in pregnancy. *Clin. Perinatol.* 2:221–232, 1975.

31. Kaminetzky, H. A., and Baker, H.: Micronutrients in pregnancy. *Clin. Obstet. Gynecol.* 20:363–380, 1977.

32. Thomson, A. M.: Pregnancy in adolescence, Chap. 13, *Nutrient Requirements in Adolescence,* McKigney, J. I., and Munro, H. N. (eds.). M.I.T. Press, Cambridge, 1976, pp. 245–256.

33. Widdowson, E. M.: Pregnancy and lactation: The comparative point of view, *Early Nutrition and Later Development,* Wilkinson, A. W. (ed.). Year Book Medical Publishers, Chicago, 1976.

34. Jelliffe, D. B.: World trends in infant feeding. *Am. J. Clin. Nutr.* 29:1227–1237, 1976.

35. Jelliffe, D. B., and Jelliffe, E. F. P.: The volume and composition of human milk in poorly nourished communities. *Am. J. Clin. Nutr.* 31:492–515, 1978.

36. Hambraeus, L.: Proprietary milk versus human breast milk in infant feeding: A critical appraisal from the nutritional point of view. *Pediatr. Clin. North Am.* 24:17–36, 1977.

37. Alfin-Slater, R. B., and Jelliffe, D. B.: Nutritional requirements with special reference to infancy. *Pediatr. Clin. North Am.* 24:3–16, 1977.

6
Physiologic Changes During Pregnancy: The Mother

Chester Martin, M.D.

Alterations occur in the functioning of most maternal organ systems during pregnancy. There are also significant changes in maternal body composition. Some of these changes are clearly advantageous in supporting the pregnancy or later during lactation, but the benefit of other alterations is not so evident. A few of the maternal adaptations to pregnancy have their basis in the presence and mechanical effects of the enlarging uterus and conceptus. The majority, however, appear to be induced or modulated by ovarian and placental hormones, either directly or through secondary effects on maternal regulatory mechanisms. An appreciation of the nature and magnitude of these maternal physiologic adaptations to pregnancy is important for the appropriate counseling and management of the woman with either normal or complicated pregnancy.

REPRODUCTIVE TRACT

The endocrine changes during pregnancy and the series of events involved in the initiation of labor are described in other chapters. There remain, however, a number of noteworthy features of the adaptation of the female reproductive tract to the actuality of pregnancy.

The Uterus

The uterus increases quite remarkably in size during human pregnancy: in terms of weight, nearly 20-fold, from approximately 60 g before pregnancy to 1000 to 1200 g at term (Fig. 1). This increase is especially notable in comparison with that in some other animals: 3½-fold in mice, 4½-fold in rabbits, about 10-fold in rhesus monkeys. The uterine cavity enlarges from a triangular potential space measuring about 3 by 5 cm to contain 4.5 to 5 liters normally at term. Greater volumes are achieved with multiple pregnancy and polyhydramnios. The expansile capacity of the uterus is limited, however, as demonstrated by the tendency for it to expel its contents at progressively earlier times as the number of fetuses per pregnancy increases. Uterine growth accounts for about 5% of the total nitrogen retention during human pregnancy (1).

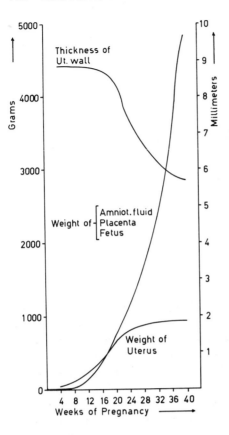

Figure 1. Growth in weight of the uterus and products of conception, and changes in thickness of the uterine wall during pregnancy, based on published data from several sources. Reproduced with permission from Stolte, L. A. M., and Eskes, T. K. A. B., in *Proc. 5th World Cong. Gynaecol. Obstet.* Sydney, Butterworth, 1967.

Hyperplasia, hypertrophy, and stretching all contribute to the uterine enlargement and accommodation to the products of conception. Formation of new cells is quite prominent during the early weeks. Until about 6 weeks after conception, uterine enlargement is due almost entirely to hyperplasia, some hypertrophy, and considerable hyperemia, since the volume of the conceptus contributes little to the uterine size at this time and almost equivalent enlargement occurs with extrauterine implantations. The wave of hyperplasia decreases late in the first trimester. Hypertrophy and, later, stretching account for most of the remaining increase in uterine size. The relative importance of the latter factors in uterine enlargement remains unsettled. Gillespie (2) suggested that there was very little increase in uterine weight after midpregnancy and that enlargement during the second half of gestation was accomplished chiefly by stretching. Uterine measurements and weights collected from the literature by Stolte and Eskes (3) support this view. Hytten and Cheyne (1), on the other hand, interpreted their data as being most compatible with a continuing smooth growth curve for uterine weight. In either case, the incremental growth rate of the uterus, expressed as a proportion of attained weight, declines over the course of pregnancy.

The growth stimuli for this uterine enlargement are both endocrine and mechanical. Estrogen evokes protein synthesis, an increase in the water content, and some mitotic activity in uterine cells. Progesterone, acting after estrogen priming, greatly enhances uterine mitotic activity. The effect is not sustained, for with continued progesterone administration there is a decrease in cell division. Moderate mechanical distension is a potent stimulus to hyperplasia, hypertrophy, and increased vascularity of the uterus in laboratory animals. The effect is greatest in the absence of estrogen and progesterone; however, progesterone increases the degree of mechanical distension at which the growth response will still occur (4).

From about the sixth week after conception onward, the products of conception contribute increasingly to the uterine volume. After about the twelfth week, they predominate. The uterus enlarges in a generally globular configuration until about this time. Thereafter, the uterus and its contained gestational sac gradually assume an ovoid shape with the long axis oriented cephalocaudally, although this may not be clearly appreciated from the physical examination until about the fifteenth to sixteenth postconceptional week, i.e., the seventeenth to eighteenth menstrual week. Expansion of the uterine fundus is relatively greater than that of the corpus. This can be readily appreciated from the location of the insertions of the round ligaments and Fallopian tubes into the term uterus in comparison with those in the nonpregnant state. This disproportionate expansion of the fundal segment is an important factor in the progressive change of uterine configuration from pear-shaped to globular to elongate oval. In consequence also of these changes in uterine shape, the predominant direction of the major myometrial fiber bundles remains a diagonal spiral in the upper segment, whereas the bundles in the lower corpus are drawn into a more vertical, though still diagonal, course. This arrangement favors fundal dominance of tension during uterine contractions and facilitates dilatation and retraction of the cervix and lower uterine segment during labor.

The connective tissue surrounding and supporting the myometrium, through which the myometrial cells transmit the tension they develop during contraction, also hypertrophies during pregnancy. There is also expansion of the uterine vascular and lymphatic beds and hypertrophy of the uterine nerve supply.

It is not clear that the changes in shape of the human uterus during pregnancy are related to the phenomenon of "conversion" described by Reynolds (4) in litter-bearing animals, although the comparison has been suggested. Conversion refers to the change in shape of the conceptus sites from spherical to nearly cylindrical in a short time at a rather consistent point in pregnancy. The occurrence of conversion is dictated by physical factors. With growth of the conceptuses, the tension in the uterine walls increases in the areas of distention. Eventually, the tension exceeds the resistance to stretching of the uterine walls between the implantation sites. The latter areas are then opened up, allowing the gestational sacs to assume an elongated shape and simultaneously reducing uterine wall tension at the former sites of maxiumum distention. A similar phenomenon can be created in blowing up a tubular balloon. Concurrent with conversion there is acceleration of blood flow to the implantation sites. Following conversion, there is little or no further uterine hypertrophy, the balance of uterine enlargement being accomplished by stretching.

Ultrasonographic measurements of the gestational sac (5) and the entire uterus (6) indicate that there is no comparable change in uterine shape during human pregnancy. Growth of all uterine dimensions continues throughout pregnancy (Fig. 2). The length of the cephalocaudal axis exceeds the other dimensions from shortly after 12 weeks onward. Growth of the transverse diameter slows during the last third of pregnancy, and the anteroposterior diameter increases more rapidly during this time. Thus the uterus becomes more rounded in transverse cross section in late pregnancy, a change to be expected from increasing distention of a hollow organ. The ratio of the greatest transverse cross-sectional area to uterine length increases steadily. The pattern of uterine growth in human pregnancy therefore seems to reflect the basic shape of the organ and the predominating arrangement of its fibers in a diagonal spiral rather than a circular-longitudinal arrangement. If a change occurs in the mechanism of uterine accommodation to growth of the products of conception, it cannot be identified from the uterine configuration.

Uterine contractions, which occur as often as three to four per minute at the time of ovulation (7), are suppressed during pregnancy. Although contractions continue to occur, they are much reduced in frequency and intensity and are infrequently

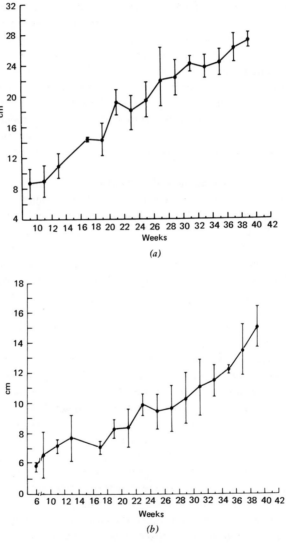

(a)

(b)

Figure 2. Ultrasound measurements of uterine size throughout pregnancy. (*a*) longitudinal measurements; (*b*) anterioposterior dimensions; (*c*) transverse dimensions. From Gohari, P., Berkowitz, R. L., and Hobbins, J. C. *Am. J. Obstet, Gynecol.* 127:255, 1977, by permission.

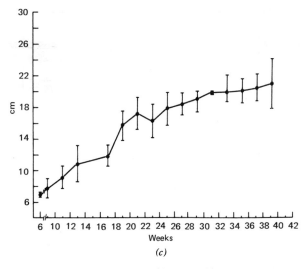

Figure 2. (Continued.)

appreciated by the gravida. Uterine contractility may be enhanced during febrile states, in association with urinary tract infections (8) and orgasm (9). There is a circadian periodicity in uterine contractility in nonpregnant women and rhesus monkeys, and this has been shown to persist during pregnancy in the monkeys (10).

The factor presumed to be responsible for the quieting of myometrial activity during pregnancy is progesterone (the "progesterone block"). The inhibition of myometrial contractility is greater at the placental sites than elsewhere in rabbits (11), and even in subhuman primates the uterus can be seen to bulge outward over the placentas during contractions induced by manipulation at laparotomy. The frequency and intensity of uterine contractions increase as labor approaches, as does the sensitivity of the myometrium to many oxytocic agents. The factors responsible for the overriding of the progesterone block are dealt with elsewhere (Chapter 4).

Uterine Blood Flow (UBF)

Increased uterine blood flow is another prominent feature in the accommodation of the reproductive tract to pregnancy. UBF fluctuates during the ovarian cycle in the nonpregnant female. In sheep, there is a remarkable increase in UBF coincident with the estrogen surge at ovulation, with a decrease to lower levels thereafter (12). Thermal conductance studies (13) indicate a similar midcycle flow peak in women, but there are no direct measurements.

With the occurrence of pregnancy, the decreasing trend of UBF during the luteal phase is reversed. Human UBF has been measured at the time of hysterotomy between 10 and 28 weeks' amenorrhea (14) and at the time of cesarean section at term (15–17). UBF increased progressively from approximately 50 ml/min at 10 weeks to 75 ml/min at 16 weeks, 185 ml/min at 28 weeks, and averaged approximately 500 ml/min at term (Fig. 3). The range of values at term was quite wide, with more than a fourfold variation being found in one study. Calculated in relation to the weight of the uterus, fetus, placenta, and membranes, UBF averaged 89 ml/(min) (kg) in the 10- to 28-week

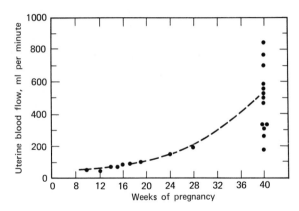

Figure 3. Uterine blood flow in human pregnancy. Reproduced with permission from Hytten, F. E., and Leitch, I. *Physiology of Human Pregnancy,* ed. 2. Oxford, Blackwell, 1971.

patients (14) and 110 (17) and 124 (16) ml/(min) (kg) in the women at term. The variation in UBF related to weight was somewhat smaller, but there was still a twofold or greater difference between the highest and lowest values in each series. Because of the range of flow rates observed, there is no statistically significant change in UBF in relation to the weight of the uterus and conceptus over the course of pregnancy. On the other hand, these data may also be interpreted as suggesting a rising trend. Since maternal placental blood flow is greater per unit of weight than myometrial blood flow and since the ratio of placental to uterine weights is greater at term than at 10 or 20 weeks, one might expect some increase in relative UBF as pregnancy advances. Unfortunately, direct measurements of placental perfusion are not presently possible in human subjects. In monkeys, the intervillous space receives approximately 90% of the total UBF in late pregnancy (18).

The data from human pregnancy were obtained with the subjects anesthetized and lying supine during surgery. Since both anesthesia and the supine position can reduce cardiac output significantly, the true basal UBF may be greater than the measurements have indicated, especially in the patients at term.

Despite the shortcomings of the available data, these values indicate that the blood flow to the pregnant human uterus increases at least as rapidly as the growth of the organ and its contents. This situation has also been demonstrated quite clearly in pregnant sheep, where UBF per kilogram of pregnant uterus, fetus, and placenta remains essentially constant over the last half of pregnancy (19). The mechanisms responsible for matching blood flow to growth of the pregnant uterus have not been fully defined. There is clearly a major decrease in uterine vascular resistance, for UBF rises despite only minor changes in maternal blood pressure. In women, expansion of the uterine vascular beds, especially the intervillous space and uteroplacental arteries and veins, is undoubtedly an important factor. The uteroplacental (spiral) arteries, microscopic at the time of implantation, have reached lumen diameters on the order of 1.5 to 2 mm at term (Fig. 4). The cross-sectional area of the intervillous space must also increase as the placenta grows, contributing to the decrease in overall uteroplacental vascular resistance. The magnitude of this change cannot be established with certainty, for the delivered placenta, or even one fixed in situ after hysterectomy or post mortem, is much collapsed from its condition in life when it is distended by maternal blood.

Ultrasonographic measurements (20) indicate that the average placental volume increases from about 60 ml at 10 weeks to approximately 140 ml at 16 weeks, 500 ml at 28 weeks, and 950 ml at 38 weeks. If the relative proportion of villi and intervillous space in the placenta does not change greatly during the last two trimesters of pregnancy, there is reasonably good agreement between the increase in the maternal blood space in the placenta and the available data on the increase in UBF from 16 weeks to term.

Another factor probably contributing to the decrease in uterine vascular resistance is the replacement of the muscular and elastic elements in the walls of the distal segments of the uteroplacental arteries by epithelioid cells of trophoblastic origin (21,22). The change involves the endometrial parts of the vessels and even extends for a distance into the intramyometrial segments. These parts of the arteries thus lose their contractile components and presumably their ability to maintain any resting vasoconstrictor tone. Vasoconstrictive capabilities are retained by the more proximal segments of the uteroplacental arteries.

Lest the situation be considered a simple matter of growing vascular beds in an enlarging organ, it should be pointed out that the increase in UBF with fetal growth in

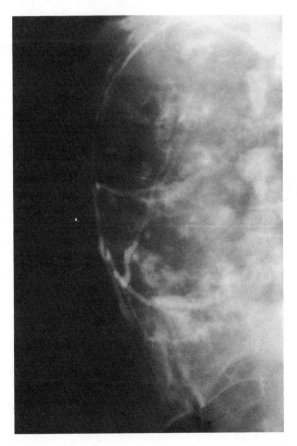

Figure 4. Radioangiogram of the human uteroplacental circulation. Note the relatively large size of the vessels supplying the intervillous space. Photograph courtesy of Prof. T. K. A. B. Eskes, Catholic University, Nijmegen, The Netherlands.

the last half of pregnancy in sheep occurs during a time when there is no growth of the placental cotyledons (23). A fetal or fetoplacental influence is suggested by the observation that the UBF of pregnant sheep fell by 50% within 30 min following fetal death (24). The decrease in flow occurred well after the fall in oxygen consumption, which was nearly immediate, but preceded any change in maternal plasma estrogen or progesterone levels.

The different uterine vascular beds have been shown to behave differently as pregnancy advances in sheep (25). In early pregnancy, both the myometrial and caruncular (maternal placental) vascular beds exhibited pressure-flow curves that were significantly convex toward the flow axis, indicating an autoregulatory capability. The myometrial bed retained this pattern in late pregnancy; however, the pressure-flow characteristics of the vessels supplying the caruncles changed markedly at about one-third of term. After this time, the pressure-flow relationship for the maternal placental vessels became nearly linear, with a slight convexity toward the pressure axis (Fig. 5). This pattern is consistent with a widely dilated vascular bed having little or no resting vasoconstrictor tone. The time of this change corresponds to the establishment of the definitive placental structure in sheep. It is also a time when maternal placental blood flow increases rapidly. These findings suggest a specific dilator effect on the caruncular arteries that does not affect the myoendometrial vessels. Greiss (26) has recently described a uterine vasodilator effect of glucosamine, a substance present in the Wharton's jelly of the fetal placental cotyledons in sheep, that might account for such a localized, differential vasodilatation.

The nonplacental vascular beds are more sensitive to the constrictor effects of epinephrine and norepinephrine than are the caruncular vessels in pregnant sheep (27,28), demonstrating another aspect of differential reactivity of the uterine vasculature in this species. An even greater difference seems to exist in the response to vasodilators,

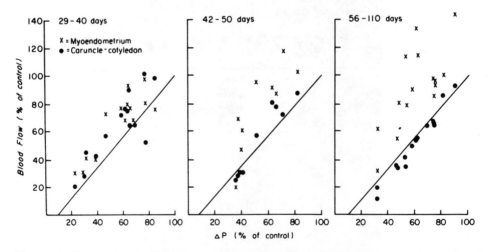

Figure 5. Changes in the blood pressure–blood flow relationship in the myoendometrial and caruncle-cotyledonary vascular beds during pregnancy in the sheep. Up to 40 days, the relationship in both beds is convex toward the flow axis, indicating the presence of a degree of autoregulation. This configuration is preserved or even accentuated in the myoendometrial circulation later in pregnancy, whereas it is progressively lost in the maternal placental vasculature. From Greiss, F. C., Anderson, S. G., and Still, J. G. *Am. J. Obstet. Gynecol.* 126:799, 1976, with permission.

for virtually all the decrease in uterine vascular resistance observed with several agents could be accounted for by dilatation in the myoendometrial beds (29). In primates, also, the likelihood of differential reactivity is suggested by the finding that myometrial blood flow increased during uterine contractions and that to the placenta was markedly decreased (18).

Endocrine factors probably contribute to the increase in uterine blood flow during pregnancy. This is especially true for the uterine hyperemia in early gestation. It was noted earlier that UBF increases with the preovulatory estrogen surge in sheep, and estrogens have been shown to be potent uterine vasodilators in oophorectomized sheep (30). The dilatation involves all parts of the uterine vasculature, and there is no preferential redistribution of flow to the caruncles (31). Estrogens also evoke a modest (25 to 40%) increase in UBF in pregnant ewes (32,33). Flow to the caruncles increases (25%), but proportionately less than myometrial or endometrial flow (33). Estrogens may not be essential for the maintenance and increase in uterine flow in established pregnancy, however, for the placental blood flow in rabbits ovariectomized on day 7 of pregnancy and given supplemental progesterone was as high, per gram of tissue, as that of the intact animals (34).

The UBF does not increase immediately in response to estrogen administration. Rather, the rise begins between 30 and 60 min following the injection, and maximal flow is attained after about 2 hr (30). This pattern suggests that estrogen itself is not the vasoactive agent but that one or more intermediary substances are involved in the response. The estrogen effect on UBF can be blocked by cycloheximide (30), an inhibitor of protein synthesis, but not by actinomycin D, which inhibits RNA production (35). The mechanism awaits further clarification.

Progesterone reduces the magnitude of the uterine vasodilator response to estrogen but favors redistribution of flow in favor of the caruncles (potential placental sites) in nonpregnant ewes (36).

Prostaglandins seem to be involved importantly in the regulation of UBF. E-series prostaglandins are potent uterine vasodilators in nonpregnant dogs (37) and sheep (38). PGE's are present in increased levels in uterine vein blood of pregnant rabbits (39) and dogs (40). Inhibition of PG synthesis in these animals decreases UBF (39,40). potentiates the uterine vasoconstrictor response to sympathetic nerve stimulation (41), and blunts the vasodilator response to exogenous estrogens (42). $PGF_{2\alpha}$ antagonized both the vasodilator action of PGE's (43) and the increase in UBF following estrogens (38). These observations, together with findings in other vascular beds, strongly suggest that locally produced prostaglandins are involved in regulation of flow in the myoendometrial vascular beds. To what extent these findings apply to the uteroplacental arteries in late pregnancy remains to be shown.

Some observations suggest an interaction between prostaglandins, the renin-angiotensin system, and adrenergic receptors in the regulation of UBF. A reninlike enzyme is present in the placenta or endometrium of several species, including man (44). Plasma renin activity of uterine vein blood was found to increase greatly during experimental uterine ischemia in nephrectomized pregnant rabbits (45). In the same animals, infusion of angiotensin in low dosage resulted in uterine vasodilatation. The effect was blocked by pretreatment with the beta-adrenergic blocker propranolol. In monkeys, angiotensin II infusions resulted in increased levels of PGE in uterine vein blood and decreased plasma renin activity (45). These findings have led to the suggestion (45,46) that uterine renin is released in increased quantities in response to a reduction in uterine perfusion. The elevated plasma renin activity catalyses increased production of angiotensin II, which in turn effects a redistribution of cardiac output in favor of the uterus by constricting cutaneous and splanchnic beds while dilating vessels in the uterus. PGE is thought to be involved as a mediator of the angiotensin effect on the uterine vessels, perhaps with intermediate activation of beta-adrenergic receptors.

The role of the autonomic nervous system in the accommodation of the uterine vascular beds to pregnancy is not clear. It has already been noted that there is little if any resting vasoconstrictor tone in the uteroplacental arteries of sheep after midpregnancy, although the nonplacental parts of the uterine vasculature retain their tone. Thus, isoproterenol (29,47) and acetylcholine (48) and their respective blockers (48,49) have been found to cause only minor changes in uterine vascular resistance during pregnancy in this species. The small changes observed in some studies are probably attributable to the nonplacental vasculature. Bell (50) has presented evidence of the existence of cholinergic vasodilator nerves in the parametrial segments of the uterine vessels in several species, including man, and argues for a role of these fibers in maintaining the hyperemia of pregnancy. These nerves were said to be absent in sheep (51), perhaps explaining the inability to demonstrate significant cholinergic influences on the pregnant UBF in this species in which so much of the investigation of UBF has been carried out.

The uterine vasculature retains its ability to constrict in response to sympathetic nerve stimulation (52) or alpha-adrenergic agonists. The reactivity to exogenous catecholamines is reduced, as noted previously. Neurally mediated vasoconstriction may also be attenuated, for there is reduced catecholamine fluorescence associated with arteries in the human uterus during pregnancy (53).

Although the changes in UBF over the latter half of pregnancy are such that the uterine arteriovenous differences for O_2 and CO_2 are relatively constant, the predominating evidence is that the uteroplacental vessels do not respond to changes in the tensions of the respiratory gases in blood with significant dilatation or constriction.

The Cervix and Lower Reproductive Tract

These structures also experience considerable hyperemia during pregnancy. Early, this accounts for softening and cyanosis of the cervix, prominent vaginal artery pulsations, and transudation of fluid into the vaginal lumen. Later there may be mucosal edema with a decrease in the vaginal rugations, and even the development of varicosities of the vagina and vulva. Estrogen has been shown to increase blood flow to the cervix and vagina, and it has been suggested that the prelabor estrogen surge, in sheep, may serve to prepare the lower tract for parturition (54).

The cervix also undergoes considerable hypertrophy in pregnancy. There is increased mitotic activity of the endocervical cells, and the squamocolumnar junction moves out onto the vaginal part. This "eversion" is also promoted by edema and softening of the cervix and by increased secretion and retention in the cervical clefts of thick, viscid mucus. With the onset of of cervical dilatation, much of the former endocervical glandular tissue is expelled along with the mucus plug.

The cervix in late pregnancy contains less collagen per gram of tissue than in the nonpregnant state, and the collagen fibers are swollen and loosely associated (55). The further softening and increased distensibility that normally occur prior to the onset of labor are familiar to every obstetrician. In the absence of these changes, the cervix dilates poorly, if at all. Cervical compliance increased abruptly prior to the onset of uterine contractions in spontaneous or dexamethasone-induced labor in sheep (56), demonstrating that this change in the maternal organism is a definite part of the sequence of events initiated by the fetus and leading to parturition. The prelabor change in cervical compliance is probably mediated by prostaglandins. There is similar but less pronounced softening of pelvic ligaments and fascias.

CARDIOVASCULAR SYSTEM

The cardiovascular system has been aptly described as "hyperdynamic" during pregnancy. There are major changes in cardiac output and regional blood flow distribution and lesser alterations in heart rate and blood pressure.

The Heart

Elevation of the diaphragm during pregnancy displaces the heart into a more transverse position. The cardiac apex is moved upward and to the left and rotated slightly forward. The electrical axis is rotated clockwise an average of 15°. Cardiac volume increases about 75 ml (57,58). This increase could result from greater cardiac filling, for both blood volume and cardiac stroke volume are increased in pregnancy. An element of cardiac hypertrophy has also been suggested (58).

Systolic heart murmurs are present in a large proportion of gravidas, probably produced by increased flow rates in the cardiac outflow tracts plus reduced blood viscosity. A continuous murmur with systolic accentuation may sometimes be heard, arising from increased flow in the arteries supplying the breasts.

Premature beats are more frequent in pregnancy, and pregnancy may increase the susceptibility to paroxysmal supraventricular tachycardias (59). The mechanisms behind these effects have not been established, but it is likely that they represent some aspect of steroid hormone activity on the myocardium.

Cardiac performance during pregnancy has been evaluated by measurements of the systolic time intervals (60,61). The findings of two studies were in disagreement with regard to changes during the first two trimesters; however, both groups of investigators observed a prolongation of the preejection period (PEP) and shortening of ventricular ejection time (VET) during the last trimester. The alterations in the systolic time intervals were accentuated in the supine position but were present with the subjects on their side as well (60). This pattern of change in systolic time intervals could be produced by either reduced cardiac filling or impaired cardiac contractility. Cardiac stroke volume is smaller in late pregnancy than earlier and is further reduced in the supine position (see below). On the other hand, altered cardiac filling does not entirely explain the prolongation of PEP and shortening of VET as compared with nonpregnant subjects. Moreover, the ratio of PEP/VET remained elevated after delivery. Thus, some change in myocardial contractility may occur during pregnancy, particularly in the last trimester. Both estrogens and progesterone have been reported to affect myocardial contractility. The subject warrants further study.

Cardiac Output

Cardiac output increases by 30 to 40% from nonpregnant values on the order of 4.5 to 5 liters/min to levels of 6.5 to 7 liters/min during much of pregnancy. The major part of the increase is present by the end of the first trimester. Cardiac output is sustained at high levels throughout the second and early third trimesters, but there is disagreement still about the course of cardiac output in late pregnancy.

Early investigators failed to take into account the effect of posture on circulatory dynamics during pregnancy. As a result, their studies, which were definitely or presumably carried out with the subjects supine, tended to show a variable decline in cardiac output beginning late in the second or early in the third trimester. But when the gravida in late pregnancy lies supine, the uterus compresses the inferior vena cava, interfering with venous return to the heart and reducing cardiac filling and cardiac output (62–64). If collateral pathways are inadequate, the effect may be severe enough to cause syncope (62). The uterus also impedes flow through the iliac veins in the sitting or standing position, but the interference with circulatory dynamics is less than in the supine position.

Three more recent studies of cardiac output have been carried out with attention to patient position (Table I) (65–67). Two of the studies, the ones of Pyörälä (65) and Lees et al. (66), showed that the increase in cardiac output measured with the subject in the lateral position was sustained throughout the latter two-thirds of pregnancy, with no decrease at term. In contrast, Ueland et al. (67) observed a decline of nearly 20% in the cardiac output between 28 and 32 weeks and 38 and 40 weeks in their subjects even when the measurements were carried out in the lateral position (Fig. 6). Their late pregnancy values were still approximately 15% greater than cardiac outputs measured 6 to 8 weeks postpartum. The reason for the persisting discrepancy in these observations of cardiac output in late pregnancy is not clear. Pyörälä's study was cross-sectional, that of Lees et al. included both serial and cross-sectional measurements, and the measurements of Ueland et al. were semiserial in that all subjects were studied during each time period. Abdominal wall tension does not seem to have been a factor, for the patients studied serially by Lees et al. were all primigravidas. Gestational age is a possible explanation, though weak; for the late pregnancy measurements of Ueland et al. were carried out between 38 and 40 weeks, whereas the third trimester observations of Lees et al. were made between 34 weeks and term (mean not given) and those of Pyörälä, between 33 and 40 weeks (mean 35.9 weeks). Thus the question of a late pregnancy fall in cardiac output is not entirely settled.

Table I. Cardiac Output During Pregnancy

Source	Early	Mid		Late	Nonpregnant
		Time			
Pyörälä (65)		6.78*	6.97	6.76	5.04
		(17–24)†	(25–30)	(33–40)	
Lee et al. (66):					
Serial 5 subjects	6.10	6.18		6.26	
All subjects	5.92	6.18		5.93	
	(10–13)	(24–27)		(34–41)	
Ueland et al. (67)		6.9	7.0	5.7	5.0
		(20–24)	(28–32)	(38–40)	

* Values in liters per minute.

† Numbers in parentheses denote period in weeks' gestation.

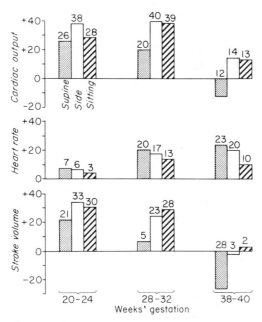

Figure 6. The effect of maternal position and gestational age on three parameters of cardiac function. Values are expressed as percent changes from nonpregnant measurements. The terminal decrease in cardiac output and stroke volume in lateral recumbency shown here has not been observed by some other investigators (see text). Reproduced by permission from Ueland, K., and Metcalfe, J. *Clin. Obstet. Gynecol.* 18:42, 1975.

Effect of Position and Exercise

Obviously, pregnant women do not spend all their time in lateral recumbency. Thus, data relating to cardiac output in other positions and during exercise are also relevant. There is agreement that during late pregnancy cardiac output in the supine position is less than that in the lateral position. But whereas Lees et al. (66) found a significant difference (20%) only in the third trimester, Ueland and coworkers (67) observed a discrepancy of 10% at midpregnancy increasing to 30% at term (Fig. 6). In fact, cardiac output in the supine position at term was lower than that measured after pregnancy. Cardiac output in the sitting position is intermediate between the supine and lateral recumbency values during the third trimester (67). Interestingly, Pyörälä (65) found that the decrease in cardiac output from the lateral recumbent to standing position was less in subjects in late pregnancy than in nonpregnant controls or in patients earlier in gestation. This may be related to the expanded blood volume of the pregnant woman.

Cardiac output rises to a higher level in response to a standard sitting exercise during pregnancy than in the nonpregnant state, and the absolute increment (in liters/min) is greater except perhaps in late pregnancy (67,68). Expressed as a proportion of the resting cardiac output, the response to mild exercise does not seem to vary greatly either over the course of pregnancy or between pregnancy and 6 to 8 weeks post partum. The proportionate response to moderate exercise appeared to be slightly greater in early pregnancy and somewhat less at term than in the nonpregnant state (67).

The energy cost of exercise is similar to nonpregnant (postpartum) values up until about 28 weeks. In late pregnancy, however, the energy expenditure of the pregnant woman is increased by 17% for standard bicycle exercise and 24% during level walking

(69). This extra energy expenditure of the pregnant woman is due only in part to her greater weight. The increase during non-weight-bearing exercise, such as on the bicycle exerciser, demonstrates that other factors also contribute. These include the increased cardiac work and greater ventilatory response to exercise during pregnancy, both of which represent additional energy costs to the gravida.

Arteriovenous O$_2$ Difference

The arteriovenous difference for oxygen between the aorta and right heart is reduced in early and midpregnancy to about 0.8 to 0.9 of the nonpregnant value. The arteriovenous difference increases progressively to equal or exceed nonpregnant levels at term, probably varying according to position. After mild exercise, the arteriovenous difference was less during pregnancy even at term than in the same subjects with equivalent exercise postpartum (67,68). Thus the increase in cardiac output during pregnancy, except perhaps just at term, appears to exceed the increased whole body need for oxygen associated with pregnancy, whether at rest or with mild exercise. The exaggerated cardiovascular responses to pregnancy and to exercise during pregnancy may perhaps be regarded as a mechanism for minimizing the likelihood of inadequate tissue oxygenation during this vital time.

Heart Rate and Stroke Volume

The increase in cardiac output during pregnancy is brought about by increases in both heart rate and stroke volume. It appears that in early pregnancy the contribution of stroke volume is the greater factor and near term increase of heart rate predominates.

The data of Pyörälä (65) and Ueland et al. (67) show stroke volume to be 20 to 30% above nonpregnant levels, depending on the subject's position, at 20 to 24 weeks. There was a slight decline to 28 to 32 weeks in Ueland's subjects and a further decrease in late pregnancy to nonpregnant levels, or even below nonpregnant values in the supine position (Fig. 6). Pyörälä's subjects exhibited a decline only in the 33- to 40-week period, when stroke volume was still about 18% above that of the nonpregnant controls.

Heart rate is generally reported to increase by about 8 bpm by the end of the first trimester, with a further gradual increase to about 15 bpm above nonpregnant levels by late pregnancy. Ueland et al. (67) found the rise to be somewhat slower, with an average increase of 4 bpm by 20 to 24 weeks, 12 bpm at 28 to 32 weeks, and 14 bpm at 38 to 40 weeks in the lateral position.

Blood Pressure and Vascular Resistance

Arterial blood pressure decreases somewhat during pregnancy. In most studies, average values for the decrease have been in the range of 3 to 5 mm Hg for systolic pressure and 5 to 10 mm Hg for diastolic pressure. Individual women may exhibit a much greater decline. The lowest readings are obtained in the second trimester, with a rise toward prepregnant levels during the last 2 lunar months. The pulse pressure is widened slightly during the first and second trimesters and narrows to nonpregnant values at term. There is a diurnal variation in blood pressure in pregnancy as in the nonpregnant woman (70), the lowest pressures occuring during sleep. The nocturnal fall is greater in hypertensive gravidas than in normotensives. Blood pressure in the supine or erect position is somewhat lower than that in lateral recumbency (65,71), especially in late pregnancy.

Since cardiac output increases during pregnancy and blood pressure decreases slightly, there is obviously a decrease in total peripheral vascular resistance. Furthermore, the decrease is greater in early pregnancy than at term (65), thus demonstrating that the vasodilatation involves vascular beds other than the uterus.

Venous pressures in the legs increase progressively during pregnancy, whereas arm and central venous pressure do not. The effect is due to compression of the pelvic veins and inferior vena cava by the uterus (64). The elevated femoral venous pressure drops abruptly at delivery.

Regional Redistribution of Blood Flow

Throughout most of pregnancy, the increment in cardiac output greatly exceeds the increase in uterine blood flow. Only in the final weeks of pregnancy does the uterus receive a major fraction of the extra blood pumped: about one-third, if the data of Pyörälä (65) and Lees (66) are correct, and essentially all, if the terminal fall in cardiac output observed by Ueland (67 is the true pattern. Other sites where increased blood flow has been measured during pregnancy include the kidneys, about 400 ml/min, and skin, estimated as high as 500 ml/min (72). The gut has also been suggested as a recipient of increased blood flow during pregnancy (72); however, there are no data on this point.

Blood flow to the pelvic organs other than the uterus and to the breasts also increases during pregnancy, although the amount has not been quantitated in human subjects. The physical evidence of hyperemia of the cervix and vagina beginning early in the first trimester is familiar to every obstetrician. Increased blood flow to the breasts is reflected in engorgement, and edema in early pregnancy and later is suggested by the increased prominence of the subcutaneous veins. Animal data on mammary blood flow is probably not applicable to human pregnancy, for in goats udder blood flow increased only on the last day of pregnancy (73), whereas the presumptive evidence of breast hyperemia is present in women from an early stage of pregnancy.

Blood flow to the extremities has been studied by means of plethysmography and [133]xenon clearance from muscles. Total forearm blood increased progressively from 16 to 20 weeks to term, whereas muscle flow remained constant (74). The increase was thus taken to represent perfusion of the skin. It is of interest that Spetz and Jansson (74) found no significant increase above nonpregnant values in total forearm flow until after the twentieth week of pregnancy. If this reflects to any extent the pattern of cutaneous blood flow in general, it raises anew the question of destination of the increased cardiac output in the late first and early second trimesters. Blood flow to the lower extremities was found to decrease in late pregnancy (75), thus supporting the suggestion of Hytten and Leitch (76) that the increase in uterine blood flow in late pregnancy occurred largely at the expense of leg flow.

Measured blood flow to the brain, liver, and skeletal muscle does not increase during pregnancy.

Figure 7 summarizes schematically the distribution of the extra cardiac output during pregnancy according to present concepts.

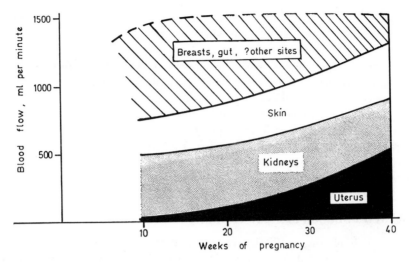

Figure 7. Distribution of the increased cardiac output in pregnancy. From Hytten, F. E., and Leitch, I. *Physiology of Human Pregnancy,* ed., 2. Oxford, Blackwell, 1971, by permission.

Mechanism of the Circulatory Changes

The occurrence of increased cardiac output, elevated renal blood flow, and decreased total peripheral resistance early in pregnancy, together with other extrareproductive tract changes later on, strongly suggests that hormonal mechanisms are responsible. Estrogens administered to nonpregnant sheep have been found to produce an increase in cardiac output, heart rate, and plasma volume and a decrease in peripheral vascular resistance (77). The dilator action of estrogens on vascular beds in the reproductive tract was discussed earlier, and similar effects have also been described in other vascular beds, e.g., skin. Prolactin has also been shown to cause a decrease in blood pressure and increase in blood volume in rats (78). Animals receiving high doses of prolactin also became hyporesponsive to angiotensin (see below). Prolactin is elevated during pregnancy and also in response to estrogen administration.

The pregnant patient becomes hyporesponsive to the vasopressor effects of infused angiotensin, but not to those of norepinephrine (79). This appears to be due more to a change in arteriolar responsiveness than to elevated baseline levels of circulating angiotensin in pregnancy or to changes in blood volume (80). Maintenance of vascular tone and blood pressure is more dependent on activity of the autonomic sympathetic nerves during pregnancy than at other times, for there is an exaggerated hypotensive response to the sympathetic effects of ganglionic blockade (81) or a conduction anesthesia. The increased sympathetic activity might be compensating for either the effects of a circulating vasodilator (72) or inhibition of vascular responsiveness to other vasotonic mechanisms.

Thus, although there are indications of some of the factors affecting the cardiovascular system during pregnancy, there remains much to be learned about the interactions of, for example, steroid and other hormones, catecholamines, angiotensin, and prostaglandins in bringing about the circulatory changes of pregnancy.

CHANGES IN THE BLOOD

Plasma Volume

Plasma volume increases, starting about the midpoint of the first trimester, and reaches values that average 1250 to 1300 ml above nonpregnant levels by 32 to 34 weeks (82–88). This represents an expansion of plasma volume of about 50% (Fig. 8). There is some uncertainty about the further course of the plasma volume in pregnancy. Some studies have shown a decline of 200 to 300 ml during the last 4 to 6 weeks (82–84), whereas others have not (85–88). In the latter studies, however, the rate of increase was slower during the terminal weeks of pregnancy than earlier. As with cardiac output, postural factors may have influenced the studies of plasma volume. Chesley and Duffus (89) have confirmed that the apparent plasma volume is greater in the lateral than in the supine position in late pregnancy; however, the effect seemed to be as great at the end of the second trimester as later on.

The variation among individual subjects in the absolute plasma volume and the amount of rise during pregnancy has been large in most studies, although the average values are fairly consistent. The absolute increase does not seem to be particularly related to nonpregnant plasma volume. Multiparas probably experience a greater increase (by 200 to 250 ml) than do primagravidas (72). The increase in plasma volume is about 50% greater in women with twins than with single pregnancies (85). A positive correlation has been observed between the amount of increase in plasma volume and the birthweight of the baby (84,88,90), and a few observations suggest that the plasma volume increase is low in women with poor reproductive performance (72,90). Plasma volume increase thus appears to reflect in a general way the competence of the placenta (or fetoplacental unit).

HEMATOCRIT AND HEMOGLOBIN

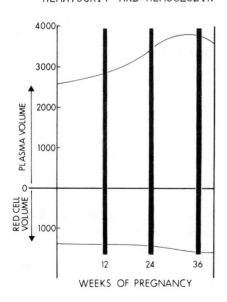

Figure 8. Schematic illustration of changes in plasma volume and total red cell volume during pregnancy. Hematocrit changes may be judged from the relative contribution of each compartment to the total vertical dimension, as at the three bars. From *Physiologic Changes in Pregnancy*. Raritan, N.J., Ortho Pharmaceutical Co., 1974, by permission.

Red Cell Volume, Hemoglobin and Hematocrit

The total volume of red blood cells also increases during pregnancy; however, the proportionate increase is less than that in plasma volume. As in the case of plasma volume, there is considerable variation in individual values. There is, further, the question of whether a small decrease in total red blood cell volume occurs in late pregnancy. The most reasonable estimate at present is that the gravida who does not take supplemental iron increases her red blood cell volume by an average of 250 ml by late pregnancy. When supplemental iron is taken, the average increase is closer to 400 to 450 ml (72). These values represent an increase of 17 and 30%, respectively, above the average nonpregnant values.

Since neither the amount of hemoglobin per erythrocyte nor the volume of individual erythrocytes changes significantly during pregnancy, the total body hemoglobin rises in parallel with the total red blood cell volume, that is, approximately 85 g without iron supplementation and 150 g with supplemental iron.

Expansion of the red blood cell volume is brought about by increased production rather than prolongation of red blood cell life span (92). The stimulus to increased erythrocyte production has been attributed to elevated levels of erythropoietin (93) and to potentiation of erythropoietin by human placental lactogen (94).

Erythrocyte 2,3-diphosphoglycerate (2,3-DPG) is increased during pregnancy (e.g., 95,96). This decreases the affinity of maternal hemoglobin for oxygen, thus favoring dissociation of hemoglobin-bound oxygen in peripheral tissues, including the intervillous space of the placenta.

Both the hemoglobin concentration and hematocrit of peripheral blood tend to fall during pregnancy. This is a dilution effect, because the proportional increase in plasma volume is greater than that in red cell mass, especially before the thirtieth gestational week. Thus in the absence of supplemental iron, but in previously well-nourished women, the hemoglobin concentration averages about 1.5 to 2.0 g per 100 ml below nonpregnant levels at 30 to 32 weeks. The corresponding figure for hematocrit is a drop of about 5 to 6%. The decrease can be reduced substantially by iron supplementation; however, even with supplemental iron, the early third trimester hemoglobin and hematocrit are likely to be somewhat below prepregnant levels in healthy gravidas.

From 32 to 34 weeks until term, the trend is reversed. Red blood cell mass increases more, or decreases less, than plasma volume, and hemoglobin and hematocrit rise by about 0.5 g and 1 to 2%, respectively, toward term.

White Blood Cells

The total white blood cell count increases to about 10,500 per mm^3 in late pregnancy. This is due predominantly to a rise in the number of polymorphonuclear leucocytes.

Platelets

The platelet count is reduced somewhat during pregnancy as a result of hemodilution. Platelet production and life span are normal in women with normal pregnancies; but platelet life span has been found to be shortened, and platelet turnover accelerated, in association with fetal growth retardation and placental infarcts (97). This may result from injury to the platelets in the uteroplacental circulation in the abnormal pregnancies.

Electrolytes and Osmolality

The concentrations of most electrolytes in serum are slightly lower during pregnancy than in the nonpregnant state (98). Plasma osmolality also decreases from nonpregnant values around 290 mOsm/l to the range of 280 mOsm/l (99). These alterations occur in the first trimester. There are no significant changes from 12 weeks to term (100).

Plasma Proteins and Colloid Osmotic Pressure

The total concentration of serum proteins decreases by about 1 g per 100 ml during pregnancy. Most of the decrease occurs during the first trimester, with variable but minor changes reported by different investigators during the rest of pregnancy.

The degree and pattern of fall in plasma proteins reflects mainly the decrease in serum albumin, which also amounts to about 1 g per 100 ml (e.g., 99,100,101). Alpha-1, alpha-2, and beta-globulin rise slowly and progressively. Gamma-globulin probably decreases slightly, although differing results have been reported. The IgG component, which is the major immunoglobulin transferred to the fetus, falls progressively (102).

Colloid osmotic pressure decreases in parallel with serum albumin levels (99,100). The small increases in the relatively inactive globulin fractions affect colloid osmotic pressure only minimally.

Fibrinogen increases progressively throughout pregnancy, with the term values being 30 to 50% above nonpregnant levels. As a result, the erythrocyte sedimentation rate is elevated during normal pregnancy and is thus of no diagnostic value.

Serum Lipids

The total serum lipid concentration rises progressively from the end of the first trimester and is 40 to 50% above nonpregnant levels at term (103). There may be a slight decrease early in the first trimester. All components of the serum lipids are increased, with the triglyceride fraction showing the largest proportionate rise (104).

Blood Coagulation

The large increase in fibrinogen concentration and small decrease in platelet count were noted above. Of the other principal clotting factors, VII, VIII, IX, and X are increased during pregnancy (105,106), whereas prothrombin and factors V and XII are reduced (106,108). From the clinical laboratory standpoint, the Quick one-stage prothrombin time and the partial thromboplastin time are shortened slightly, and bleeding and clotting time are unchanged.

The components of the fibrinolytic system are also altered during pregnancy. Plasminogen levels are probably increased, although this has not been a uniform finding. The level of circulating plasminogen activator is decreased (109), and clot lysis is prolonged. Levels of fibrin degradation products rise progressively in normal pregnancy (109), an observation suggesting that the fibrinolytic system is compensating for an accelerated rate of intravascular coagulation. It is not clear whether the increased fibrin formation is a widespread phenomenon in multiple vascular beds or limited mainly to the intervillous space. The reduced levels of plasminogen activator in pregnancy would seem to enhance the likelihood of significant obstruction of microcirculatory beds during episodes of greatly increased intravascular coagulation, as, for example, with eclampsia, abruptio placentae, or severe sepsis.

The alterations in the levels of clotting factors and plasminogen are probably brought about by the action of estrogens on the liver. The placenta has been implicated in the reduced fibrinolytic activity, for this increases promptly after delivery (110).

THE RESPIRATORY SYSTEM

Anatomic Changes

During pregnancy the diaphragm rises about 4 cm, the lower ribs flare outward, and the subcostal angle widens. The transverse diameter of the lower thorax increases by about 2 cm. The excursion of the diaphragm increases, and the abdominal muscles are less active in breathing movements. These changes occur early in pregnancy, well in advance of any possible mechanical effects from the enlarging uterus. The changes in the shape of the thorax and in the mechanics of breathing have the effect of reducing somewhat the pulmonary residual volume and enhancing the efficiency of mixing of the tidal air volume in the alveoli (Fig. 9).

There is increased prominence of the pulmonary vasculation in chest radiographs during pregnancy because of the increased central vascular volume.

Functional Changes

Respiratory muscle volume is increased early in pregnancy and rises progressively to about 40% above nonpregnant levels at term. The increase in ventilation is due almost

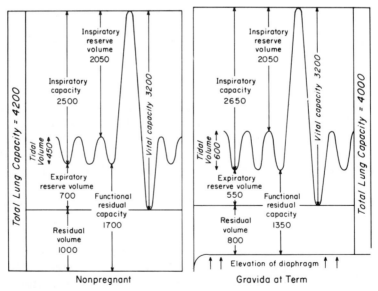

Figure 9. Lung volumes and capacities in the nonpregnant woman and the gravida at term. Reproduced with permission from Bonica, J. J. *Principles and Practice of Obstetric Analgesia and Anesthesia.* Philadelphia, Davis, 1972.

entirely to an increase in the tidal volume, since respiratory rate does not change significantly (111). Maximum breathing capacity and timed vital capacity are normally unchanged. Lung compliance and specific airway conductance are also unchanged in pregnancy (112).

Just as the change in the configuration of the thorax precedes significant uterine enlargement, so also does the rise in respiratory minute volume exceed at all stages the increase in oxygen consumption. These changes in the minute volume and mechanics of breathing are the result of enhanced sensitivity of the respiratory center to CO_2, caused by progesterone, perhaps with some synergism from estrogens (113). As a result, alveolar and arterial blood CO_2 tensions are reduced from about 39 mm Hg in the nonpregnant woman to near 31 mm Hg in pregnancy. This is compensated by a reduction in plasma bicarbonate levels, so that arterial blood pH does not change. The changes in respiratory function thus become interrelated with those in blood composition, for the reduction in bicarbonate (about 2 mEq/liter) requires a decrease in serum sodium and adjustments for maintaining the lowered plasma osmolality (72).

Another consequence of the enhanced respiratory center sensitivity is a heightened awareness of the desire to breath and an exaggerated breathlessness on exertion experienced by some gravidas. Laboratory observations have confirmed the augmented ventilatory response to exercise in pregnancy (114). These symptoms should not be mistaken for pathologic dyspnea when no other evidence of cardiac of pulmonary decompensation is present.

Oxygen Consumption

The increase in oxygen consumption in late pregnancy has been estimated by Hytten and Leitch (72) to be approximately 31 ml/min, or about 15% more than the basal O_2 uptake in the nonpregnant state. Several published studies have shown much greater differences between late pregnancy and postpartum values (111,115). At term, the fetus and placenta account for about half of the extra oxygen consumption. Increased cardiac work and breathing effort account together for 30%, and the remainder probably represents largely the increased uterine and breast tissue (72).

RENAL FUNCTION AND THE URINARY TRACT

Anatomic Changes

The kidneys enlarge somewhat during pregnancy, as judged from intravenous pyelograms. The enlargement probably represents hyperemia and perhaps a degree of hypertrophy, since it is highly unlikely that new nephrons are added during pregnancy.

The changes in the ureter during pregnancy—dilatation, elongation, and often tortuosity—are well known. The increased volume of urine contained in the ureters and renal pelves results in a relative slowing of urine flow in these parts of the urinary tract and contributes to the predisposition of pregnant women to ascending urinary infections. The cause of ureteral dilatation now seems to be largely mechanical obstruction by the enlarging uterus (116) and ovarian veins (117). Resting intraureteric pressure above the pelvic brim has been found to be elevated during pregnancy, especially in the supine position, and to decrease to nonpregnant levels immediately after emptying of the uterus (118). The frequency and intensity of ureteral contractions were not reduced in the pregnant subjects. Such evidence contradicts the view that progesterone-induced hypotonia of the ureteral smooth muscle is a significant favor in the ureteral dilatation during pregnancy.

The bladder is progressively elevated by the enlarging uterus during the last two trimesters of pregnancy. The trigone area undergoes moderate hyperplasia and hypertrophy. In later pregnancy, the trigone may be stretched to the point of incompetence of the ureterovesical valves, with resultant vesicoureteral reflex, another factor predisposing to ascending urinary infections. The vesical wall and mucosa are also affected by the general pelvic hyperemia during pregnancy.

Changes in Renal Function

Renal blood flow and glomerular filtration rate are much elevated during pregnancy. The classic studies of Sims and Krantz (119) showed that effective renal plasma flow (RPF) was elevated 45% above nonpregnant levels to an average of about 725 ml/min by the beginning of the second trimester and was maintained near this level through the first half of the third trimester. RPF thereafter decreased to approximately 15% above nonpregnant values in the last weeks of pregnancy. It is likely that this terminal fall in RPF represented the effects of the supine position on cardiovascular dynamics. Chesley and Sloan (120) observed a difference of 20% in the RPF measured in the supine and lateral positions. If this amount is added to the late pregnancy values of Sims and Krantz, the terminal fall is largely eliminated (72).

Glomerular filtration rate (GFR) is elevated about 60% above nonpregnant levels (119,121). As with RPF, the increase in GFR is present by the end of the first trimester. Sims and Krantz did not observe a terminal fall in GFR, although a fall might have been expected from the late decline in their RPF values. The findings of other investigators in this regard have been inconsistent. Postural changes in GFR similar to those in RPF were confirmed by Chesley and Sloan (120). Davison and Hytten (121) found a late pregnancy decrease from 155 to 135 ml/min in the 24-hr endogenous creatinine clearance, whereas inulin and creatinine clearances measured in the sitting position during specific clearance studies changed insignificantly (Fig. 10). They concluded that GFR measurements are valid only for the conditions under which the measurements are made and that a late pregnancy fall in GFR may "truly represent the real life situation where the woman spends much of her time in positions that may not allow maximum clearance" (121).

Since GFR increases by a greater proportion during pregnancy than RPF (60 as compared to 45%), the proportion of plasma flow that is filtered (filtration fraction) increases.

The mechanism behind the increased RPF and GFR during pregnancy has not been defined. Estrogens do not appear to affect RPF (122). Sustained elevations of RPF and GFR are present in early diabetes and in acromegaly, both characterized by increased levels of growth hormone. The growth hormone-like actions of HPL have been suggested as a basis for the pregnancy changes in renal hemodynamics (72,123,130); however, the concept has not been proved.

Because of the increased RPF and GFR, the renal clearance of many substances is elevated during pregnancy. This accounts for a fall of serum concentrations of urea and creatinine, for example, to about two-thirds of their normal nonpregnant levels. The normal decrease in BUN and creatinine levels during pregnancy must be taken into

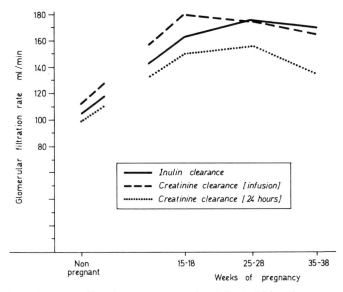

Figure 10. Mean glomerular filtration rate measured serially in 10 healthy women during pregnancy and at 8 to 12 weeks postpartum. There is a substantial decrease in the 24-hr endogenous creatinine clearance in late pregnancy, whereas the changes in inulin clearance and creatinine clearance (infusion) measured in the sitting position were not significant. From Davison, J. M., and Hytten, F. E. *J. Obstet. Gynaecol. Brit. Commonw.* 81:588, 1974, by permission.

account when these measurements are used as clinical screening tests for renal impairment. Results must be assessed by pregnancy norms and not by standard nonpregnant values.

Increased amounts of amino acids, water-soluble vitamins, glucose and several other sugars are lost in the urine during pregnancy. The pattern of excretion of different amino acids varies according to the stage of pregnancy (72). Thus it is likely that changes in tubular function are involved, as well as the effect of greater filtered loads presented to the renal tubules.

Glycosuria

The renal handling of glucose during pregnancy is of particular interest because of the frequent appearance of clinical glycosuria in normal gravidas and the necessity to differentiate this "renal glycosuria" from that of pregnancy-aggravated diabetes mellitus. The increase in glycosuria during pregnancy has usually been attributed to an increase in the filtered glucose load, reflecting the elevated GFR. This mechanism undoubtedly contributes; however, it does not entirely explain the increasing incidence of glycosuria in late pregnancy nor the variability of pattern. Although Christensen (124) and Welsh and Sims (125) found no change in the tubular reabsorptive ability for glucose during pregnancy, Davison and Hytten (126) have recently shown a decrease in this function in both glycosuric and nonglycosuric gravidas (Fig. 11). Moreover, the women who excreted increased amounts of glucose during pregnancy reabsorbed less glucose, in relation to the amount filtered, both during pregnancy and afterward, when they were not clinically glycosuric, than those women without pregnancy glycosuria. Thus, it would

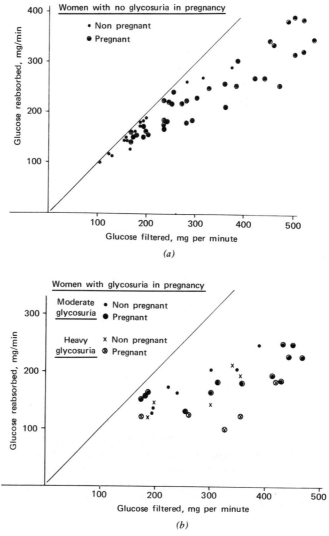

Figure 11. Relationship between the amount of glucose filtered and the amount reabsorbed during and after pregnancy in healthy women without (*a*) and with (*b*) glycosuria in pregnancy. No glycosuria indicates less than 150 mg/24 hr; moderate glycosuria, 150 to 600 mg/24 hr; heavy glycosuria, over 600 mg/24 hr. The proportion of glucose reabsorbed was decreased in all subject groups during pregnancy, and women with pregnancy glycosuria tended to reabsorb a smaller fraction of filtered glucose when nonpregnant than did women without glycosuria. From Davison, J. M., and Hytten, F. E., in *Carbohydrate Metabolism in Pregnancy and the Newborn.* Edinburgh, Churchill Livingston, 1975.

seem that "renal glycosuria" in pregnancy results from a preexisting deficiency in tubular function that is aggravated during gestation.

Excretion of Water and Sodium

The ability of the kidneys to excrete a sodium or water load is not impaired by normal pregnancy. In fact, the ability to excrete free water is enhanced during the middle trimester (127). Maximum urine flows in response to water diuresis are depressed in late pregnancy when measured in the sitting position (127), probably as a result of movement of the water into the extravascular space of the lower extremities (72). As might be expected, the excretion of both sodium and water is markedly reduced in the supine position (120,128). This is probably brought about both by a reduction in renal blood flow and by alterations in the factors regulating tubular reabsorption as a result of changes in the central blood volume. The normal nocturnal reduction in sodium and water excretion is reversed in pregnancy as a result of mobilization of interstitial fluid from the legs during the hours of recumbency. Hence, the frequent occurrence of nocturia in pregnant women.

The Renin Angiotensin System and Aldosterone

The production and circulating levels of renin, renin substrate, angiotension I and II, and aldosterone are all increased during pregnancy (129–133). On the other hand, the levels do not exhibit parallel trends, and the correlation among the levels of renin, angiotension II, and aldosterone that is observed in the nonpregnant state is absent during pregnancy. The highest levels of plasma renin, or plasma renin activity, have been observed in the first trimester, with a gradual decrease toward term. Plasma levels of renin substrate and angiotension II exhibit the opposite trend with a progressive rise over the three trimesters. Both the plasma levels and urinary excretion of aldosterone increase progressively during pregnancy. A decrease has been reported in the 24-hr urinary excretion of aldosterone after 34 weeks, but the late pregnancy values remained well above nonpregnant levels (133). Even though the trends for angiotension II and aldosterone appear grossly similar, concurrent measurements of plasma levels showed no correlation (132).

It is clear from the changes described above, plus those in plasma volume and composition, that the control of water and electrolyte balance is modified during pregnancy; however, the functional interrelationships of the various mechanisms involved are not so clearly understood. The elevation in aldosterone secretion rates and plasma levels is believed to occur to counteract the natriuretic effect of progesterone. Aldosterone levels increased markedly during sodium restriction (134), a finding further linking aldosterone to the control of sodium balance. However, a positive correlation has been observed between the 24-hr urinary levels of aldosterone and sodium in gravidas on unrestricted diets (133). Angiotensin II levels have been found to be correlated with plasma osmolality (132), but angiotensin does not seem to play an important role in the control of aldosterone secretion in pregnancy. Further, the effects of angiotensin II on urine flow and sodium excretion in pregnancy are blunted to a greater degree than is the vascular reactivity to this agent (130). The interactions of other hormones such as ACTH, glucocorticoids, and prolactin with the renin-angiotensin system and aldosterone during pregnancy have not been extensively explored.

THE ALIMENTARY SYSTEM

The Mouth

Edema and increased vascularity of the gums are frequent during pregnancy and often produce minor bleeding. There is an increase in gingivitis, some loosening of attachment, and an increase in tooth mobility (135). The acidity of saliva and frequency of dental caries may also increase, but the evidence is not strong. Increased salivation is a frequent subjective complaint in gravidas with nausea and vomiting. Measurements of saliva flow rates tend to confirm this symptom, for, although mean saliva flow was found to be somewhat decreased in pregnancy, it was elevated in women with nausea (136).

Esophagus

During pregnancy the lower esophageal sphincter may be displaced into the thorax, with consequent reduction of its competence. This, plus delayed gastric emptying, favors the reflux of acidic gastric contents into the distal esophagus, causing the symptom of heartburn. Upward displacement of the stomach may also contribute to the gastro-esophageal reflux.

Stomach

Gastric tone and motility are reduced during pregnancy. Although not all studies agree (72), there is probably also a small decrease in gastric acid secretion during most of pregnancy. Thus food is retained longer in the stomach as a result of both slowed motility and retarded digestion. This increases the danger of regurgitation and aspiration of food or acid gastric contents whenever general anesthesia is used during pregnancy.

Small and Large Intestines

Motility is reduced throughout the intestinal tract during pregnancy. The decrease in large bowel motility often leads to a complaint of constipation. There is no good evidence that digestion or absorption in the small intestine is altered during pregnancy (72). Water and electrolytes may be absorbed in increased amounts from the large intestine (137), and this may add to the difficulties with defecation by promoting dryer, firmer stools.

Hemorrhoids may develop or worsen as part of the general pelvic hyperemia, and these may be aggravated by the hard stools and straining with constipation.

Liver and Biliary Tract

Liver size does not change in human pregnancy, although significant enlargement occurs in many laboratory animals (138). Very minor alterations have been described in liver histology (139). The ultrastructural features are unaltered in normal pregnancy (140). Hepatic blood flow does not increase (141), and thus the fraction of the cardiac output perfusing the liver decreases.

That some changes in liver function occur during pregnancy is shown by alterations in the levels of serum albumin, some globulin fractions, and several clotting factors, as described above. The capacity of the liver cells to excrete bilirubin and BSP dye into the bile may be somewhat impaired in the second half of pregnancy (138). Serum bilirubin levels are normal, however, and the proportion of gravidas with elevated BSP retention is small. The changes in liver function appear to be hormone-induced, for similar alterations have been observed in nonpregnant women receiving estrogens or estrogen-progestin combinations.

The serum levels of alkaline phosphatase and leucine aminopeptidase are elevated during pregnancy; however, the increase in both instances appears to result from release of placental enzymes into the maternal circulation. Transaminase levels are normal during pregnancy but may be mildly increased in some patients during labor (142).

The gallbladder is hypotonic and empties poorly during pregnancy (143). Aspirated bile has been described as viscous and tarry, although aside from increased concentration, no significant chemical changes have been found (144). It is generally believed that pregnancy predisposes to gallstone formation as a result of the increased bile concentration and incomplete gallbladder emptying.

INTEGUMENTARY SYSTEM

The Skin

Blood flow to the skin increases considerably in pregnancy, as stated in the section on blood flow distribution. Local increases in cutaneous vasodilatation give rise in some gravidas to prominent palmar erythema, a tendency toward flushing of the face and upper trunk, and spider angiomas. The local vascular effects are believed to be related to elevated plasma estrogen levels. Palmar erythema and spider angiomas also occur in patients with liver disease; however, these findings have no such implication in pregnancy.

There is a tendency toward darkening of skin pigmentation during pregnancy. In some gravidas, irregular light brown patches appear on the face, especially the malar areas and forehead (chloasma gravidarum, or mask of pregnancy), and on the neck and top of the shoulders. Nevi may become darker, and new ones may develop. Pigmentation may appear or darken along the midline of the abdominal skin (linea nigra). The areolae of the breasts and the genital skin also tend to become darker and more brownish during pregnancy. These pigmentation changes usually fade markedly after pregnancy, although there is often some residual darkening of the linea nigra and areolae. The increase in skin pigmentation is believed to be caused by the elevated levels of melanocyte stimulating hormone (MSH) that are present during the latter two-thirds of pregnancy (145). Estrogen and progesterone may also play a role, for similar though less marked changes occur in susceptible women taking the oral contraceptive pill.

"Stretch marks" (striae gravidarum) may develop in the skin of the abdomen and to a lesser extent over the breasts, hips, and thighs during the latter months of pregnancy. These are the result of distension of the skin in these areas by the uterus, breast growth, and fat deposition, together with softening and relaxation of the dermal collagenous and elastic tissue. There is marked individual variation in the tendency to develop these stretch marks and in their degree of persistence after pregnancy. There does, however, appear to be some correlation with the amount of uterine enlargement—e.g., multiple pregnancy, polyhydramnios—and with excessive weight gain.

Many women note thickening of the scalp hair and increased prominence of facial and body hair during pregnancy. Conversely, an increase in the rate of shedding of hair, most notable for the scalp hair, occurs during the puerperium. These symptoms are produced by changes in proportion of hair follicles in the actively growing and resting phases, perhaps as a result of the elevated skin blood flow. During pregnancy, the active growth phase is prolonged, and fewer hairs are shed (146). The overaged hairs then fall out during the puerperium, sometimes quite rapidly, when the stimulus to prolonged growth is removed. There does not seem to be any change in the rate of hair growth during pregnancy.

Breasts

The enlargement, increased firmness, and sensitivity of the breasts during the early weeks of pregnancy is probably the result of hyperemia and some interstitial edema. Similarly, the straw-colored nipple discharge at this time probably represents to a large extent transudation of plasma into the duct system. There is often a reduction in breast size as these changes subside late in the first trimester (72).

During the second and third trimesters there is a progressive increase in breast size as a result of glandular growth. There is considerable variability in the degree of breast enlargement, especially in primigravidas. Hytten observed a range from an increase of 880 ml in one breast to a small decrease, with an average of 200 ml per breast (72). The average increase was similar in multiparas, though the range was less extreme. The degree of breast enlargement in primigravidas also decreased with advancing age. The nipples enlarge and become more erectile during pregnancy. The tissue behind the nipple becomes looser, increasing mobility of the nipple and its ability to be pulled outward and grasped during suckling. The areolae of the breasts enlarge, and the glands of Montgomery (modified sebaceous glands thought to represent rudimentary mammary glands) increase in size and prominence.

Growth of the breasts and preparation for lactation is a multihormonal affair involving estrogens, progesterone, prolactin, placental lactogen, insulin, and cortisol. The initiation of lactation appears to be triggered in some fashion by the decline in estrogen and progesterone levels that occur with separation of the placenta. Lactation is sustained by repeated suckling or nipple stimulation that stimulates release of prolactin (147). Suckling also causes release of oxytocin from the posterior pituitary, in turn resulting in contraction of myoepithelial cells around the alveoli and milk ducts and ejection or "let down" of milk.

MUSCULOSKELETAL SYSTEM

Growth of the uterus and its contents progressively adds mass anterior to the usual axis of weight bearing. To maintain balance, especially in late pregnancy, the gravida develops a posture of increased lumbar lordosis with, secondarily, anterior flexion of the neck and more forward carriage of the shoulder girdle. In addition, there is softening and relaxation of the interosseous ligaments of many joints, resulting in an increase in the mobility of the sacroiliac and sacrococcygeal joints and symphysis pubis, and a tendency to develop flat feet.

The postural changes and increased weight place additional stress on the joints of the low back at the same time their ligamentous support is weakened. Thus, low back pain is frequent in late pregnancy, and occasionally lumbar or sacral nerve root irritation may occur. Paresthesias, hypesthesias, and less often discomfort may also occur in the arms and hands as a result of the increased flexion of the lower cervical spine and slumping of the shoulders. Infrequently, pelvic instability resulting from excessive mobility of the pubic symphysis and sacroiliac joints may produce a pronounced waddling gait or even prevent the gravida from walking.

WEIGHT GAIN AND CHANGES IN BODY COMPOSITION

It has been difficult to establish the "normal" pattern of weight gain during pregnancy because of medical and cultural prejudices that have encouraged pregnant women to limit their weight increase, sometimes by rigorous dietary measures. The best evidence, however, is that a healthy gravida may be expected to gain an average of 10 to 12.5 kg (22 to 27 lb) over the course of an uncomplicated pregnancy (72,148,149). These are average figures, not upper limits; and thus approximately half of normal pregnant women will show greater degrees of weight gain. In the "average" case, only about 1 to 1.5 kg of the total is gained in the first trimester, and this is almost entirely due to growth of maternal tissues: uterus, blood volume, breasts, and perhaps some fat storage. The large balance of weight gain is distributed rather evenly over the second and third trimesters, with the maximum rate of just under 1 lb/week occurring in the latter half of the second trimester. The weekly increment in weight gain contributed by the fetus, placenta, and amniotic fluid increases with successive time periods until the last lunar month, when there is a decrease in the rates of fetal and placental growth and an absolute decrease in amniotic fluid volume. Even so, the products of conception account for, at most, about half of the total maternal weight gained by term (Table II). Other obvious components of weight gain include the uterus (about 1 kg), breasts (400 g), and increased plasma and red cell volume (together about 1.5 to 1.7 kg). Increased maternal fat stores and accumulation of water in the extravascular interstitial space account for the remaining 3 to 3.5 kg of an average 11-kg total weight gain. Although there is a correlation between the amount of maternal weight gain and the birthweight of the infant, it is not close. Most of the variation in weight gain between individuals reflects differences in the expansion of maternal body fluids and fat stores. In general

Table II. Components of Maternal Weight Gain by Term*

Products of conception:		
Fetus	3400 g	
Placenta and membranes	650	
Amiotic fluid	800	
	————	4,850
Increase in maternal tissues:		
Uterus	1000	
Breasts	400	
Blood volume	1600	
Extravascular, extracellular water	2000	
Fat	1500	
	————	6,500
Total		11,350 g

* Values are approximations derived from comparison of several published sources.

the maternal weight gain in excess of about 8.5 to 9 kg at term is attributable to one or both of the latter compartments.

Body Fluid Volume

Expansion of all three body fluid compartments occurs during pregnancy. The increase in plasma volume to levels around 1250 to 1300 ml above nonpregnant values by about 34 weeks, with a smaller change thereafter, was described earlier. The expansion of total body water and extracellular, extravascular fluid follows a somewhat different course.

In gravidas without edema, total body water was found to increase by an average of 1.7 liter at 20 weeks, 4.3 liters at 30 weeks, and 7.5 liters at term (150). The increase in total body water was little different in women who developed leg edema, averaging only 0.3 liter more at term. Women who developed generalized edema, however, were found to have accumulated 0.5 liter of extra water as early as 20 weeks, and a total of 10.8 liters, nearly 3 liters more than the nonedematous gravidas, by term. Figure 12 shows that the measured increase in total body water up through 30 menstrual weeks in women without edema correspondends closely with the calculated water content of the products of conception and added maternal tissues and blood (72,150). At term, however, the measured total body water exceeds the theoretical amount by approximately 2 liters. In women with generalized edema, the excess is nearly 5 liters.

Measurements of extracellular fluid volume are less reliable than those of total body water, and the problem is accentuated during pregnancy by apparent changes in the distribution of tracers and incomplete equilibration with the fetus and amniotic fluid (72).

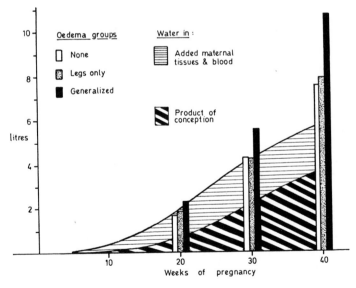

Figure 12. The measured gain in body water during pregnancy in three edema groups compared with the calculated water accumulation in the products of conception and added maternal blood and tissues. At term, there is a surplus of measured body water above the theoretical amount in all groups, suggesting retention of water in a form other than classical edema fluid. From Hytten, F. E., and Leitch, I. *Physiology of Human Pregnancy.* Oxford, Blackwell, 1971.

Despite these uncertainties, 6 to 6.5 liters would seem to be a reasonable estimate of the increase in extracellular fluid volume by term in patients without unusual edema. Since this figure is 2 to 2.5 liters greater than the calculated extracellular fluid volume of the added tissue (72), it appears that the extra body water added by term is contained in the extracellular, extravascular space.

The calculated surplus of extracellular water in women without edema appears to represent increased hydration of connective tissue ground substance, especially in the skin (72,151,152). This is an estrogen effect resulting from depolymerization of connective tissue mucopolysaccharides, with consequent increased binding of water and sodium. Transudation of edema fluid into the subcutaneous tissues of the ankles and lower legs accounts for part of the greater fluid retention in gravidas with clinical edema; but even in these women the average late pregnancy increase in leg volume was only 200 to 250 ml greater than in women without swelling (152). Thus even in clinically edematous women, most of the extra water is not retained as dependent edema fluid.

Edema

The occurrence of clinical edema during pregnancy deserves comment, for edema has been linked closely in obstetrical thought with hypertensive toxemia. This concept must be modified, for, in most cases, edema appears to be only a somewhat exaggerated expression of the normal pregnancy changes in body fluid compartments, and the association between edema and hypertension is quite inconsistent.

In a retrospective study of over 24,000 patient records, Thompson et al. (153) found that edema was noted to be present in 40% of the cases. Leg edema only was recorded in 25%, and the remainder were classified as having generalized edema. Thirty-five percent of women who remained normotensive showed edema. With hypertension, the incidence of edema was 60%; with hypertension plus albuminuria it was 85%. The prematurity rate was lower in patients with edema than in those without, and the mean infant birthweights, when compared within groups of similar parity and maternal weight and height, were greater in the edematous patients.

An even higher incidence of edema, 83%, was found by Robertson (152) in a prospective study of 83 healthy gravidas. Over 40% of the women reported generalized swelling by 38 weeks. Hypertension developed in 3 out of the 14 patients who had no edema at any stage and 8 out of 34 who developed continuous swelling. Looked at in another way, 63 out of 72 women who remained normotensive had edema, compared with 8 out of 11 who became hypertensive. Interestingly, none of the 35 women who had only sporadic edema became hypertensive. This study also confirmed an increased birthweight of infants born to women who developed persistent edema late in pregnancy, but the infants of mothers who had early (before 34 weeks) persistent edema were lighter than those of women with no or sporadic edema.

It is unreasonable to regard a symptom or finding that occurs in such large percentages of healthy pregnant women as anything other than normal. This is especially true when the finding appears to be associated with higher birthweight and a lower incidence of premature delivery. Although edema may be more common, or perhaps more exaggerated, in gravidas with preeclampsia, still the majority of patients with generalized edema do not become hypertensive. Sporadic or leg edema is clearly not an ominous finding. Perhaps further studies will demonstrate differences in the mode of occurrence or other aspects of the edema associated with preeclampsia. At present, however, the occurrence of mild to moderate generalized edema, in the absence of hypertension, albuminuria, or other abnormalities, must be accepted as a rather frequent and even physiologic occurrence in normal pregnancy.

Fat Storage

There can be no doubt that some women accumulate fat, sometimes in very large quantities, during pregnancy, but the extent to which fat storage is a normal feature of the maternal adaptation to pregnancy is not clear. The concept that there is normally an increase in body fat during pregnancy is derived mainly from comparison of the sum of the individually measurable components of weight gain, i.e. products of conception, uterus, increased blood volume, increased body water, etc., with the average total weight gained at various stages of pregnancy (72,150). Thus, Hytten and Leitch (72) have estimated that an average gravida gains about 3.5 kg of fat. Most of this storage of calories occurs by the thirtieth menstrual week, and an actual loss of fat in late pregnancy was calculated for those women who developed generalized edema. Measurements of skin-fold thickness have also suggested an accumulation of fat, chiefly over the abdomen, upper back, hips, and thighs (154). The increase in skin-fold thickness was greatest between 20 and 30 weeks with little change thereafter, a pattern that agrees well with the calculated estimates of fat storage. Progesterone has been shown to induce accumulation of fat in rats (155) and by analogy has been suggested to promote fat storage during human pregnancy as well.

Other studies have indicated that fat storage is not a regular feature of human pregnancy. Seitchik (156) found no significant change in body density during pregnancy and from this concluded that there is no metabolic trend for fat gain or loss. Emerson and coworkers (115) observed a small loss of total body fat in two pregnant subjects in "caloric equilibrium." Comparison of changes in body composition with caloric intake in these two patients and three others led these authors to the conclusion that storage of body fat during pregnancy depends on food intake, just as it does in the nonpregnant individual. In contrast, the increase in body cell mass in these patients was found to be independent of the caloric intake as long as the dietary protein was adequate.

The key to these differing conclusions regarding fat storage in human pregnancy lies in the amount of weight gained by the patients and accepted as normal by the authors. Thus, Hytten and Leitch base their calculations on an average weight gain of 12.5 kg by the normal gravida, whereas three out of the five normal women studied by Emerson et al. gained less than 9 kg and the maximum gain was 10.6 kg. The majority of these patients were said to have restricted their calories voluntarily because of fear of obesity. Seitchik does not give values for the average weight gain of his patients; however, he regarded weight increases of 12.4 and 13.1 kg by two patients as "somewhat excessive."

It seems reasonable to conclude that fat storage is not a necessary part of successful adaptation of the human female to pregnancy but instead represents an "optional" storage of excess calories. It also seems reasonable to assume that the appetite of the normal gravida is readjusted so as to provide some caloric excess, since most studies of healthy pregnant women on unrestricted diets have shown average weight gains exceeding the obligatory value by 1 to 3 kg. Fat storage of this degree may thus be regarded as a normal accompaniment of pregnancy in a substantial proportion of women, perhaps originally serving as a buffer against dietary deficits during late pregnancy and the early puerperium. Even though this fat storage may now be physiologically unnecessary, it would seem unwise to attempt to eliminate it by dietary restriction during pregnancy. The excessive degrees of fat accumulation observed in some gravidas may represent the effects of other than physiologic factors on appetite and food intake. Excessive weight gain due to overeating and consequent fat storage appears to have little effect on the course of pregnancy beyond a small increase in fetal weight; however, the long-term implications with regard to obesity would seem to provide adequate grounds for some dietary restriction in the latter women.

REFERENCES

1. Hytten, F. E., and Cheyne, G. A.: The size and composition of the human pregnant uterus. *J. Obstet. Gynaec. Brit. Commonw.* 76:400, 1969.

2. Gillespie, E. C.: Principles of uterine growth in pregnancy. *Am. J. Obstet. Gynecol.* 59:949, 1950.

3. Stolte, L. A. M., and Eskes, T. K. A. B.: Cervical incompetence, in Wood, C. (ed.): *Proc. 5th World Cong. Gynaecol. and Obstet.* Butterworth, Sydney, 1967, p. 729.

4. Reynolds, S. R. M.: *Physiology of the Uterus.* Hafner, New York, 1965.

5. Reinold, E.: Ultrasonics in early pregnancy: Diagnostic scanning and fetal motor activity, *Contrib. Gynecol. and Obstet.,* Vol. I. Karger, Basel, 1976.

6. Gohari, P., Berkowitz, R. L., and Hobbins, J. C.: Prediction of intrauterine growth retardation by determination of total intrauterine volume. *Am. J. Obstet. Gynecol.* 127:255, 1977.

7. Hendricks, C. H.: Inherent motility patterns and response characteristics of the human uterus. *Am. J. Obstet. Gynecol.* 96:824, 1966.

8. Mitchell, J. C., and Benson, R. C.: Pyelonephritis during pregnancy. *Obstet. Gynecol.* 10:555, 1957.

9. Goodlin, R. C., Keller, D. W., and Raffin, N.: Orgasm during late pregnancy. *Obstet. Gynecol.* 38:916, 1971.

10. Harbert, G. M., Jr.: Diurnal patterns in uterine dynamics, in Comline, K. S., Cross, K. W., Dawes, G. S., and Nathanielsz, P. W. (eds.): *Foetal and Neonatal Physiology: Proceedings of the Barcroft Centenary Symposium.* Cambridge University Press, 1973, p. 279.

11. Csapo, A.: Defense mechanism of pregnancy, in *Ciba Foundation Study Group No. 9.* Churchill, London, 1961, p. 3.

12. Greiss, F. C., and Anderson, S. G.: Effect of ovarian hormones on the uterine vascular bed. *Am. J. Obstet. Gynecol.* 107:829, 1970.

13. Prill, H., and Götz, F.: Blood flow in the myometrium and endometrium of the uterus. *Am. J. Obstet. Gynecol.* 82:102, 1961.

14. Assali, N. S., Rauramo, L., and Peltonen, T.: Measurement of uterine blood flow and uterine metabolism: VIII. Uterine and fetal blood flow and oxygenation in early human pregnancy. *Am. J. Obstet. Gynecol.* 79:86, 1960.

15. Assali, N. S., Douglass, R. A., Jr., Baird, W. W., Nicholson, D. B., and Suyemoto, R.: Measurements of uterine blood flow and uterine metabolism: IV. Results in normal pregnancy. *Am. J. Obstet. Gynecol.* 66:248, 1953.

16. Metcalfe, J., Romney, S. L., Ramsey, L. H., and Burwell, C. S.: Estimation of uterine blood flow in normal human pregnancy at term. *J. Clin. Invest.* 34:1632, 1955.

17. Blechner, J. N., Stenger, V. G., and Prystowsky, H.: Uterine blood flow in women at term. *Am. J. Obstet. Gynecol.* 120:633, 1974.

18. Lees, M. H., Hill, J. D., Ochsner, A. J., III, Thomas, C. L., and Novy, N. J.: Maternal placental and myometrial blood flow in the rhesus monkey during uterine contractions. *Am. J. Obstet. Gynecol.* 110:68, 1971.

19. Huckabee, W. E.: Uterine blood flow. *Am. J. Obstet. Gynecol.* 84:1623, 1962.

20. Hellman, L. M., Kobayashi, M., Tolles, W. E., and Cromb, E.: Ultrasonic studies on the volumetric growth of the human placenta. *Am. J. Obstet. Gynecol.* 108:740, 1970.

21. Harris, J. W. S., and Ramsey, E. M.: The morphology of the human uteroplacental vasculature. *Contrib. Embryol. Carnegie Inst. Wash.* 38:43, 1966.

22. Beck, A. J., and Beck, F.: The origin of intra-arterial cells in the pregnant uterus of the macaque (Macaca mulatta). *Anat. Rec.* 158:111, 1967.

23. Rosenfeld, C. R., Morriss, F. H., Jr., Makowski, E. L., Meschia, G., and Battaglia, F. C.: Circulatory changes in the reproductive tissues of ewes during pregnancy. *Gynecol. Invest.* 5:252, 1974.

24. Caton, D., Lackore, L. K., Thatcher, W. W., and Barron, D. H.: Uterine blood flow, oxygen consumption, and maternal plasma estradiol and progestins following fetal death. *Am. J. Obstet. Gynecol.* 125:624, 1976.

25. Greiss, F. C., Jr., Anderson, S. G., and Still, J. G.: Uterine pressure-flow relationships during early gestation. *Am. J. Obstet. Gynecol.* 126:799, 1976.

26. Greiss, F. C., Jr., and Still, J. G.: A uterine vasoactive property of glucosamine. *Gynecol. Invest.* 8:57, 1977.

27. Rosenfeld, C. R., Barton, M. D., and Meschia, G.: Effects of epinephrine on distribution of blood flow in the pregnant ewe. *Am. J. Obstet. Gynecol.* 124:156, 1976.

28. Rosenfeld, C. R., and West, J.: Circulatory response to systemic infusion of norepinephrine in pregnant sheep. *Am. J. Obstet. Gynecol.* 127:376, 1977.

29. Greiss, F. C., Jr.: Differential reactivity in the myoendometrial and placental vasculations: Vasodilatation. *Am. J. Obstet. Gynecol.* 111:611, 1971.

30. Killam, A. P., Rosenfeld, C. R., Battaglia, F. C., Makowski, E. L., and Meschia, G.: Effect of estrogens on the uterine blood flow in oophorectomized ewes. *Am. J. Obstet. Gynecol.* 115:1045, 1973.

31. Anderson, S. G., and Hackshaw, B. T.: The effect of estrogen on uterine blood flow and its distribution in nonpregnant ewes. *Am. J. Obstet. Gynecol.* 119:589, 1974.

32. Greiss, F. C., Jr., and Marston, E. L.: The uterine vascular bed: Effect of estrogens during ovine pregnancy. *Am. J. Obstet. Gynecol.* 93:720, 1965.

33. Rosenfeld, C. R., Morriss, F. H., Jr., Battaglia, F. C., Makowski, E. L., and Maschia, G.: Effect of estradiol 17β on blood flows to reproductive and nonreproductive tissues in pregnant ewes. *Am. J. Obstet. Gynecol.* 124:618, 1976.

34. Bruce, N. W.: Effect of oestrogens on placental and myometrial blood flows in rabbits, in Comline, K. S., Cross, K. W., Dawes, G. S., and Nathanielsz, P. W. (eds.): *Foetal and Neonatal Physiology: Proceedings of the Barcroft Centenary Symposium.* Cambridge University Press, 1973, p. 288.

35. Resnik, R., Battaglia, F. C., Makowski, E. L., and Meschia, G.: The effect of actinomycin D on estrogen-induced uterine blood flow. *Am. J. Obstet. Gynecol.* 122:273, 1975.

36. Anderson, S. G., Hackshaw, B. T., Still, J. G., and Greiss, F. C.: Uterine blood flow and its distribution after chronic estrogen and progesterone administration. *Am. J. Obstet. Gynecol.* 127:138, 1977.

37. Clark, K. E., Ryan, M. J., and Brody, M. J.: Effect of prostaglandin E_1 and $F_{2\alpha}$ on uterine hemodynamics and motility. *Adv. Biosci.* 9:779, 1973.

38. Resnik, R., and Brink, G. W.: Modulating effect of prostaglandins on the uterine vascular bed. *Gynec. Invest.* 8:10, 1977.

39. Venuto, R. C., O'Doriso, T., Stein, J. H., and Ferris, T. F.: Uterine prostaglandin E (PGE) secretion and uterine blood flow in the pregnant rabbit. *J. Clin. Invest.* 55:193, 1975.

40. Torberto, N., Terrango, A., and McGiff, J. C.: The uterine circulation, pregnancy and prostaglandin synthesis. *Clin. Res.* 22:307A, 1974.

41. Clark, K. E., Farley, D. B., van Orden, D. E., and Brody, M. J.: Role of endogenous prostaglandins in regulation of uterine blood flow and adrenergic neurotransmission. *Am. J. Obstet. Gynecol.* 127:455, 1977.

42. Ryan, M. J., Clark, K. E., van Orden, D. E., Farley, D., Edvinsson, L., Sjöberg, N. O., van Orden, L. S., III, and Brody, M. J.: Role of prostaglandins in estrogen-induced uterine hyperemia. *Prostaglandins* 4:629, 1973.

43. Clark, K. E., and Brody, M. J.: Competitive antagonism of prostaglandins (PG) E_1, E_2 and A_1 by $PGF_{2\alpha}$ in the canine uterus. *Pharmacologist* 16:197, 1974.

44. Skinner, S. L., Lumbers, E. R., and Symonds, E. M.: Renin concentration in human fetal and maternal tissues. *Am. J. Obstet. Gynecol.* 101:529, 1968.

45. Ferris, T. J., Stein, J. H., and Kauffman, J.: Uterine blood flow and uterine renin secretion. *J. Clin. Invest.* 51:2827, 1972.

46. Franklin, G. O., Dowd, A. J., Caldwell, B. V., and Speroff, L.: Effect of angiotensin II intravenous infusion on plasma renin activity and prostaglandins A, E, and F levels in the uterine vein of the pregnant monkey. *Prostaglandins* 6:271, 1974.

47. Ladner, C., Brinkman, C. R., III, Weston, P., and Assali, N. S.: Dynamics of uterine circulation in pregnant and nonpregnant sheep. *Am. J. Physiol.* 218:257, 1970.

48. Greiss, F. C., Jr., Gobble, F. L., Jr., Anderson, S. G., and McGuirt, W. F.: Effect of acetylcholine on the uterine vascular bed. *Am. J. Obstet. Gynecol.* 99:1073, 1967.

49. Oakes, G. K., Walker, A. M., Ehrenkrantz, R. A., and Chez, R. A.: Effects of propranolol infusion on the umbilical and uterine circulations of pregnant sheep. *Am. J. Obstet. Gynecol.* 126:1038, 1976.

50. Bell, C.: Control of uterine blood flow in pregnancy. *Med. Biol.* 52:219, 1974.

51. Bell, C.: Distribution of cholinergic vasomotor nerves to the parametrial arteries of some laboratory and domestic animals. *J. Reprod. Fertil.* 27:53, 1971.

52. Greiss, F. C., Jr., and Gobble, F. L.: Effect of sympathetic nerve stimulation on the uterine vascular bed. *Am. J. Obstet. Gynecol.* 97:962, 1967.

53. Nakanishi, H., McLean, J., Wood, C., and Burnside, G.: The role of sympathetic nerves in the control of the nonpregnant and pregnant uterus. *J. Reprod. Med.* 2:20, 1968.

54. Rosenfeld, C. R., Worley, R. J., and Gant, N. F.: The effect of systemic infusions of dehydroisoandrosterone on the distribution of uterine blood flow in ovine pregnancy. *Gynec. Invest.* 8:37, 1977.

55. Danforth, D. N., and Buckingham, J. C.: Connective tissue mechanisms and their relation to pregnancy. *Obstet. Gynecol. Survey* 19:715, 1964.

56. Stys, S. J., Clewell, W. H., and Meschia, G.: Changes in cervical compliance at parturition independent of uterine activity. *Gynec. Invest.* 8:58, 1977.

57. Gemzell, C. A., Robbe, H., and Ström, G.: Total amount of haemoglobin and physical working capacity in normal pregnancy and the puerperium. *Acta Obstet. Gynecol. Scand.* 36:93, 1957.

58. Ihrman, K.: A clinical and physiological study of pregnancy in material from Northern Sweden: VII. The heart volume during and after pregnancy. *Acta Soc. Med. Upsal.* 65:326, 1960.

59. Barnes, C. G.: *Medical Disorders in Obstetric Practice,* ed. 4. Blackwell, Oxford, 1974.

60. Burg, J. R., Dodek, A., Kloster, F. E., and Metcalfe, J.: Alterations in systolic time intervals during pregnancy. *Circulation* 49:560, 1974.

61. Liebson, P. R., Mann, L. I., Evans, M. I., Duchin, S., and Arditi, L.: Cardiac performance during pregnancy: Serial evaluation using external systolic time intervals. *Am. J. Obstet. Gynecol.* 122:1, 1975.

62. Quilligan, E. J., and Tyler, C.: Postural effects on the cardiovascular status in pregnancy: A comparison of the lateral and supine postures. *Am. J. Obstet. Gynecol.* 78:465, 1959.

63. Vorys, N., Ullery, J. C., and Hanusek, G. E.: The cardiac output changes in various positions in pregnancy. *Am. J. Obstet. Gynecol.* 82:1312, 1961.

64. Kerr, M. G., Scott, D. B., and Samuel, E.: Studies of the inferior vena cava in late pregnancy. *Brit. Med. J.* 1:532, 1964.

65. Pyörälä, T.: Cardiovascular response to the upright position during pregnancy. *Acta Obstet. Gynecol. Scand.* 45(Suppl.):5, 1966.

66. Lees, M. M., Taylor, S. H., Scott, D. B., and Kerr, M. G.: A study of cardiac output at rest throughout pregnancy. *J. Obstet. Gynaecol. Brit. Commonw.* 74:319, 1967.

67. Ueland, K., Novy, M. J., Peterson, E. N., and Metcalfe, J.: Maternal cardiovascular dynamics: IV. The influence of gestational age on the maternal cardiovascular response to posture and exercise. *Am. J. Obstet. Gynecol.* 104:856, 1969.

68. Ueland, K., Novy, M. I., and Metcalfe, J.: Cardiorespiratory responses to pregnancy and exercise in normal women and patients with heart disease. *Am. J. Obstet. Gynecol.* 115:4, 1973.

69. Blackburn, M. W., and Calloway, D. H.: Basal metabolic rate and work energy expenditure of mature, pregnant women. *J. Am. Diet. Assn.* 69:24, 1976.

70. Seligman, S. A.: Diurnal blood-pressure variation in pregnancy. *J. Obstet. Gynaecol. Brit. Commonw.* 78:417, 1971.

71. Ginsberg, J., and Duncan, S.: Direct and indirect blood-pressure measurements in pregnancy. *J. Obstet. Gynaecol. Brit. Commonw.* 76:705, 1969.

72. Hytten, F. L., and Leitch, I.: *The Physiology of Human Pregnancy,* ed. 2. Blackwell, Oxford, 1971.

73. Linzell, J. L.: Mammary blood flow and methods for identifying and measuring precursors of milk, Ch. 3, in Larson, B. L., and Smith, V. R. (eds.): *Lactation,* Vol. I. Academic Press, New York, 1974, p. 143.

74. Spetz, S., and Jansson, I.: Forearm blood flow during normal pregnancy studied by venous occlusion plethysmography and [133]xenon muscle clearance. *Acta Obstet. Gynecol. Scand.* 48:285, 1966.

75. Sandström, B.: Calf blood flow during normal primipregnancy. *Acta Obstet. Gynecol. Scand.* 52:199, 1973.

76. Hytten, F. E., and Leitch, I.: *The Physiology of Human Pregnancy,* ed. 1. Blackwell, Oxford, 1964.

77. Parer, J. T., Metcalfe, J., and Jones, W. D.: The effect of estrogen on the circulation in nonpregnant ewes. *Fed. Proc.* 23:462, 1964.

78. Bryant, E. E., Douglas, B. H., and Ashburn, A. D.: Circulatory changes following prolactin administration. *Am. J. Obstet. Gynecol.* 115:53, 1973.

79. Chesley, L. C., Talledo, E., Bohler, C. S., and Zuspan, F. P.: Vascular reactivity to angiotensin II and norepinephrine in pregnant and nonpregnant women. *Am. J. Obstet. Gynecol.* 91:837, 1965.

80. Gant, N. F., Chand, S., Whalley, P. J., and MacDonald, P. C.: The nature of pressor responsiveness to angiotensin II in human pregnancy. *Obstet. Gynecol.* 43:854, 1974.

81. Assali, N. S., Vergon, J. M., Tada, Y., and Garber, S. T.: Studies on autonomic blockade: VI. The mechanisms regulating hemodynamic changes in pregnant women and their relation to the hypertension of toxemia of pregnancy. *Am. J. Obstet. Gynecol.* 63:978, 1952.

82. Caton, W. L., Roby, C. C., Reid, D. E., Caswell, R., Maletskos, C. J., Fluharty, R. G., and Gibson, J. G.: The circulating red cell volume and body hematocrit in normal pregnancy and the puerperium. *Am. J. Obstet. Gynecol.* 61:1207, 1951.

83. Berlin, N. I., Goetsch, C., Hyde, G. M., and Parsons, R. J.: The blood volume in pregnancy as determined by P[32] labelled red blood cells. *Surg. Gynec. Obstet.* 97:173, 1953.

84. Hytten, F. H., and Paintin, D. B.: Increase in plasma volume during normal pregnancy. *J. Obstet. Gynaecol. Brit. Commonw.* 70:402, 1963.

85. Rovinsky, J. J., and Jaffin, H.: Cardiovascular dynamics in pregnancy: I. Blood and plasma volumes in multiple pregnancy. *Am. J. Obstet. Gynecol.* 93:1, 1965.

86. Flanagan, B., Muldowney, F. P., and Cannon, P. J.: The relationship of circulating red cell mass, basal oxygen consumption and lean body mass during normal human pregnancy. *Clin. Sci.* 30:439, 1966.

87. Lund, C. J., and Donovan, J. C.: Blood volume during pregnancy. *Am. J. Obstet. Gynecol.* 98:393, 1967.

88. Pirani, B. B. K., and Campbell, D. M.: Plasma volume in normal first pregnancy. *J. Obstet. Gynaecol. Brit. Commonw.* 80:884, 1973.

89. Chesley, L. C., and Duffus, G. M.: Posture and apparent plasma volume in late pregnancy. *J. Obstet. Gynaecol. Brit. Commonw.* 78:406, 1971.

90. Duffus, G. M., MacGillivray, I., and Dennis, K. J.: The relationship between baby weight and changes in maternal weight, total body water, plasma volume, electrolytes and proteins and urinary estriol excretion. *J. Obstet. Gynaecol. Brit. Commonw.* 78:97, 1971.

91. Gibson, H. M.: Plasma volume and glomerular filtration rate in pregnancy and their relation to differences in fetal growth. *J. Obstet. Gynaecol. Brit. Commonw.* 80:1067, 1973.

92. Pritchard, J. A., and Adams, R. H.: Erythrocyte production and destruction during pregnancy. *Am. J. Obstet. Gynecol.* 79:750, 1960.

93. Manase, B., and Jepson, J.: Erythropoietin in plasma and urine during human pregnancy. *Can. Med. Assoc. J.* 100:687, 1969.

94. Jepson, J. H., and Friesen, H. G.: The mechanism of action of human placental lactogen on erythropoiesis. *Brit. J. Haematol.* 15:465, 1968.

95. Bauer, C., Ludwig, M., Ludwig, L., and Bartels, H.: Factors governing the oxygen affinity of human adult and foetal blood. *Resp. Physiol.* 7:271, 1969.

96. Mac Donald, R. G., and Mac Donald, H. N.: Erythrocyte 2,3-diphosphoglycerate and associated haematological parameters during the menstrual cycle and pregnancy. *Brit. J. Obstet. Gynecol.* 84:427, 1977.

97. Wallenburg, H. C. S., and van Kessel, P. H.: Platelets and poor intrauterine fetal growth, in Salvadori, B., and Bacchi-Modena, A. (eds.): *Poor Intrauterine Fetal Growth.* Minerva Medica, Rome, 1977, p. 107.

98. Newman, R. L.: Serum electrolytes in pregnancy, parturition and puerperium. *Obstet. Gynecol.* 10:51, 1957.

99. Robertson, E. G.: Increased erythrocyte fragility in association with osmotic changes in pregnancy serum. *J. Reprod. Fertil.* 16:323, 1968.

100. Robertson, E. G., and Cheyne, G. A.: Plasma biochemistry in relation to oedema of pregnancy. *J. Obstet. Gynaecol. Brit. Commonw.* 79:769, 1972.

101. MacDonald, H. N., and Good, W.: Changes in plasma total protein, albumin, urea and α-amino nitrogen concentrations in pregnancy and the puerperium. *J. Obstet. Gynaecol. Brit. Commonw.* 78:912, 1971.

102. Studd, J. W., and Wood, S.: Serum and urinary proteins in pregnancy, in Wyun, R. M. (ed.): *Obstetrics and Gynecology Annual.* Appleton Century Crofts, New York, 1976, p. 103.

103. De Alvarez, R. R., Gaiser, D. F., Simkins, D. N., Smith, E. K., and Bratvold, G. E.: Serial studies of serum lipids in normal human pregnancy. *Am. J. Obstet. Gynecol.* 77:743, 1959.

104. Peters, J. P., Heineman, M., and Man, E. B.: The lipids of the serum in pregnancy. *J. Clin. Invest.* 30:388, 1951.

105. Todd, M. E., Thompson, J. H., Bowie, E. J. W., and Owen, C. A.: Changes in blood coagulation during pregnancy. *Mayo Clin. Proc.* 40:370, 1965.

106. Nossel, H. L., Lanzkowsky, P., Levy, S., Mibashan, R. S., and Hansen, J. D. L.: A study of coagulation factor levels in women during labour and in their newborn infants. *Thrombes. Diath. Hemorrh.* 16:185, 1966.

107. Ratnoff, O. D., and Holland, T. R.: Coagulation components in normal and abnormal pregnancies. *Ann. N.Y. Acad. Sci.* 75:626, 1959.

108. Talbert, L. M., and Langdell, R. D.: Normal values of certain factors in the blood clotting mechanism in pregnancy. *Am. J. Obstet. Gynecol.* 90:44, 1964.

109. Woodfield, D. G., Cole, S. K., Allan, A. G. E., and Cash, J. D.: Serum fibrin degradation products throughout normal pregnancy. *Brit. Med. J.* 4:655, 1968.

110. Ratnoff, O. D., Colopy, J. E., and Pritchard, J. A.: The blood clotting mechanism during normal parturition. *J. Lab. Clin. Med.* 44:408, 1954.

111. Cugell, D. W., Frank, N. R., Gaensler, E. R., and Badger, T. L.: Pulmonary function in pregnancy: I. Serial observations in normal women. *Ann. Rev. Tuberc.* 67:568, 1953.

112. Milne, J. A., Mills, R. J., Howie, A. D., and Pack, A. I.: Large airways function during normal pregnancy. *Brit. J. Obstet. Gynaecol.* 84:448, 1977.

113. Wilbrand, U., Porath, Ch., Matthaes, P., and Jaster, R.: Der Einfluss der Ovarialsteroide auf die Funktion des Atemzentrums. *Arch. Gynäk.* 191:507, 1959.

114. Pernoll, M. L., Metcalfe, J., Kovach, P. A., Wachtel, R., and Dunham, M. J.: Ventilation during rest and exercise in pregnancy and post partum. *Resp. Physiol.* 25:295, 1975.

115. Emerson, K. M., Jr., Poindexter, E. L., and Kothari, M.: Changes in total body composition during normal and diabetic pregnancy: Relation to oxygen consumption. *Obstet. Gynecol.* 45:505, 1975.

116. Harrow, B. R., Sloane, J. A., and Salhanick, L.: Etiology of the hydronephrosis of pregnancy. *Surg. Gynecol. Obstet.* 119:1042, 1964.

117. Bellina, J. H., Dougherty, C. M., and Mickal, A.: Pyeloureteral dilatation and pregnancy. *Am. J. Obstet. Gynecol.* 108:356, 1970.

118. Rubi, R. A., and Sala, N. L.: Ureteral function in pregnant women: III. Effect of different positions and of fetal delivery upon ureteral tonus. *Am. J. Obstet. Gynecol.* 101:230, 1968.

119. Sims, E. A. H., and Krantz, K. E.: Serial studies of renal function during pregnancy and the puerperium in normal women. *J. Clin. Invest.* 37:1764, 1958.

120. Chesley, L. C., and Sloan, D. M: The effect of posture on renal function in late pregnancy. *Am. J. Obstet. Gynecol.* 89:754, 1964.

121. Davison, J. M., and Hytten, F. E.: Glomerular filtration during and after pregnancy. *J. Obstet. Gynaecol. Brit. Commonw.* 81:588, 1974.

122. Dignam, W. J., Voskian, J., and Assali, N. S.: Effects of estrogens on renal hemodynamics and excretion of electrolytes in human subjects. *J. Clin. Endocr.* 16:1032, 1956.

123. Berman, L. B.: The pregnant kidney (Editorial). *J.A.M.A.* 230:111, 1974.

124. Christensen, P. J.: Tubular reabsorption of glucose during pregnancy. *Scand. J. Clin. Lab. Invest.* 10:364, 1958.

125. Welsh, G. W., III, and Sims, E. A. H.: The mechanisms of renal glycosuria in pregnancy. *Diabetes* 9:363, 1960.

126. Davison, J. M., and Hytten, F. E.: Renal handling of glucose in pregnancy, in Sutherland, H. W., and Stowers, J. M. (eds.): *Carbohydrate Metabolism in Pregnancy and the Newborn.* Churchill Livingston, Edinburgh, 1975, p. 2.

127. Hytten, F. E., and Klopper, A. I.: Response to a water load in pregnancy. *J. Obstet. Gynaecol. Brit. Commonw.* 70:811, 1963.

128. Lindheimer, M. D., and Weston, P. V.: Effect of hypotonic expansion on sodium, water, and urea excretion in late pregnancy: The influence of posture on these results. *J. Clin. Invest.* 48:947, 1969.

129. Helmer, O. M., and Judson, W. E.: Influence of high renin substrate levels on renin-angiotensin system in pregnancy. *Am. J. Obstet. Gynecol.* 99:9, 1967.

130. Chesley, L. C.: Disorders of the kidney, fluids and electrolytes, Ch. 5, in Assali, N. S., and Brinkman, C. R. (eds.): *Pathophysiology of Gestation,* Vol. I. Academic Press, New York, 1972, p. 355.

131. Gordon, R. D., Symonds, E. M., Wilmshurst, E. G., and Pawsley, G. C. K.: Plasma renin activity, plasma angiotensin and urinary electrolytes in normal and toxemic pregnancy including a prospective study. *Clin. Sci. Mol. Med.* 45:115, 1973.

132. Wier, R. J., Brown, J. J., Fraser, R., Lever, A. F., Logan, R. W., McIlwaine, G. M., Morton, J. J., Robertson, J. I. S., and Tree, M.: Relationship between plasma renin, renin-substrate, angiotensin II, aldosterone and electrolytes in normal pregnancy. *J. Clin. Endo. Metab.* 40:108, 1975.

133. Lammintausta, R., and Erkkola, R.: Renin-angiotensin-aldosterone system and sodium in normal pregnancy: A longitudinal study. *Acta Obstet. Gynecol. Scand.* 56:221, 1977.

134. Watanabe, M., Meeker, C. I., Gray, M. J., Sims, E. A. H., and Solomon, S.: Secretion rates of aldosterone in normal pregnancy. *J. Clin. Invest.* 42:1619, 1963.

135. Cohen, D. W., Friedman, L., Shapiro, J., and Kyle, G. C.: A longitudinal investigation of the periodontal changes during pregnancy. *J. Periodont.* 40:563, 1969.

136. Kullander, S., and Sonesson, B.: Studies on saliva in menstruating, pregnant and postmenopausal women. *Acta Endocr. (Kbh)* 48:329, 1965.

137. Parry, E., Shields, R., and Turnbully, A. C.: The effect of pregnancy on the colonic absorption of sodium, potassium and water. *J. Obstet. Gynaecol. Brit. Commonw.* 77:616, 1970.

138. Combes, B., and Adams, R. H.: Pathophysiology of the liver in pregnancy, Ch. 6, in Assali, N. S., and Brinkman, C. R. (eds.): *Pathophysiology of Gestation,* Vol. I. Academic Press, New York, 1971, p. 479.

139. Ingerslev, M., and Teilum, G.: Biopsy studies on the liver in pregnancy: II. Liver biopsy on normal pregnant women. *Acta Obstet. Gynecol. Scand.* 25:532, 1946.

140. Adlercreutz, H., Svanborg, A., and Ånberg, A.: Recurrent jaundice in pregnancy: A clinical and ultrastructural survey. *Am. J. Med.* 42:335, 1967.

141. Munnell, E. W., and Taylor, H. C., Jr.: Liver blood flow in pregnancy: Hepatic vein catheterization. *J. Clin. Invest.* 26:952, 1947.

142. Stone, M. L., Lending, M., Slobody, L. B., and Mestern, J.: Glutamic oxalacetic transaminase and lactic dehydrogenase in pregnancy. *Am. J. Obstet. Gynecol,* 80:104, 1960.

143. Potter, M. G.: Observations of the gall bladder during pregnancy. *J.A.M.A.* 106:1070, 1036.

144. Large, A. M., Johnston, C. G., Katsuki, T., and Fachnie, H. L.: Gallstones and pregnancy: The composition of gall bladder bile in the pregnant woman at term. *Am. J. Med. Sci.* 239:713, 1960.

145. Ances, I. G., and Pomerantz, S. H.: Serum concentrations of β-melanocyte stimulating hormone in human pregnancy. *Am. J. Obstet. Gynecol.* 119:1062, 1974.

146. Lynfield, Y. L.: Effect of pregnancy on the human hair cycle. *J. Invest. Derm.* 35:323, 1960.

147. Tyson, J. E., Friesen, H. G., and Anderson, M. S.: Human lactational and ovarian response to endogenous prolactin release. *Science* 177:897, 1972.

148. *Maternal Nutrition and the Course of Pregnancy.* National Academy of Sciences, Washington, 1970.

149. Pitkin, R. M., Kaminetzky, H. A., Newton, M., and Pritchard, J. A.: Maternal nutrition: A selected review of clinical topics. *Obstet. Gynecol.* 40:773, 1972.

150. Hytten, F. H., Thompson, A. M., and Taggart, N.: Total body water in normal pregnancy. *J. Obstet. Gynaecol. Brit. Commonw.* 73:553, 1966.

151. Gersh, I., and Catchpole, H. R.: The nature of ground substance of connective tissue. *Perspectives Biol. Med.* 3:282, 1960.

152. Robertson, E. G.: The natural history of oedema during pregnancy. *J. Obstet. Gynaecol. Brit. Commonw.* 78:520, 1971.

153. Thomson, A. M., Hytten, F. E., and Billewicz, W. Z.: The epidemiology of oedema during pregnancy. *J. Obstet. Gynaecol. Brit. Commonw.* 74:1, 1967.

154. Taggart, N., Holliday, R. M., Billewicz, W. Z., Hytten, F. E., and Thomson, A. M.: Changes in skinfolds during pregnancy. *Brit. J. Nutr.* 21:439, 1967.

155. Galletti, F., and Klopper, A.: The effect of progesterone on the quantity and distribution of body fat in the female rat. *Acta Endocr.* 46:379, 1964.

156. Seitchik, J.: Total body water and total body density of pregnant women. *Obstet. Gynecol.* 29:155, 1967.

7
Fetal Pathophysiology

William H. Clewell, M.D.
Stanley J. Stys, M.D.
Frederick C. Battaglia, M.D.

Placentation is characteristic of the eutherian and marsupial orders of mammals. While lower vertebrate development is characterized by a large store of yolk with each egg produced, mammalian development is characterized by a phase of intrauterine development during which the fetus depends upon a continuous supply of nutrients from the placenta. The term "placenta" describes an organ composed of tissues of fetal and maternal derivation the function of which is the exchange of nutrients and waste products. The term has become more general than its original meaning in mammals, which described the functional union between fetal membranes and the uterus. Placental functions include all physiologic activities depending directly or indirectly upon diffusion and interaction of the fetal and uterine tissues during prenatal life.

Placentation has been categorized among mammals in several ways, including classifications based upon the number of tissue layers separating the two circulations, uterine and umbilical, and by the fetal membranes specifically involved. For example, the fetal constituent of the chorionic placenta is limited to the true, avascular chorionic membrane. In the chorioallantoic placenta, the fetal part consists either of the allantochorionic membranes or, in the absence of a vesicular allantois, the chorion vascularized by allantoic vessels. The yolk sac placenta consists of the vascularized splanchnopleuric wall of the yolk sac, everted against the bilaminar omphalopleure, or against the endometrium directly. Chorionic, chorioallantoic, and yolk sac placentation are the three basic types of placentation that occur in eutherian mammals. Choriovitelline placentation is the principal means of fetal–maternal exchange in most marsupials.

One of the striking differences between development in marsupial mammals and in eutherian mammals is that marsupial development is characterized by a very short period of intrauterine development and the delivery of a newborn of quite small size compared with intrauterine development in eutherian mammals. For example, in the red kangaroo, the largest of the marsupials, weighing 40 kg, the weight of the newborn at birth is approximately 750 mg. The birthweight of the infant, as a percentage of maternal body weight, is approximately 0.002%. Even if one considers development in the larger eutherian mammals, the contrast with marsupial development is striking. For example, the elephant, with an adult weight of approximately 2,500 kilograms, produces a young of approximately 90 kg, or 3.5% of maternal weight.

Another interesting difference between marsupial and eutherian intrauterine development is the diapause phenomenon. Essentially, this phenomenon consists of an arrest in growth and development, occurring after fertilization and before implantation. It is a characteristic of marsupial development, although it does occur in eutherian mammals. In the mink and sable, for example, it is an obligatory part of development; in other eutherian mammals it is variably present, but never to the extent demonstrated in marsupials. Development usually proceeds to the unilaminar blastocyst stage (approximately 80-cell stage). The length of the diapause can be as long as one year in certain marsupials, when the quiescent phase produced by lactation is followed by a quiescent phase triggered by the season of the year. At the end of this long phase of developmental arrest, implantation can then occur and development proceed normally.

The basic arrangement of a placenta consisting of a trophoblast separating two circulations occurs in all mammals. The belief held in the past that one could have fetal endothelial vascular tissue in direct contact with maternal blood was disproved as electron microscopy techniques permitted more thorough investigation of placental morphology.

Chorioallantoic placentation is the principal mechanism of feto-maternal exchange in most higher mammals, including man. A fundamental step of chorioallantoic placentation is the formation of vascular chorionic villi. The villi may interdigitate with vascular outfoldings of the endometrial surface, or may penetrate directly into the endometrium. The chorionic villi occur in ungulates, cetaceans and man, producing a villous placenta, but in other mammals the villi fuse and assume a more labyrinthine configuration. The shape of the chorioallantoic placenta is determined by the distribution of villi over the chorionic surface. In some species, the villi persist over most of the chorionic surface, and the placenta represents a rather thick but continuous membrane of tissue, such as in the placenta diffusa of the pig, horse, and porpoise. In other species, such as cattle and sheep, the villi are restricted to areas identified as caruncles over the uterus, even in the nonpregnant state. These caruncles define potential implantation sites and, with the development of placentation, the chorion produces tufts of villi confined to those areas. The zonal placenta of most carnivores has villi grouped in bands around the equator of the chorioallantoic sac. In man, apes, rodents, bats, and most insectivores, placentas are disc-shaped.

The number of tissue layers constituting the placental membrane forms the basis of Grosser's classification of chorioallantoic placentas. The minimal histologic barrier between maternal and fetal circulations is represented by the hemochorial placenta found in most rodents, higher primates, and some insectivores. The hemochorial placenta is comprised of only three fetal components—the trophoblast, connective tissue, and fetal endothelium—with the trophoblast being exposed directly to the maternal blood. Grosser's approach to the classification of placental morphology has stood the test of time; however, its shortcomings include the lack of description for the structural complexity of the placental membrane, the changes accompanying placental maturation, and the accessory placental organs.

The implication in any classification of placental types based upon the number of tissue layers in the placental membrane is that membrane thickness determines the rate of transfer of compounds across the placenta. This would certainly be true for those compounds crossing by simple diffusion; however, it may or may not be true for compounds transported by a carrier-mediated mechanism or by active transport. Within these limitations, however, there are suggestions that, for various solutes, placental

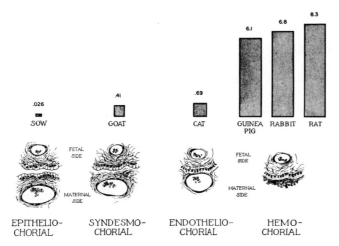

Figure 1. Variation of transfer rate per unit weight of placenta with the morphologic type of placenta. The numerical values give the milligrams of Na transferred across a unit weight of placenta per hour as observed in each instance at the middle of the ninth-tenth of pregnancy. The relative magnitudes of the transfer rates are indicated by the relative areas of the dotted rectangles. The diagrams indicate the number and kind of tissue layers interposed between maternal and fetal circulations in each of Grosser's four groups. From Flexner, L. B., and Gellhorn, A. The comparative physiology of placental transfer. *Am. J. Ob. Gyn.* 43:965–974, 1942.

permeability does correlate with placental type and, specifically, with a placental classification based upon the number of tissue layers. The transfer rate of sodium across various types of placentas is shown in Figure 1. Note the inverse relationship between the number of placental tissue layers and the transfer rate of sodium, the placental transfer of which is limited by the permeability of the placental diffusing membrane. If one considers the transfer of carbohydrates, a group of solutes believed to be transferred by specific carrier-mediated pathways, there is still a suggestion of increasing glucose permeability with decreasing placental thickness. Figure 2 presents a comparison of the relationship between umbilical arterial glucose concentration and maternal arterial glu-

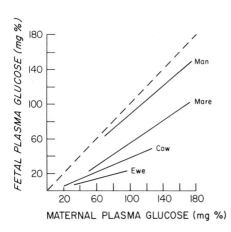

Figure 2. The relationship of fetal umbilical arterial and maternal arterial glucose concentration. The slope of the regression line for fetal versus maternal glucose concentration approaches the dashed identity line with the hemochorial placenta of man. The slope of the regression line decreases with thicker placental types. Redrawn from Coltart, T. M. Beard, R. W., Turner, R. C., and Oakley, N. W. Blood glucose and insulin relations in the human mother and fetus before onset of labour. *Brit. Med. J.* 4:17–19, 1969, and Silver, M., Steven, D. H., and Comline, R. S. Placental exchange and morphology in ruminants and mare, in Comline, R. S. (ed.): *Foetal and Neonatal Physiology: Barcroft Centenary Symposium.*

cose concentration, with an identity line shown for comparison. As Figure 2 demonstrates, the slope of the regression line for umbilical arterial versus maternal arterial glucose concentration is less with thicker placentas, and approaches an identity line with the hemochorial placenta of the rhesus monkey or man. Thus, for electrolytes, for compounds moving by simple diffusion, and even for some of the compounds whose transfer is regulated by specific carrier systems, there appears to be increasing placental permeability as the number of placental tissue layers is decreased.

GROSS STRUCTURE OF THE PLACENTA

Although the human placenta resembles an amorphous tissue mass with little intrinsic organization, it is, in fact, a highly structured organ. The gross anatomy of the placenta is dominated by its vascular organization. Its structure brings the maternal and fetal circulations into such close apposition that exchange between them is efficient. The relationship between the two circulations is also dynamic, enabling the placenta to meet the progressive demands of the growing fetus.

In man the umbilical cord is composed of one umbilical vein and two umbilical arteries. Its length is variable, measuring as little as 10 cm. or as much as 150 cm. Functionally, the umbilical vein can be regarded as a composite of pulmonary and portal veins, for it contains the most highly oxygenated blood of the fetus and that richest in nutrients. The umbilical vein terminates within the fetal abdomen at its junction with the ductus venosus. The umbilical arteries are the main continuation of the fetal internal iliac arteries and carry the deoxygenated blood to the placenta. Usually the umbilical arteries are equal in size, each supplying one half of the placenta. But variations in which the arteries supply unequal portions of the placenta are common.

The cotyledons of the human placenta comprise the terminal portions of the fetal circulation. The peripheral surface of the cotyledon displays the capillary bed which forms the functional unit for exchange by diffusion within the placenta. The average placenta is formed from approximately 200 cotyledons of varying size. The cotyledon develops with progressive divisions of the primary trunks and formation of villi, each containing a single artery and vein separated from the intervillous space by trophoblastic tissue. The shape of the cotyledon is globular, with the broader peripheral end toward the decidua. Cotyledons interdigitate with each other, grouping themselves around the largest cotyledon. This grouping and interdigitation produces the characteristic lobes of the maternal surface of the placenta. Twenty to 40 lobes can usually be recognized, although the grooves between the lobes are often indistinct. Even though there is an impression of continuity of cotyledonary substance throughout the placenta, anastomosis between vessels in the same or contiguous cotyledons apparently does not occur.

The placenta's growth depends on the enlargement of those cotyledons established early in gestation through further branching of villi; new cotyledons are not formed after the first several weeks of placental development. Through continuing formation of new villi, the volume of a cotyledon at term may be 500 times its volume at 12 weeks.

DEVELOPMENT AND MATURATION OF THE PLACENTA

Implantation and subsequent development of the human placenta depend upon the maturation of the endometrial lining to form a receptive state for the blastocyst. Attachment of an implanting blastocyst normally occurs between openings of the enlarged endometrial glands of the luteal phase. The glands adjacent to the site of nidation are compressed and occluded by the circumferential growth of the blastocyst and dilate markedly with the accumulation of secretions. After the erosion of the endometrial stroma and glandular epithelium by the actively proliferating trophoblast, the endometrial glands are able to contribute directly to the nourishment of the conceptus before a placental circulation develops.

By the eighth day, the blastocytic trophoblast has differentiated at the implantation pole into a thick plaque of proliferating syncytium and cytotrophoblast. The primitive syncytium is primarily responsible for the local destruction and invasion of maternal tissues. The syncytium shows marked vacuolation soon after its first appearance. The vacuoles become confluent by the twelfth day, forming lacunar spaces throughout the syncytium. Dilated maternal sinusoids open and communicate with the lacunae, filling them with maternal blood. During the next week of placental development, the trophoblast proliferates radially around the chorion, taking on a villous appearance, while the maternal circulation becomes well established within the intervillous space.

The villous cores are established when mesenchymal elements invade the primary villi, converting them into secondary villi. Tertiary villi are formed with vascularization of the stroma of secondary villi. Tertiary villi first appear in the late presomite embryo, but new villi continue to develop throughout all of gestation. The surface area of the placenta is increased by this continued growth of new villi (Fig. 3), contributing to the increased permeability of the placenta with advancing gestation.

Age differences are recognizable among villous structures. In general, the older the villi the smaller are their average diameters. The terminal villi of mature placentas are more richly vascularized than villi of younger placentas, with blood vessels closer to the overlying trophoblast in older placentas. Maturational alterations occur in the trophoblast, its basement membrane, and the villous stroma. These changes include thinning of the syncytial trophoblast, decrease in cytotrophoblastic cell numbers with interruption of Langhans' layer, attentuation of the basement membrane, and increased stromal fibrosis. And even though these structural changes suggest degeneration histologically,

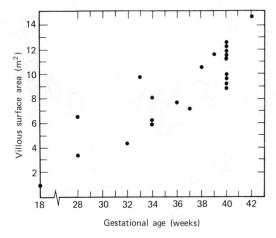

Figure 3. Villous surface area of the human placenta versus gestational age. From Aherne, W., and Dunnill, M. S. Quantitative aspects of placental structure. *J. Path. Bact.* 91:123–139, 1966.

they coincide and most likely contribute to the increasing permeability which the placenta shows with increasing gestation.

Early in gestation the cytotrophoblast forms a continuous layer of cells known as Langhans' layer between the syncytium and the fetal vessels. In the second half of pregnancy, Langhans' cells are progressively reduced. The cytotrophoblast of the terminal villi may be found in full-term placentas as isolated cells, as small groups of cells, or even as a continuous layer. The progressive reduction of cytotrophoblast with advancing gestation is illustrated in Figures 4 and 5. As gestation advances, the syncytium is renewed from cytotrophoblast. The gradual disappearance of the Langhans' layer without obvious cellular degeneration and the presence of frequent mitosis in cytotrophoblast with none in the syncytium support the contention that disappearing cytotrophoblast is transformed into syncytium. A brush border is a prominent feature of the syncytial villous surface. The brush border is present on large areas of villous syncytium at all stages of gestation. Electron microscopy has demonstrated that the brush border of syncytium is composed of a complex of microvilli, as illustrated in Figure 6. These microvilli further increase the surface area of the villi and increase the permeability of the placental membrane. By the fourth month of gestation, the thickness of the syncytium shows considerable regional variation, ranging from 2 μ on the trunci to 10 μ, or more, on the terminal villi. As gestation advances, there is progressive thinning of the syncytial layer, as illustrated in Figures 4 and 5. The combined effect of the

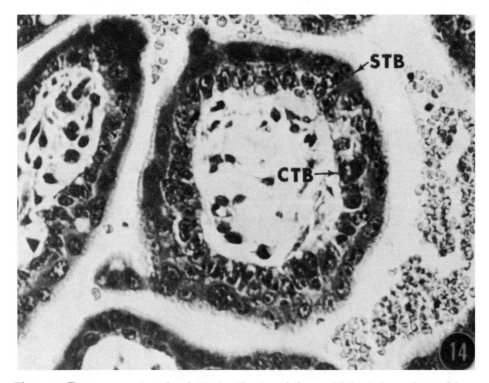

Figure 4. Transverse section of a chorionic villus branch from a 26-day baboon placenta showing the double nature of the villus wall. CTB, cytotrophoblast; STB, syncytiotrophoblast. From Houston, M. L. The villous period of placentogenesis in the baboon. *Am. J. Anat.* 126:1–16, 1969.

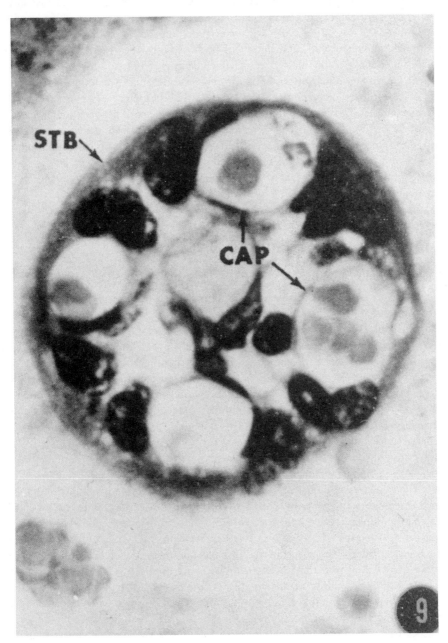

Figure 5. A photomicrograph taken late in the fetal period. Note the lack of cytotrophoblast, the diminished diameter of the villus, the close proximity of the fetal capillary (CAP) to the villus wall, and the thinned syncytial wall (STB). From Houston, M. L. The development of the baboon placenta during the fetal period of gestation. *Am. J. Anat.* 126:17–30, 1969.

disappearance of the cytotrophoblast and the thinning of the syncytium with advancing gestation is to decrease the diffusing distance between the maternal and fetal circulation, increasing the permeability of the placenta. Thus, the increase in placental permeability to a wide variety of substances with advancing gestation can be related to the placenta's maturational changes of villi, and microvilli proliferation which increases surface area, and to thinning of the trophoblastic layers which decreases diffusion distance.

The early events of fertilization, implantation, and placental development can greatly influence the ultimate outcome of the pregnancy. The frequency of spontaneous abortion, for example, increases significantly as the time span between ovulation and fertilization increases (1). This suggests that aging of spermatozoa or ova can have deleterious effects, more subtle than unsuccessful fertilization, which become apparent long after successful fertilization has occurred. Similarly, the number of cotyledons formed during the earliest phase of placental development can be a limiting factor of both placental and fetal size at term (2).

PHYSIOLOGY OF TRANSPLACENTAL DIFFUSION

The Exchange Function of the Placenta

Although the placenta has invasive and regulatory functions, its most obvious function is that of an exchanger. The placenta exchanges respiratory gases, metabolic fuels, and excretory products between the maternal and fetal circulations. The efficiency of this exchange process varies among species, among substances and with gestational age. Several indices have been proposed to evaluate the placenta's performance as an exchanger: the transfer rate across the placenta; transplacental concentration gradients, a reflection of placental permeability; and placental clearance. Because the measure of the efficiency of placental exchange is important to an understanding of the physiology of transplacental diffusion, transfer rate, permeability, and clearance are discussed in some detail in the following text.

The relative directions of flow of the two streams of an exchange organ such as the placenta are an important determinant of the efficiency of transfer of matter or heat between the two streams. There is significant physiological evidence indicating that the placenta resembles a concurrent exchanger functionally, at least in some species such as primates and sheep. In other species this pattern of perfusion has not been demonstrated. Characteristically, a concurrent exchanger is one in which the blood flows on either side of the placenta are in the same direction. The transfer rate of a substance across the placenta can be calculated by an application of the Fick principle, which states that the quantity transfered across the organ is the product of the arterial and venous concentration differences and the rate of blood flow to the organ. Thus, the quantity leaving the uterine circulation and entering the umbilical circulation can be determined by an application of the Fick principle to either side of the membrane. It is important to emphasize that whole blood concentrations must be determined in order to apply the Fick principle to a calculation of a quantity of substance entering or leaving an organ. If the blood flow on either side of the placenta were altered, the transfer rate of the substance across the placenta might or might not change proportionately, depending upon whether the placenta permeability was limiting the rate of transfer. Two extremes are possible. In one case the rate of transfer would be a function only of the rate of perfusion of the organ, the placenta being sufficiently permeable to the substance

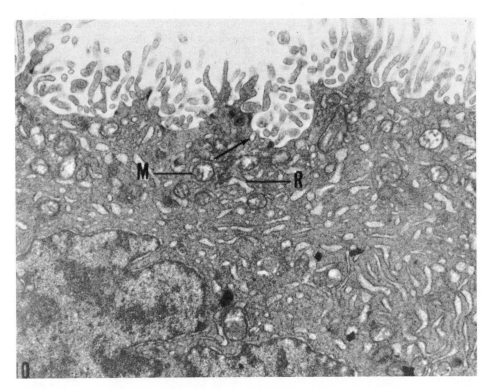

Figure 6. Syncytial surface at term, showing well-developed vesicular and tubular endoplasmic reticulum (R). Small promontories and numerous microvilli project from the surface, beneath which are numerous pinocytotic vesicles (arrow) and mitochondria (M). From Wynn, R. M., Pinigel, M., and MacLennan, A. H. Fine structure of placental and fetal membranes of the baboon. *Am. J. Ob. Gyn.* 109:638–648, 1971.

that it provides no barrier to transfer. Such substances would be flow limited in their rates of transfer. Another extreme would be represented by the exchange of a substance across the placenta in which a doubling of blood flows produces no change in the rate of transfer. In this instance, the rate of transfer would be entirely permeability-limited. For most substances crossing the placenta their rates of transfer fall between these two extremes and are altered by placenta permeability and by blood flow. For example, glucose, a substance crossing the placenta by a specific carrier-mediated system is primarily permeability-limited across the sheep placenta. Thus, marked alteration in uterine and umbilical blood flow produce little change in the rate of transfer of glucose.

It should be emphasized that a system simulating a concurrent exchanger has, as a characteristic, equilibration of the outflow streams. In the case of the placenta, this means the uterine veins and umbilical veins tend to equilibrate. This is an important point when we come to consider fetal oxygenation since it limits the most arterialized blood of the fetus to the oxygen tensions of the uterine venous circulation.

Placental Clearance

The concept of placental clearance has been as useful in fetal physiology as that of renal clearance has been in renal physiology. The placental clearance of a compound is equal to the ratio of the quantity crossing per unit time divided by the concentration difference between two arterial streams into the placenta, namely, the uterine arterial and umbilical arterial concentrations:

$$C = \frac{q}{c_A - c_a}$$

Placental clearance will be a function of both perfusion (uterine blood flow and umbilical blood flow) and permeability of the placenta. The clearance by an organ of a compound measures some functional property of that organ; the functional property measured depends upon the characteristics of the test substance. For example, inulin clearance across the kidney measures glomerular filtration rate, while PAH clearance measures renal blood flow, and urea clearance measures a complex combination of functional properties of the kidneys. Similarly in the placenta, depending upon the test substance chosen for the clearance measurement, placental clearance may reflect the combined effects of perfusion or may reflect placental permeability or the characteristics of both.

The placental clearance can be determined in the following way: A constant infusion of a substance is introduced into the fetal circulation and eventually reaches a state in which the transplacental diffusion rate becomes equal to the infusion rate of the substance with minor corrections. Because the infusion rate of the substance is known and the concentrations of this substance in the two arterial streams can be measured, the placental clearance can be calculated.

The Placental Clearance of Specific Substances

If a constant infusion of a substance is introduced into the fetal circulation, eventually a steady state develops in which the transplacental diffusion rate is equal to the infusion rate of the substance, with minor corrections. Then, the placental clearance can be calculated and the uterine and umbilical blood flows can be determined experimentally by measuring the concentration of the substance in the inflow and outflow streams of the placenta. Data for three substances from such an experiment, using the sheep model, are presented in Figure 7. If the placenta is highly permeable to the substance, clearance will be flow-limited and the uterine and umbilical vein concentrations will be nearly identical. Such is the case for both antipyrine and tritiated water in this example. In contrast, the concentration difference of urea between the uterine and umbilical veins is large, indicating that clearance of urea is far from maximum and, therefore, must be limited by the permeability of the sheep placenta to urea.

If the clearances of antipyrine and tritiated water are calculated, they are found to be identical. In vitro measurements, however, indicate that the permeability of tritiated water is three times greater than that of antipyrine. These data indicate that the transplacental clearance of water and antipyrine represent the maximal clearance of inert molecules. For the concurrent exchanger, this is a flow-limited clearance. Figure 8 presents in vivo data comparing the relationship between antipyrine clearance across the ovine placenta and maximal clearance for an ideal concurrent exchanger. Antipyrine clearance is not quite identical to the maximal clearance of a totally efficient concurrent exchanger.

Defining a maximal clearance across the placenta has the value of providing a fixed reference point by which to compare the clearances of other substances. For this com-

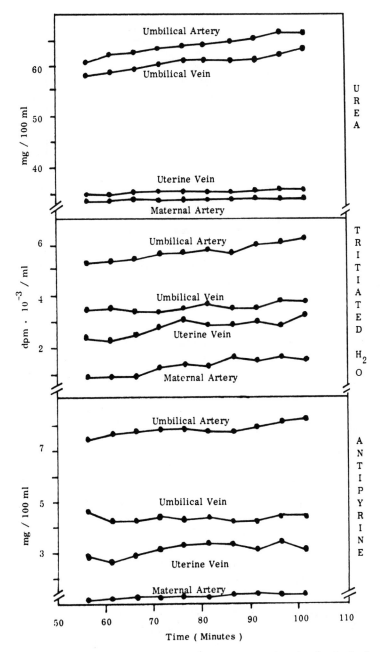

Figure 7. The blood concentrations of urea, tritiated water, and antipyrine in the four placental vessels are plotted against time. Time zero represents the beginning of constant infusion of these three substances in the fetus. From Meschia, G., Battaglia, F. C., and Bruns, P. D. Theoretical and experimental study of transplacental diffusion. *J. Appl. Physiol.* 22:1171–1178, 1967.

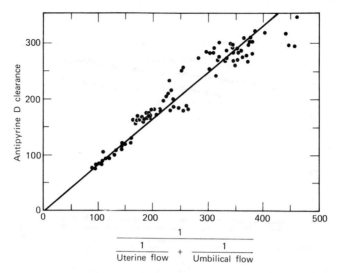

Figure 8. Relationship between the placental diffusion clearance of antipyrine and the uterine and umbilical flows. From Meschia, G., Cotter, J. R., Makowski, E. L., and Barron, D. H. Simultaneous measurement of uterine and umbilical blood flows and oxygen uptakes. *Quart. J. Exper. Physiol.* 52:1–18, 1967.

parison of clearances, the degree of diffusion limitation (L_D), can be defined as the relative decrease in clearance that occurs when the permeability of the substance is low enough to become a determinant of clearance. The diffusion limitation is defined by the simple equation

$$L_D = \frac{C_{max} - C}{C_{max}}$$

where C_{max} represents the clearance of the flow-limited substance. In this scheme, the diffusion limitation for flow-limited, maximal clearance will equal zero, while the diffusion limitation for a substance totally impermeable to the placenta will equal one.

The diffusion limitations of five substances across the placenta for sheep and rhesus monkeys are shown in Table I. Clearance is maximal for tritiated water and antipyrine in both species; therefore, the diffusion limitation equals zero. The placental clearance of urea for both animals is only 30 per cent of the antipyrine or tritiated water clearance, indicating urea clearance is permeability-limited in sheep and monkeys. The clearances of sodium and chloride in sheep are determined principally by the permeability of the placenta to these substances and are virtually independent of blood flow. A striking difference between the syndesmochorial placenta of the sheep and the hemochorial placenta of the primate is shown by the fact that clearances of sodium and chloride approach 20 per cent of the maximal flow limited clearance for the primate placenta. Thus, the primate placenta, while similar to the sheep placenta in other respects, is much more permeable to sodium and chloride.

Both flow-limited and permeability-limited clearances increase with advancing gestation, indicating an increase in the efficiency of the exchange mechanism of the placenta during a period when the metabolic and respiratory demands of the fetus continue to

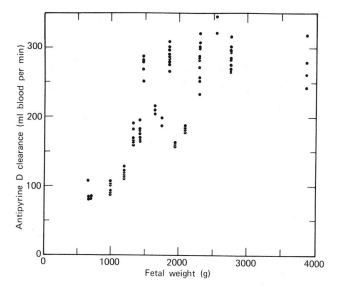

Figure 9. Plot of the placental diffusion clearance of antipyrine against fetal body weight. From Meschia, G., Cotter, J. R., Makowski, E. L., and Barron, D. H. Simultaneous measurement of uterine and umbilical blood flows and oxygen uptakes. *Quart. J. Exper. Physiol.* 52:1–18, 1967.

increase. The increase in antipyrine clearance with continued fetal growth is shown in Figure 9. Since antipyrine clearance is flow-limited, its increase reflects an increased flow to the placenta from umbilical and uterine circulations. Microsphere studies of uterine and umbilical blood flows indicate that the flows of both streams increase as the fetus increases in size and that the increased flows are primarily to the cotyledons (Figs. 10 and 11).

The clearance of substances limited by placental permeability also increases with advancing gestation. The permeability, or diffusing capacity, of urea increases linearly

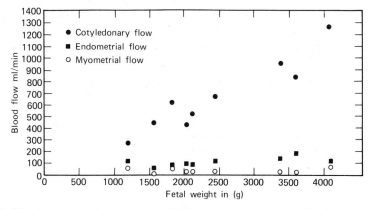

Figure 10. Blood flow to various segments of the uterus versus fetal weight. From Makowski, E. L., Meschia, G., Droegemueller, W., and Battaglia, F. C. Distribution of uterine blood flow in the pregnant sheep. *Am. J. Ob. Gyn.* 101:409–412, 1968.

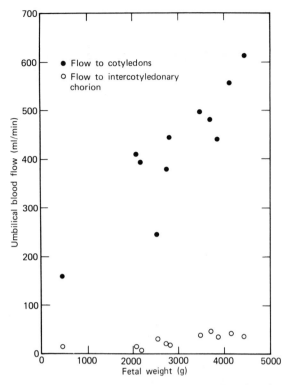

Figure 11. Cotyledonary and intercotyledonary blood flows plotted against fetal weight. From Makowski, E. L., Meschia, G., Droegemueller, W., and Battaglia, F. C. Measurement of umbilical arterial blood flow to the sheep placenta and fetus in utero. *Circ. Res.* 23:623–631, 1968.

in the sheep placenta with fetal weight, as is shown in Figure 12. This rise in placental permeability continues until term in spite of the cessation in placental growth, measured in placental weight and DNA content, which occurs during midgestation in the sheep. Similarly, Hellman et al. (3) noted an increase in the sodium permeability of the human placenta with advancing gestation. The increase in permeability with gestation corresponds to maturational changes in the morphology of the placenta described earlier.

Table I. Diffusion Limitation L_D of Various Solutes

Solute	L_D for Sheep	L_D for Rhesus Monkey
THO	0.00	0.00
Antipyrine	0.00	0.00
Urea	0.72	0.73
Sodium 22	0.90	0.83
Chloride 36	0.90	0.78

SOURCE: Battaglia, F. C., Meschia, G., and Makowski, E. L. Comparison of in vitro and in vivo placental permeability measurements. *Am. J. Physiol.*, **216**:1540–1544 (1969).

Histologic changes in the placenta with advancing gestation, interpreted by some as aging, and the decreased rate of growth of the placenta relative to fetal growth have been used to support the concept that an increasing placental insufficiency develops late in pregnancy which compromises fetal growth near term. The functional studies of the placenta just presented, however, indicate that the placenta increases its efficiency of exchange with advancing gestation, though not necessarily its weight, to keep pace with the increasing metabolic and respiratory demands of the growing fetus.

Oxygen Transfer Across the Placenta

The exchange of the protein-bound substance oxygen across the placenta is more complex than for an inert, unbound substance such as antipyrine. The rate of transfer of oxygen depends on the flow rates of the uterine and umbilical streams, the permeability of the placental membrane to oxygen, and the concentration and oxygen affinity of hemoglobin in the two streams. Furthermore, placental O_2 consumption tends to lower uterine venous P_{O_2} and thus umbilical venous P_{O_2}. Since oxygen transfer is primarily flow-limited under normal conditions, the umbilical venous P_{O_2}, while tending to equilibrate with uterine venous P_{O_2}, will never exceed it. This relationship between umbilical and uterine venous P_{O_2} is illustrated in Figure 13.

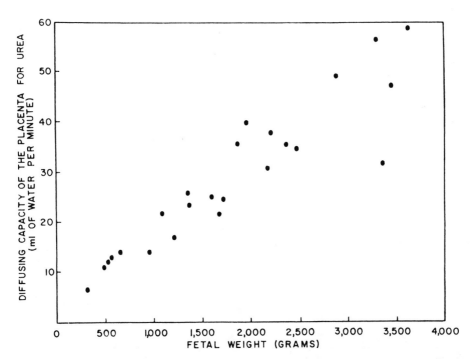

Figure 12. The milligrams of urea that cross the placenta in 1 min for a transplacental difference of concentration of 1 mg/ml of water are plotted against the fetal body weight. From Meschia, G., Breathnach, C. S., Cotter, J. R., Hellegers, A., and Barron, D. H. The diffusion of urea across the sheep placenta in the last 2 months of gestation. *Quart. J. Exper. Physiol.* 50:23–41, 1965.

Both the permeability of the placenta to oxygen and the flow rates of the perfusing streams of the placenta increase with advancing gestation and contribute to an increase in the efficiency of exchange for oxygen. Nevertheless, the increase with advancing gestation in total oxygen uptake by the umbilical circulation is very large, and also results in a wider concentration difference of oxygen across the uterine circulation.

Because the umbilical venous Po_2 cannot exceed the uterine venous Po_2, the fetus must maintain adequate oxygen uptake in the presence of very low oxygen tensions. The higher O_2 affinity of fetal blood is one mechanism contributing to the ability of the fetus to accomplish this task, demonstrated by the maternal and fetal oxyhemoglobin dissociation curves shown in Figure 14. Since fetal red cells bind more oxygen at a given Po_2 than do maternal cells, the fetal oxyhemoglobin dissociation curve is to the left of the maternal curve.

An understanding of the physiology of transplacental oxygen exchange and of the oxygen affinity relationship of fetal and maternal blood leads to an accurate interpretation of the fetal benefits of maternal oxygen therapy. When the mother inhales 100 per cent oxygen, her arterial Po_2 may approach 600 mmHg. Uterine venous Po_2 rises also, but much less than the arterial Po_2.

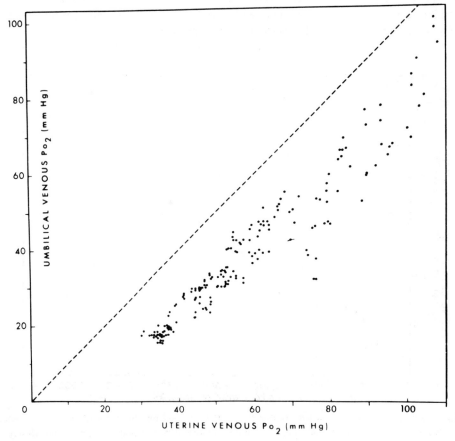

Figure 13. Umbilical venous Po_2. From Rankin, J. H. G., Meschia, G., Makowski, E. L., and Battaglia, F. C. Relationship between uterine and umbilical venous Po_2 in sheep. *Am. J. Physiol.* 220:1688–1692, 1971.

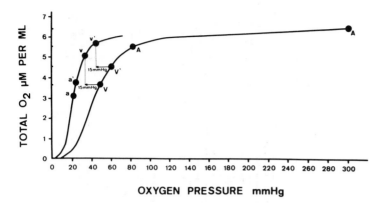

Figure 14. Effect of maternal O_2 inhalation in the normal animal. A plot of O_2 content versus P_{O_2} for ovine fetal and maternal blood. Maternal arterial points, A (normal) and A' (hyperoxia); uterine venous points, V (normal) and V' (hyperoxia); umbilical venous points, v (normal) and v' (hyperoxia); umbilical arterial points, a (normal) and a' (hyperoxia). From Meschia, G. *Physiology of transplacental diffusion*, in Wynn, Ralph M. (ed.): *Obstetrics and Gynecology Annual: 1976*. New York, Appleton-Century-Crofts, 1976.

The increase in maternal arterial P_{O_2} does not cause any significant change in uterine blood flow or an increase in oxygen consumption. Thus, the arterial–venous difference of oxygen content per milliliter of blood before and during oxygen therapy remains constant. Because of the shape of the oxyhemoglobin dissociation curve (Fig. 14), an equal vertical shift of the maternal arterial point, A to A', and venous point V to V', results in a much smaller P_{O_2} change in the vein than in the artery. The P_{O_2} change in the umbilical vein, v to v', will also be small because of the relationship of umbilical venous P_{O_2} to uterine venous P_{O_2}. Furthermore, the increase of umbilical arterial P_{O_2}, a to a', will be even smaller than in the umbilical vein because the umbilical arterial point is positioned on the steepest part of the fetal oxyhemoglobin dissociation curve. The critical fact to note is that the increase in umbilical arterial P_{O_2} of only a few mmHg results in nearly a 30 per cent increase in oxygen content in the blood supplying the fetal tissues. Thus, even a small increase in fetal arterial P_{O_2} can lead to a substantial and at times life-saving increase in fetal oxygen content.

FETAL GROWTH

The Relationship of Fetal and Placental Weight

The relationship of placental weight and infant birthweight has been studied in many mammals, including man. Thomson et al. (6) looked at this relationship in their study of more than 52,000 pregnancies in Aberdeen. At any gestational age large placentas are associated with larger mean birthweights, as can be seen in Figure 15. The fetal weight-to-placental weight ratio increases from 32 weeks of gestation onward, indicating that while both the fetus and placenta increase in weight as gestation progresses, the fetal growth rate is greater than that of the placenta.

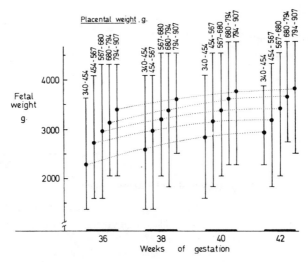

Figure 15. Means and ranges of birthweights at certain weeks of gestation by placental weight. The values at each stage of gestation have been "staggered" for the sake of clarity. From Thomson, A. M., Billewicz, W. Z., and Hytten, F. E. The weight of the placenta in relation to birthweight. *J. Obstet. Gynaecol. Brit. Commwlth.* 76:865–872, 1969.

The relationship between the growth rates of placenta and fetus varies with gestational age and with species. The relationship is similar in the rhesus monkey and man, as is shown in Figure 16. Early in gestation the placental and fetal growth rates are similar. Later, the fetal growth rate increases substantially while the placenta continues to grow until term at a fairly constant rate. In contrast, the sheep placenta achieves its maximal weight at 90 days of gestation, and shows no further weight increase during the period of maximal fetal growth, as is demonstrated in Figure 17.

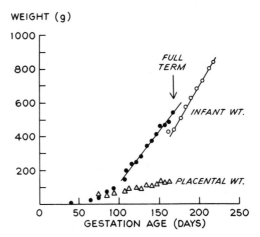

Figure 16. Prenatal and postnatal growth in the rhesus monkey. From Dawes, G. S. The placenta and foetal growth, in *Fetal and Neonatal Physiology*. Chicago, Yearbook Medical Publishers, Inc., 1968, pp. 42–59.

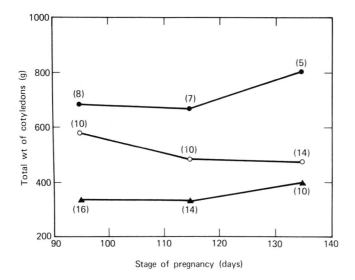

Figure 17. Total weight of intact cotyledons in ewes killed between the 95th and 135th day of pregnancy. The numbers of animals are shown in parentheses. ●'s, ditocous ewes (total per ewe); ▲'s ditocous ewes (total per fetus); O's, monotocous ewes. From Alexander, G. Studies on the placenta of the sheep. *J. Reprod. Fertil.* 7:289–305, 1964.

There are three stages of placental development: implantation, growth, and organ maturation. The studies by Alexander (3a) in sheep illustrate the potential impact of the implantation phase in determining the size of the placenta at the end of gestation. The separate cotyledons of the sheep placenta are formed during the implantation stage of development when the blastocyst makes contact with the caruncles of the uterine mucosa. Cotyledons are usually formed at only 70 to 80 per cent of the uterine caruncles, the number being fixed by the fiftieth day of gestation. The second stage of placental development is growth of the individual cotyledons, and is complete by the ninetieth day of gestation. Functional maturation of the placenta continues until term despite a plateau in placental weight.

Kulhanek et al. (2) have demonstrated a realtionship between placental size and placental functional capacity. In sheep, fetal growth in the last third of gestation takes place without any significant increase in placental weight and DNA content. However, the permeability of urea per gram of DNA increases fivefold in the last 50 days of gestation, as is shown in Figure 18. Thus, advancing gestation is accompanied by increasing placental function, even though cellular growth of the placenta has ceased.

Cotyledon number varies widely in sheep, though usually 70 to 80 per cent of the 100 caruncles present are used. Fetal weight does not correlate well with cotyledon number because of the wide variation in cotyledonary size. In fact, the mean weight of cotyledons is inversely related to their number. This indicates compensatory growth at each implantation site when relatively few cotyledons develop, although compensatory growth is inadequate to reach a normal placental size. Thus, the placenta with fewer total cotyledons is smaller and contains less total DNA than one with the usual complement of cotyledons. The smaller placenta will, therefore, show a relative functional

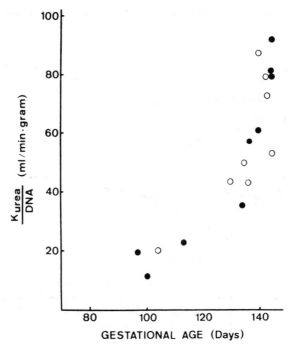

Figure 18. Urea permeability per gram of placental DNA rises steeply the last 2 months of gestation. ●'s, singletons; O's, twins. From Kulhanek, J. F., Meschia, G., Makowski, E. L., and Battaglia, F. C. Changes in DNA content and urea permeability of the sheep placenta. *Am. J. Physiol.* 226:1257–1263, 1974.

impairment compared with a placenta of normal cotyledon number, as is illustrated in Figure 19.

The placenta in normal rhesus monkeys continues to increase in weight, DNA, RNA, and protein content until term, as shown in Figure 20. In studies of the human placenta, Dayton (3b) found a similar linear increase of DNA content until term. The importance of placental size to placental function and fetal development is also substantiated by the morphometric data of Aherne and Dunnill (3c). The chorionic villous surface area relates directly to placental volume, as demonstrated in Figure 21. It is likely that the correlation of placental and fetal weight reflects the functional relationship of chorionic villous surface area to the efficiency of transfer of metabolic substrates to the fetus.

It is important, therefore, when attempting to sort out the relationship of placental function to placental size, that one compare placentas of the same gestational age. Otherwise, the marked maturational changes will obscure the relation of size to function.

Other Determinants of Fetal Growth

In addition to the direct effects of placental weight and function, fetal growth is influenced by a large number of other factors. Some of these are discussed below.

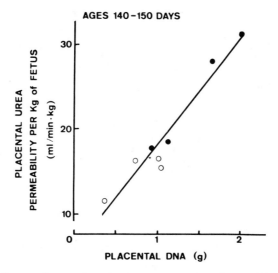

AGES 140–150 DAYS

Figure 19. Among fetuses of approximately the same age, there is a positive correlation between urea permeability per kilogram of fetal weight and total placental DNA (first-order regression analysis). ●'s, singletons; O's, twins. From Kulhanek, J. F., Meschia, G., Makowski, E. L., and Battaglia, F. C. Changes in DNA content and urea permeability of the sheep placenta. *Am. J. Physiol.* 226:1257–1263, 1974.

The sex of the fetus influences birthweight during the last few weeks of pregnancy in both man and animals. At 32 weeks of gestation in the human, the weights of male and female fetuses are essentially the same. But, thereafter, males grow at a more rapid rate. After 38 weeks, males are about 150 grams heavier than females, with little or no compensatory increase in placental weight.

Infant birthweight is also related to parental height and weight. The paternal contribution to birthweight is mediated solely through the father's contribution to the genetic makeup of the fetus. The maternal contribution is more extensive and includes

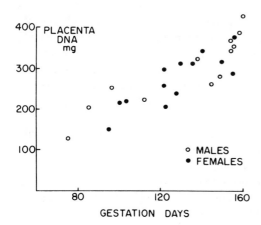

Figure 20. The change during gestation in the total placental DNA in the macaque. From Hill, D. E. Cellular growth of the rhesus monkey placenta, in Cheek, D. B. (ed.): *Fetal and Postnatal Cellular Growth.* New York, John Wiley & Sons, 1975.

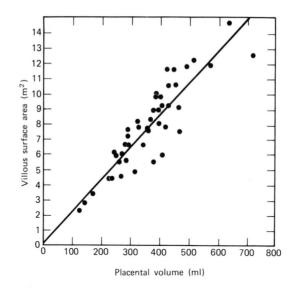

Figure 21. Chorionic villous surface area plotted against placental volume. From Aherne, W., and Dunnill, M. S. Morphometry of the human placenta. *Brit. Med. Bull.* 22:5–8, 1966.

both the genetic influence and the influence of the untrauterine environment of the fetus, the latter being much more significant. The classic demonstration of the relationship between fetal growth and intrauterine environment was made by Walton and Hammond (4). In this study, large Shire horses were crossed with small Shetland ponies. At birth the foals were very similar in size and birthweight to foals of the pure breeds to which the mothers belonged, with the cross-foals from the Shire mare approximately three times the size of the cross-foals from the Shetland mares. Maternal nutrition and weight gain during pregnancy have also been shown to relate to birthweight and placental weight in both animals and man. A significant decrease in birthweight and placental weight was noted, for example, during the Dutch wartime famine, but the effects were limited to mothers who experienced famine during the third trimester, the period of most rapid fetal growth.

The effect of birth order on birthweight can be a useful measure in the multiparous patient to distinguish an impaired intrauterine growth pattern from physiologic growth. The second baby is approximately 130 grams heavier than the first, with smaller weight increments in subsequent pregnancies. These differences do not appear to be related to maternal age or stature. Although an initial spontaneous abortion seems to have no effect on subsequent birthweight, the effect of an initial stillbirth is to decrease the average weight of a second baby by 250 grams compared with second babies with a liveborn first sibling.

There is also a highly significant correlation between length and birthweight of siblings, indicating that mothers have a distinct tendency to have babies of similar birthweights. Thus, intrauterine fetal growth and birthweight are better evaluated against the fetal growth pattern of earlier pregnancies than against a standardized growth chart. This was demonstrated in the study of Turner (5), in which the birthweights of infants with congenital rubella and their siblings were compared.

LGA and SGA Infants

Deviations from normal intrauterine growth are associated with increased perinatal morbidity and mortality. Large-for-gestational-age infants are often the product of mothers with diabetes mellitus of varying degrees of severity and duration. Presumably, the abnormal glucose metabolism of these mothers provides an environment of excessive substrate to the fetus, stimulating insulin secretion in the fetus, resulting in growth of both fetus and placenta. The large size of these infants does not imply organ maturity, which is much better correlated with gestational age than with size.

Small-for-gestational-age infants result from a reduction of the normal growth potential of the fetus or from inadequate maternal or placental support for fetal growth. Reduced growth potential of the fetus can result from chromosomal or genetic abnormalities of the fetus or from viral infections such as rubella or cytomegalic inclusion disease.

The exact mechanisms of inadequate maternal and placental support of the fetus that lead to growth retardation are poorly understood. A number of theories have been proposed and indicate our overall uncertainty about the maternal and placental causes of intrauterine growth retardation.

As already alluded to, an early mechanism by which placental development, and thus, fetal development may be impaired occurs early in pregnancy at the time of implantation. During this critical time, the cotyledonary number of the placenta is established. Later in pregnancy, more obvious pathology such as multiple small infarcts of the placenta may reduce placental function. A limitation in placental function from any cause might then impose on the fetus the dilemma of curbing its own rate of growth and metabolism in order to avoid hypoxia and hypoglycemia or, on the other hand, maintaining normal rates of growth at the risk of hypoxia or inadequate nutrition. The solution achieved is a compromise by which the fetus is growth-retarded, yet relatively large with respect to the functional capacity of the placenta.

Fetal growth may be affected by maternal pathology, often attributed to the imprecise, "wastebasket" term, "uteroplacental vascular insufficiency." These diseases include pregnancy-induced and essential hypertension, severe diabetes mellitus, chronic renal disease, or collagen vascular disease, all of which can lead to inadequate uterine blood flow. Presumably the supply of a variety of nutrients may then be restricted, both to the placenta and to the fetus. It is interesting that it is in association with chronic vascular disease in the mother that one finds a small placenta as well as a growth-retarded fetus. In contrast, in some clinical conditions, such as preeclampsia occurring late in the pregnancy, the fetal/placental weight ratio is low (6). This is probably related to a limitation in the supply of nutrients from the maternal circulation occurring at a time when fetal growth is much faster than that of the placenta.

In addition to the metabolic building blocks supplying carbon and nitrogen for growth, a restriction of oxygen supply to the fetus seems to have a growth-retarding effect. Studies of both man and sheep at elevations greater than 10,000 feet indicate that hypoxia is an important factor in the etiology of fetal-growth retardation (7,8).

Small-for-gestational-age infants have increased perinatal morbidity and mortality in comparison with their gestational-age peers. Furthermore, the type of morbidity and the causes of death in these infants differ from normally grown infants. Many SGA infants are more susceptible to hypoglycemia, hypocalcemia, symptomatic polycythemia, and pulmonary hemorrhage. Later growth and development of SGA infants is quite variable and reflects the heterogeneity of possible etiologies.

Assessment of Fetal Growth

The assessment of intrauterine growth is an important measure of fetal well-being with significant prognostic value. It is unfortunate, therefore, that estimations of body weight in utero, either by measurements of fundal height or by abdominal palpation, are so imprecise (9). Similarly, the estimation of gestational age from the menstrual history or by endocrinologic tests is also imprecise, further confusing the assessment of intrauterine growth. The use of ultrasonic measurements of fetal size has proven to be a safe and useful tool in the assessment of both fetal growth patterns and gestational age.

Mammalian Growth Potential

The determinants of the growth rate and the length of gestation of the mammalian fetus have long puzzled biologists. By 1951, Huggett and Widdas (10) found that there was a close linear relationship between gestational age and the cube root of the fetal weight:

$$\text{Weight}^{1/3} = \alpha(t - t_0)$$

where t is gestation time from conception, t_0 is some finite but undefined time after insemination, and the intercept on the time axis, and α is the slope or growth rate. Both t_0 and α are constants unique to each species. Figure 22 is a plot of the cube root of birth weight against gestation time; the fan of lines through the origin indicates the range of fetal growth rates seen in placental mammals. Clearly there are remarkable differences in the velocity of growth between primates and other mammals.

Recently, Sacher and Staffeldt (11) reexamined the data of Huggett and Widdas and noted a large variance of growth rates both between and within orders, thus challenging the conclusion of Huggett and Widdas that the growth rate is constant within but variable between orders. Concluding that the mass growth of the fetus is not the controlling factor in fetal growth, they examined the hypothesis that the rates of fetal growth in mammals are governed by a common limiting factor, the rate of growth of neural tissue. Specifically, they studied the relationship of brain weight at birth and gestation times among mammals, which is shown in Figure 23. There is a good linear relation between these variables, both overall and within orders, with the majority of species falling within a twofold range of variation. Sacher and Staffeldt suggested, therefore, an association between the rate of growth of the brain, its size at birth, and the length of gestation.

Fetal Growth and Subsequent Intelligence

Many attempts have been made to relate intelligence to various parameters of intrauterine growth. However, there are no simple relationships between brain size, head circumference, brain cell number, and intelligence in humans. Later intelligence is so heavily influenced by environmental factors such as maternal educational level, socioeconomic factors, and birth order, that it is difficult to demonstrate an effect of intrauterine growth retardation upon later intelligence. Stein et al. (12), in their study of the offspring of mothers exposed to the Dutch famine, concluded that mental performance was

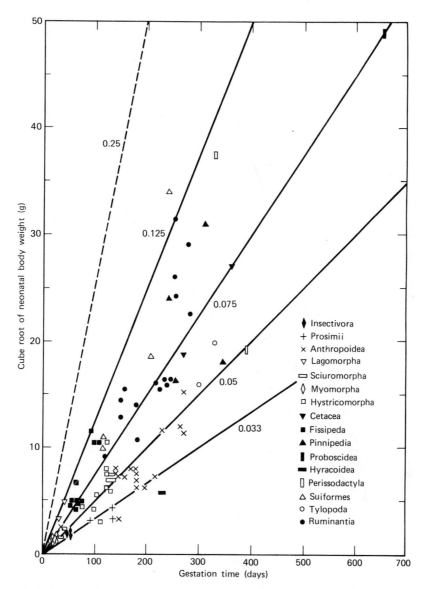

Figure 22. Cube root of neonatal body weight versus gestation time. Lines are drawn for visual guidance to the range of growth rates observed. From Sacher, G. A., and Staffeldt, E. F. Relation of gestation time to brain weight for placental mammals: Implications for the theory of vertebrate growth. *Amer. Natur.* 108:593–615, 1974.

more closely related to social class than to birthweight or exposure to starvation during the intrauterine growth phase.

CARDIOVASCULAR PHYSIOLOGY OF THE FETUS

If one considers the high metabolic requirements of growing tissues and the rapid growth of the fetus, it becomes apparent that the establishment of a functional cardio-

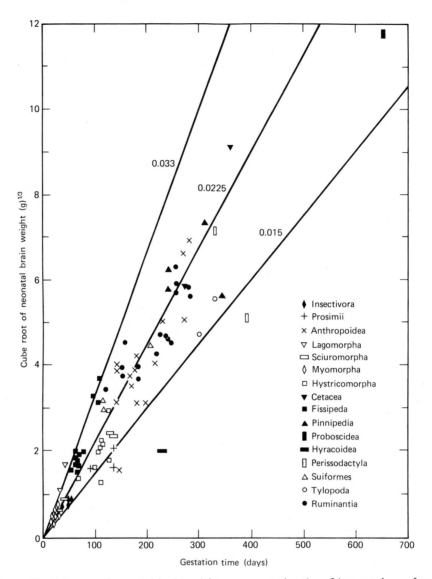

Figure 23. Cube root of neonatal brain weight versus gestation time. Lines are drawn for visual guidance to the range of growth rates observed. From Sacher, G. A., and Staffeldt, E. F. Relation of gestation time to brain weight for placental mammals: Implications for the theory of vertebrate growth. *Amer. Natur.* 108:593–615, 1974.

vascular system is one of the first developmental tasks of the embryo. Warburg (13) derived a theoretical model for predicting the maximal radius of a cylindrical organism relying on diffusion for gas exchange. Bartels and Baumann (14) used this formula to predict a maximal radius of a chick embryo prior to cardiac function:

$$r_{\max} = \frac{4K_{O_2} \times P_{O_2}}{\dot{V}_{O_2}}$$

K_{O_2} = diffusion constant for oxygen
$\dot{V}_{O_2}$ = rate of oxygen consumption in tissue
P_{O_2} = partial pressure of oxygen

They found a value of approximately 1 mm, which correlated reasonably well with embryologic observations. This calculation would predict an upper limit for size, since it assumes a P_{O_2} of zero in the center of the organism and an ambient P_{O_2} of 100 mm Hg. Certainly a P_{O_2} of zero is below the lower limit for tissue survival. The mammalian embryo develops in an atmosphere of lower ambient P_{O_2} than the 100 mm Hg assumed in their calculations. Thus the radius representing an upper limit for a mammalian embryo would be much less than 1 mm. Therefore, it is not surprising that the cardiovascular system is one of the first organ systems to become functional, with a rudimentary circulation established at 4 weeks after conception.

The circulatory system in the fetus has two sorts of physiologic adjustments to make. First, it must adjust to changes in availability of oxygen, such as periods of relative hypoxia. Second, it must continuously adjust to the changing demands of rapidly growing and developing fetal tissues.

For obvious technical reasons, cardiovascular physiology has not been studied in embryologic and early fetal life. In later stages of fetal development, cardiac output and the distribution of blood flow have been studied as functions of both gestational age and fetal oxygenation. Before discussing the physiology of the fetal circulation, we should review the unique features of fetal cardiovascular anatomy. Because of the interatrial communication via the foramen ovale and the arterial communication via the ductus arteriosus the two ventricles of the fetal heart can be considered to function in parallel rather than in series, as in the adult heart. Thus the cardiac output of the fetus is the sum of the left and right ventricular outputs. In view of this arrangement, the output of the two ventricles need not be equal.

Most of the blood returning via the inferior vena cava passes through the foramen ovale into the left atrium. However, a variable part of this blood passes into the right ventricle. Blood from the superior vena cava enters the right ventricle, where it mixes with a variable part of the inferior vena cava blood. The return from the umbilical circulation may pass to the left or right lobe of the liver or via the ductus venosus to the inferior vena cava. This inferior vena cava blood, which contains the umbilical venous return, has the highest oxygen content of any blood in the fetus. This oxygen-rich blood is ejected from the left ventricle into the ascending aorta to supply the coronary and carotid arteries.

The changes in fetal cardiac output and its distribution as a function of maturity have been studied by Rudolph and Heymann (15). They observed that the combined ventricular output increased with gestational age in parallel with fetal weight. Expressed in terms of output per gram of fetal weight, there was no change throughout gestation. The distribution of blood flow changes significantly with fetal maturity. The proportion of cardiac output going to the placenta fell from 50% at midpregnancy to 40% at term. There were slight increases in the proportion going to the lung, gut, brain, and perhaps myocardium in the older fetuses. This redistribution of blood flow represents changes in the relative vascular resistance of various beds. Teasdale (16) has shown that the marked increase in placental blood flow occurring in late gestation can be related to an increase in the number of fetal capillaries in the placenta (see Fig. 24). Part of the increase in blood flow to some fetal organs may be due to vasodilation as these organs

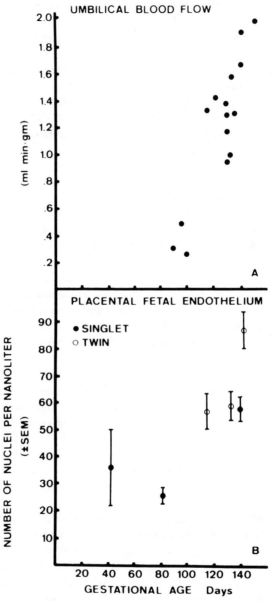

Figure 24. Comparison of umbilical blood flow per gram of placenta with the numerical density of fetal endothelial nuclei (mean ± SEM). From Teasdale, F. Numerical density of nuclei in the sheep placenta. *Anat. Rec.* 185:187–196, 1976.

begin to function. Teasdale found that the increase in maternal blood flow to the placenta was not accompanied by an increase in the number of maternal capillaries. This implies that the increase in uterine blood flow occurs principally by vasodilatation on the maternal side of the placenta.

The changes in distribution of cardiac output with maturation are relatively minor when compared with circulatory adjustments in response to changes in fetal oxygenation. Recent work by Peeters et al. (17) has clarified some of the circulatory adjustments in response to hypoxia. The fetal arterial pressure does not change with varying degrees of arterial oxygenation. It is interesting to note that fetal cardiac output also does not vary significantly with oxygenation over a wide range of oxygen contents. Thus, vasodilatation in certain beds, in response to hypoxia, must be rather precisely compensated by vasoconstriction in other vascular beds.

In considering the response of fetal circulation to changes in oxygenation, the various vascular beds respond differently. For example, the brain and myocardium show a marked vasodilatation with hypoxia. Teleologically, it would seem advantageous to maintain adequate oxygenation of these organs in times of stress. In fact, their blood flow changes in such a way as to maintain constant oxygen delivery to these organs over a very wide range of arterial oxygen contents. Since cardiac output of the fetus is kept constant in mild to moderate hypoxia, other organs must decrease blood flow as flow increases to the brain and heart. At some point the total tissue mass receiving a reduced blood flow containing a lower oxygen content produces a sufficient lactic acid load for metabolic acidosis to appear in the general circulation. In part, this is the basis for the observations that scalp pH and bicarbonate measurements are useful in signifying a fairly severe degree of fetal hypoxia in clinical obstetrics.

The autonomic nervous system control of the heart is present in late gestation regardless of the species studied. On the other hand a number of studies have shown that the release of catecholamines into the maternal circulation under conditions of maternal stress does not lead to the transplacental passage of catecholamines and an increase in the fetal circulation. The maternal uterine circulation responds with marked vasoconstriction to an increase in epinephrine or norepinephrine. The dose response curves for a reduction in uterine blood flow with increasing epinephrine or norepinephrine concentration are the same in pregnant and nonpregnant animals. At one time it was thought that the uterine vascular bed during pregnancy was relatively resistant to the vasoconstrictor effects of catecholamines. However, recent studies have shown that this apparent difference was because the same amount of drug was given on a body weight basis to both pregnant and nonpregnant animals. Thus, a far lower concentration of the drug was present in the uterine arterial blood of the pregnant animals, since uterine blood flow in pregnant animals would be much higher than in nonpregnant animals. Even in pregnant animals uterine blood flow can be reduced virtually to zero by sufficiently high concentrations of catecholamines. Thus, maternal stress would lead to the following chain of events with ultimate effects on the fetus: First, catecholamine concentrations in the maternal circulation would increase. This would lead to a fall in uterine blood flow, which, in turn, would lead to a reduction in uterine venous Po_2. The lower uterine venous Po_2 would lead to a lower umbilical venous Po_2 and oxygen content. If severe enough, this would lead to significant fetal hypoxia, which would then trigger the changes in distribution of fetal cardiac output previously described.

Currently, there is considerable debate whether the stroke volume of the fetal heart is constant at different fetal heart rates. If this were true, it would imply that changes in fetal heart rate would be reflected in proportional changes in fetal cardiac output. However, the bulk of the evidence is against this hypothesis, and it seems likely that stroke volume changes with heart rate minimize any changes in cardiac output induced by the fetal bradycardia.

FETAL RENAL FUNCTION

Since the fetal kidney cannot serve as a final excretory organ in utero, its function in fetal life has been obscure. Urine produced by the fetal kidney is excreted into the amniotic cavity. It does not directly escape from the uterine cavity. As with other fetal organs that are not fully functional by adult standards, it seems unlikely that they remain nonfunctional in utero and then abruptly assume a vital role in neonatal physiology.

The clearance of inulin is accepted as a valid measure of glomerular filtration rate in postnatal life. Using chronically instrumented sheep fetuses, Rankin et al. (18) studied the inulin clearance of late gestation fetuses. They collected fetal urine by catheterization of the urachus and maintained a constant negative pressure on this catheter. They showed that in the fetus, as in the adult, the inulin clearance is reproducible from day to day and appears to be a valid measurement of renal function.

Gresham et al. (19) studied fetal renal function in chronic animal preparations for up to 28 days following surgery. They found that, after a period of recovery from surgery, the urine flow rate was quite stable at 0.14 ml/(min)(kg). This is a relatively high flow rate, comparable with that found in an adult animal with water diuresis. The glomerular filtration rate per kilogram of body weight was approximately 30 to 50% of that of a newborn lamb. Through most of gestation, fetal urine is hypotonic with respect to amniotic fluid. Its composition, however, parallels that of the amniotic fluid with respect to sodium, potassium, and chloride. Mellor and Slater (20) have reported that the osmolality of urine rose sharply with approaching parturition. Based on the observation that there is a low sodium-to-potassium ratio in the urine immediately following surgery, Mellor and Slater (20) suggested that this effect was due to increased glucocorticoid secretion. It is one more physiologic change that occurs in the fetus long before the onset of labor.

The parallelism of urine and amniotic fluid composition is particularly interesting when combined with the observation of Gresham et al. (19) that, with the continuous drainage of urine from the fetal bladder, the volume of amniotic fluid was severely reduced. In these experiments, the chronic drainage of urine from the fetus represented an enormous loss of water and electrolytes from the fetal compartment. This loss produced no significant change in the fetal plasma concentrations and did not have any obvious deleterious effect on the fetus.

From these observations, it appears that the fetal kidney is the principal site of amniotic fluid production in late gestation. This is consistent with the observation that in cases of fetal renal agenesis there is very little amniotic fluid. Wladimiroff and Campbell (21) have measured fetal urine production rates in normal and complicated human pregnancies using ultrasound techniques. Their observations indicate that the growth-retarded fetus has a reduced urine production rate. This suggests that the oligohydramnios often encountered in complicated pregnancies with intrauterine growth retardation may be a reflection of decreased urine flow rate. This decreased flow rate may reflect a stress response on the part of the fetus, similar to that observed after surgery.

The kidneys are similar to the lungs in that they do not appear to play a vital role in fetal life. After birth, however, they assume a vital role for postnatal survival, since excretory functions can no longer be carried on by the placenta. Glomerular filtration rate (GFR) increases with gestation (21). However, this increase has been correlated with fetal size and kidney weight rather than with gestational age. The simplest interpretation is that the increase in function is a reflection of growth. Although this is a reasonable assumption, the explanation may be more complicated.

In postnatal life there is a dramatic increase in GFR and renal blood flow (23). This is accompanied by a marked fall in both the relative and absolute renal vascular resistance. Thus, a greater proportion of the cardiac output is diverted to the kidneys with advancing postnatal age. By 1 year of age the proportion of cardiac output perfusing the kidney is at adult levels (15 to 25%) (23). The pronounced increase in blood flow to the kidney appears to represent both vasodilatation of existing vascular beds and the development of new, low-resistance paths through the kidney. Aschenberg et al. (24) have shown that a rapidly perfused cortical zone appeared in the kidney following birth. The perfusion of this low-resistance, glomerular-rich zone accounts for much of the observed increase in renal blood flow and GFR over the first year of life.

Thus, the kidney appears to function in fetal life in ways that are qualitatively similar to its role in adult life. There are, however, substantial maturational changes in intrarenal blood flow distribution and function that occur after delivery.

FETAL CNS

The relationship between cerebral blood flow and cerebral metabolism has been studied extensively in both adult and fetal animals. In general, cerebral metabolism reflects the size differences one finds in metabolic rate among adult mammals; that is, the cerebral oxygen consumption for the adult rat brain would be higher than the cerebral oxygen consumption of a larger mammal such as the adult sheep. Blood flow to the brain is carefully regulated in both adult and fetal animals to maintain a constant oxygen delivery over a wide range of arterial oxygen tensions and oxygen contents. Johnnsson and Siesjo (25) found a constant cerebral oxygen consumption over a range of arterial P_{O_2}'s from 140 to 23 mm Hg and of arterial oxygen content from 9.9 to 2.1 millimol. Cerebral blood flow in their adult rat studies increased four to six times during hypoxia (25). Similarly, Jones et al. (26) found that fetal cerebral oxygen consumption stayed constant in the fetal lamb over a wide range of arterial oxygen contents, from 5.3 to 0.8 millimol (Fig. 25 from their report, showing cerebral O_2 consumption versus arterial oxygen content). Blood flow to the fetal brain thus was controlled during hypoxia, so that oxygen delivery (blood flow × oxygen content) could be kept constant over a wide range of arterial oxygen content. Obviously, the enormous vasodilatation in the cerebral circulation and the increased blood flow could be accomplished only by either an increase in fetal cardiac output with hypoxia or a decrease in organ blood flow to some other fetal tissues. Since fetal cardiac output has been shown in independent studies to stay constant over this range of arterial oxygen contents, the increase in cerebral blood flow was accomplished by vasoconstriction in the vascular bed to other fetal tissues. The

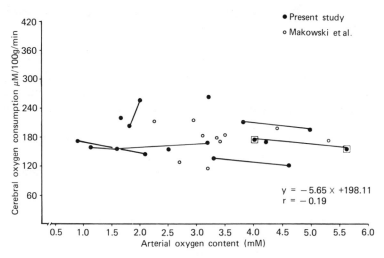

Figure 25. Relationship of cerebral oxygen consumption to arterial oxygen content. Measurements in the same animal are connected. ● = present study; ○ = Makowski et al.; □ = catheter in the confluence of sinuses. From Jones, M. D., Jr., Sheldon, R. E., Peeters, L. L., Meschia, G., Battaglia, F. C., and Makowski, E. L. Fetal cerebral oxygen consumption at different levels of oxygenation. *J. Appl. Physiol.* 43:1080–1084, 1977.

normal cerebral blood flow in the sheep fetus is approximately 120 ml/100 g/min. This is more than double the comparable figure for the adult brain (53 ml/100 g/min). The higher cerebral blood flow of the fetus reflects the relatively low oxygen content of fetal blood and is an adaptation consistent with the response of the adult cerebral circulation to a lower arterial oxygen content. It involves vasodilatation and an increase in blood flow to maintain a constant oxygen delivery to the brain. The increased cerebral blood flow, together with a much higher oxygen affinity of fetal blood, preserves oxygen delivery. Thus, at a low oxygen tension, the high oxygen affinity permits a much higher oxygen content in fetal blood than in adult blood. This, coupled with the higher cerebral blood flow, preserves oxygen delivery to the brain.

All these studies imply that oxidative metabolism is very important to the fetal brain. At first glance, this appears to be a surprising result, since other in vitro studies have suggested that anaerobic glycolysis is a major energy source in the mammalian fetal brain. However, it is unlikely that anaerobic metabolism is of major importance in the fetus. Fetal oxygen consumption is high, and, although fetal arterial lactate concentrations are elevated, two separate studies (27,28) have shown that arterial lactate/pyruvate ratios are normal in the fetus and not different from adult blood. In addition, no significant arterial-venous differences for lactate could be found across the cerebral circulation of the fetal lambs studied in vivo. Lactate production by the brain of the newborn infant and that of newborn animals is also quite low (28). The fuel requirements for the brain to meet its need for oxidative metabolism are met at least in part by the metabolism of glucose. Tsoulos et al., in measurements across the cerebral circulation of the fetal lamb, found a glucose/oxygen quotient of 1.0. Similarly, a number of studies in newborn animals and man have found glucose/oxygen quotients across the cerebral circulation of 1.0. Some of the carbon represented by glucose consumption may be used for synthesis rather than for aerobic metabolism. Some newborn animals develop a significant ketoacidemia during the neonatal period when they are suckling on breast milk containing a high fat concentration. In these newborns there is a significant ketoacid uptake by the developing brain. Even in these species, glucose uptake is significant, and the glucose/oxygen quotient remains greater than 1. The effects of cerebral metabolism on total body caloric requirements are different in the different mammalian fetuses and newborns, primarily as a reflection of differences in the brain-to-body-weight ratio. In the newborn sheep, with approximately the same birthweight as that of man, the brain is one-eighth the size of the brain of the newborn infant. Thus, restriction in oxygen or glucose supply in man, with a much larger brain-to-body-weight ratio at birth, may present a far greater challenge for the human newborn infant to overcome.

FETAL METABOLISM

Fetal metabolism is a field of active research at this moment. Many of the concepts that have developed in metabolism as it applies to adults are still to be tested for their applicability to the fetus. However, two cardinal features of fetal metabolism should be stressed: the first is that the fetus relies on the placenta for the transport of a continuous supply of nutrients for both growth and fuel requirements. In mammals there is no large store of calories in the form of yolk or other materials found in other vertebrates. At any point in gestation, the fetus must rely on the transport each day across the placenta of sufficient carbon and nitrogen to meet its requirements for growth and fuel. The second characteristic that imposes itself on all aspects of fetal metabolism is that the fetus is effectively buffered from the marked fluctuation in blood concentrations that the adult liver sees in the portal venous blood, with the intermittent feeding patterns characteristic of most adult mammals. One can consider this relatively constant concentration of solutes in fetal arterial blood, which the growing organs of the fetus "see," as a reflection of a cascade phenomenon. The maternal liver imposes the first dampening on the oscillations in solute concentration that appear in the portal venous blood of the mother after feeding. After the maternal liver, the placenta further alters maternal arterial concentrations to produce a different spectrum of concentrations of solutes in umbilical venous blood. Again, the variation in solute concentrations in umbilical venous blood has been further reduced from that seen in maternal arterial blood. Finally, the fetal liver imposes still another buffer between both the maternal gastrointestinal tract and the fetal organs that are growing and developing.

The total caloric requirements of the fetus are a reflection of both the fetus' need to meet its fuel requirements, that is, maintain its oxygen consumption, and to meet the requirements reflected by the carbon and nitrogen deposited as new tissue each day. These carbon and nitrogen growth requirements vary among fetuses, depending on their rate of growth. In general, because of a short gestation, the smaller mammals have a much higher rate of growth than the larger mammals. In addition, the smaller mammals have a larger litter size. Thus, their carbon requirements as a percentage of maternal body weight are much larger each day of gestation.

Fetal Oxygen Consumption and Respiratory Quotient

First, let us consider the needs of the fetus for calories to meet its total fuel requirements as reflected by fetal oxygen consumption. The metabolic rate of the fetus has been studied under a number of conditions and in a wide variety of fetal mammals. The oxygen consumption has varied even within the same species from approximately 5 to 9 ml of oxygen/kg/min at STP. The explanation for this variation is not apparent at this time. The O_2 consumption is met in an environment in which the arterial oxygen tension is quite low by adult standards, that is, approximately 30 mm mercury. This has led people to suggest that some fetal organs might function by anaerobic glycolysis to meet their energy requirements. However, a variety of data from several studies speak strongly against this possibility. First of all, the lactate/pyruvate ratios in fetal blood are identical with that of adult blood. There is no evidence of "excess lactate" in fetal blood. Second, there is no evidence in any mammalian fetus of a reduction in standard bicarbonate concentration or the presence of a persistent metabolic acidosis. Third, when oxygen concentration and oxygen content in arterial blood are increased, there is no increase in fetal oxygen consumption, supporting the fact that organs of the fetus are metabolizing aerobically. The CO_2 production rate of the fetus has been approximately equal to the O_2 consumption rate, giving a respiratory quotient (RQ) of approximately 1. The fact that the RQ has been found to be 1 in several mammalian fetuses has been interpreted to mean that carbohydrate, specifically glucose, has been the sole metabolic fuel of the fetus. It should be stressed, however, that RQ measurements cannot be used to reflect the kinds of substrates being used as metabolic fuels in a rapidly growing organism. The reason for this is that during growth a significant percentage of the total carbon intake of the organism appears as new carbon deposited in tissues of the animal and thus does not appear as carbon dioxide. The RQ can then vary from extremely low values to very high values (greater than 1) depending on whether fat or carbohydrate is being deposited in tissues or burned as fuel. The oxygen consumption of the fetus has been reported to be lower, on a per kilo basis, in growth-retarded fetuses, including twins, and in those with idiopathic growth retardation.

Growth Requirements

The total caloric requirements of the organism can be described by calculating the caloric requirements for fuel from the oxygen consumption and the caloric requirements for new tissue growth by measuring the amount of new tissue accretion each day in the fetus and determining the caloric equivalent of that tissue by bomb calorimetry. The combination of both measurements has not yet been done in any mammalian fetus. However, the caloric equivalent of new tissue growth has been determined by bomb calorimetry in the newborn of several species, and the results have been remarkably similar. If one applied these values to the lamb fetus, a species in which fetal O_2 consumption has been measured in several laboratories, in the latter third of gestation, when growth is occurring at approximately 3 to 3½% per day, one can then calculate the proportion of the total calories needed as fuel and growth. Through the latter third of gestation this figure is approximately 50%. That is, about half the total calories required are represented by new tissue accretion.

For nutritional and metabolic studies, it is important to examine the net quantity of a substance such as glucose or amino acids appearing in the umbilical circulation; that is, one must measure directly umbilical uptake. Such measurements require an umbilical venous as well as an umbilical arterial catheter for determining the whole blood arterial-venous differences and an independent measurement of umbilical blood flow. Then, using the Fick principal, $Q = AV$ difference $\times$ flow, the umbilical uptake can be calculated. Alternately, one can measure simultaneously the arterial-venous differences in whole blood content of two substances, one serving as a reference point for the determination of metabolic quotients. (In metabolism, the arterial-venous differences of other substances have been compared in terms of their oxygen equivalents if those compounds were completely metabolized aerobically.) In the lamb fetus the glucose/oxygen quotient is approximately 0.5 across the umbilical circulation. Thus, if all the glucose delivered to the fetus were used as fuel, it could still account for no more than 50% of the fetal oxygen consumption. Considering the total carbon required by the fetus each day, that is, that required for CO_2 production, urea production, and as new carbon deposited in the tissues, glucose uptake in the lamb fetus would provide approximately 20 to 25% of these total carbon requirements. The glucose uptake by the sheep fetus is approximately 3 mg/(kg)(min). When compared with the oxygen uptake, this gives a glucose/oxygen quotient of 0.46:

$$\text{Glucose} + \text{oxygen} = \text{carbon dioxide} + \text{water}$$
$$C_6H_{12}O_6 + 6O_2 = 6CO_2 + 6H_2O$$

$$\text{Glucose/oxygen quotient} = \frac{\text{glucose consumed} \times 6}{\text{oxygen consumed}}$$

A number of different studies in various mammals have shown that free fatty acid uptake varies among the different mammalian fetuses. However, in none of the mammals has a rapid utilization of free fatty acids as fuel been demonstrated. In the lamb fetus, despite a relatively low glucose/oxygen quotient, no appreciable uptake of carbon in the form of free fatty acids or fructose can be demonstrated.

However, Burd et al. (29) recently demonstrated that lactate provides a significant source of carbon to the lamb fetus. As early as 1925, lactate production under aerobic conditions had been demonstrated in the rat placenta. Subsequently, these observations were confirmed in human placenta studied in vitro by Hagemann and Villee. More recently, in chronic animal preparations, Burd demonstrated that lactate appeared in higher concentrations in both the umbilical venous and uterine venous circulations. Thus, lactate production could be demonstrated by the placenta in three different mammalian species. The quantity of lactate produced was very high and could account for approximately 10 to 12% of the total carbon requirements of the fetus. In newborn rats during a rapid phase of postnatal growth, and in the lamb fetus during an equally rapid phase of intrauterine growth, a high rate of urea production per kilo has been demonstrated. Miller estimates that approximately 25% of the total calories required by the newborn rat could be met by the catabolism of amino acids from the measured urea excretion rates. A similar calculation was made on the basis of measurements of the urea production rate of the fetus, and it was found that approximately 25% of the O_2 consumption in the lamb fetus could be met by catabolism of amino acids. More recently the direct measurement of umbilical uptake of each amino acid has been determined in the lamb. The observations of a high urea production rate have been supported by the findings that the transport rate for most amino acids across the placenta was far greater than needed for new tissue growth (30–32). The observations in newborn infants reflect a different pattern of metabolism from that in newborn rats and fetal lambs. In the nursery it has been documented many times that newborn infants have a low urea excretion rate (33). At this time the explanation for this discrepancy between the human newborn infant and studies in other mammals is not clear. It may reflect differences in dietary intake, that is, in the quantity of nitrogen supplied in the diet to the newborn infant and in the spectrum of compounds supplying this total nitrogen to the infant.

In summary, glucose, lactate, and amino acids can account for virtually all the fuel required to meet the O_2 consumption of the fetal lamb. These compounds would not account for the total caloric requirement of the lamb, which includes the caloric requirements of tissue accretion. It should be cautioned that such a balance sheet has been described thus far for only one mammalian fetus; the extent to which this will apply to other mammalian fetuses is conjectural. However, the similar O_2 consumption rates in a wide variety of mammalian fetuses and the documentation of a high rate of lactate production by the placenta under aerobic conditions in several different mammals supports the hypothesis that many of the general characteristics of fetal metabolism are shared among mammals. The metabolic profile of individual organs of the fetus has not been thoroughly studied. It is quite possible, in fact, likely, that a metabolic profile of individual organs will be quite different from that of the fetus as a whole.

The effect of alterations in maternal diet on fetal metabolism has been studied in a few situations. During maternal fasting the glucose/oxygen quotient falls to values of approximately 0.2. Under these conditions in the lamb fetus, glucose represents a rather minor source of carbon to the fetus. The fall in the glucose/oxygen quotient is accompanied by a fall in the fetal glucose concentration and a rise in fetal urea concentration, suggesting an increase in amino acid catabolism by the fetus during maternal starvation. The endocrinologic mechanisms involved in many of the adaptations of the fetus to changes in maternal nutritional state or substrate availability have not been well studied. However, in general the patterns of change seem to be similar to those in the adult with certain important differences. The fetal pancreas, for example, responds to elevations in fetal arterial glucose concentration by increasing insulin release. However, at any given arterial glucose concentration, the fetal plasma insulin concentration is considerably higher than that of the adult, or, alternately, at the same plasma insulin concentrations in the fetus and mother, the fetal glucose concentration is lower. These differences cannot be explained by placental transfer of insulin, since essentially no placental transfer occurs.

A number of studies have demonstrated that glycogen deposition in fetal liver is a phenomenon that occurs in the latter part of gestation (approximately the last 20% of gestation). This is clearly demonstrated in Fig. 26 taken from Ballard's review (34). The deposition of glycogen in other organs of the fetus has not been so thoroughly studied in many mammals. However, a recent study (35) in the pig fetus clearly demonstrated striking differences in the pattern of glycogen deposition in fetal tissues. This is shown in Fig. 27 taken from that report. It demonstrates that skeletal muscle and liver glycogen deposition occur mainly during the latter part of gestation. On the other hand, myocardial glycogen concentration was relatively constant throughout gestation, and lung glycogen concentration fell in the latter part of gestation. The significance of these differences in the pattern of glycogen deposition requires further study. Additionally, it is not clear at this time what sources are used for the glycogen formation. Glinnsman et al., in a series of studies with perfused fetal liver obtained from rhesus monkeys, have demonstrated that the fetal liver does not take up glucose at any appreciable rate; this finding strongly suggests that plasma arterial glucose concentration is not the source of the rapid glycogen deposition in fetal liver. This suggestion that other carbon sources are being used for gluconeogenesis and glycogen deposition by the fetal liver remains to be confirmed in other mammalian species.

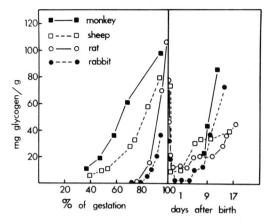

Figure 26. Glycogen content in livers of fetal and neonatal animals expressed as milligrams per gram liver. From Ballard, F. J., Hanson, R. W., and Kronfeld, D. S. Gluconeogenesis and lipogenesis in tissue from ruminant and nonruminant animals. *Fed. Proc.* 28:218–231, 1969.

In conclusion, the fetus clearly uses a variety of substrates other than glucose to meet both its growth and fuel requirements for metabolism. Glucose remains a major source of carbon for the fetus and presumably represents a major oxidative fuel. Likewise, amino acid uptake by the fetus is very great, and the carbon represented by the total amino acid uptake in the umbilical circulation far exceeds the carbon represented by the

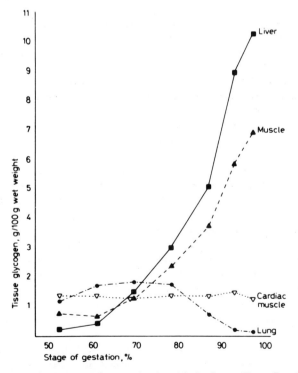

Figure 27. Changes in fetal tissue glycogen levels with fetal age. From Randall, G. C. B., and L'Ecuyer, C. L. Tissue glycogen and blood glucose levels in the pig fetus during the second half of gestation. *Biol. Neonate* 28:74–82, 1976.

glucose uptake. Lactate represents a significant carbon source to the fetus. Free fatty acid and ketoacid uptake by the umbilical circulation varies among the different mammalian fetuses. The role of these compounds as oxidative and synthetic substrates has not been clearly defined.

REFERENCES

1. Guerrero, R., and Rojas, O. I.: Spontaneous abortion and aging of human ova and spermatozoa. *NEJM* 293:573-575, 1975.

2. Kulhanek, J. F., Meschia, G., Makowski, E. L., and Battaglia, F. C.: Changes in DNA content and urea permeability of the sheep placenta. *Am. J. Physiol.* 226:1257-1263, 1974.

3. Hellman, L. M., Flexner, L. B., Wilde, W. S., Vosburgh, G. J., and Proctor, N. K.: The permeability of the human placenta to water and the supply of water to the human fetus as determined with deuterium oxide. *Am. J. Obstet. Gynecol.* 56:861-868, 1948.

3a. Alexander, G.: Studies on the placenta of the sheep. *J. Reprod. Fertil.* 7:289-305, 1964.

3b. Dayton, D. H., Filer, L. J., and Canosa, C.: Cellular changes in the placentas of undernourished mothers in Guatemala. *Fed. Proc.* 28:488, 1969.

3c. Aherne W., and Dunnill, M. S.: Morphometry of the human placenta. *Brit. Med. Bull.* 22:5-8, 1966.

4. Walton, A., and Hammond, J.: The maternal effects on growth and conformation in Shire horse–Shetland pony crosses. *Proc. Roy. Soc. London* 125B:311-335, 1938.

5. Turner, G.: Recognition of intrauterine growth retardation by considering comparative birth-weights. *Lancet* 2:1223-24, 1971.

6. Thomson, A. M., Billewicz, W. Z., and Hytten, F. E.: The weight of the placenta in relation to birthweight. *J. Obstet. Gynaecol. Brit. Commwlth.* 76:865-872, 1969.

7. Lichty, J. A., Ting, R. Y., Bruns, P. D., and Dyar, E.: Studies of babies born at high altitude. *Am. J. Dis. Child.* 93:666-678, 1957.

8. Metcalfe, J., Meschia, G., Hellegers, A., Prystowsky, H., Huckabee, W., and Barron, D. H.: Observations on the growth rates and organ weights of fetal sheep at altitude and sea level. *Quart. J. Exper. Physiol.* 47:305-313, 1962.

9. Beazley, J. M., and Underhill, R. A.: Fallacy of the fundal height. *Brit. Med. J.* 4:404-406, 1970.

10. Huggett, A. St G., and Widdas, W. F.: The relationship between mammalian foetal weight and conception age. *J. Physiol.* 114:306-317, 1951.

11. Sacher, G. A., and Staffeldt, E. F.: Relation of gestation time to brain weight for placental mammals: Implications for the theory of vertebrate growth. *Amer. Natur.* 108:593-615, 1974.

12. Stein, Z., Susser, M., Saenger, G., and Marolla, F.: Nutrition and mental performance. *Science* 178:708-713, 1972.

13. Warburg, O.: Versuche an uberlebendem carcinomgewebe. *Biochem. Zeitschr.* 142:317-333, 1923.

14. Bartels, H., and Baumann, F.: Preplacental gas exchange, in *Respiratory Gas Exchange and Blood Flow in the Placenta.* U.S. Department of Health, Education and Welfare, Bethesda, Md., 1972.

15. Rudolph, A. M., and Heymann, M. A.: The circulation of the fetus in utero: Methods for studying distribution of blood flow, cardiac output and organ blood flow. *Circ. Res.* 21:163-184, 1967.

16. Teasdale, F.: Numerical density of nuclei in the sheep placenta. *Anat. Rec.* 185:187-196, 1976.

17. Peeters, L. L. H.: *Fetal Blood Flow at Various Levels of Oxygen,* thesis. Katholieke Universiteit te Nijmegen, February 16, 1978.

18. Rankin, J. H. G., Gresham, E. L., Battaglia, F. C., Makowski, E. L., and Meschia, G.: Measurement of fetal renal inulin clearance in a chronic sheep preparation. *J. Appl. Physiol.* 32:129-133, 1972.

19. Gresham, E. L., Rankin, J. H. G., Makowski, E. L., Meschia, G., and Battaglia, F.: An evaluation of fetal renal function in a chronic sheep preparation. *J. Clin. Invest.* 51:149-156, 1972.

20. Mellor, D. J., and Slater, J. S.: Daily changes in foetal urine and relationships with amniotic fluid and maternal plasma during the last two months of pregnancy in conscious, unstressed ewes with chronically implanted catheters. *J. Physiol.* 217:573, 1971.

21. Wladimiroff, J. W., and Campbell, S.: Fetal urine-production rates in normal and complicated pregnancy. *Lancet* 1:151–154, 1974.

22. Robillard, J. E., Kulvinskas, C., Sessions, C., Burmeister, L., and Smith, F. G., Jr.: Maturational changes in the fetal glomerular filtration rate. *Amer. J. Obstet. Gynec.* 122(5):601–606.

23. Gruskin, A. B., Edelmann, C. M., Jr., and Yuan, S.: Maturational changes in renal blood flow in piglets. *Pediat. Res.* 4:713, 1970.

24. Aschinberg, L. C., Goldsmith, D. I., Olbing, H., Spitzer, A., Edelmann, C. M., Jr., and Blaufox, M. D.: Neonatal changes in renal blood flow distribution in puppies. *Amer. J. Physiol.* 228(5):1453–1461.

25. Johannsson, H., and Siejo, B. K.: Cerebral blood flow and oxygen consumption in the rat in hypoxic hypoxia. *Acta Physiol. Scand.* 93:269–276, 1975.

26. Jones, M. D., Jr., Sheldon, R. E., Peeters, L. L., Makowski, E. L., Meschia, G., and Battaglia, F. C.: Fetal cerebral oxygen consumption at different levels of oxygenation. *J. Appl. Physiol.*, in press.

27. Huckabee, W. E., Metcalfe, J., Prystowsky, H., and Barron, D. H.: Insufficiency of O_2 supply to the pregnant uterus. *Am. J. Physiol.* 202:198–204, 1962.

28. Jones, M. D., Jr., Burd, L. I., Makowski, E. L., Meschia, G., and Battaglia, F. C.: Cerebral metabolism in sheep: A comparative study of the adult, the lamb, and the fetus. *Amer. J. Physiol.* 229(1):235–239, 1975.

29. Burd, L. I., Jones, M. D., Jr., Simmons, M. A., Makowski, E. L., Meschia, G., and Battaglia, F. C.: Placental production and foetal utilisation of lactate and pyruvate. *Nature* 254(5502):710–711, 1975.

30. Lemons, J. A., Adcock, E. W., III, Jones, M. D., Jr., Naughton, M. A., Meschia, G., and Battaglia, F. C.: Umbilical uptake of amino acids in the unstressed fetal lamb. *J. Clin. Invest.* 58:1428–1434, 1976.

31. Battaglia, F. C., and Meschia, G.: Foetal metabolism and substrate utilization, in *Foetal and Neonatal Physiology,* Proceedings of the Sir Joseph Barcroft Centenary Symposium. Cambridge University Press, 1973, pp. 272–278.

32. Gresham, E. L., James, E. J., Raye, J. R., Battaglia, F. C., Makowski, E. L., and Meschia, G.: Production and excretion of urea by the fetal lamb. *Pediatrics* 50:372–379, 1972.

33. Jones, M. D., Jr., Gresham, E. L., and Battaglia, F. C.: Urinary flow rates in newborn infants. *Biol. Neonate* 21:321–329, 1972.

34. Ballard, F. J., Hanson, R. W., and Kronfeld, D. S.: Gluconeogenesis and lipogenesis in tissue from ruminant and nonruminant animals. *Fed. Proc.* 28:218–231, 1969.

35. Randall, G. C. B., and L'Ecuyer, C. L.: Tissue glycogen and blood glucose levels in the pig fetus during the second half of gestation. *Biol. Neonate* 28:74–82, 1976.

8
Pulmonary Surfactant and the Respiratory Distress Syndrome

Philip M. Farrell, M.D., Ph.D.
Richard D. Zachman, M.D., Ph.D.

A number of significant developments in this decade have vastly improved our understanding of the physiology and biochemistry of the lung surfactant system. These advances have arisen from studies initiated by both clinical and basic scientists concerned with fundamental aspects of lung differentiation and respiratory mechanics. As a result, the pathophysiology of neonatal respiratory distress syndrome (RDS) is much better understood than in the 1960s, when intensive perinatal care began. This in turn has permitted development of more rational approaches to therapy and the discovery of seemingly effective means of prenatal intervention. Thus, in the short span of 5 to 10 years, our approach to managing infants with, or at risk for developing, RDS has undergone almost complete revision. Such rapid and meaningful advances could only have been achieved through coordination of efforts by obstetricians and pediatricians working together toward a longstanding, common goal—to lower the mortality and morbidity associated with RDS.

The purpose of this chapter is to review current knowledge concerning lung surfactant and RDS. Our aim is not to present an exhaustive survey of research observations, for this information is available elsewhere in a variety of comprehensive reviews (1–3). Rather, we wish to summarize selected advances of major importance and describe a number of general concepts and insights that have come to be appreciated in recent years. In so doing, we have deliberately chosen to emphasize developments of a perinatal nature and experimental results that have truly bridged the gap between the laboratory bench and the bedside.

PULMONARY SURFACTANT AND THE PROCESS OF FETAL LUNG DEVELOPMENT

General

At birth, interruption of the fetal-placental unit requires the newborn infant to assume vital functions that were previously sustained by the maternal circulation. Among the major demands are respiration and nutrition, the first of which must be met within a few minutes following delivery if the newborn is to survive undamaged. Because of the immediate need to achieve effective gas exchange, the lung is called on as the critical organ in early adaptation to extrauterine life. It is a curious phenomenon, therefore, that this vital organ is completely untested until birth and further must begin to carry out air exchange from a fluid-filled state. Thus, sufficient differentiation or maturation of the fetal lung is an essential aspect of intrauterine development.

Differentiation of the lung must bring about complete structural remodeling, ensure the presence of surface-tension-lowering material (pulmonary surfactant), and provide the capacity for rapid resynthesis and renewal of this phospholipid-rich substance lining the alveoli. Fetal lung development, therefore, requires coordination of anatomic, physiologic, and biochemical processes, the timing of which must be carefully regulated. The ultimate product of these changes in structure, function, and metabolism is an organ with alveoli having adequate surface area and capable of sustained ventilatory excursions for efficient gas exchange. The surfactant system, as discussed subsequently, plays a major role in development of the fetal lung and in postnatal respiratory function.

The Physiology and Biochemistry of Surfactant

The function and composition of pulmonary surface active material (SAM) have been the subject of several comprehensive reviews (1,2,4) and thus require only brief definition herein. Some authors have simply termed this material the "anti-atelectasis factor." Others recognize or postulate roles for surfactant that extend beyond those of a mechanical nature. There are two functions that are particularly relevant for the newborn: (1) maintenance of alveolar stability or prevention of diffuse collapse of the terminal respiratory units and (2) reduction of the pressure needed to distend the lung initially. Both of these are attributable to the capacity of this material for lowering surface tension. More specifically, the presence of surfactant along the air-water interface of the alveolar surfaces ensures a low and variable surface tension such that the "hysteresis" requirement for stable alveolar excursions is met (2).

The composition of the surfactant system has been carefully studied by several investigators (5,6). On a mass basis, the principal components are phospholipids, especially lecithins* with highly saturated fatty acid substructures. Indeed, it may be calculated that lecithins account for nearly three-quarters of the organic compounds in surface active material obtained by lung lavage. Approximately 60% of this fraction is dipalmitoyl lecithin, and monounsaturated species comprise at least 30%. Not only are pulmonary lecithins important in terms of quantity, but, as has long been appreciated, they can account for the surface-tension-lowering capacity of isolated surfactant, i.e., the quality of the material relative to respiratory mechanics. In addition to highly saturated lecithins, other potentially important constituents of the surfactant system that have come under more recent study include phosphatidylglycerol (6,7) and "surfactant apoprotein" (8).

* Lecithin is the trivial name for the choline phosphoglyceride known systematically as 1,2-diacyl-sn-glycero-3-phosphoryl-choline; the recommended generic term is 3-sn-phosphatidylcholine or, as generally used, phosphatidylcholine (PC). Because "lecithin" enjoys widespread clinical usage and is permitted by the Combined Commission on Nomenclature (IUPAC-IUB), it is used herein to designate the compound, along with dipalmitoyl lecithin (DPL) for 1,2-dipalmitoyl-sn-glycero-3-phosphorylcholine.

Studies on the biosynthesis and renewal of surfactant have focused to date on its principal phospholipid component. Pathways for de novo formation of lecithin are depicted in Figure 1. Despite an earlier hypothesis to the contrary, abundant evidence now exists to support the conclusion that pathway I, the choline incorporation mechanism, is predominant in both fetal and postnatal lung lecithin biosynthesis (Table I). As indicated in Figure 1, there are three enzymes in this pathway, all of which might conceivably play a role in regulating DPL production (9). Other enzymes of potential importance in supporting pulmonary phospholipid synthesis through formation of the diglyceride substrate are lipoprotein lipase (10), glycerol phosphate acyltransferase (11), and phosphatidic acid phosphohydrolase (12).

The major site of all these metabolic activities is thought to be the large alveolar epithelial cell, known as the type II pneumonocyte. This cell type comprises approximately 10% of the lung's cells and contains osmiophilic lamellar bodies, the presumed storage granules of the surfactant complex. A triad of functions has therefore been proposed for these cells—*synthesis, storage,* and *secretion* of the pulmonary surfactant. Their secretory activity may be of great importance in adaptation of the newborn to breathing air but has not been carefully studied to date.

From the foregoing considerations, the following definition emerges: Pulmonary surfactant is a unique complex lipoprotein, particularly rich in highly saturated lecithins, that is produced in type II pneumonocytes and secreted onto the alveolar surfaces; by providing a low and variable interfacial surface tension, it serves to facilitate maintenance of alveolar stability.

The Process of Prenatal Lung Development

As indicated previously, pulmonary maturation involves a sequence of coordinated events affecting the anatomy, physiology, and biochemistry of the fetal lung. The architecture and histology of the developing lung can be appreciated from Figure 2, which shows morphologic changes in fetal rat lung from 16 days of gestation to term (22 days) and at birth, as reported by Blackburn et al. (13). A glandular phase is shown to be present at 16, 17, and 18 days' gestation; canaliculi are evident at 20 to 21 days and

Table I. Evidence that the Choline Pathway is the Primary *de novo* Mechanism of Lung Lecithin Biosynthesis

Rate of conversion of radioactive choline to lecithin greatly exceeds that of ethanolamine and methionine as measured in:
  Lung slices
  Tissue-cultured type II pneumonocytes
  Whole lung (in utero)
Relative enzyme activities
Kinetic properties of isolated enzymes
The pattern of augmented choline pathway rates in late gestation
The correlation between increases in pathway I activity and the PC concentration in:
  Fetal lung
  Amniotic fluid

SOURCE: References 1, 16, 50, and 51.

alveoli at 21 to 22 days. In the human fetus, the *glandular stage* is reported to be present from 5 to 16 weeks and the *canalicular stage* from 16 to 24 weeks; the *alveolar stage* is then evident beyond 24 weeks of gestation (3). Electron microscopic studies have demonstrated that during the "alveolarization" phenomenon in late gestation, cytologic and subcellular changes occur with appearance of osmiophilic lamellar bodies in the cuboidal-shaped, type II alveolar pneumonocytes.

Physiologic studies performed with the classical pressure-volume apparatus have revealed that adequate retention of air, or stability on deflation of the lung, is first achieved during the last 10 to 20% of gestation; this signals the presence of increased alveolar surfactant. During this time, the residual volume maintained under experimental conditions of zero transpulmonary pressure increases dramatically (14), corresponding to the infant's ability to maintain a functional residual capacity. In addition to an increased amounts of alveolar surfactant, other readily detectable physiologic indices of lung development include the appearance of surface-tension-lowering material in lung extracts, producing minimum surface tension values of less than 10 dyn/cm, and increased lung distensibility.

Biochemical features of lung development include increased enzyme activities, augmented choline pathway rates, and an increase in the concentration of lecithin in lung tissue and fluids derived from the respiratory epithelium, such as fetal pulmonary fluid and amniotic liquid. Although these changes have been identified in several species, most of the comprehensive studies dealing with the biochemistry of lung maturation have been carried out in lower animals having short gestational periods. The rat fetus has been an especially useful model in this regard and has provided valuable insights. It has been observed, for instance, that each of the enzymes of the choline pathway shows increased activity at approximately 85% of gestation (15). As illustrated in Figure 3, a peak of activity is reached at 18.5 to 19 days of gestation, and this is followed by a decline. Figure 3 also demonstrates that the overall conversion of choline to phosphatidylcholine is augmented after 20 days of gestation. Subsequently, the concentration of lecithin is likewise increased in the fetal rat lung. A similar increase in the conversion of choline to pulmonary lecithin has been detected in lung samples from fetal rhesus monkeys (16). This is followed by an increase in the concentration of lecithin and a surge in the lecithin/sphingomyelin (L/S) ratio of amniotic fluid. Curiously, however, the lung of the fetal rhesus monkey does not show increased activites of choline pathway enzymes in late gestation (17). This, as well as other evidence, indi-

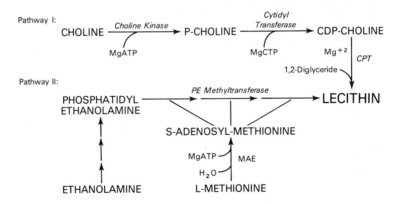

Figure 1. Pathways of de novo lecithin biosynthesis.

| GESTATIONAL AGE (days) | 16 | 17 | 18 | 19 | 20 | 21 | 22-BIRTH |

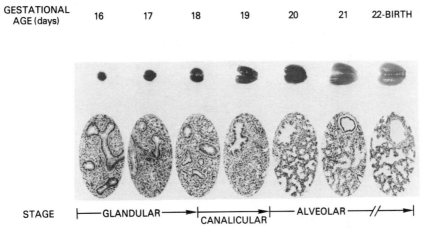

STAGE |———GLANDULAR————►|———————|——ALVEOLAR——/ /——►|
                        CANALICULAR

Figure 2. The growth and development of the fetal rat lung. Term gestation is 22 days. Illustration modified from that kindly provided by Dr. Will Blackburn, Departments of Pediatrics and Pathology, University of South Alabama.

cates that species specificity exists with respect to mechanisms operating to regulate metabolic processes important in fetal lung development. Further study is thus needed to clarify our understanding of the biochemistry of pulmonary maturation.

SURFACTANT AND THE RESPIRATORY DISTRESS SYNDROME

The intimate association between lung surfactant and the respiratory distress syndrome was first discovered by Avery and Mead (18). They reported in 1959 that surface-tension-lowering material was absent in lungs removed at autopsy from infants succumbing to RDS. In the ensuing years, an imposing body of evidence has accumulated supporting the hypothesis that RDS is in most cases an expression of underlying *pulmonary surfactant deficiency*. Observations in favor of this proposal include (1) the abnormal mechanical properties of isolated lungs, (2) the abnormal surface-tension characteristics of lung extracts, (3) the low concentration of saturated lecithin in lung, (4) the predictability of amniotic fluid lecithin concentration as L/S ratio, (5) the predictability of amniotic fluid surfactant titers ("shake test"), (6) the low lecithin concentration in tracheal effluent, and (7) the clinical effectiveness of continuous distending airway pressure. Very little evidence arguing against the primacy of diminished surfactant in RDS has appeared and withstood the test of time. Therefore, it is reasonable to assert that in most cases RDS occurs as a consequence of the relative inability of the lung to synthesize or secrete surfactant in amounts sufficient for normal neonatal respiratory adaptation (1).

PRENATAL IDENTIFICATION OF FETAL LUNG MATURITY

Background

As listed in Table II, several properties of amniotic liquid can be used for establishing diagnoses in utero. One of the more important recent advances in perinatal medicine

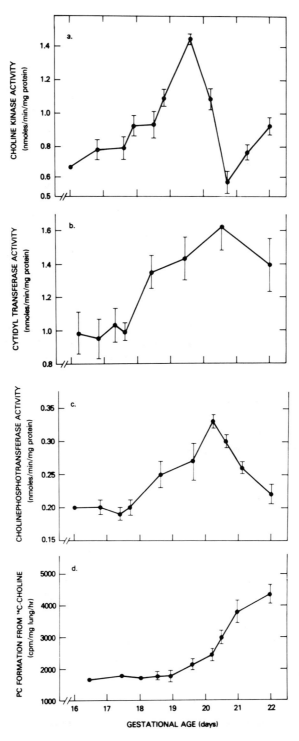

Figure 3. Specific activities of choline pathway enzymes in developing fetal rat lung (*a,b,c*) compared with the apparent rate of the overall pathway (*d*). Adapted from Farrell (15).

Table II. Conditions and Diagnoses Possible Through Amniotic Fluid Analysis

Amniotic Fluid Character Analyzed	Method of Analysis	Examples of Predicted Diagnoses or Claimed Relationship to Pregnancy
Volume:	Clinical	Maternal diabetes; multiple
Excess	inspection	pregnancy; erythroblastosis; fetal anencephaly; gastro-intestinal atresia
Diminution		Fetal renal agenesis; leaking membranes
Color:		
Yellow (bilirubin)	Spectroscopic analysis	Erythroblastosis fetalis
Meconium-stained		Fetal defecation (? distress)
Cells:		
Cultured cells	Cytologic—karyotyping	Trisomy 21, D,E; hemophilia A and B; Duchenne muscular dystrophy
	Enzymatic	Fabry disease; Tay-Sachs disease glycogen storage disease
Neutrophiles	Cytologic—staining (Wright's)	Intrauterine infection
Composition:	Chemical	
Alpha-fetoprotein—elevated		Fetal spina bifida, anencephaly
Creatinine—elevated		Fetal size and maturity
Osmolarity—elevated		Perinatal death
Cortisol—elevated		Absence of RDS
Phospholipids—low		Respiratory distress syndrome
Glucose—low		Placental insufficiency
Albumin—low		Respiratory distress syndrome
Reverse T_3—low		Fetal hypothyroidism

concerns the measurement of amniotic fluid phospholipids to estimate the probability of an infant's developing RDS. Since the report by Graven in 1968 (19) demonstrating the presence of phospholipids in human and monkey amniotic fluid, there have been over 200 studies published on the analysis of amniotic fluid in relation to fetal lung maturation. The work with the most significant clinical impact has been that of Gluck and associates (20). Their studies suggested that (1) both sphingomyelin and lecithin present in amniotic liquid originate from the fetal lung; (2) an increase occurs in the concentration of lecithin during late gestation, and this change correlates with the appearance of functional pulmonary surfactant; and (3) the ratio of lecithin to sphingomyelin (L/S) provides an index of the risk of neonatal respiratory distress syndrome.

Since RDS is related to inadequate pulmonary surfactant and amniotic fluid phospholipid determinations can predict the risk of RDS, the clinician now has an invaluable tool to help him manage high-risk pregnancies. In many instances, finding an amniotic fluid L/S ratio indicating an immature fetal respiratory system compels the obstetrician to use more aggressive and intensive care of the mother in order to prolong her pregnancy and allow time for attainment of fetal lung maturity before delivery. The importance of this approach was recently pointed out in an article by Goldenberg and Nelson (21). Their survey of hospital records from 1970 to 1974 disclosed that approximately 30% of RDS admissions at the Yale Special Care Nursery were related to untimely or unwarranted delivery of a premature infant with immature lungs. Many of these problems could have been anticipated or avoided by the use of an amniotic fluid L/S analysis.

Phospholipid Analysis in Amniotic Fluid

Techniques

The L/S ratio methods use extraction of lipids from amniotic fluid with a mixture of chloroform and methanol. The chloroform phase containing the phospholipids is separated from the water-soluble part of the amniotic fluid and then concentrated by evaporation. Small samples of the extract are then applied to glass plates coated with silica gel. The plates are placed upright in a solvent of chloroform, methanol, and water (usual proportions: 65/25/4) and the various lipids separated by the ascending solvent front; separation is based on polarity and charge properties of the phospholipids. Isolated compounds on the silica gel plate are then charred by strong acid and heat, and the concentration of each "spot" determined by reflectance densitometry using a scanner and recorder. From the observed char densities of the lecithin and sphingomyelin, the L/S ratio is calculated.

Other methods have also been developed to measure the L/S ratio. A review featuring a comparison of some of these techniques has been published by Olson and Graven (22). In addition, approaches other than the L/S methods have been described for analyzing amniotic fluid to assess fetal pulmonary maturity, including measurement of total lecithin concentration, evaluation of alkaline-labile versus alkaline-stable phospholipids, and demonstration of the presence of surface-tension-lowering material in concentrated amniotic fluid.

The shake test, or bubble-stability test as it is often called, is a more rapid and less expensive procedure than extraction and quantitation of amniotic fluid phospholipids. To perform this test, one mixes amniotic fluid with one volume of 95% ethyl alcohol and shakes the mixture, causing formation of bubbles. The stability of these bubbles or "foam" depends on the surface-tension-lowering properties of the lipids contained in the amniotic liquid. Major disadvantages of the shake test include its subjectivity and semiquantitative nature. Since the orginal findings of Clements and associates (23), the shake test has been compared with the L/S approach and clinical outcome by several investigators, as reviewed by Farrell and Avery (1). In essence, the shake test has proved valuable as a screening procedure to identify fetuses with mature lungs. However, when the shake test results are not clearly positive, i.e., the "foam" generated is unstable, the L/S value is a more reliable predictor of RDS.

Clinical Use of Amniotic Fluid Phospholipid Analyses in Relation to RDS

The indications for amniotic fluid analysis to assess fetal lung maturity are several. Included among these are premature labor at less than 37 weeks of gestation and various high-risk pregnancies such as those complicated by diabetes, Rh sensitization, and hypertension. Most obstetricians feel that amniotic fluid phospholipid data should also be obtained when planning for an elective cesarean section in circumstances where the dates are uncertain or the clinical impression differs from the gestational age given by history. Some studies suggest that maternal disease might alter the rate of fetal lung maturation, such as acceleration with intrauterine growth retardation or slowing with some diabetic pregnancies.

Since 1971, the L/S ratio procedure has been the major method used to predict fetal lung maturity in high-risk pregnancies. In regard to interpreting results, the first proposal by Gluck et al. (20) was that an L/S ratio greater than 2.0 indicated fetal pulmonary maturation and virtually eliminated the possibility of neonatal RDS. Many others subsequently reported similar results (1). However, a substantial number of patients have developed RDS with the presence of an L/S ratio of 2 or greater (2). Olson et al. (24) found that the critical L/S value calculated from the absolute amounts of the two phospholipids was 3.5, rather than 2.0.

It has become clear, therefore, that, regardless of the method used, an infant might be born with a "mature" L/S ratio and still develop RDS. One possible reason for this could be laboratory error. There are also other factors such as maternal diabetes and asphyxia neonatorum that predispose to development of RDS, even in the face of a "mature" L/S value. Another important aspect of interpreting results is the recognition that an "immature" L/S value may change to a "mature" ratio between the time of amniocentesis and the time of delivery. Hence, the results of many studies relating RDS incidence to "mature" or "immature" L/S ratios need to be defined with such additional data. Finally, recent evidence suggests that other surface-active lipids, such as phosphatidylglycerol (25) and possibly the type of fatty acids on the lecithin (26), are important in imparting stable surface activity to the alveolar lining layer, hence lowering the risk for RDS. Laboratories performing L/S ratio procedures must constantly update their results in comparing L/S data with neonatal outcomes. Only then can the clinician use the test with confidence.

In the practice of perinatology, it is important to strike a balance between the determined L/S value and the total clinical situation. For example, even though an amniotic fluid analysis at 32 weeks' gestation might show a L/S ratio indicating pulmonary maturity, an infant of that gestation frequently has more problems than the 37-week-gestation infant, including a higher incidence of patent ductus arteriosus, necrotizing enterocolitis, sepsis, hyperbilirubinemia, and feeding difficulties. Hence, the maternal indication for delivery must be seriously evaluated in light of the other potential risks of prematurity when one is faced with a "mature" L/S ratio and an otherwise immature fetus.

CLINICAL FEATURES OF THE RESPIRATORY DISTRESS SYNDROME

Epidemiology and Statistics

Recently, national mortality statistics for RDS were examined over a 5-year period by Farrell and Wood (27). The data indicated that the disease was involved in the death of nearly 12,000 neonates per year, or approximately 20% of all neonatal deaths. A review of several studies has concluded that the incidence in babies with a birthweight less than 2500 g is approximately 14% (1). This means that, in the United States, there are about 40,000 cases per year. Even though these calculations were based on birthweight alone, rather than a more strict criterion of birthweight and gestational age combined (to eliminate small-for-gestational-age infants), these are probably the most accurate estimates of the incidence of RDS and of the mortality associated with it.

Small studies have shown a definite correlation between RDS incidence figures and gestational age (28). While the syndrome is rare in the term neonate ($<0.5\%$), data from our hospital have indicated an incidence of 75% in preterm infants born at less than 30 weeks of gestation. Neonates delivered between 30 and 32 weeks show a 45% incidence, whereas 22% of those born at 33–34 weeks develop RDS at the Southcentral Wisconsin Perinatal Center. RDS seems to have a worldwide occurrence, and males contribute more to death totals than do females.

Recognition of RDS and Differential Diagnosis

Signs and Symptoms
The main clinical features of RDS include tachypnea, expiratory grunting, poor air exchange, and cyanosis. Although some neonates have a respiratory rate of greater than 60/min for 1 or 2 hr after birth without major pulmonary disease, those with RDS show tachypnea prolonged beyond that time. Accompanying this is evidence of diffusely atelectatic lungs, assessed clinically by noting retractions of the chest. These can vary from mild "seesawing" of the chest and abdomen with respirations to a tracheal tug and deep substernal retractions. Another helpful finding that can be noted clinically if the baby has required resuscitation is that the lungs in RDS "feel stiff" when one is bagging by hand to establish respiration. Poor alveolar air entry detected by auscultation with the stethoscope is also a convenient sign of inadequate chest expansion and hypoventilation. It should be stressed that the above signs and symptoms can worsen rapidly to produce a gasping, ashen-gray infant with apnea and bradycardia if oxygen supplementation and other therapies have not been initiated immediately after suspecting the respiratory distress syndrome.

The diagnosis of RDS can usually be confirmed shortly after birth with a chest radiograph. Classically, this reveals hypoinflation ("seven to eight ribs" expansion during inspiration on a frontal projection), a reticulogranular pattern, and small air bronchograms extending throughout the lung fields. Sequential chest x-rays are of help in distinguishing RDS from diseases that occasionally mimic this disorder.

Differential Diagnosis
Although the likelihood of RDS is high in a premature infant with early respiratory difficulty, many other diseases can lead to respiratory distress in the first few hours of life. One must carefully differentiate these diseases to arrive at optimum therapeutic decisions. The physical examination may lead one to suspect certain disorders and offers one the opportunity to rule out others. For example, if the heart tones are shifted significantly to one side or the other, it is possible that the infant has a pneumothorax or diaphragmatic hernia that has forced the mediastinum laterally. The chest radiograph serves to confirm or rule out problems such as these which call for immediate surgical intervention. Intrauterine congenital pneumonia can present soon after birth with signs of marked respiratory distress. The disease with special virulence causing considerable neonatal mortality in recent years is streptococcal pneumonitis due to nongroup A, beta-hemolytic organisms. This infection can have an early onset, with signs, symptoms, and even radiographic findings similar to RDS. Recently, Ablow and colleagues (29) summarized their experience with cases of streptococcal pneumonia in comparison with RDS. The major points in the differential diagnosis for streptococcal disease included a gastric aspirate positive for gram-positive cocci, asphyxia at birth, gestational age close

to term, and more compliant lungs requiring less pressure for ventilation, as compared with infants with RDS.

In addition to diaphragmatic hernia and pneumothorax, other surgical emergencies must also be ruled out, usually by the chest radiograph. Some common neonatal cardiac problems presenting with cyanosis from anatomic right-to-left shunts in the first hours of life can often be differentiated from RDS by increasing the inspired oxygen concentration and observing no improvement in the neonate's color and degree of hypoxemia.

Treatment

Optimum treatment of RDS demands a *perinatal approach*. Anticipation of the risk for developing RDS by determination of the amniotic fluid L/S ratio, expert neonatal resuscitation, early recognition of the afflicted neonate, and transfer to a facility equipped to deal with the disease are all of great importance in decreasing the mortality and morbidity associated with RDS.

In recent years, the concept of regionalization of perinatal health care has become increasingly popular as an approach aimed at reducing neonatal mortality and morbidity. Some preliminary reports have attributed a significant decline in infant mortality rates to implementation of newborn intensive care units and perinatal care centers (30,31). One report states that the fatality rate for 100 neonates with RDS was almost halved among infants transported to regional centers compared with those who were not (32). After a baby with RDS is stabilized postnatally, a decision must quickly be made as to whether the hospital facilities are adequate to deal effectively with the patient. As discussed subsequently, the treatment of neonatal respiratory distress may require extended and complex supportive measures. Swyer (33) has listed some factors that might influence one's decision as to whether or not transfer of an infant with RDS is indicated. Among these criteria are hypoxia and acidosis in 100% O_2 and a birthweight of less than 2000 g. Swyer, however, only dealt with indications for transfer of the neonate. As modern perinatal care develops further, consideration must be given to transport of the high-risk mother with the baby in utero, i.e., prenatal referral.

The transport of a patient from a community hospital to a tertiary care center involves some "sacrifice" on the part of the referring hospital and physician. Some clinicians feel that patient rapport suffers when responsibilities for care during an acute illness are passed on to others. However, if the mother and infant can obtain more effective and intensive care at another facility and the transport risk is low, it is clear that the patient should be transferred. The referring physician, therefore, must recognize the importance of this approach and the fact that it may offer the best possible treatment for his patient.

Management of RDS involves maximum supportive measures for the infant. A critical balance of essential, interacting components is necessary to maintain normal pulmonary metabolism, ventilation, and perfusion. Adequate surfactant production depends on active metabolic processes in type II alveolar cells. Surfactant synthesis and secretion allow lung expansion, thereby facilitating ventilation. Satisfactory ventilation and continued lung expansion allow normal oxygenation, which in turn helps to ensure good blood flow through the pulmonary arteries. Adequate lung perfusion ensures delivery of oxygen, glucose, fatty acids, and other nutrients to the alveolar cells, thus completing the cycle and permitting synthesis of abundant surfactant.

The situation is much different in RDS, as shown schematically in Figure 4. The normal metabolism-ventilation-perfusion cycle is converted into an abnormal, and

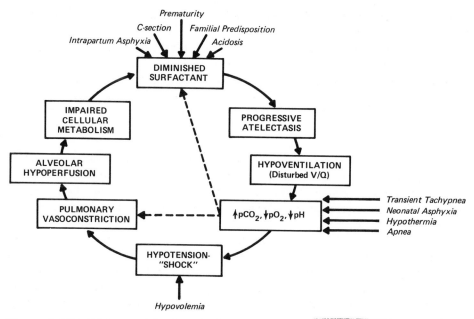

Figure 4. The "vicious cycle" in neonatal respiratory distress syndrome. Hypothetical, simplified representation of factors presumed to play key roles in the pathophysiology of the disease.

potentially malignant, cycle. Early atelectasis and loss of a satisfactory functional residual capacity due to surfactant deficiency results in hypoventilation, right-to-left shunts, hypoxia, and acidosis. This leads to constriction of pulmonary arteries and increased right-to-left shunting both on an intrapulmonary level and through the foramen ovale and ductus arteriosus. The constriction of the pulmonary arteries may lead to reduced lung perfusion, poor alveolar cell metabolism, and diminished surfactant synthesis. This aggravates the atelectasis and completes the "vicious cycle." If the cycle is not interrupted, the most likely consequence of RDS is a fatal outcome.

A variety of insults can thrust a neonate into the cycle characterized by hypoxia and respiratory insufficiency. A deficiency of surfactant from any of several possible causes may lead directly to atelectasis. Asphyxia at birth, apnea, and other neonatal problems might result in severe hypoventilation and hypoxia; this would cause constriction of the pulmonary arteries and thereby compromise lung perfusion and metabolism, leading to development of prolonged respiratory distress. Although little is known from direct studies about specific mechanisms operating to impair alveolar cell metabolism, the possibility of a lack of sufficient substrate, such as glucose deprivation in hypoglycemia, would theoretically be another way of entering the "vicious cycle."

The design of immediate and long-term supportive therapy for RDS follows from consideration of the metabolism-ventilation-perfusion cycle. Maintenance of a normal body temperature and a neutral thermal environment is an important component in the supportive treatment of any ill neonate. This helps to ameliorate increased oxygen consumption and peripheral vasoconstriction; the latter tends to promote generation of metabolic acids, which then contribute to pulmonary hypoperfusion. The temperature of the neonate should be 98.6°F as soon as possible after birth. While maintaining body temperature, one must be certain that the inspired oxygen concentration is raised sufficiently in an attempt to support tissue oxygenation, regardless of what therapeutic maneuvers are being carried out. Inspired oxygen should be adequate to maintain a PaO_2 of 50 to 70 mm Hg. Frequently, the ambient oxygen content does not rise above 60% in ordinary incubators, and some form of a head box must be used to facilitate adequate oxygen delivery. Also, inspiratory efforts must be adequate. The patient breathing rapidly and regularly is much better off than one who is gasping and periodically apneic.

It is not satisfactory merely to supply increased amounts of inspired oxygen to a neonate with signs of RDS. The care team is obligated to determine the PaO_2, $PaCO_2$, and pH frequently. The most useful way of obtaining blood for this is by the insertion of an umbilical arterial catheter. Some institutions have also routinely used blood samples from temporal and radial arteries for the blood gas determinations. Finally, a reliance on "arterialized" capillary blood for gas determinations must sometimes be accepted if procedures for obtaining arterial samples have failed. New instrumentation using oximeters has produced hope that in the future external oxygen monitoring can be performed continuously. As yet, however, this approach is not sufficiently well established for widespread acceptance.

Along with a concern for oxygenation, the physician caring for neonates with RDS must use intravenous nutrition to ensure maintenance of blood glucose and to facilitate production of lung surfactant. Premature infants exhaust hepatic glycogen stores rapidly and have inadequate gluconeogenic mechanisms. They must, therefore, have early intravenous glucose to preserve a normoglycemic state. The intravenous access line can also be useful as a route for administration of blood, plasma, or albumin in case of hypotension.

If oxygenation cannot be maintained by increasing the inspired oxygen concentration, continuous distending airway pressure must be applied. This is frequently done with the use of nasal prongs or a nasopharyngeal catheter to attain a positive end expiratory pressure of 6 to 10 cm H_2O. Such an approach helps maintain the functional residual capacity, prevent further atelectasis, and facilitate oxygen uptake. If the nasal route does not suffice, the baby must be intubated. Respiratory assistance to improve oxygenation and ventilation may be necessary if respiratory acidosis, apnea, or hypoxia persists. Intermittent positive pressure with various types of respirators is now common practice in neonatal intensive care units and has been associated with increased survival from RDS. Detailed discussion of the intensive respiratory care approach to treatment of RDS is available in several reviews (1–3,33) but is beyond the scope of this chapter.

Frequent chemical assessment of ventilation, oxygenation, and the acid-base status of the infant must be made. Respiratory acidosis is treated with ventilatory assistance. If the blood pressure is marginal or low and metabolic acidosis supervenes, consideration should be given to expanding the blood volume, since inadequate perfusion could contribute to the acidosis. Persistent and severe metabolic acidosis is sometimes treated with alkali infusions, but care must be taken that these infusions are of dilute bicarbonate and given into major blood flow areas. Before using bicarbonate to neutralize hydrogen ions and organic acids, the physician must ascertain that ventilation is sufficient to permit removal of the CO_2 generated and prevent hypercapnia and aggravation of the acidosis.

Mortality and Morbidity Associated with RDS

Reprts now indicate that the survival rate for RDS treated in an intensive care nursery is approximately 80% for babies of greater than 1000-g birthweight. The mortality for babies less than 1000 g is probably much higher. The usual complication causing death in severe RDS is a persistence of hypoxia and acidosis. One-half of the patients who die have an associated central nervous system hemorrhage, particularly of the ventricular system. Complications from assisted ventilatory therapy, such as pneumothorax or pneumopericardium, can also contribute to the mortality. High inspired oxygen concentrations, intubation, and positive pressure have been implicated as factors contributing to pulmonary oxygen toxicity, termed bronchopulmonary dysplasia. This disease, if severe, may have a high fatality rate.

A premature infant with RDS is at risk for other potentially devasting diseases. One of these is patent ductus arteriosus with congestive heart failure. As the pulmonary vasculature relaxes with improvement of RDS, the ductus arteriosus might remain open and allow left-to-right shunting, leading to increased pulmonary blood flow, pulmonary edema, and congestive failure. The pulmonary edema may decrease lung compliance, impair oxygenation, and prolong the need for assisted ventilation with supplemental oxygen. This can, in turn, lead to an increased risk for development of pulmonary oxygen toxicity.

Necrotizing enterocolitis (NEC) is another complication of RDS that has occurred with an increased frequency during recent years, particularly in infants of birthweight less than 1500 g who have suffered hypoxia. This disease usually has its onset with abdominal distention and gastric retention followed by traces of blood in the stool. Later, *pneumatosis intestinalis* might appear on abdominal x-rays. Infants with NEC have a fairly good prognosis if medical intervention is instituted early enough. Antibiotics, discontinuation of oral feedings, gastric suction, and maintainance of good nutrition through hyperalimentation are the recommended approaches to treatment. If the disease progresses to such an extent that the necrotic bowel breaks down and causes perforation, survival is less than 20%.

Hyperbilirubinemia occurs frequently in the premature infant and is an added concern in the presence of hypoxia and acidosis. Under these conditions, the central nervous system may be vulnerable to bilirubin levels not generally considered toxic, especially in term neonates.

Infants with severe RDS need hospitalization in an intensive care setting and require constant surveillance with monitoring equipment and frequent laboratory studies. This may well lead to a problem of delayed social development and impaired "parenting." It has been shown that early parental contact leads to improved parent-infant relationships in future years (34). A serious illness in the premature infant, dissociating him from his mother because of transfer to an intensive care nursery, as well as the subsequent long-term hospitalization, might hinder this attachment. Some of the difficulties can be overcome by physicians, nursing staff, and paramedical personnel attempting to bring the parents in close contact with the sick neonate as early and frequently as possible.

NEW HORIZONS IN THE PREVENTION OF RDS

General

The prevention of the respiratory distress syndrome, particularly in very immature infants of less than 32 weeks, would relieve society of a substantial socioeconomic burden. Indeed, it may be calculated that the cost of this disease for primary care alone in the United States exceeds 400 million dollars. It is encouraging, therefore, that recent clinical studies have suggested that pharmacologic agents such as glucocorticoids, when given at least 24 hr prior to delivery, can lower the incidence of RDS (35). Consistent with this observation is evidence from studies with sheep, rabbits, and monkeys indicating that glucocorticoids are capable of promoting maturation of the lung with respect to both structure and production of surfactant (1).

Role of Glucocorticoids in Fetal Lung Development

Using the anatomic approach, several investigators have demonstrated that 48 to 72 hr following administration of glucocorticoids, increased potential air space and greater "alveolarization" is apparent (1,2). As listed in Table III, this is manifested primarily by attenuation of alveolar cells and narrowing of septae. In the rabbit, for instance, instead of the usual phenomenon of complete "alveolarization" at day 28, these maturational changes can be demonstrated at day 26 if steroids are injected at 23 to 24 days of gestation. In addition, prominent type II alveolar pneumonocytes are also evident within 2 days of corticosteroid injection to immature fetuses.

Physiologic evidence of maturation following fetal corticosteroid administration includes greater lung distensibility, greater deflation stability, and an earlier appearance of surface-active material. In other words, there is an acceleration in the appearance of surfactant and a shifting of the time when alveolar stability is evident. Hormonal influences on alveolar stability were originally studied in fetal rabbits by Kotas et al. (14,36). They found markedly improved deflation stability after glucocorticoid treatment such that the percent volume remaining at 10 cm pressure (% V_{10}) was more than twofold higher in the lungs of 27-day steroid-treated animals as compared with control lungs. The retention of air was twice as great during an experimental maneuver simulating expiration.

Table III. Effects of Glucocorticoid on Lung Development

Anatomic:
    Increased potential airspace:
        Attenuation of alveolar cells
        Narrowing of septae
        Greater "alveolarization"
    Increased prominence or numbers of type II pneumonocytes

Physiologic:
    Greater distensibility
    Greater deflation stability
    Earlier appearance of SAM

Biochemical:
    Increased concentration or degree of saturation of lecithin in:
        Lung parenchyma
        Lung lavage fluid
    Increased conversion of choline to lecithin, i.e., the apparent rate of the choline pathway is enhanced
    Increased activities of cholinephosphotransferase, glycerolphosphate phosphatidyltransferase, and lipoprotein lipase

The biochemical effects of glucocorticoids with respect to lung development are also listed in Table III. Following the demonstration in 1971 that alveolar surfactant is augmented in rabbits given exogenous glucocorticoid in utero (14), a number of investigators have measured the concentration or fatty acid composition of lung lecithin. Farrell and Zachman (37), for instance, reported in 1973 that the amount of lecithin present in fetal rabbit lung was increased 72 hr after administration of 9α-fluoroprednisolone acetate. More recently, Ekelund et al. (38) reported that cortisol promotes the accumulation of phospholipids in cultured human fetal lung. In addition, Rooney and associates (39) have observed that pulmonary fluid obtained by saline lavage contains increased amounts of lecithin when fetal rabbits are given cortisol. Measurements of the lecithin concentration in amniotic fluid also suggest, but have not conclusively demonstrated, that lung-derived phospholipids in the amniotic space are increased following glucocorticoid treatment.

A further, and more primary, biochemical effect of glucocorticoid on lung development is an increased conversion of choline to phosphatidylcholine, i.e., an enhanced rate of choline pathway activity. Such an effect was first demonstrated by Farrell and Zachman (37) when lung slices were used to measure the incorporation of ^{14}C-choline into lecithin, as well as the conversion of ^{14}C-methionine to the final product. With this approach, it was found that lungs of corticosteroid-treated rabbit fetuses are approximately 50% more active in terms of choline pathway rates than those of controls. In contrast, phosphatidylethanolamine methylation rates were not influenced significantly by injection of glucocorticoid. Subsequently, the finding of augmented choline pathway rates after steroid treatment has been independently confirmed by numerous investigators working with a variety of animals and lung systems. For instance, Barrett and associates (40) in rabbits, Russell et al. (41) in rats, Ekelund et al. (38) working with lung explants from human fetuses, and Smith and Torday (42) using lung cells in tissue culture have all reported that corticosteroids enhance choline incorporation rates.

The list of biochemical effects of glucocorticoid on lung development presented in Table III gives an indication of enzymes reported to show increased activities in lung tissue on corticosteroid administration. These include (1) *choline phosphotransferase* (37,43), the terminal enzyme of the choline pathway; (2) *glycerolphosphate phosphatidyltransferase* (10), a key enzyme in phosphatidylglycerol production; and (3) *lipoprotein lipase* (11), which, through hydrolysis of circulating triglyceride, may play an important role in supplying fatty acid for phospholipid synthesis.

The net biochemical effect of glucocorticoid, through apparent induction of these enzymes, is to enhance the capacity of the fetal lung to produce the surface-active phospholipids of the alveolar lining layer. Because of exogenous corticosteroid, this capacity is developed at an earlier time in gestation than would normally be found. The hormone therefore acts as a stimulus capable of changing the timing of lung development such that the maturation process is accelerated.

Clinical Trials

The most extensive controlled study of antepartum corticosteroid treatment to date was conducted by Liggins and Howie (35,44) in New Zealand between December, 1969, and February, 1975. They administered a potent glucocorticoid intramuscularly in a randomized, double-blind fashion to pregnant women in premature labor. The preparation, consisting of a mixture of 6 mg betamethasone phosphate and 6 mg betamethasone acetate, was injected on admission to the trial and 24 hr later, unless delivery had occurred. An attempt was made to delay parturition in all women for a period of 48 to 72 hr with intravenous infusion of ethanol or salbutamol; neither of these agents was found in the final analysis to influence the incidence of RDS when comparison was made with a group of patients receiving no uterine relaxant.

A total of 431 infants resulted from the steroid-treated pregnancies and 42%, or 182, were delivered more than 1 but less than 7 days after entry into the trial. Reflecting the obstetrician's inability to establish perfect control over uterine activity, 18% of the neonates were delivered less than 24 hr from the time of the first betamethasone injection. The other 40% were delivered more than 7 days after the mother entered the protocol. In comparison with the corresponding control group, no differences in the incidence of RDS were found in infants treated antenatally with betamethasone for less than 1 or more than 7 days.

The composition and outcome of the control and steroid-treated groups in which the interval from "entry to delivery" was between 1 and 7 days are described in Table IV. Of 59 infants of less than 32 weeks gestation whose mothers received betamethasone, 20% developed the respiratory distress syndrome. This incidence is significantly lower than the control group of 51 prematures who showed an RDS incidence of 57%. Significant, though less striking, improvement in the rate of RDS was also noted in steroid-treated infants of 32 to 34 weeks gestation, whereas the group greater than 34 weeks was not statistically different from corresponding controls. The total group of premature infants born between 1 and 7 days after initiation of maternal betamethasone injections showed an RDS incidence of 8.8%, as compared with 23.7% in the control group ($p < .001$).

Relative to clinical problems associated with prenatal corticosteroid treatment, Liggins and Howie found that pregnant diabetics have greater difficulty with carbohydrate

Table IV. The Glucocorticoid Trial of Liggins and Howie: Composition and Outcome of Control and Betamethasone-Treated Groups of Premature Infants Delivered between 1 and 7 Days after the Initial Dose

	Control Group	Betamethasone Treated Group	Significance
Number of infants	164	186	NS
Mean gestational age	32.4 weeks	32.3 weeks	NS
Mean birth weight	1882 g	1797 g	NS
Premature rupture of membranes	46.3%	45.7%	NS
Mean Apgar score	6.3 at 1 min	6.4 at 1 min	NS
Sex: male	52.2%	52.4%	NS
Perinatal deaths	22.6%	8.6%	$p < .001$
Intraventricular hemorrhage	9%	3.3%	$p < .05$
RDS incidence:			
Total	23.7%	8.8%	$p < .001$
By gestational age:			
<30 weeks	57.7%	27.8%	$p < .04$
30–32 weeks	56.0%	8.7%	$p < .001$
32–34 weeks	12.9%	0%	$p < .04$
>34 weeks	5.4%	5.5%	NS

SOURCE: Reference 44.

metabolism and require increased insulin after betamethasone injections. A more significant obstetrical problem was encountered in women with severe hypertension-edema-proteinuria syndromes. Fetal death occurred in 25.6% of these cases after betamethasone treatment, whereas intrauterine demise was noted in 7% of controls ($p <$ .04). Thus, if the placenta is dysfunctional, administration of betamethasone seems to compromise the fetus further. Aside from this, no complication of pregnancy, labor, delivery, or the postpartum period was detected by Liggins and Howie that could have been attributed to the corticosteroid preparation. In addition, there was no added risk of fetal or postnatal infection, particularly neonatal pneumonia.

In addition to the New Zealand study, a number of subsequent clinical investigations have been, and are being, conducted around the world to assess the possible prophylactic role of glucocorticoids. Although some of these trials suffer from either faulty design or improper control, they have all provided data in support of the original observations by Liggins and Howie. One recent study conducted in Czechoslovakia (45), for instance, which was controlled with randomization at entry, reported that infants averaging 31 weeks gestation show a decrease in RDS incidence from 45 to 16% ($p <$ .001), if maternal administration of 100 mg of hydrocortisone occurred at least 24 hr prior to delivery.

In the majority of clinical trials, betamethasone has been the agent administered intramuscularly to pregnant women in premature labor. This potent steroid crosses the placenta, as demonstrated by Ballard and associates (46), and raises circulating glucocorticoid in fetal plasma to approximately three times that found prior to injection, expressed on the basis of cortisol equivalents. Thus, it may be inferred that in terms of circulating corticosteroid levels, betamethasone in the dosage of Liggins and Howie mimics a physiologic stress response. Noteworthy is the fact that such concentrations saturate or "fill" the high affinity lung cell corticosteroid receptors, as determined by Ballard and Ballard (47), and thus presumably give an optimum response.

With regard to side effects of glucocorticoids on the developing fetus, Taeusch (48) has reviewed the toxicity studies published before 1975. He and others have concluded that the purported adverse effects of short-duration, near-physiologic doses of glucocorticoid given to the human fetus during the third trimester of pregnancy were not well documented. He concluded, therefore, that no fetal or maternal risks have been reported that would preclude the use of this therapy in cases where there is high potential for benefit. Studies in rats that have uncovered central nervous system pathology must be evaluated on the basis of the relatively high steroid doses administered and must take into account the stage of neurological development at the end of a short gestation period. Ballard et al. (46), in fact, have been able to offer evidence arguing that the studies of concern in rats are not applicable to the human situation because (1) the doses used are approximately 10 to 100-fold greater than those used effectively by Liggins and Howie to prevent RDS and (2) lowering the dose to a more comparable level eliminates the CNS toxicity.

The most useful studies regarding possible adverse effects in humans are those which evaluate infants and children exposed in utero to exogenous glucocorticoids for the purpose of promoting lung maturation. Results available from such studies are limited but sound an encouraging note thus far. All investigators reporting on growth indicate that infants feed and gain weight normally during both the neonatal and subsequent periods. In addition, Denver Developmental Screening Tests have disclosed normal patterns for acquisition of developmental milestones (49). Finally, Liggins and Howie (44) have recently noted that 46 betamethasone-exposed children show a normal Stanford-Binet IQ at a mean age of 4 years 3 months (mean $\pm$ SD = 100 $\pm$ 15.7; IQ in 35 matched controls = 98.9 $\pm$ 20.2).

CONCLUSION: UNANSWERED QUESTIONS AND CONTINUED CONCERNS

Despite the major advances of the past decade in diagnosis and treatment of acute neonatal disease in general, and the respiratory distress syndrome in particular, the United States still ranks unacceptably low (fifteenth) among developed countries in overall neonatal mortality rates. A large proportion of newborn fatalities are attributable to premature birth, and, of this group, approximately half result from respiratory disease. Thus, the recent observations with glucocorticoids offer exciting promise and strengthen the hopes of those whose primary concern is prevention of RDS, rather than salvaging neonates once the disease has developed. It must be emphasized, however, that the potential for adverse side effects secondary to exposure of the fetus to potent corticosteroid hormones has not been adequately explored. There is no doubt that steroids influence numerous organs and that even short-term hormonal treatment during gestation can significantly alter metabolic processes throughout the body, with many possible ramifications, both good and bad. Until complete information is available on the risk/benefit ratio, therefore, it is necessary to withhold final judgment and recommendations on the general use of antenatal corticosteroids for the prevention of RDS. Hopefully, the comprehensive clinical trial now being conducted in the United States, under the sponsorship of the National Heart, Lung and Blood Institute, will provide the definitive data on both efficacy and toxicity of steroids. In the meantime, a cautious attitude is warranted while this issue is being settled and while other agents, with less generalized effects, are being explored.

REFERENCES

1. Farrell, P. M. and Avery, M. E.: Hyaline membrane disease. *Am. Rev. Resp. Dis.* 111:657, 1975.

2. Farrell, P. M., and Kotas, R. V.: The prevention of hyaline membrane disease: New concepts and approaches to therapy, *Adv. Pediatr.* 23:213, 1976.

3. Avery, M. E., and Fletcher, B. D.: *The Lung and Its Disorders in the Newborn Infant*, ed. 3. Philadelphia, W. B. Saunders Company, 1974.

4. Clements, J. A.: Surfactant in pulmonary disease. *New Eng. J. Med.* 272:1336, 1965.

5. King, R. J., and Clements, J. A.: Surface active materials from dog lung: II. Composition and physiological correlations. *Am. J. Physiol.* 223:715, 1972.

6. Body, G. R.: The phospholipid composition of pig lung surfactant. *Lipids* 6:625, 1971.

7. Godinez, R. I., Sanders, R. L., and Longmore, W. J.: Phosphatidylglycerol in rat lung: II. Comparison of occurrence, composition, and metabolism in surfactant and residual fractions. *Biochem.* 14:835, 1975.

8. Gikas, E. G., King R. J., Mescher, E. J., et al.: Radioimmunoassay of pulmonary surface-active material in the tracheal fluid of the fetal lamb. *Am. Rev. Resp. Dis.* 115:587, 1977.

9. Farrell, P. M., and Morgan, T. E.: Lecithin biosynthesis in the developing lung, in Hodson, W. A. (ed.): *The Development of the Lung.* New York, Marcel Dekker, 1977.

10. Hamosh, P., Hamosh, M., Yeager, H., et al.: Effect of dexamethasone on lipoprotein lipase activity of the rat lung. *Biochim. Biophys. Acta* 431:519. 1976.

11. Rooney, S. A., Gross, I., Gassenheimer, L. N., et al.: Stimulation of glycerolphosphate phosphatidyl-transferase activity in fetal rabbit lung by cortisol administration. *Biochem. Biophys. Acta* 398:433, 1975.

12. Schultz, F. M., Jimenez, J. M., MacDonald, P. C., et al.: Fetal lung maturation: I. Phosphatidic acid phosphohydrolase in rabbit lung. *Gynecol. Invest.* 5:222, 1974.

13. Blackburn, W. R., Travers, H., and Potter, D. M.: The role of the pituitary-adrenal-thyroid axes in lung differentiation: I. Studies on the cytology and physical properties of anencephalic fetal rat lung. *Lab. Invest.* 26:306, 1972.

14. Kotas, R. V., and Avery, M. E.: Accelerated appearance of pulmonary surfactant in the fetal rabbit. *J. Appl. Physiol.* 30:358, 1971.

15. Farrell, P. M.: Fetal lung development and the influence of glucocorticoids on pulmonary surfactant. *J. Steroid Biochem.,* 8:463, 1977.

16. Epstein, M. F., and Farrell, P. M.: The choline incorporation pathway: Primary mechanism for *de novo* lecithin synthesis in fetal primate lung. *Pediatr. Res.* 9:658, 1975.

17. Kotas, R. V., Farrell, P. M., Ulane, R. E., et al.: Fetal Rhesus monkey lung development: Lobar differences and discordances between stability and distensibility. *J. Appl. Physiol.,* 43:92, 1977.

18. Avery, M. E., and Mead, J.: Surface properties in relation to atelectasis and hyaline membrane disease. *Am. J. Dis. Child.* 97:517, 1959.

19. Graven, S. N.: Phospholipids in human and monkey amniotic fluid. *Pediatr. Res.* 2:318, 1968.

20. Gluck, L., Kulovich, M. V., Borer, R. C., et al.: Diagnosis of the respiratory distress syndrome by amniocentesis. *Am. J. Obstet. Gynecol.* 109:440, 1971.

21. Goldenberg, R. L., and Nelson, K.: Iatrogenic respiratory distress syndrome. *Am. J. Obstet. Gynecol.* 123:617, 1975.

22. Olson, E. B., and Graven, S. N.: Comparison of visualization methods used to measure the lecithin/sphingomyelin ratio in amniotic fluid. *Clin. Chem.* 20:1408, 1974.

23. Clements, J. A., Platzkar, A. C., Tierney, D. F., et al.: Assessment of the risk of the respiratory distress syndrome by a rapid test for surfactant in amniotic fluid. *N. Eng. J. Med.* 286:1077, 1972.

24. Olson, E. B., Graven, S. N., and Zachman, R. D.: Amniotic fluid lecithin to sphingomyelin ratio of 3.5 and fetal pulmonary maturity. *Pediat. Res.* 9:65, 1975.

25. Hallman, M., Kulovich, M., Kirkpatirck, E., et al.: Phosphatidylinositol and phosphatidylglycerol in amniotic fluid: Indices of lung maturity. *Am. J. Obstet. Gynecol.* 125:613, 1976.

26. Maclenran, A. H., Roxburgh, D., Thornton, C., et al.: Palmitic acid levels in amniotic fluid and the shake test. *Brit. J. Obstet. Gynaec.* 82:199, 1975.

27. Farrell, P. M., and Wood, R. E.: Epidemiology of hyaline membrane disease in the United States. *Pediatrics* 58:167, 1976.

28. Usher, R. H., Allen, A. C., and McLean, F. H.: Risk of respiratory distress syndrome related to gestational age, route of delivery, and maternal diabetes. *Am. J. Obstet. Gynec.* 111:826, 1971.

29. Ablow, R. C., Driscoll, S. G., Effmann, E. L., et al.: A comparison of early onset group B streptococcal neonatal infection and the respiratory distress syndrome of the newborn. *N. Eng. J. Med.* 294:65, 1976.

30. Graven, S. N., Howe, G., and Callon, H.: Perinatal health care studies and program results in Wisconsin, 1964–1970. Presented at the spring session of the American Academy of Pediatrics, San Diego, April 24–27, 1972.

31. Butterfield, I. J.: Regional newborn care. *Rocky Mt. Med. J.* 69:53, 1972.

32. Meyer, H. B., and Daily, W. J.: A report to the Maricopa County Pediatric Society on the current status of the Arizona State Newborn Intensive Care and Transport Program. Phoenix, Ariz., February, 1972.

33. Swyer, P. R.: Further management and disposal of the high risk newborn, in Swyer, P. R. (ed.): *The Intensive Care of the Newly Born.* New York, S. Karger, 1975, p. 75.

34. Klaus, M., and Kennell, J.: Care of the mother, in Klaus, M., and Fanaroff, A. A. (eds.): *Care of the High Risk Neonate.* Philadelphia, W. B. Saunders, 1973, p. 98.

35. Liggins, G. C., and Howie, R. N.: A controlled trial of antepartum glucocorticoid treatment for prevention of the respiratory distress syndrome in premature infants. *Pediatrics* 50:515, 1972.

36. Kotas, R. V., Fletcher, B. D., Torday, J., et al.: Evidence for independent regulations of organ maturation in fetal rabbits. *Pediatrics* 47:57, 1971.

37. Farrell, P. M., and Zachman, R. D.: Induction of choline phosphotransferase and lecithin synthesis in the fetal lung by corticosteroids. *Science* 179:297, 1973.

38. Ekelund, L., Arvidson, G., and Astedt, B.: Cortisol-induced accumulation of phospholipids in organ culture of human fetal lung. *Scand. J. Clin. Lab. Invest.* 35:419, 1975.

39. Rooney, S. A., Gobran, L., Gross, I., et al.: Studies on pulmonary surfactant: Effects of cortisol administration to fetal rabbits on lung phospholipid content, composition, and biosynthesis. *Biochem. Biophys. Acta* 450:121, 1976.

40. Barrett, C. T., and Sevanian, A.: Cyclic AMP and surfactant production: New means for enhancing lung maturation in the fetus. *Pediatr. Res.* 9:394, 1975.

41. Russell, B. J., Nugent, L., and Chernick, V.: Effects of steroids on the enzymatic pathways of lecithin production in fetal rats. *Biol. Neonat.* 24:306, 1974.

42. Smith, B. T., and Torday, J. S.: Factors affecting lecithin synthesis by fetal lung cells in culture. *Pediatr. Res.* 8:848, 1974.

43. Farrell, P. M., Blackburn, W. R., and Adams, A. J.: Lung phosphatidylcholine synthesis and cholinephosphotransferase activity in anencephalic rat fetuses with corticosteroid deficiency. *Pediatr. Res.*, 11:770, 1977.

44. Liggins, G. C.: The prevention of RDS by maternal betamethasone administration, in Stern, L. (ed.): *Lung Maturation and the Prevention of Hyaline Membrane Disease.* Columbus, Ohio, Ross Laboratories, 1976, p. 189.

45. Dluholucký, S., Babic, J., and Taufer, I.: Reduction of incidence and mortality of respiratory distress syndrome by administration of hydrocortisone to mothers. *Arch. Dis. Child.* 51:420, 1976.

46. Ballard, P. L., Granberg, P., and Ballard, R.: Glucocorticoid levels in maternal and cord serum after prenatal betamethasone therapy to prevent the respiratory distress syndrome. *J. Clin. Invest.* 56:1548, 1975.

47. Ballard, P. L., and Ballard, R. A.: Cytoplasmic receptor for glucocorticoids in lung of the human fetus and neonate. *J. Clin. Invest.* 53:477, 1974.

48. Taeusch, H. W.: Glucocorticoid prophylaxis for respiratory distress syndrome: A review of potential toxicity. *J. Pediatr.* 87:617, 1975.

49. Killiam, A. P.: Comparison of two glucocorticosteroid regimens for acceleration of fetal lung maturation, in Stern, L. (ed.): *Lung Maturation and the Prevention of Hyaline Membrane Disease.* Columbus, Ohio, Ross Laboratories, 1976, p. 199.

50. Farrell, P. M., Epstein, M. F., Fleischman, A. R., et al.: Lung lecithin biosynthesis in the nonhuman primate fetus: Determination of the primary pathway *in vivo. Biol. Neonate* 29:238, 1976.

51. Douglas, W. H. J., Jones, R. M., and Farrell, P. M.: Isolation of cells that retain differentiated functions *in vitro*: Properties of clonally isolated type II pneumonocytes. *Environ. Health Perspect.,* 16:83, 1976.

9

Infant Development Viewed in the Mother-Infant Relationship

Evelyn B. Thoman, Ph.D.

An infant's behavior is the ultimate expression of its biological functioning. At the time of birth, the infant is closest to its biological heritage, and thus the neonatal period can be considered the most appropriate time for exploring its biological programming for survival. Since the infant is dependent for survival on successful social relations, typically with the mother, the clearest view of this earliest programming can be obtained from observing the baby in the context of the mother-infant interaction. The coping behaviors expressed in this relationship most fully reflect the infant's capabilities as designed by the evolutionary process. A growing emphasis on this perspective for the study of early development has led to research that is much more closely connected with reality than has been the case in the past.

An example from the literature illustrates this point. In contradiction to the generally held notion that the newborn infant "couldn't learn," Gunther, at a 1961 CIBA Conference (1) showed films of newborn infants during their first postnatal feeding. Some of these infants experienced moments of smothering when their noses were occluded by the mother's breast. At subsequent feedings, these infants persistently fought and struggled against being put to the breast. Gunther's films provided a dramatic documentation of the newborn's adaptive modification to the circumstances of its environment. The feeding interaction with the mother in the early days of life is clearly a biologically relevant circumstance for exploring the infant's adaptive capabilities. Gunther's pioneering work in the study of newborns with their mothers marked the beginning of a blooming interest in this stage of life, as well as a recognition of the necessity for using ethologically relevant conditions for such study.

Both our perspective on infancy and the procedures considered most appropriate for its study are undergoing major changes. The direction of some of these changes are

The research described in this chapter was supported by the William T. Grant Foundation, NICHD Grant HD-08195-01A2, and NIMH Predoctoral Fellowship 5268-81-13645.

243

described in this chapter, illustrated by recent findings that may be of interest to medical clinicians. Research in this area is considered from the point of view that the most meaningful empirical findings about early development are those which are closely connected with reality. This position is not necessarily taken because it is felt that we need "applied" research but rather reflects a philosophical position that research provides insights into the nature of early development only by investigating real babies developing in their real worlds. Thus, it turns out that studies that are aimed at answering basic questions about development can, and we take the position that they also should, have relevance for the interests of parents and clinicians. The alliance between these two directions of interest is a major theme of this chapter.

A brief look at past views of infants, mostly views that still have not been completely relinqushed, is given to put the newer conceptualizations in bold relief.

Changing Views of the Infant

A major form of mythology in the not too distant past has been that the infant, especially during the neonatal period, is an incomplete, relatively incompetent and inadequate organism and that by a series of linear progressions, the infant becomes a complex, competent, and complete organism—an adult. Such a view was the logical and emotional heritage of the supposedly discarded notion that the infant is a miniature adult with a *tabula rasa,* helpless and passive, dependent initially on genetically programmed maturation and subsequently on an imprint from the mature caretaker who provides both the model for the infant to imitate and the stimulus for the infant to learn adult modes of thinking and behaving. Early on, maturation was seen as the primary mode of change, as the newborn infant was not considered to be capable of learning. This "deficit" view of infancy was based on claims that, at birth and for sometime thereafter, the human infant was functionally decorticate, largely a reflexive organism, controlled primarily by its internal environment and organic processes and responsive to only a small number of external inputs. As Stone, Smith, and Murphy pointed out in 1973 (2), only the baby biographers and mothers knew better.

The recent history of the study of infancy has made major changes in this deficit mythology, with a burgeoning number of studies exploring numerous facets of the infant's competence and behavior. Highly sophisticated experimental laboratory studies have demonstrated the infant's sensitivity to stimuli in all sense modalities. From birth, the infant is not only responsive to patterns of sound but is selectively sensitive to the characteristics of human speech (3,4); the newborn is selectively attentive to patterns of visual stimuli, especially those patterns characteristic of the human face (5); and the infant can attend to and be entrained by the temporal patterning of events (6–8). Likewise, from the time of birth, the infant is demonstrably capable of learning. Gunther's work, referred to earlier, inspired many researchers to rush to the laboratory in search of additional learning capabilities of the mysterious newborn.

In fact, the human infant, like the college sophomore and the laboratory rat, has become a favorite laboratory subject. In commenting on the numerous and diverse studies of early infancy, Stone, Smith, and Murphy (2) say, ". . . from our perch overlooking that vast new landscape of infancy, a landscape thrown up like a new volcanic island in the past decade and a half, we have come not only to marvel at how much new information has been produced, but also to see how badly it needs to be digested . . . particularly needed now is research that links and relates specific, sometimes atomistic findings" (p. 9). Their statements articulately describe the state of research in infancy not only in terms of its progress but also in terms of its limitations. They recognize that something is missing. That something is actually the human infant—or rather, the infant as a total human being. The atomistic nature of the accumulated findings from the vast number of studies of infants render those findings indigestable. Developmentalists, like many other psychologists, have striven for scientific respectability by modeling their field after the physical sciences, by exploring molecular systems without due consideration for their integration. They have, in fact, missed the lessons to be learned from the biological sciences, which have developed methods for investigating large and complex systems (9). Consequently, we have accumulated innumerable bits and pieces of knowledge that could only be assembled into a tinker-toy baby, rather than a live organism adapting to its environment.

Segmentation in science is a necessity for rigorous analytical study, but in the process of integration, the complete system is never seen. For example, as a possible consequence of the intensely empirical and molecular approach to the study of infants, a rather detached view of the infant's subjective experience is prevalent. The infant's competence as a perceiver and a performer has received a great deal of attention; the infant's competence as a feeling being has received little attention. The possibility that the infant may have a rich affective life has been virtually overlooked. In fact, casual observation rather than scientific investigation has been accepted as evidence that the infant has little affect, particularly of a positive nature. For example, although the infant's smiles during the newborn period are no longer considered to be "gas produced," they are taken into account only as reflexes occurring during drowsiness or active (REM) sleep. Yet, in 1966, Wolff (10) reported that neonates smile in response to mild and unexpected stimuli. This is a very human response.

The bland view of the infant's emotional life is now being challenged by an accumulation of other research findings. Cairns and Butterfield (11) have shown that 2-day-old infants can express an auditory preference for vocal instrumental music by modifying their sucking patterns. The infants not only indicate a positive preference for vocal music but also selective avoidance of white noise. Lipsitt (12) describes changes in sucking patterns as a function of taste and discusses the newborn's responses in terms of "pleasure" and "annoyance." Eisenberg (13) has recorded smiling as a response to auditory sounds characteristic of human speech. These studies lend support to the view that the infant's competence as a feeling being and complexity as a social being are only beginning to be explored. The first step, however, has been taken—a recognition of the need for such study.

Evidence of the infant's responsiveness to characteristics of the human face, voice, and movement suggests that the infant is preprogrammed to respond to certain kinds of sensory stimuli that are not only pleasurable but also are embodied in the person of the caregiver, usually the mother. She is the most ubiquitous object in the infant's environment and as such an amalgam of prepotent stimuli to which the infant, by virtue of his neuronal organization, is programmed to respond. Her voice, which constitutes a stimulus pattern, is the most important sound the infant hears because it is presented under highly relevant conditions: at close quarters and during feeding and other caretaking activities. Her face, which can also be considered a stimulus pattern, is the object of closest regard during these activities. Thus, the infant emerges from the womb rather neatly equipped to organize his sensory world. His sensory perceptions, beginning at birth, constitute the roots of both his social and intellectual development (13).

The Need for New Models of Early Development

The question of early adaptation and development is now being seriously explored in the context of changing interpersonal relationships. Research on early development today is in the process of creating new paradigms for exploring infancy, a process that will not only supplement existing paradigms but, more important, replace those which have been based on mythology—the mythology that the newborn infant is incomplete or incompetent; the mythology that the newborn infant can be explored using adult models; the mythology that the functioning of the total infant can be comprehended by the study of isolated behavioral processes; and the mythology that development can be understood by isolated study of either the baby or the mother.

A number of investigators are searching for ways to study early behavioral processes without oversimplifying the nature of the problems or the nature of the baby. Papousek and Papousek (14), for example, say explicitly that their aim is to investigate the biological-social-behavioral organization of infants from the time of birth. Their research is carried out in both the laboratory and the home, and in either case the circumstances for observation are designed to be as natural as possible. An example is a study of 3-month-old infants observed in interaction with their mothers. At specified times the mother suddenly and unexpectedly disappeared from the infant's view. This violation of the infant's expectancies with respect to the mother was found to produce marked changes in autonomic functions, as well as in the infant's behavioral state; moreover, if the intervention was repeated over successive trials, the baby began to avoid looking at the mother and gradually exhibited more withdrawal behavior. Eventually the baby reached a point of actually rejecting the mother's approach on her return. Once these dramatic changes were observed, further explorations using this particular intervention paradigm were discontinued. However, even milder violations of typical maternal responsiveness can produce distress in babies at this age. Papousek has asked the mothers simply to close their eyes or to maintain a still, unexpressive face. This maternal misbehavior also produces distress and rejection on the part of the infants.

A variety of research strategies are being used in the search for new approaches to the study of development. These include naturalistic observations in the home and laboratory observations that are ever more carefully designed both to provide conditions that are as natural as possible and to elicit "typically" occurring behaviors. The findings are impressive, but their major message is that the adaptive capabilities of infants are still grossly underestimated and unexplored. For example, a remarkable degree of temporal responsiveness is demonstrated in a study by Condon and Sander (15). Microanalysis of filmed sequences show that the rhythm of an adult's spoken words, in Chinese or English, is immediately reflected in synchronous motor movements by the infant. The vocalization is presented while the adult is out of visual range of the infant. Furthermore, Condon reports that by 2 weeks of age, if the infant is exposed to a language that is different from the one heard during the first 2 weeks, the "foreign" language causes distress. Condon's findings are consistent with the very elegant studies of speech sound discrimination by Eimas (4), who finds that neonates can perceive very fine differences in the time relationships between the vocal and nonvocal parts of speech sounds. They can make discriminations that are basic to all human spoken languages. Significantly, this exquisite discrimination is lost over time and is not present in adults. Adults are capable of making only those temporal discriminations which are characteristic of their native language.

Sander, who has long combined clinical and research interests in exploring development in the context of care-giver–infant interaction, expresses his frustration with the segmental nature of developmental study as follows:

> The bulk of the new information [about infants] has been won as a result of a step by step process of teasing apart influences, defining functions, and narrowing causality by ever more precise specification. As it comes now, however, to the *application* of such information as a means of facilitating development in particular instances, the worker is faced with a necessity to adopt quite a different orientation for the *use* of the information than that which led to its discovery. The research orientation is traditionally analytic; the developmental process is essentially integrative, a process of synthesis of highly complex determinants. . . . [In order] to augment the clinical perspective, it is to be expected that research strategies aimed at clarifying mechanisms of synthesis and integration in the coordinations between infant and caregiver will be forthcoming (7).

Sander's work is an excellent illustration of research with infants that integrates biobehavioral and environmental variables, primarily in the mother-infant relationship. Sander has made continuous recordings of the infant's states and activity rhythms by means of a sensor mattress whenever the baby is in the crib and direct observations of mother and infant when the baby is out of the crib. In this way, he has identified the physiological rhythms of the infant as the infant and mother gradually achieve a coordination in terms of their temporal organization around the clock. Sander considers the mutual temporal regulation of maternal and infant activities as one of the earliest tasks of their mutual adaptation.

Temporal patterning in the interactive system is also a focus of Stern's (6,16–18) research with mothers and infants. Stern (16) considers the relatively brief moments of social interaction, or "free play," between mother and infant as among the most crucial experiences in the infant's first phase of participation in human events. A most important early experience for the infant is simply observing whatever the mother may do with her face, voice, body, and hands. "The ongoing flow of her acts provides for the infant his emerging experience with the stuff of human communication and relatedness. This choreography of maternal behaviors is the raw material from the outside world with which the infant begins to construct his knowledge and experience of all things human . . ." (p. 9). Stern and others have described the variety of ways in which mothers or caregivers use the face and voice differently when they interact with infants from the way they do in other situations. Face movements are exaggerated and prolonged; vocalizations are repeated, drawn out, and varied on an intonation theme.

Stern has extensively studied face-to-face interactions with a specific emphasis on mutual gazing and vocalization exchanges. He notes that mothers can be intrusive simply by gazing intensively at the infant and from a very early age infants can respond to such intrusiveness with gaze aversion. Another form of caregiver intrusion is that of looming toward the infant's face. Bower and others have shown that the infant has an aversive response to objects that loom toward the face, deriving from reflexes evolved for protection of the face and eyes (16,19). Yet mothers, and other adults, and older children are generally careless about zooming in to talk, kiss, or otherwise touch the baby.

Stern (16) talks about the "split-second" world of the mother and infant and describes frame-by-frame film analyses of play interaction, where the great majority of maternal and infant behavior was in the range of 0.3 to 1.0 sec in duration. Behavior may be either sequential or simultaneous, and these characteristics have implications for the nature of their mutual "dance". His detailed filmed analyses depict a choreography of mother-infant behavior in which the visual gaze and other behavior are so completely matched that it must be assumed that the joint performance requires anticipatory "knowledge" each of the other's behavioral flow. The data suggest that the infant must have an ability to form temporal expectancies of the mother's vocalizations in order for this synchrony to occur. ". . . [H]is ability to form expectancies and to evaluate deviations from the expected will remain intact across the wide range of behavioral tempos a caregiver must use. Furthermore, unless the infant were equipped with this timing process, or a similar one, he could only react to —follow or lead—the caregiver but never dance *with* her" (p. 92).

For Stern, as for the other researchers just described, the infant's temporal organization and the capacity to perceive, respond to, and integrate his own behavior with the temporal organization in the environment are some of the biologically programmed capabilities that have only begun to be explored. Each of these investigators, and others concerned with early development, are exploring the mother-infant relationship with a recognition of the complexities inherent in the interaction between a growing, changing, modifiable young organism and an organism that, although adult, is also subject to change by the relationship.

A number of researchers interested in the early parent-infant relationship are expressing dissatisfaction with simple, unidirectional models. In part, this dissatisfaction has derived from a failure to find any specific caretaking practices by mothers, or fathers, or other caretakers that have an identifiable effect on the infant's development. Likewise, studies focused on the infant's behavior have not been successful in specifying the impact of the child's characteristics on the parent. Additionally, and even more important, is the growing recognition that simplistic, single-factor models for the parent-infant relationship are not isomorphic with the complex and dynamic interplay of forces and events that go into any interaction. Thus, we are still searching for models and concepts that may provide the basis for research on the nature of the parent-infant relationship and how this ongoing interaction influences the development of the child.

More recently, process models of mother-infant interaction have been proposed. For example, Sameroff and Chandler (20) have suggested the concept of transactional analysis for the ongoing interaction between a mother and infant. They stress the importance of the transactional process as an influence on the infant's development, an influence that is generally not predictable and, therefore, is a source of apparent discontinuity in the behavioral changes of the infant during the course of development.

Sander (21,22) has for some time conceptualized the mother-infant relationship as process. For example, he states: "The interplay of active tendencies in infant and mother in reaching a reciprocal quality of relationship forms the unifying thread around which interactional accounts will be organized. The reciprocal quality in interaction is an achievement which is marked by harmony. It represents a fit or fitting together of active tendencies in each partner" (21, p. 233).

Similarly, Jaffe, Stern, and Peery (18) have focused on the flow and mutuality of the mother and infant behavior, although with a much more molecular approach. They describe gazing and verbalizing by mother and infant as "conversational" coupling of the pair and propose that there may be a universal property of dyadic communication that can be identified by the study of mutuality in behaviors. Theirs is a model of interpersonal constraint applied to the gross temporal patterning of mutual behavior.

Along with new views of interaction, a number of creative approaches and methodologies are currently being used. Brazelton's eloquent descriptions of the flow of mother and infant interaction focus on the waxing and waning in intensity of mutually attentive behavior (23,24). Tronick and Brazelton (24) have developed a procedure for molecular analyses of mother and infant behavior from film, quantitatively depicting the matching, or mismatching, of behavior patterns.

And again, Stern (6,17) has used film to depict the mutuality of the mother-infant system, obtaining a very fine-grained analysis of instant-by-instant events in play interaction. In the analysis of his data, he has used transitional matrices to show patterns of probabilities for sequences of dyadic states, described as mother attending to baby; baby attending to mother; both attending; neither attending. Individual mother-infant pairs have very different patterns of such sequences. Lewis and Lee-Painter (25) have also used sequential analyses of mother-infant data obtained from film, and they eloquently emphasize the limitations of our current models, which cannot yet adequately depict the non-static flow of interaction apart from its elements.

General Systems Theory as Applicable to the Mother-Infant Relating Process

Each of the researchers referred to thus far has used the term "system" in describing the mother-infant relationship, and although the term has been applied very loosely, it points to a new conceptual framework for this area of study. Sander, Thoman, and Denenberg have each independently proposed general systems theory as a way of taking systems notions seriously (7,21,26,17). General systems theory, as presented by Bertalanffy (28,29) and Weiss (30,31), provides a perspective derived from biology that may ultimately enable us to understand and analyze the complexities of the interactive process.

In 1933 Bertalanffy (28) proposed that any theory of development and life in general must be a systems theory, applicable to social relationships as well as other levels of biological organization. Systems notions have since been applied at a range of levels, from aggregates of inanimate particles to aggregates of living organisms. Although there are many approaches to systems theory, we can consider briefly some general characteristics of systems and how they may provide a framework for early interaction.

As summarized by Fowler, ". . . a system is a whole or a unit composed of hierarchically organized and functionally highly interdependent subunits that may themselves be systems" (32, p. 26). Within a system, the component units, by "systematic" coordination, preserve an integral configuration after nondestructive disturbances (31). An important characteristic of a system is that the variability of the whole is less than the sum of the variability of the component parts. Thus, more generally, a system is an organization whose overall state is stable relative to the states of its components (32). This stability, in turn, provides constraints within which the subunits function. As with any system, the overall organization has characteristics that are not apparent in the behavior of any of the components.

A primary implication of the application of systems theory is that one can no longer focus on single main effects, or direct causal factors, but must be concerned with the interplay of numerous interacting factors. Nonlinear relations are of the essence, and nonstatic models are required. As Ashby says, "Today science is developing along the lines not included in the 'classic' form. The classic method . . . dealt essentially with parts alone: the difficulties of 'interaction' were evaded. . . . 'Modern' science however is characterized by an uninhibited advance into the nonlinear. It not merely studies systems with high internal interaction but also confidently tackles systems in which it is the interactions themselves that are of interest" (33, p. 80).

The relevance of systems notions for the study of the infant's early development and the development of the mother-infant relationship may be apparent, but it has not until very recently been considered seriously by developmental researchers. Sander has been the one long-time proponent of this view. To quote him once again:

> The study of the infant and caregiving environment from the systems perspective . . . opens the way for the application of *methods* to early developmental research which . . . allow the examination of 'process' and of change in the system. This is a different domain of investigation than that based on traditional correlative methods and on the concept of a linear causality in development, wherein one searches for an effect of a variable measured at point A in time on a second, or outcome, variable measured at point B in time. The difference between the two approaches lies in the acknowledgment of and appreciation of 'organization' in the biological system and of the great complexity of variables which represent the interface of exchange between the living, actively adapting elements making up the system. The infant and caregiver are already highly organized; each, as organisms with a degree of relative autonomy, are already actively 'running' so to speak; each is actively self-regulating; and each is capable of a degree of modification as a result of encounter with the other. . . . 'Organization' here means that the infant-caregiving system moves towards some optimal solution to the configuration of relationships between interfaced functions commensurate with the particular characteristics of interacting constitutents making up the system (7).

As Sander points out, systems notions may be of particular importance where there are disturbances, or disruptions, in the ongoing self-righting tendencies that may enable the systems components to maintain an equilibrium despite perturbation.

IMPLICATIONS OF GENERAL SYSTEMS THEORY

The application of general systems theory to early development has implications not only for methods used in research but also for problems of assessment and for issues with respect to intervention.

Development of Interaction Viewed as a Process

The interactive system of a mother and baby can be depicted and understood only as it develops over time. This point is made most clearly by reference to the problems of early assessment. It has generally been found that prediction of mental and motor performance is most reliable for babies with scores at the very low end of the continuum (34), and, in fact, it is the extreme values that are most responsible for the predictive relationships reported in some studies. In extreme cases, of course, the biological damage to an infant from prenatal, perinatal, or early postnatal events is sufficiently evident that assessment for screening purposes is practically superfluous. The major challenge for assessment is posed by the infant without apparent anomaly who has nevertheless been exposed to stressful circumstances such as anoxia or prolonged labor in isolation or in combination with prematurity. As Parmelee, Kopp, and Sigman (35) point out, some of these infants may develop normally, whereas others may have developmental difficulties at a later age.

It is known that the obstacles to prediction of developmental dysfunction derive from several sources of variation: (1) Some infants may have been subject to an early insult with only transient consequences; such infants may appear deficient during the newborn period but recover sufficiently for their development to proceed uneventfully. (2) Some pregnancy and perinatal problems may cause central nervous damage that is not apparent during the neonatal period, the consequences becoming more serious as the behavioral repertoire becomes more complex (35). (3) It is now generally recognized that prediction is complicated by the influences of the infant's transactions with the environment between the time of the first testing and later assessment. It should be noted that there is abundant evidence in the animal literature to indicate that the effects of an early trauma, including stress and malnutrition, may be ameliorated or abolished as a consequence of subsequent environmental interactions (36).

Thus, longitudinal study of infants is a requisite for understanding the early developmental processes as they occur within the infant's environmental transactions and as they are influenced by these transactions. Longitudinal study is not only important for an understanding of developmental mechanisms but is also a means of assessing the developmental course for individual infants and mother-infant pairs. It is in the study of the mother-infant relationship that the interests of basic researchers and clinicians intersect. The need is for an understanding of the infant's progress in adaptation, which includes the development of synchrony with the mother's temporal rhythms and her interactive behavior. This interweaving of mutuality constitutes a process of its own, a process that can only be studied or assessed longitudinally, with observations sufficiently close together to capture the special qualities of the process.

Clinicians have generally been most keenly aware of the importance of the cumulative interactive effects of experience. Emde, Gainsbauer, and Harmon (37) explain that, although it is sometimes possible during therapy to thread out important events in the life history of a person retrospectively, it is not possible to predict from a multiplicity of factors which ones will be relevant at some future time. As Denenberg has pointed out in recent theoretical papers (27,38), it is precisely these interactive effects which are the essence of the developmental process; yet the major preoccupation of experimental researchers at both the animal and human level is to exclude these complexities from study. Unfortunately, for developmental scientists, the interacting events are not always the same for every subject, nor are they always identifiable. Thus, the development of each individual baby has its own unique course.

A New Emphasis on the Study of the Individual

Over the years of vigorous experimental laboratory research, the idea of studying an individual has fallen into disrepute. This is the case despite the remarkable success of Skinner's studies of learning in individual pigeons and despite the comprehensive theory of development derived from Piaget's observations of three individual children. In an experimental study, individual variation is a source of error, highly objectionable because group differences may not be significant as a result of within-group variability. Likewise, predictions from correlations are based on group means. Thus, although strategies for dealing with group data are appropriate for identifying highly potent factors affecting development, they give minimal information on the individual within the group and no information on developmental processes, which can only occur within the individual system.

Study of the individual has most often been associated with case studies or baby biographies that were not truly observational. Dismissal of this mode of study has been hastened by a rejection of the enormous numbers of abstractions that were made without any rigorously obtained empirical data base. It can reasonably be asked whether it is possible to study the interaction of individual mothers and infants without a return to the old "case study" approach. The answer is clearly affirmative. First of all, new methodologies permit the collection of empirical data by recording behavior with minimal interpretive loading. Second, process analyses based on such data are very different from the judgmental or qualitative interpretations that were the basic research strategy used in the historical case studies. And, finally, computer technology makes it possible to deal with large quantities of empirically obtained bits of data.

The major point of concern here is that development is a process, and process can only occur within an individual unit. In the mother-infant relationship, the process is the ongoing interaction. New statistical approaches and methods are being designed for analyzing data on individual subjects, or dyads, as the basis for investigating developmental processes. These approaches promise new and more realistic directions in the study of early development.

A major issue for single-subject study is the generalizability of the results. This is a serious issue that must be confronted. It is certainly not possible to generalize from a single subject to the effects of demographic characteristics such as sex, socioeconomic level, and race. However, generalization may be possible with respect to the individual baby or the individual mother-infant pair, and, ultimately, the objective of developmental research is to have a sufficient understanding to predict for the individual baby or mother-baby pair. Thus, once again the practical and the theoretical objectives intersect.

With respect to further uses of data from individuals, the promises are important. Although the patterns exhibited in each mother-infant pair may differ, as Einstein describes in *The Meanderings of Rivers* (39), it is assumed that different patterns of behavior reflect some common processes or functions. After examining patterns in individuals singly, it is possible to group pairs that have commonality in their interactive qualities. There is no reason to assume that a single, or even a limited number, of interactive processes must be applicable to all developing mother-infant relationships. The variability in patterns of relationships is a source of richness in life. As researchers, our responsibility is to account for variability, rather than to force behaving humans into look-alike prototypes.

A noncausal view of the mother-infant relationship is a very important aspect of the general systems view. McKearney (40) pointed out that, "Human behavior is complexly and multiply determined, and if we chose to ignore this, it is at our own peril both as scientists and individuals" (p. 118). Behavioral processes occur over time, and causation must inevitably be cumulative or historical. Thus, everything that happens is a function of all that has previously occurred within the system. McKearney argues that biological phenomena may not have simple and direct "causes" in the same sense that gravity causes objects to fall, or a rock causes glass to shatter, and proposes as more appropriate the concept of "equifinality," which means that the same thing can be arrived at in many different ways.

McKearney emphasizes that medical research must recognize the complexity of interactive relationships, pointing out as an example that the effects of any particular drug are dependent on a variety of situational details. His examples come from the administration of drugs to children and adults. There are similar examples in the study of early infancy. Attempts have been made to relate specific events in the prenatal or perinatal period to later development, events such as prematurity per se, relatively mild anoxia, and length of labor. The results of such studies have generally been mixed, and therefore their effects have not been firmly established. One aspect of this problem is the difficulty in empirically establishing a measurable level for the independent variable. For example, in the case of medication during labor and delivery, the specific drug used for medication, the quantity administered, mode of administration, time of administration with respect to delivery, and combination of drugs administered are all factors that may interact to produce a potency of effect (41). Thus, drug dosage per se cannot meaningfully be considered a cause of any specific behavioral effect. Furthermore, the consequence to the neonate may vary as a function of the subsequent interactive system.

AN APPLICATION OF GENERAL SYSTEMS THEORY TO THE STUDY OF MOTHER-INFANT INTERACTION

The Mother-Infant Relationship as a Communication System

A reasonable assumption about the earliest mother-infant interaction is that all modalities are involved in a communication system from the time of birth. Obviously, communication with a newborn baby is not linguistic. Furthermore, we have maintained (42) that linguistic models are not applicable for understanding this early communication.

Because of a great interest in the emergence of language, it has been very natural for researchers to impose on the earliest mother-infant interaction models that have been derived for linguistic development, presuming that the very early period constitutes a precursor for language and therefore the same rules hold. But there are subtle and complex characteristics of the early nonverbal communication that have no analogy in later verbal exchanges. Two primary differentiating characteristics separate verbal from nonverbal communication. The first is the totality of mutual involvement, which has no analogy in linguistic exchange. For example, if the mother picks the baby up and holds it close to her, she may feel the infant's soft skin against her cheek, the baby's motor movements, and its clinging to her body. She may be aware of the infant's skin odor or attend to the infant's visual gaze, grimacing, and various limb or body movements. At the same time, she may move the infant about in space, as she talks, touches, smiles, and makes other facial movements. On the infant's part, there may be the sensation of being moved about in space, the visual image of the mother's mobile face, auditory stimulation from the mother's vocalization; the infant may receive tactile, kinesthetic, and proprioceptive stimulation from her movements; and the infant may smell the mother and feel her body warmth. All sensory modalities and response systems are involved as mother and infant communicate with each other with their entire bodies.

In the study of very complex communication, the simultaneity of behavior defies sequential analysis, although many of us have tried this approach. The simultaneity of behavior has no parallel in linguistic exchange. In fact, if two partners attempt to speak simultaneously, communication "breaks down," and the interaction becomes disorganized. Thus, a more complex model than that of simple turn taking is necessary for depicting the early nonverbal communication.

There is another unique aspect of this early nonverbal communication, namely, the pervasiveness of affect. Clearly, "information" in the traditional sense is not being transmitted between mother and infant, whether communication takes the form of vocalization, or gesture, or body movement. The early interaction certainly includes vocalization, but its characteristics are very different from later verbal patterns. Mothers talk to their babies, but without an expectation of their words being comprehended. In fact, some mothers even respond, with change of intonation, for their babies and thus carry on a "conversation" with themselves. At this stage, it is undoubtedly the intonation that is most relevant for affective communication. Eisenberg (13) speculates that the early programming of the infant's nervous system accounts for the discrimination of those auditory stimuli which are most "pleasant" and "unpleasant" to the neonate. Thus, the affective nature of the interaction is an inherent quality that expresses itself in the flow of behaviors and is very closely integrated and expressed with great subtlety. A variety of research techniques may be needed to thread out the related patterns and their changes over age. A number of investigators have been engaged in fruitful research in this area (43–45).

The Problem of Recording Interaction Behavior

The systems approach will be illustrated with data from our laboratory describing the mother-infant relationship during the first 5 postnatal weeks. Mothers and infants are observed in their natural habitats, first in the hospital and subsequently in the home, under circumstances that are as natural as possible. Our purpose is to describe the process of mutual adaptation during this period.

Rather than focus on a single mode of communication, such as gestural, vocal, or visual, we have chosen to record as many behaviors as possible in all modalities. Over the past 2 years, we have developed a coding scheme that is very much like a shorthand notation, and it is possible for a trained observer to record the occurrence of any of 75 kinds of behavior exhibited by the mother or infant, making such notations continuously for each successive 10-sec epoch throughout an observation. The code system itself is like a language, with nouns, action words, and modifiers. Some simple examples used in the coding of infants' state will illustrate the simplicity of the types of codes used:

   o The baby is in the waking active state (the eyes are open but not alert).
   ℰ The baby is alert, but the body is relatively quiet.
   ℰ The baby is alert and engaged in gross motor movements.

The significance of this coding system is that it is designed to solve the methodological problem of codifying and notating behavior as it occurs simultaneously and sequentially. Such a methodological solution was called for 10 years ago by Gajdusek at the XIIth International Congress of Pediatrics (46), when he said, "I wish to develop the theme of a critical problem of methodology (the annotation of behavior) which must be solved if we are ever to leave the confines of long-winded and crude verbal discussion of what the environment 'does' to a child, and become more specific and penetrating in our observation and analysis." He expresses his view even more dramatically: "If pediatric research gives us a new notation and representation for 'those first affections' of perception, it will have contributed to more than the remedy of the ailments of man, but, as the arts, to the joys and meaning of his existence!'' (p. 14). Our claims to solutions would not be so sweeping; however, our claims for the importance of having a reliable description of much of the behavior that occurs in the course of a mother-infant day permit the exploration of patterning across modalities and across partners within the system.

Very generally, the kinds of behavior we record in the home are designed to give information on the infant's behavioral states throughout any observation; the infant's sleep states, state-related behavior, and respiration during periods of time in the crib; maternal behavior that describes her location with respect to the infant, the position in which she holds or places the infant; and stimulation given to the infant, including tactile, movement, vocal, gestural, and visual attention; and the nature of her activities during periods of caretaking interaction, including feeding, changing, and bathing the baby.

It should be noted that all behavior recorded is regarded as characteristics of the mother-infant system, even though it is necessary to record some as mother behavior and some as infant behavior. The activities of each member of the dyad are considered a function of the total interactive system. Even when the infant is asleep, as indicated above, there may be an exchange between the partners. And characteristics of the sleep states may reflect the immediately previous interaction during the infant's wake period, as well as the ongoing rhythmicity attained in the relationship.

Golani (47) has provided very dramatic evidence of the importance of relating multiple behavior in the identification of patterns. He has examined in great detail the motor movement patterns in a variety of species and has found that measures of behavior may not reveal regularity, whereas the patterning of combinations of movements may reveal regularities of behavior that are characteristic of an organism, animal or human. He has referred to this patterning as the "orchestration" of behavior. Golani provides a working model for the search for the infant's adaptive behavior and the orchestration of the adaptive behavior of mother and infant. A major objective of this search is to identify that behavior which constitutes units that may show regularities in patterning and thus provide information on the interactive process.

One major premise for our research is that we can identify individual patterns of infant and mother behavior. A second premise is that these patterns will either persist over time or serve as the basis for later patterns of behavior in the infant or the mother-infant relationship.

Patterning of Interaction for a Group of Normal Babies and Three with Developmental Delay at 1 Year

The data for mother-infant interaction during the first 5 weeks was examined for three babies who were found to be developmentally slow at 1 year—Mental Development level 80, using the Bayley Scales of Infant Development (48). All three were initally in our normal group (49). The three special subjects showed similar patterns of interaction during the first 5 weeks: there was overall less interaction of a purely social nature, that is, when the infants were awake and the mothers were not engaged in caretaking activities; and, during social interaction, there was much less visual attention to the infants and less stimulation, including patting, rocking, caressing, and moving the infants. Figure 1 presents the comparisons between the three pairs and the total group, summed over the first 5 weeks. It should be noted that the special infants did not differ from the entire group in the amount of wakefulness or fussing and crying during these weeks.

In interpreting these data, we do not attribute the distinctive qualities of the three individual pairs primarily to differences in the mother's behavior. Consistent with the systems approach, the behavior patterning is viewed as an expression of the ongoing adjustment that each member of the dyad is making to the other. These patterns are therefore truly mutual, and the developmental outcome for the infant is considered a consequence of the earlier developing system.

The three mother-infant pairs had similarities in their patterns of interaction, but there were also differences—they were not necessarily three of a kind. Detailed analyses of the individuality in the interaction of these three pairs reveals other basic aspects of their relationships that may be differentially implicated in the developmental dysfunction observed at 1 year. These results must also be interpreted cautiously with respect to their implications for the infants' later development, which may possibly be within the normal range. However, at 1 year, the babies were not functioning at the same level as other babies of similar age.

Patterning of Sleep-Wake States for a Group of Normal Infants and an Infant with CNS Dysfunction

Figure 2a presents the distribution of waking and sleep states for 20 infants from observations on weeks 2, 3, 4, and 5. These distributions are based on the percentage of

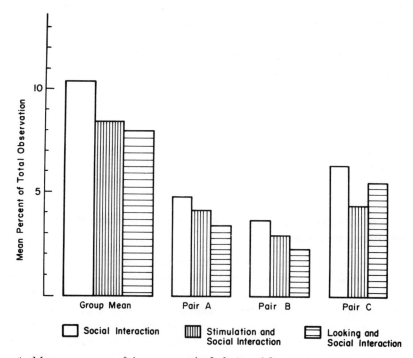

Figure 1. Mean percentage of time over weeks 2, 3, 4, and 5 spent in social interaction, stimulation with social interaction, and looking with social interaction: group mean (20 infants) and mother-infant pairs A, B, and C.

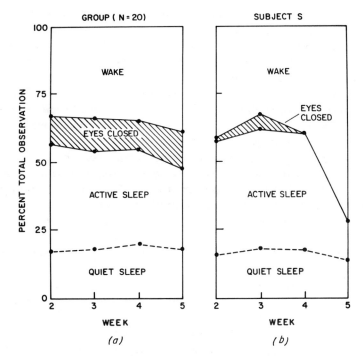

Figure 2. Distribution of states during 7-hr observation at 2, 3, 4, and 5 weeks of age. (*a*) Mean values for group of normal infants; (*b*) individual values for subject S.

the total 7-hr observation for each week. The "eyes closed" category occurs when the mother is holding the baby, the eyes are closed, and it is not possible to judge accurately whether the baby is actually asleep, or, if asleep, what state of sleep the baby is in. Such periods occur most frequently during feedings.

The data in Figure 2*a* represent mean values for the group of 20 babies on each week. However, these variables reliably describe individual babies within the group, as indicated by assessment for individual differences using a repeated measures analysis of variance. It is also possible to establish confidence limits for any measure in order to assess whether a single subject deviates from the mean for the group more than would be expected by chance (49). Thus, the profile for the normal group of infants provides a base line for evaluating individual variations. As with the mother-infant comparisons above, it is also possible to use the baseline group to identify aberrant patterns that may suggest the possibility of risk status. An example of this strategy for identifying possible risk patterns is described.

One baby proved to be of special interest because of a developmental problem that was not at all apparent during the early months of life—to the parents, to those of us making home observations, or to the pediatrician in charge of the infant. We had described this baby in clinical notes following observations as "bright-eyed and alert much of the time." It was therefore a surprise when at 7 months the baby appeared to be somewhat slow developmentally, had begun to experience seizures, and was soon thereafter diagnosed as having infantile seizures with a hypsarrhythmia of the EEG. At 1 year of age, the child is markedly delayed, and the prognosis is uncertain.

Because of the dramatic change in the developmental picture of this baby—the infantile seizure syndrome typically is not diagnosed until around 6 months of age—it was of great interest to explore the early data retrospectively to determine whether there were any possible clues to the later course of events. And in fact there were. They were primarily apparent in the state organization and respiratory characteristics of the infant.

Figure 2b presents the distributions of states over the 5 weeks for this subject, S. It can be seen that the overall organization of states is quite different from that for the total group. The differences become most marked on the fifth week of age, with the amount of wakefulness being dramatically increased; likewise, the level of "eyes closed" is very low during the first 2 weeks and virtually disappears during weeks 4 and 5. No infant in the normal group approximated this pattern.

In order to depict what was going on during wakefulness, Figure 3a presents the percentage of wakefulness spent in alert, fussing or crying, waking active, and drowse for the total group; and Figure 3b presents the data for subject S. Throughout the 5 weeks of observations, subject S was significantly more alert during wakefulness than the mean of the total group of babies. The other waking states were proportionately reduced.

Another way of describing the baby's alertness is to look at the total amount of time spent alert as a percentage of the 7-hr period. These data are presented in Figure 4, where it can be seen that the absolute portion of time spent alert by baby S is also consistently deviant from the group. It must be said that if we had had these data analyses available soon after making the observations of baby S, we certainly might have wondered, but we would not have necessarily worried about this infant.

More worrisome data appeared with respect to the baby's respiratory characteristics. These data are presented elsewhere (49). In summary, the baby showed extraordinarily

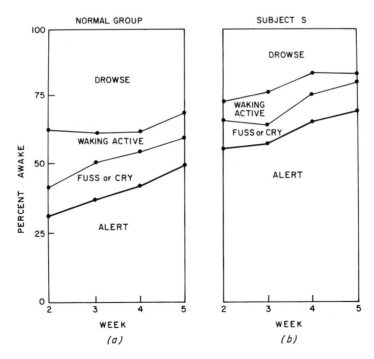

Figure 3. Distribution of wake states during 7-hr observation at 2, 3, 4, and 5 weeks of age. (a) Mean values for total group of normal infants; (b) individual values for subject S.

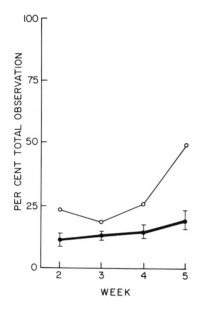

Figure 4. Percentage of total observation spent in alert state at 2, 3, 4, and 5 weeks of age: mean for total group of normal infants and individual values for subject S (normal infants O—O, subject S ●—●).

high levels of brief apneic pauses during the first 2 weeks and equally deviant low levels on the last weeks, and respiration rates were generally high and variable.

A Strategy for Identifying Risk Status from Developing Patterns

The approach described involved intensive study of a single subject. However, it is assumed that any one infant is not totally unique and that other infants with developmental dysfunction will show similarities in patterns, even though with individual variations. Thus, the findings are a source of working hypotheses for predicting risk status. The strategy for this longitudinal research project is to continue to add full-term normal subjects to the base-line group in order to expand and maintain an ongoing data bank of normative measures on mother-infant interaction, behavioral state, and respiration. Any infant with a known risk condition during the prenatal, perinatal, or postnatal period is not included in this base-line group but can be observed for comparison with the normal group as we have done with the subject just described. In this way, it should be possible to specify behavior patterns that indicate deviancy from the total group. It is equally important to be able to determine that an infant does not differ.

The patterning of deviancy for any subject may be in terms of a specific constellation of behavior that is extremely different from normal; developmental changes over successive observations that differ; or some combination of these two expressions of deviancy.

The findings from comparing this subject with the total group clearly do not assure us that the deviancies we observed during the early weeks are necessary antecedents to the developmental difficulties observed later for this one infant. Their significance lies in the fact that the patterning of deviancy, derived from a large number of measures taken from a wide variety of behavior and over successive observations, provides us with hypotheses for future study. For example, an interesting aspect of baby S's state organization was the very high level of wakefulness and especially of alertness. The generally held view of alertness is "the more the better" because of the great importance of this state for attentiveness to the environment and especially social interaction. The increased wakefulness of baby S over weeks was not accompanied by an increase in crying; he therefore gave the appearance of being an alert and contented baby. In retrospect, it now appears possible that the infant's waking characteristics, as well as the distribution of sleep states, reflected an ongoing endogenous stress. Papousek and Papousek (51) have described a waking-state response to temporary environmental stress conditions; they and other investigators have described sleep changes consequent to stressful interventions (52–57). Evidence of the susceptibility of state to various exogenous stressors leads to the speculation that some forms of neurological damage, including that seen in baby S, may be associated with state changes of an analogous sort. In fact, Monod and Guidasci (58) report that infants with early and obvious neurological damage show increased wakefulness. This is an important question, but a difficult one to investigate at the human level because only correlational data are available. An initial approach can be made at the animal level, however. The state categories used for human infants have been adapted for observation of behavioral states in the rabbit (59–62), so that the effects on state development of stressing conditions for the young can be investigated using an animal model (63).

Another example of the use of data from a single subject is provided by a recent report (64) of the state, respiration, and apnea patterns of a baby who subsequently died of sudden infant death syndrome (SIDS) at 3 months of age. From these patterns, derived post hoc, we are able to identify another infant with very similar characteristics as one who might also be susceptible to SIDS. The second baby was placed on an apnea monitor at 3 weeks of age and did have prolonged apneic episodes over a period of 2 months from 5 to 7 months of age. The data from the subject who died provided a hypothetical risk syndrome consisting of extremely low levels of apnea and high and variable respiration rates during the early weeks of life. Previous studies of early brief apnea and later prolonged apnea, with relevance to SIDS, have been based on correlational analyses of groups of babies that have suggested that very high levels of apnea are the primary predictors of subsequent prolonged apneic episodes. The results from only a single subject were sufficient to suggest that both ends of the continuum may be relevant for identifying risk status in this respect. Furthermore, the data from the single subject also suggested that respiratory rates as well as apnea are implicated in the identification of respiratory instability. These data have found support from a study of siblings of SIDS infants (65), who were found to have less apnea and higher respiratory rates than the siblings of a control group of infants.

The Liaison Between Developmental Study and Assessment for Developmental Status

It is clear that the complexities of development require multiple criteria obtained from successive observations. But even more important, these complexities mean that it is not enough to discriminate simply between normal and nonnormal groups of infants. A very simple example can be given from screening for hearing loss. Because of an almost exclusive interest in identifying those babies with auditory deficiencies, the concern for individual differences in auditory thresholds has received virtually no attention. Individual differences among infants in this and other sensory modalities, however, can have a major impact on the infant's subsequent development (66). Variations in the infant's sensitivities may interact with initial status as well as subsequent events to account for the cross-over between the normal and nonnormal categories, as depicted in Figure 5.

The search for refined assessment measures is most appropriate for the ultimate objective of relating changes in patterns of reliable measures at an early age to patterns of reliable measures at a later age. A major reason that the pattern approach is essential is that central nervous deficits may not always be expressed by the same syndrome of deficiencies. Again, the issue is individuality among infants. The reasonableness of this statement is apparent if one realizes the reductionistic implications of assuming a one-to-one relationship between any specific form of neural damage and its behavioral expression.

In the conventional medical model for disease entities, a specific neural deficiency would be expected to have a specific behavioral concomitant. However, awareness of the individual expression of disease is suggested in a very recent book entitled *Toward a Man-Centered Medical Science* (67), based on a conference that brought together ". . . scientists who are interested in a science of man for man—a science which, instead of excluding man as conventional science does, develops his unique and special position in all fields" (67, p. i). As expressed by Dubow (68) ". . . the components of a human body machine naturally react to external stimuli in much the same way as do similar components in any other living system. But the human organism as a whole responds to all challenges, real or imagined, in a more personal manner than is suggested by the purely biological view of organism-environment relationship. Furthermore, the response is usually more inventive than could be expected from the usual processes of biological determinism" (p. ix). Thus, the behavioral manifestations of any given disease syndrome represent an interaction among the disease process, the individual, and the envi-

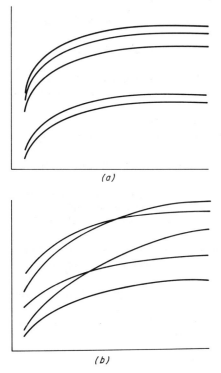

(a)

(b)

Figure 5. Developmental curves for two groups of infants. (*a*) Idealized curves for two normal infants (lower group) and three abnormal infants (upper group); (*b*) curves showing crossover from normal to abnormal status.

ronmental context. It is the "inventive nature" of the human infant's responses to stressful conditions, either endogenous or exogenous, that accounts for the variations in patterning of individual behavior. Both individual patterns and commonalities within groups must be studied to understand normal and deviant developmental processes.

All the principles that apply to the study of development apply equally to the problems of developmental assessment. Any understanding of the factors that influence the development of the infant requires a conceptual scheme that accounts for the ongoing process of mutual modification of mother and infant. Thus, process assessment, rather than specific behavioral assessment at any point in time, is needed to understand the factors that are influencing the developmental course of any individual infant. Developmentally relevant research will ultimately provide the basis for decisions as to the age at which any group of measures may be meaningful, as well as the ages over which such measurements must be taken.

There is a growing awareness of the need for intervention at earlier and earlier ages. Such intervention cannot be devised to meet the "average" problem; it has to be designed for the individual infant. Research is beginning to provide information that has greater relevance for the development of individuals in their environment, information that will make effective intervention possible. An ongoing exchange between clinicians and researchers offers the opportunity for developmental study that is humanistic because it is realistic.

REFERENCES

1. Gunther, M.: Infant behaviour at the breast, in B. M. Foss (ed.): *Determinants of Infant Behaviour.* London, Methuen and Company, Ltd., 1961.

2. Stone, L. J., Smith, H. T., and Murphy, L. B. (eds.): *The Competent Infant: Research and Commentary.* New York, Basic Books, 1973.

3. Eisenberg, R. B.: *Auditory Competence in Early Life.* Baltimore, University Park Press, 1976.

4. Eimas, P. D.: On the processing of speech: Some implications for language development, in C. L. Ludlow and M. E. Doran-Quine (eds.): *The Neurological Bases of Language Disorders in Children: Methods and Directions for Research.* NINCDS Monograph, Washington, D.C., Government Printing Office, in press.

5. Bower, T. G. R., and Wishart, J. G.: Towards a unitary theory of development, in E. B. Thoman and S. Trotter (eds.): *Origins of the Infant's Social Responsiveness.* Hillsdale, N.J., Lawrence Erlbaum Associates, Inc., 1978.

6. Stern, D. N.: A micro-analysis of mother-infant interaction. *J. Am. Acad. Child Psychiatry* 10:501–517, 1971.

7. Sander, L. W., Stechler, G., Burns, P., and Lee, A.: Changes in infant and caregiver variables over the first two months of life: Regulation and adaptation in the organization of the infant-caregiver system, in E. B. Thoman and S. Trotter (eds.): *Origins of the Infant's Social Responsiveness.* Hillsdale, N.J., Lawrence Erlbaum Associates, Inc., 1978.

8. Watson, J. S.: Perception of contingency as a determinant of social responsiveness, in E. B. Thoman and S. Trotter (eds.): *Origins of the Infant's Social Responsiveness.* Hillsdale, N.J., Lawrence Erlbaum Associates, Inc., 1978.

9. Blurton-Jones, W. (ed.): *Ethological Studies of Child Behavior.* Great Britain, Cambridge University Press, 1974.

10. Wolff, P. H.: The causes, controls, and organization of behavior in the neonate, *Psychological Issues,* 5(1), Monogr. 17. New York, International University Press, 1966.

11. Cairns, G. F., and Butterfield, E. C.: Assessing infants' auditory function, in B. F. Brieflander, G. M. Sterritt, and G. Kirk (eds.): *The Exceptional Infant, Vol. 3, Assessment and Intervention.* New York, Brunner-Mazel, 1975.

12. Lipsitt, L. P.: The pleasures and annoyances of infants: Approach and avoidance behavior of babies, in E. B. Thoman and S. Trotter (eds.): *Origins of the Infant's Social Responsiveness.* Hillsdale, N.J., Lawrence Erlbaum Associates, Inc., 1978.

13. Eisenberg, R. B.: Stimulus significance as a determinant of infant responses to sound, in E. B. Thoman and S. Trotter (eds.): *Origins of the Infant's Social Responsiveness.* Hillsdale, N.J., Lawrence Erlbaum Associates, Inc., 1978.

14. Papousek, N., and Papousek, M.: The infant's fundamental adaptive response system in social interaction, in E. B. Thoman and S. Trotter (eds.): *Origins of the Infant's Social Responsiveness.* Hillsdale, N.J., Lawrence Erlbaum Associates, Inc., 1978.

15. Condon, W. S., and Sander, L. W.: Neonate movement is synchronized with adult speech: Interactional participation and language acquisition. *Science* 3:99–101, 1974.

16. Stern, D. N.: *The First Relationship: Mother and Infant.* Cambridge, Harvard University Press, 1977.

17. Stern, D. N.: The goal and structure of mother-infant play. *J. Am. Acad. Child Psychiatry* 13:402–421, 1974.

18. Jaffe, J., Stern, D. N., and Peery, J. C.: Conversational coupling of gaze behavior in prelinguistic human development. *J. Psycholinguistic Res.* 2:321–329, 1973.

19. Bower, T. G. R.: Stimulus variables determining space perception in infants. *Science* 149:88–89, 1965.

20. Sameroff, A. J., and Chandler, M. J.: Reproductive risk and the continuum of caretaking casualty, in F. D. Horowitz, M. Hetherington, S. Scarr-Salapatek, and G. Siegel (eds.): *Review of Child Development,* Vol. 4. Chicago, University of Chicago Press, 1974, pp. 187–244.

21. Sander, L. W.: Adaptive relationships in early mother-child interaction. *J. Am. Acad. Child Psychiatry* 3:231–264, 1964.

22. Sander, L. W., Stechler, C., Burns, P., and Julia, H.: Early mother-infant interaction and 24-hour patterns of activity and sleep. *J. Am. Acad. Child Psychiatry* 9:103–123, 1970.

23. Brazelton, T. B., Koslowski, B., and Main, M.: The origins of reciprocity, in M. Lewis and L. A. Rosenblum (eds.): *The Effect of the Infant on Its Caregiver.* New York, John Wiley & Sons, 1974.

24. Tronick, E., Als, H. and Brazelton, T. B.: Monadic Phases: A structural descriptive analysis of infant-mother face to face interaction. *Child Dev.* 1978, in press.

25. Lewis, M., and Lee-Painter, S.: An interactional approach to the mother-infant dyad, in M. Leis and L. A. Rosenblum (eds.): *The Effect of the Infant on Its Caregiver.* New York, John Wiley & Sons, 1974.

26. Thoman, E. B., Acebo, C., Dreyer, C. A., Becker, P. T., and Freese, M. P.: Individuality in the interactive process, in E. B. Thoman and S. Trotter (eds.): *Origins of the Infant's Social Responsiveness.* Hillsdale, N.J., Lawrence Erlbaum Associates, Inc., 1978.

27. Denenberg, V. H.: Paradigms and paradoxes in the study of behavioral development, in E. B. Thoman and S. Trotter (eds.): *The Origins of the Infant's Social Responsiveness.* Hillsdale, N.J., Lawrence Erlbaum Associates, Inc., 1978.

28. Bertalanffy, L. von: *Modern Theories of Development: An Introduction to Theoretical Biology,* translated and adapted by J. H. Woodger. London, Oxford University Press, 1933.

29. Bertalanffy, L. von: *General System Theory,* rev. ed. New York, Braziller, 1968.

30. Weiss, P.: The living system: Determinism stratified, in A. Koestler and J. R. Smythies (eds.): *Beyond Reductionism.* Boston, Beacon Press, 1969.

31. Weiss, P.: The basic concept of hierarchical systems, in P. Weiss (ed.): *Hierarchically Organized Systems in Theory and Practice.* New York, Hafne, 1971.

32. Fowler, C. A.: A systems approach to the cerebral hemispheres. *Status Report on Speech Research.* Haskins Laboratories, 1975.

33. Ashby, W. R.: Systems and their information measures, in G. J. Klir (ed.): *Trends in General Systems Theory.* New York, Wiley-Interscience, 1972.

34. Honzik, M. P.: Value and limitations of infant tests: An overview, in M. Lewis (ed.): *Origins of Intelligence: Infancy and Early Childhood.* New York, Plenum Press, 1976.

35. Parmelee, A. H., Kopp, C. B., and Sigman, M.: Selection of developmental assessment techniques for infants at risk. *Merrill-Palmer Quarterly* 22:177–199, 1976.

36. Levitsky, D. A., and Barnes, R. H.: Nutritional and environmental interactions in the behavioral development of the rat: Long-term effects. *Science* 176:68, 1972.

37. Emde, R. N., Gainsbauer, T. G., and Harmon, R. J.: Emotional expression in infancy: A biobehavioral study, *Psychol. Issues,* 1976, 10(1), Monograph 37. New York, International University Press.

38. Denenberg, V. H.: Interactional effects in early experience research, in A. Oliverio (ed.): *Genetics, Environment and Intelligence.* Amsterdam, Elsevier/North-Holland Biomedical Press, 1977.

39. Einstein, A.: Die ursache der mäanderbildung der flussläufe und des sogenannten baerschen gesetzes. *Naturwissenschaften* 14:223–224, 1926.

40. McKearney, J. W.: Asking questions about behavior. *Perspect. Biol. Med.* 21:109–119, 1977.

41. Kraemer, H. C., Korner, A. F., and Thoman, E. B.: Methodological considerations in evaluating the influence of drugs used during labor and delivery on the behavior of the newborn. *Dev. Psychol.* 6:128–134, 1972.

42. Thoman, E. B., and Freese, M. P.: A model for the study of early mother-infant communication, in R. W. Bell and W. P. Smotherman (eds.): *Maternal Influences and Early Behavior.* Jamaica, N.Y., Spectrum Publications, Inc., in press.

43. Brown, J., Bakeman, R., Snyder, P., Fredrickson, W. T., Morgan, S., and Helper, R.: Interactions of black inter-city mothers and their newborn infants. *Child Dev.* 46:677–686, 1975.

44. Dunn, J. B., and Richards, M. P. M.: Observations on the developing relationship between mother and baby in the neonatal period, in N. R. Schaffer (ed.): *Studies in Mother-Infant Interaction.* New York, Academic Press, 1977.

45. Beckwith, L., Cohen, S. E., Kopp, C. B., Parmelee, A. H., and Marcy, T. G.: Caregiver-infant interaction and early cognitive development in preterm infants. *Child Dev.* 47:579–587, 1976.

46. Gajdusek, D. C.: Environmental modification of human form and function: The problem of coding in the study of patterning in infancy of nervous system function: An approach to the study of learning. A discourse at the First Plenary Session on Growth and Development, XIIth International Congress of Pediatrics, Mexico, D.F., Dec. 1–7, 1968.

47. Golani, I.: Homeostatic motor processes in mammalian interactions: A choreography of display, in *Perspectives in Ethology,* Vol. 2., P. P. G. Bateson and P. H. Klopfer (eds.). New York, Plenum Press, 1976, pp. 69–134.

48. Bayley, N.: *Bayley Scales of Infant Development.* New York, Psychological Corporation, 1969.

49. Thoman, E. B., Becker, P. T., and Freese, M. P.: Individual patterns of mother-infant interaction, in G. P. Sackett (ed.): *Observing Behavior,* Vol. I, *Theory and Applications in Mental Retardation.* Baltimore, University Park Press, 1977.

50. Thoman, E. B., and Becker, P. T.: Issues in assessment and prediction for the infant born at risk, in Tiffany Field (ed.): *The High-Risk Newborn.* Jamaica, N.Y., Spectrum Publications, Inc., in press.

51. Papousek, H., and Papousek, M.: Cognitive aspects of preverbal social interaction between human infants and adults, in M. O'Connor (ed.): *Parent-Infant Interaction.* Amsterdam, Elsevier, 1975, pp. 63–85.

52. Brown, J. L.: States in newborn infants. *Merrill-Palmer Quarterly* 10:313–321, 1964.

53. Wolff, P. H.: The causes, controls and organization of behavior in the neonate. *Psychol. Issues* 5:1–105, 1966.

54. Emde, R. N., Harmon, R. F., Metcalf, D., Koening, K. L., and Wagonfeld, S.: Stress and neonatal sleep. *Psychosom. Med.* 33:491–497, 1971.

55. Anders, T., and Chalemian, R.: Effect of circumcision on sleep-wake states in human neonates. *Psychosom. Med.* 36:174–179, 1974.

56. Brackbill, Y.: Continuous stimulation reduces arousal level: Stability of the effect over time. *Child Dev.* 44:43–46, 1973.

57. Sostek, A. M., Anders, T. F., and Sostek, A. J.: Diurnal rhythms in 2- and 8-week-old infants: Sleep-waking state organization as a function of age and stress. *Psychosom. Med.* 38:250–256, 1976.

58. Monod, N., and Guidasci, S.: Sleep and brain malformation in the neonatal period. *Neuropädiatrie* 7:229–249, 1976.

59. Denenberg, V. H., DeSantis, D., Waite, S., and Thoman, E. B.: The effects of handling in infancy on behavioral states in the rabbit. *Physiol. Behav.* 18:553–557, 1977.

60. DeSantis, D., Waite, S., Thoman, E. B., and Denenberg, V. H.: Effects of isolation rearing upon behavioral state organization and growth in the rabbit. *Behav. Biol.* 21:273–285, 1977.

61. Waite, S. P., DeSantis, D., Thoman; E. B., and Denenberg, V. H.: The predictive validity of neonatal state variables in the rabbit. *Biol. Behav.* 2:249–261, 1977.

62. Thoman, E. B., Waite, S., DeSantis, D., and Denenberg, V. H.: Ontogeny of behavioral states in rabbits. *Anim. Behav.* 1978, in press.

63. Denenberg, V. H., and DeSantis, D.: An animal model for the small-for-gestational-age infant: Some behavioral and morphological findings, in N. R. Ellis (ed.): *Aberrant Development in Infancy: Human and Animal Studies.* Hillsdale, N.J., Lawrence Erlbaum Associates, Inc., 1975, pp. 77–88.

64. Thoman, E. B., Miano, V. N., and Freese, M. P.: The role of respiratory instability in the sudden infant death syndrome. *Dev. Med. Child Neurol.* 19:729–738, 1977.

65. Hoppenbrouwers, T. T., Hodgman, J. E., Harper, R. M., McGinty, D. J., and Sterman, M. B.: Respiratory rates and apnea in infants at high and low risk for sudden infant death syndrome (SIDS). *Clin. Res.* 25:189A, 1977.

66. Korner, A. F.: Some hypotheses regarding the significance of individual differences at birth for later development, in J. Hellmuth (ed.): *Exceptional Infant,* Vol. 1, *The Normal Infant.* New York, Brunner-Mazel, Inc., 1967, pp. 191–205.

67. Schaefer, K. E., Hensel, H., and Brady, R. (eds.): *Toward a Man-Centered Medical Science.* New York, Futura, 1977.

68. Dubos, R.: Foreword, in K. E. Schaefer, H. Hensel, and R. Brady (eds.): *Toward a Man-Centered Medical Science.* New York, Futura, 1977.

10
Fetal and Neonatal Immunology

Ricardo Bernales, M.D.
Joseph A. Bellanti, M.D.

The immunologic system consists of a wide variety of cells and cell products that interact in the recognition and disposal of foreign matter (1). Cells of the immunologic system of the fetus and the neonate, once thought to be inactive, manifest a striking capacity for response to the environment despite the fact that they are not fully developed. However, the fetus and newborn appear to be particularly vulnerable to injury that is either caused directly by immunologic mechanisms or inflicted by infectious agents that take advantage of the relative state of immaturity and inexperience of the immune system. These two concepts, which overlap at times, are clearly different. Immaturity refers to the genetically programmed low response or lack of response of the fetal and newborn immune system. Inexperience refers to the fact that the newborn immune system has not yet had its first encounter. The initial response of the naïve immune system is diminished, but, because it has full potential, its future responses intensify. Moreover, responsiveness occurs only at a given age when maturation has been achieved. The immune system of the human newborn is by far more inexperienced than immature; thus it is imperative for those concerned with perinatal medicine to have a fundamental grasp of the function of the immune system in this age period. This knowledge forms the basis for the diagnosis, treatment, and prevention of disease entities that afflict the fetus and the newborn.

GENERAL DEVELOPMENT OF THE IMMUNE SYSTEM

Role of the Environment

The development of the immune system may be visualized as a series of adaptive cellular responses to an ever-changing and potentially hostile environment. Development may be considered at several levels: the species, the individual, or the cell (1) (Table I).

From the evolutionary standpoint, we may make the assumption that existing species represent certain levels of progressive or positive adaptive changes that have occurred in response to a hostile environment. It is likely that a hostile macroenvironment provided the selective pressures that led to the survival of those life forms in the species which

267

Table I. Effect of Environment on the Development of the Immune Response

Target	Inductive Environment	Process	Selection Form
Species	Macroenvironment	Phylogeny	Existing life forms
Individual	Microenvironment	Ontogeny	Immunologically mature individual "Memory" cells
Cell	Molecular environment (antigen)	Induction of immune response	

SOURCE: Bellanti, J. A. (ed.). *Immunology II.* Philadelphia, W. B. Saunders Co., 1978.

were best adapted to that environment (phylogeny). In the developing fetus, the microenvironment, such as the bursa of Fabricius or the thymic epithelium, in which undifferentiated progenitor cells exist, provides yet another type of inductive environment, permitting the full expression of immunity in the developing individual (ontogeny). Finally, the molecular environment in which immunologically reactive cells exist provides yet another type of inductive stimulus leading to the proliferative and differentiative events seen in both humoral and cellular immune responses. The establishment of memory cells may be considered the best adaptation to this environment. Thus, fetal and neonatal development of the immunological system, although very likely genetically predetermined, can be best understood against this backdrop of the developing host responding to an ever-changing and hostile environment. As we shall see, the cells and functions of the immunologic system appear very early in fetal life, but at least part of them achieve full reactivity only after they have been in contact with the external environment following birth. Under ordinary circumstances, the fetus is protected in utero from stimulation by the external environment. However, under pathologic conditions, such as intrauterine infection, the immunologic system may be challenged and respond even in utero.

The generalization that ontogeny recapitulates phylogeny applies only partially to the immunological system. This section includes a brief description of phylogeny followed by a review of the ontogenetic development of the lymphoreticular system.

Phylogeny

In evaluating the evolution of immune responses, it is important to stress that the phylogenetic tree does not represent a simple linear evolutionary progression among several animal classes. In the majority of instances, common ancestral forms have been extinct for millions of years. Therefore, one cannot build a complete phylogenetic history of the immune system based on existing life forms. One should also recognize that many immunological common denominators of various vertebrate species may reflect convergent points of evolution of immunological mechanisms that protected them against a common type of hostile macroenvironment. For ease of discussion, a simple taxonomic scheme is presented in Table II. The three major phylogenetic levels of evolution shown in Table III provide a basis for the discussion that follows (2).

Sir Macfarlane Burnet alerted us to the relevance of invertebrate immunology (3) (Table IV). He stressed the importance of deciphering the mechanism by which cells recognize the basic difference between "self" and "non-self," a capacity that is present

Table II. A Classification of Animals

Phylum Protozoa	Acellular animals, usually unicellular
Phylum Porifera	The sponges
Phylum Coelenterata or Cinidaria	Aquatic, mostly marine, tissue grade organisms; jelly fishes, sea anemones, hydra
Phylum Platyhelminthes	Flatworms
Phylum Aschelminthes	Rotifers, round worms, arrow worms, horsehair worms, gastrotrichs
Phylum Acanthocephala	Spiny-headed worms
Phylum Annelida	Segmented worms, terrestrial (earthworms); marine (Nereis)
Phylum Mollusca	Oysters, clams, snails, octapuses, squids
Phylum Arthropoda	Insects, crayfish, lobsters, crabs, spiders, scorpions
Phylum Echinodermata	Starfish, sea urchins
Phylum Chordata	Chordate animals: notochord, pharyngeal gill slits
Subphylum Hemichordata	Acorn worms
Subphylum Cephalochordata	Lancelets
Subphylum Tunicata (Urochordata)	Ascidians
Subphylum Vertebrata	
Superclass Pisces	Aquatic vertebrates (fish)
Classes:	
Agnatha	Jawless fish, lampreys
Placodermii	Now extinct
Chondrichthyes	Cartilaginous fish, sharks and relatives
Osteichthyes	Higher bony fish which constitute most of the piscine world
Superclass Tetrapida	
Classes:	
Amphibia, Reptila,	
Aves, Mammalia	

Table III. Major Phylogenetic Levels of Immunoevolution

Main Immune Mechanisms	Occurrence	Phylum or Classes Identified	Experimental Evidence
Quasi-immuno-recognition	Invertebrates and vertebrates	Coelenterates, tunicates, and mammals	Allograft incompatibility; allogeneic incompatibility; MLC reaction
Primordial cell-mediated immunity	Advanced invertebrates; vertebrates(?)	Annelids and echinoderms	Allograft incompatibility with specific memory
Integrated cell-mediated and humoral immunity	All vertebrates	Fishes, amphibians, reptiles, birds, and mammals	Very extensive

SOURCE: Modified from *Federation Proceedings,* vol. 32, no. 12, December 1973.

Table IV. Evolution of Immunity in Invertebrates*

Phylum or Subphylum	Graft Rejection	Immunologic Specificity of Graft Rejection	Immunologic Memory	Nonspecific Human Factors	Specialized Leucocytes Present	Inducible Specific "Antibodies"†
Protozoa	Yes; enzyme incompatibility	No	No	No	No	No
Porifera (sponges)	Yes; aggregation inhibition, glycoproteins	No	No	No	No	No
Coelenterata (corals, jellyfish, sea anemones)	Yes; with graft necrosis	Yes	?	No	?	No
Annelida (earthworms)	Yes	Yes; first and second set graft rejection	Yes; short-term	Yes; non specific hemagglutinins	Yes	No and yes
Mollusca	Yes	Yes	?	Yes; hemagglutinins act as opsonins	Yes	Yes
Arthropoda	Yes	Yes and no	?	Yes	Yes	Yes
Echinodermata	Yes; prolonged 4–6 months	Yes	Yes	Yes	Yes	?
Protochordata (tunicates)	Yes; genetically determined allo-immunity	Probable; tolerance possible	?	Yes	Yes	?

SOURCE: Modified from Hildemann, W. H., and Reddy, A. L. *Fed. Proc.* 322:2188, 1973.

* Several phyla not included because of available data.

† Vertebrate type of immunoglobulin has not been demonstrated in any invertebrate.

270

even in the most primitive invertebrates. The protozoan, the first major level, is capable of rejecting transplanted foreign nuclei and differentiating food or invading microorganisms from its autologous cell components. Slightly higher forms are the Porifera (sponges), the simplest metazoans, which are organized as colonies of differentiated cells. When dissociated, these colonies can reassemble spontaneously into a functional sponge, whereas cells of different species do not aggregate to form such functional groupings (4). This phenomenon, which is essentially species-specific, must require molecular specificity at cell surfaces. Nonetheless, temporary aggregation of cells from different species may also occur (5). Additional studies have marshaled evidence that species-specific adherence of sponge cells may be analogous to tissue-specific cell aggregation in higher animals (2). As can be seen in Table III, incompatibility reactions are also exhibited against foreign tissues in the tunicate. The incompatibility, although usually specific, lacks a memory component. Since it is now well known that mixed lymphocyte reactions are present in the human fetus at 10 to 14 weeks of gestational age (6), ontogeny in mammals appears to recapitulate phylogeny in the sense that mixed lymphocyte reactions precede other immunologic reactions.

Moving to the second major phylogenetic level of immunoevolution (Tables III and IV), we see the beginnings of short-term memory as exemplified in the annelids and echinoderms. The emergence of these forms of cell-mediated immunity can be attributed to the evolution of an enclosed body cavity and circulatory system, in which an immunosurveillance system of some sort obviously constitutes an evolutionary advantage. These invertebrates have a variety of leukocytes, including lymphocytelike cells, to which this immunosurveillance function can be ascribed. Although immunoglobulins are absent in the invertebrates, a variety of nonspecific humoral factors, such as bacteriolysins, hemolysins, and opsonins, serve as a humoral defense. Some of these factors are induced by immunization (7-9). It is impossible, however, from available data to conclude whether or not these molecules bear any relationship to the immunoglobulins of higher animals. Thus, there is now good evidence that cellular immunity precedes humoral immunity in the evolutionary scale.

The highest level of immunoevolution is seen in the vertebrates (Tables III and V). A full review of the immense literature in this area is beyond the scope of this chapter, and interested readers are referred to the literature (10,11). The hagfish, the most primitive of the living cyclostomes, is no longer the "negative hero of the phylogeny of immunity." The reports of Good et al. (12), which considered these vertebrates immunologically incompetent, have been conclusively disproved. These life forms can recognize and reject skin allografts and make humoral antibodies (13). Phylogenetically the immunoglobulin production in these forms precedes the appearance of plasma cells and an organized lymphoid tissue (11). These findings help to clarify a long-standing fallacy in human ontogenesis, namely, that a lack of plasma cell equates with absence of immunoglobulin production. Moreover, the recent exciting findings of T- and B-cell cooperation and T-suppressor activity also appears in these early vertebrate forms (fish and amphibians) (11). In these forms, two types of immunoglobulin classes have been described. Moreover, definitive thymuses and spleens, as well as kidney-associated lymphoid aggregates, have been detected in cartilagenous fish. The bony fish have an additional bone marrowlike hematopoietic tissue, containing numerous lymphocytes and plasma cells. Among the anuran amphibians, lymph nodelike organs, a definitive lymphopoietic bone marrow, and gut-associated lymphoid tissue (GALT) are found in addition to the thymus and spleen. The pivotal role of amphibians in immunological

Table V. An Overall View of Development of Immunity in Vertebrates

Class	Lympho-cytes	Plasma Cells	Thymus	Spleen	Bone Marrow	Lymph Nodes	Bursa	Anti-bodies	Allograft Rejection
Agnatha (jawless fish, hag fish, lampreys)	+	−	— Prim	Prim	−	−	−	+	+
Chondrichthyes (cartilaginous fish, sharks)	+	±	+	+	−	−	−	+	+
Osteichtyes (bony, fish)	+	+	+	+	+?	−	−	+	+
Amphibians	+	+	+	+	+	±?	−	+	+
Reptilia	+	+	+	+	+	+?	+?	+	+
Aves	+	+	+	+	+	+?	+	+	+
Mammalia	+	+	+	+	+	+	+?	+	+

SOURCE: Modified from Hildemann, W. H. *Fed. Proc.* 322:2188, 1973.

Prim = primitive.

? = Indicates some question regarding the presence of lymphoid structures under consideration, although such structures or their functional counterparts may have been described.

± = Indicates that only some species have presence of lymphoid structures.

1. Some homograft reactions occur in the absence of a thymus.
2. Ab production can occur in the absence of plasma cells.
3. Ab production can occur in the absence of a bursa of Fabricius or its equivalent.

evolution may reflect their emergence as terrestrial animals, shaped by the novel selective pressures operating in this new macroenvironment. The cytoarchitecture of the primary and peripheral lymphoid organs increases in complexity in the birds and mammals. Complexity of cytoarchitecture in these vertebrates is accompanied by increased diversity of immunologic cell type and interactions as well as further molecular diversification of antibodies (Table V). Lymphoid nodules in germinal centers also appear in the birds and mammals. The histocompatibility system also increases in complexity among the higher vertebrates. With regard to the phylogenesis of immediate hypersensitivity, the recent discovery of IgE and its role in human allergy have posed several interesting questions regarding the significance of this form of immunologic refinement as a recent phylogenetic addition. IgE mediates systemic anaphylaxis, an explosive response occurring within a few minutes, that can lead to shock, smooth muscle constriction, and, if death does not follow, recovery within 1 hr. When the same type of reaction takes place, but in miniature, on the skin, it is called cutaneous anaphylaxis and is characterized by transient wheal-and-erythema response within seconds to 20 min. Studies of both types of anaphylactic reactions have been controversial in teleosts. Dreyer and King (14) reported an "anaphylactic-type" reaction following a shock-inducing dose of horse serum. In contrast, Clem and his associates (10) were unable to produce systemic or cutaneous anaphylaxis in teleosts. The latter authors also failed to demonstrate one additional aspect of immediate hypersensitivity: the cutaneous Arthus type of reaction, which consists of localized skin inflammation with vasculitis, following injection of an antigen into a previously sensitized animal. The principal requirement for an Arthus reaction is the formation in tissues of antigen-antibody complexes; the antibody could be almost any class of immunoglobulins. The Arthus reaction can be clinically differentiated from cutaneous anaphylaxis because it appears after 1 to 2 hr and the changes are maximal at approximately 4 hr, disappearing by 12 hr.

In chickens, Ovary (15) and Hirata et al. (16) failed to demonstrate anaphylaxis. However, other workers (11) demonstrated reactions that resembled anaphylaxis. In addition, passive cutaneous anaphylaxislike reactions have been demonstrated in birds (17–19). However, the nature of the antibodies involved in these passive cutaneous anaphylaxislike reactions has not been determined.

Finally, it is important to stress that functional immunologic reactions or quasi-immunorecognition (Table III) is attained prior to the development of a definite, organized cytoarchitecture of the lymphoid system. Thus, in the ontogeny of the human immune system, we cannot assume that a lack of obvious morphologic development necessarily implies a lack of immunological function.

Ontogeny

The first site of hematopoiesis in birds and mammalian embryos is the mesenchymal blood islands found in the primitive yolk sac (20,21). In man (see Fig. 1 for an overview of ontogenesis of the mammalian immune system), the primitive mesenchymal cells (stem cells) from the yolk sac (22–24) appear between 2 and 6 weeks' gestation and proliferate and differentiate into precursor cells afterward. These cells differentiate into erythrocytic, megakaryocytic, granulocytic, lymphocytic, and monocytic cells (23,24). At about the sixth week, the developing liver is invaded by hematopoietic stem cells and becomes the major blood-forming organ during early fetal life (23). The hematopoietic activity of the liver precedes the establishment of hematopoiesis in the bone marrow. Although the liver was previously considered to be exclusively erythropoietic in fetal life (25), recent studies have yielded evidence of myelopoiesis and lymphopoiesis (26). In the hematopoietic cell mass of the liver, a minority of pluripotential hematopoietic stem cells is present (26). These cells probably are responsible for the success of therapy in which six patients with thymic deficiency were reconstituted with transplants of human fetal liver cells (27). As might be expected from the ontogenic sequence of development (Fig. 2), the graft-versus-host reaction is less frequently seen in fetal liver transplants than in bone marrow transplants. Fetal liver transplantation thus represents the first successful organ transplant of fully incompatible hematopoietic cells in man (27). Hepatic hematopoiesis ceases at 22 to 24 weeks of gestation. In general, at about 4 weeks of gestation, primitive erythroblasts are produced (23). Although nucleated red cells are predominant during the second month, lymphocytes, granulocytes, and megakaryocytes have also formed in the hematopoietic organs. In the fifth week of gestation, few lymphocytes are present in the fetal circulation (28). As early as the eighth week in the human fetus, nodules of lymphoid tissue have been found in the connective tissue of the neck (29).

Normally, in the absence of intrauterine infection, lymph nodes are devoid of primary follicles and usually do not contain plasma cells (30). But lymph nodes may have a few plasma cells prior to birth (31). Although the splenic anlage is present at 5 weeks, lymphopoiesis in the spleen is not evident at the eleventh gestational week (32) and is delayed until the twelfth week (33). Erythropoiesis still remains predominant until the fifth month, when lymphocyte and monocyte production are at their maximum (23,34). Between the twelfth and fifteenth weeks, central arterioles appear that, from the

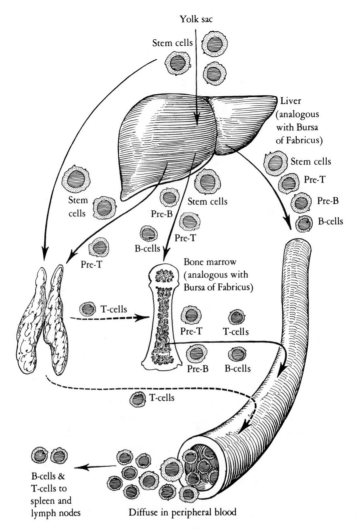

Figure 1. Current overview of lymphocyte development in mammals. Stem cells: lack markers, are multipotential, and can develop into any of the blood cells. T cells: Lymphocytes that form spontaneous rosettes with sheep red blood cells but do have human T differentiation antigens (these cells become T cells under the influence of thymic extracts). B cells: contain readily detectable surface immunoglobulins and human B differentiation antigens. Pre-B cells: negative surface immunoglobulin cells, but positive human B differentiation antigens. The dotted lines indicate those cells which do not return to the thymus.

seventeenth week on, are accompanied by cuffs of small lymphocytes (35). In the human appendix, lymphocyte aggregates and primary follicles increase in the lamina propria after the twentieth week of gestation until term. The appendix behaves like a secondary rather than a primary lymphatic organ (36). As in the case of the spleen, evidence of a functional bone marrow is found at the eleventh to twelfth week of gestation (32,37). From this time on, the lymphoid compartment of the bone marrow forms approximately 25% of the total nucleated mass (37). With the decline in erythropoietic activity of the liver and spleen seen after the eighth month, the marrow hematopoiesis assumes maximal activity (38) and becomes the major source of erythroblasts and myelocytes (22). During the first 3 months of prenatal life, bone marrow lymphoid cells show a steady rise, and at the end of the neonatal period lymphocytes form approximately 50% of all the nucleated marrow cells (39,40). Bone marrow volumes of newborns approximate 16 to 44 ml (40% of skeletal volume), or 1.4% of total body weight (41).

At the sixth week, the thymus (Figs. 1 and 3) originates from the third and fourth pharyngeal pouches, which also give rise to the parathyroid structures. The gland is originally epithelial (42). Small lymphocytes infiltrate this organ by the eighth to ninth week of gestation (43,44). The origin of these thymic lymphocytes is not known in the human, but animal studies suggest that they are formed in the primitive yolk sac or hepatic lymphoid precursor cells (45). From the fourteenth week on, a cortical zone rich in mitotically active lymphocytes and lymphocyte precursor cells appears, reaching a maximum at about 20 weeks (44). At this time, epithelial cells and Hassal corpuscles are regularly seen in the thymic medulla (46). Thus the thymus shows a dual origin with a derivation from an epithelial-mesenchymal origin. The anatomical changes in structure of the thymic gland are shown schematically in Fig. 1.

In the peripheral blood, lymphocytes are first detectable in the fetus at about the eighth to the tenth week of gestation (28,43,48). After that period, a rapid rise of lymphocytes occurs until the twenty-fifth week, when a plateau of 2500 or 3000

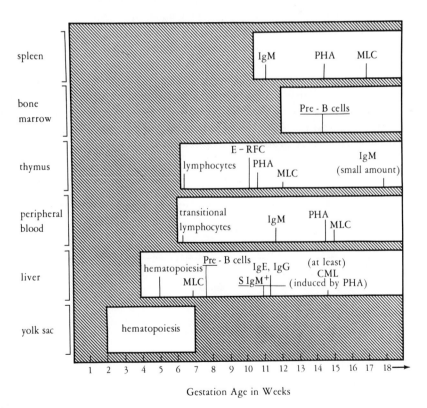

Figure 2. Time of initiation of hematopoiesis and different humoral and cell-mediated immune functions in different human lymphoid organs.

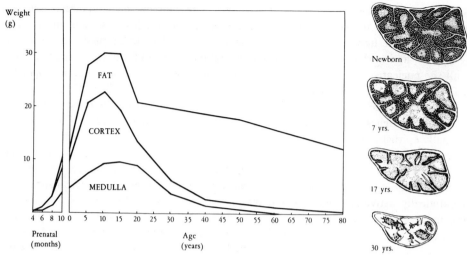

Figure 3. Schematic representation of changes in weight and composition of thymus gland during maturation. After Hammar, J. A., in Bellanti, J. A. *Immunology II.* Philadelphia, W. B. Saunders Co., 1978.

cells/mm³ is reached and maintained until birth. This plateau indicates a dynamic equilibrium between production and destruction of lymphocytes/mm³ of blood (47,49,50) (Table VI). After a transitory drop, the peripheral blood lymphocytes reach a level of 6000 per mm³. Premature newborn infants have somewhat lower levels, depending on the gestational age and birthweight. From exchange transfusion studies, the lymphocyte reserves of the newborn have been calculated as 25.4×10^7 cells per kilogram of body weight. The lymphopenia that regularly follows exchange transfusion reaches its lowest level at 17 to 40 hr, after which blood lymphocytes begin to rise again, increasing even beyond normal values after 96 hr (51,52). The reasons for this phenomenon are not clear. Circulating stem cells probably are present in the chick embryo (20,53,54) and

Table VI. The White Blood Cell Count and Differential During the First Two Weeks of Life (95% Range Expressed as Cells per cu mm $\times 10^3$)

Age	Leukocytes	Neutrophils Total	Seg	Band	Eosinophils	Basophils	Lymphocytes	Monocytes
Birth:								
Range	9.0–30.0	6.0–2.6			20–850	0–640	2.0–11.0	0.4–3.1
Mean %		61	52	9	2.2	0.6	31	5.8
7 days:								
Range	5.0–21.0	1.5–10.0			70–1100	0–250	2.0–17.0	0.3–2.7
Mean %		45	39	6	4.1	0.4	41	9.1
14 days:								
Range	5.0–20.0	1.0–9.5			70–1000	0–230	2.0–17.0	0.2–2.4
Mean %		40	34	5.5	3.1	0.4	48	8.8

SOURCE: Altman, P. D., and Dittmer, D. S. *Blood and Other Body Fluids.* Federation of American Societies for Experimental Biology, Washington, D.C., 1961.

mammals (21,55,56). Although recent evidence favors a unicentric theory, it has been pointed out that hematopoietic stem cells may also originate locally, at least during hepatic development (57). They may possibly be derived from endodermal cells that have not fully differentiated into liver cells (25,58). There is also evidence that the bone marrow contains stem cells. Similarly, we have evidence that the cord blood contains stem cells or at least T-cell precursors (59–61). Studies performed in our laboratory and by other investigators indicate that the activity of cord blood mononuclear cells, as measured by DNA incorporation of tritiated thymidine, is significantly higher than that seen in adult peripheral mononuclear cells (44,61,63–65,67). The cells at least partially responsible for this observation appear to be transitional between lymphocytes and blast cells and are present in a subset that we called "null" because it is composed of cells that lack classical B- or T-cell markers. Radioautography studies show that the number of these cells is approximately 10 times higher in cord blood than in adult peripheral blood.

DEVELOPMENT OF THE DIFFERENT COMPONENTS OF THE IMMUNE SYSTEM

For ease of discussion, the immunologic system may be considered under two major headings:

1. The nonspecific mechanisms, which include phagocytosis and the inflammatory response
2. The specific immune response, which consists of humoral (B-cell) and cell-mediated (T-cell) systems

The nonspecific mechanisms also include the activity of the complement system, coagulation system, and the kinin system. It is important to stress that the nonspecific and specific mechanisms are intimately interrelated and interdependent. For example, the activation of the complement system by immunoglobulins (IgM and IgG) or the production of chemotactic factors and other lymphokines plays a significant role in the whole inflammatory response. The monocyte or macrophage may function in both phagocytic and inflammatory responses as well as playing a significant role in the processing of antigen, steps essential for the induction of the specific immune response. Thus, the macrophage actually forms part of both the nonspecific and specific immune systems important to both the afferent and efferent limbs of the immune response. The lymphokines are other products secreted by mononuclear cells that play a role in both nonspecific and specific mechanisms.

Nonspecific Immune Mechanisms

Inflammatory Response
Inflammation is a systemic and localized complex process involving cellular as well as humoral factors and a target organ where the action takes place. The absent or diminished febrile response of the newborn to bacterial infections, a phenomenon well known to pediatricians, illustrates the functional immaturity of this system. Similarly, leukocytosis and an increase in sedimentation rate, common in bacterial infections in the adult, are not usually seen in the newborn. There is also evidence that apparently indi-

cates that newborn skin has a decreased inflammatory response (72). The cellular and humoral factors of nonspecific immunity are described separately in order to elucidate better the developmental status of this system in fetal and neonatal life.

Cellular Component of Inflammatory Response. The cellular responses are carried out primarily by polymorphonuclear leukocytes, macrophages (monocytes), eosinophils, and lymphocytes. Phagocytosis is described with each cell when pertinent. Lymphokines are described under cell-mediated immunity.

Polymorphonuclear Leukocytes. The polymorphonuclear leukocyte performs three functions (1) migration, including chemotaxis and random migration or mobility; (2) phagocytosis; and (3) microbicidal activity.

Chemotaxis and Random Migration of Polymorphonuclear Leukocytes. Chemotaxis refers to the process by which a phagocytic cell moves in an organized, specific fashion toward a stimulant (chemoattractant). This process also involves the participation of lymphocytes, macrophages, and a variety of humoral factors. One can study in vivo migration with the skin-window screening test of Rebuck (73). In this technique a 5-mm superficial abrasion is produced in the skin and covered with a coverglass. The cells that come to the abraded area attach to the glass and can be stained and counted at intervals. In adults a prominent polymorphonuclear leukocyte infiltration can be demonstrated during the first 4 to 12 hr; this is followed at 24 hr by a predominant infiltration of macrophages and lymphocytes (73). This shift is slower and less intense in the newborn (74). Neonatal polymorphonuclear leukocytes exhibit lower chemotactic activity than adult cells when both are incubated in the presence of a wide variety of chemotactic stimuli (75,76). When neonatal polymorphonuclear leukocytes are incubated with endotoxin-activated serum from umbilical cord blood, the chemotaxis is even lower (77). Moreover, replacement of human serum by diluent plus casein as a chemotactic stimulator also produced significantly lower chemotaxis in newborns than in adults (77). In brief, chemotaxis in newborns is low because of deficiencies of both intrinsic cellular factors and extrinsic humoral factors. Although other serum factors may be involved, it appears that the primary humoral deficiency is in complement components C3 and C5. Addition of IgM antibody fails to correct the humoral deficiency of chemotaxis in vitro (75).

Random mobility refers to the nondirected migration of the polymorphonuclear leukocyte. An example of a defect in random mobility and chemotaxis is the "lazy leukocyte syndrome" (78). Two families have been described with chemotactic defects but intact random mobility (79). These observations suggest that random mobility and chemotaxis might involve separate mechanisms. In the newborn, there is evidence that random mobility, as measured by the millipore filter method or capillary tubes, is normal (77). Membrane deformability of the newborn polymorphonuclear leukocyte has also been observed to be markedly decreased when compared with adult leukocytes. This increased membrane rigidity may explain in part the defective chemotaxis of the newborn leukocyte. This is supported by the observations that iodoacetate and other substances that decrease membrane deformability also appear to decrease chemotaxis (77).

Phagocytosis by Polymorphonuclear Leukocytes. Phagocytic cells are present in the fetus at the time of development of the vascular organs. Various conflicting reports have appeared concerning the adequacy of phagocytosis in the human neonate. However, some of the conflict in the literature stems from differences in methodology. In general, experiments reported thus far indicate decreased phagocytic activity in infants as compared with adults (80). A few reports, however, indicate increased or normal phagocytosis but decreased killing capacity. Other investigators (81–83) have reported normal phagocytic capacity in the newborn polymorphonuclear leukocytes when incubated in the presence of serum concentrations of 10% or greater. If the serum concentrations of 3% are used, the neonatal polymorphonuclear leukocyte exhibits a deficiency in phagocytic activity (84). Miller (85), using 2.5% pooled plasma, observed that fewer yeast particles were ingested by newborn polymorphonuclear leukocytes than by adult leukocytes. The phagocytic capacity of these leukocytes in full-term and low birthweight infants is similar when adult sera are used. However, phagocytosis by leukocytes from low birthweight infants proved to be much less efficient when their cells were tested with their own sera (82). Thus at birth phagocytosis is generally found to be decreased, provided the assay used is sensitive enough to identify the deficiency. It also appears that low birthweight newborns are deficient in humoral substances required for phagocytosis or that they have an inhibitor of phagocytosis.

Bactericidal and Metabolic Activity of Polymorphonuclear Leukocytes. The literature concerning the bactericidal activity of the polymorphonuclear leukocyte is also contradictory. It has been reported that whole blood of the premature infant has bactericidal activity similar to that of the full-term infant when tested with *Pseudomonas aeruginosa* measured at 90 min incubation but that blood from premature infants is deficient in bactericidal activity when measurements are taken at 3-hr intervals (87). The addition of serum from different sources had no apparent effect on leukocyte killing capability. Leukocytes from full-term and low birthweight infants kill *Staphylococcus aureus* equally well in the presence of adult opsonins, but killing appears to be decreased in the low birthweight infants in the presence of their own sera (82).

Dosset et al. (88) found no deficiency in bactericidal activity of newborn leukocytes using *E. coli*. Coen et al. (89) found the bactericidal activity of leukocytes from 9 out of 25 full-term infants to be decreased within the first 12 hr of life.

These studies of functional activity of neonatal polymorphonuclear leukocytes led to the study of metabolic activities of these cells. After phagocytosis, oxygen consumption increases markedly, and glucose utilization increases through the hexose monophosphate shunt (90,91). Neonatal leukocytes consume twice as much oxygen as matched maternal leukocytes in the resting phase (92). However, following phagocytosis oxygen consumption by neonatal and maternal leukocytes appears to be similar (92). In contrast, it has been reported (89,93) that the increase in the metabolic activity of the hexose monophosphate shunt that follows phagocytosis in newborn leukocytes is of less magnitude than the increase observed in adult leukocytes. A recent report by Strauss et al. (94) could explain these apparently divergent results. These investigators found that hexose monophosphate activity of newborn leukocytes is greater than that of adult leukocytes in the resting state and during phagocytosis. However, the absolute increase from resting to phagocytic values was significantly less in cord blood leukocytes. These authors observed that the kinetics of the cord blood leukocyte reactions are quite different. Cord blood leukocytes initiate a sharp postphagocytic oxidative metabolism that is comparable with that of adult leukocytes but occurs at a later time. Hexose monophosphate activity wanes in the cord blood leukocytes but it is sustained in adult leukocytes.

The postphagocytic increase in oxidative metabolism of the leukocyte has led to the development of a simple screening test of leukocyte function, the nitroblue tetrazolium (NBT) test (95). This test is based on the fact that the dye is colorless in the oxidized state and assumes an intense blue color when reduced to the blue formazan pigment. This screening test, which was originally designed for the diagnosis of chronic granulomatous disease, has been applied to the study of cord blood leukocytes. In cord blood, we found a decreased reduction of NBT dye (96). Our results were at variance with those of Park et al. (92), who found an increased rate of reduction of the dye. This discrepancy may stem in part from the fact that there were differences in the incubation times used in the analysis. Park et al. used a 30-min incubation as opposed to the 15 min that was originally recommended for the assay. In additional studies of NBT dye reduction, there appears to be an increase in reduction with increasing age (Fig. 4) (97). These values indicate the importance of considering the age of the infant in interpreting this function, particularly in the study of newborns or small infants. We have also shown that leukocyte glucose-6-phosphate dehydrogenase (G-6-PD) activity increases with age and that the activity of this enzyme has a decreased thermal stability in infants; thermal stability increases with age (97) (Fig. 5). Similar accelerated decay of G-6-PD under heating conditions has been demonstrated in three patients with chronic granulomatous disease (98). The lability appears to be related to a lack of availability of NADP, owing to a diminished or absent NADPH oxidase activity. These two observations could partially account for the increased resistance to infection that occurs with

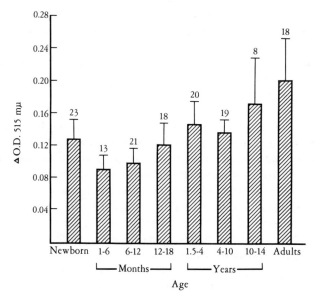

Figure 4. Change in NBT reduction occurring with age. Results express the mean ± SE of change in optical density (ΔOD) between resting and phagocytosing values. The number of cases is illustrated above each column. After Bellanti, J. A. *The Phagocytic Cell in Host Resistance.* New York, Raven Press, 1975.

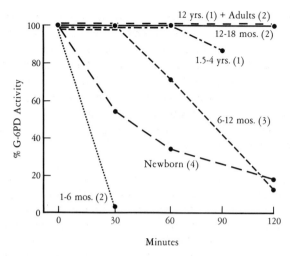

Figure 5. Thermal stability (37°C) of leukocyte G-6PD at different ages. Leukocyte homogenates were tested in the presence of 2-mercapto-ethanol and NADP. After Bellanti, J. A. *The Phagocytic Cell in Host Resistance.* New York, Raven Press, 1975.

age and may explain the susceptibility of the newborn to infections with certain microbial agents.

Monocytes (Macrophages). The macrophage appears to be a central cell type involved in several immunologic processes. Knowledge of its role may explain the fact that newborns, despite almost complete maturation of the B- and T-cell systems, remain relatively immunodeficient. Evidence obtained from experimental animals (99–103) indicates that the neonate has a deficiency in macrophage function. It is also likely that the human monocyte shows similar deficiencies. This observation could explain the newborn's inability to respond to the pneumococcus and *Hemophilus influenzae* capsular antigens.

Blaese (103), in an excellent study of neonatal monocyte function in the Lewis rat, provides clear insights into this problem and confirms previous experiments, which showed that cytomegalovirus (100) and herpes simplex (101) infection in newborn mice could be effectively prevented by injections of adult macrophages. These experiments indicated a maturation in macrophage function with age, as demonstrated by testing the specific immune response to a variety of antigens. They also showed that neonatal rats can easily be induced to develop tolerance. Development of tolerance can be prevented by activating macrophages or giving the neonatal rats adult macrophages. In the human neonate, phagocytic and bactericidal capacity against *Staphylococcus aureus* and *E. coli* has been said to be quantitatively similar to that of adults (104). These investigations used from 5 to 12% monocytes, and apparently no attempt was made to correct these different concentrations (104). Consistent with these findings are the reports of normal NBT reduction and ingestion of latex particles (105). As far as neonatal monocyte movement is concerned, there is only one report of increased random motility (106). Similar studies on chemotaxis are conflicting. Decreased chemotaxis has been reported in cells from 1- to 5-day-old newborn infants (107) and in full-term (108) infants. In contrast, normal or increased monocyte chemotaxis has been reported (107–109). These divergent results perhaps can be explained by methodologic differences. Interestingly, there is some evidence that cord blood serum inhibits chemotaxis to a lesser degree than adult serum (106). A similar inhibitor of adult lymphocyte responses to PHA and heterologous cells and of the lymphokine leukocyte inhibitory factor (LIF) production has been described (110). The antibody-dependent cellular cytotoxicity (ADCC) reaction against chicken erythrocytes, which seems to be a monocyte target, has been shown to be normal in newborns (111). At this point, no definitive conclusions can be reached. However, it may be predicted that with better techniques useful information regarding monocyte function will be forthcoming in the near future.

Eosinophils. In general, little is known about the eosinophils. At birth and during the immediate neonatal period, levels of peripheral blood eosinophils are lower than in the adult. Studies performed with the skin-window technique of Rebuck have produced some indications of unusually great numbers of eosinophils in newborns older than 24 hr but not in those less than 24 hr old (74). However, Bullock et al. (112) did not find this consistently higher percentage of eosinophils in the early exudate. There is also evidence in animals that lymphocytes may play a role in regulating eosinophilia. In the human, eosinophilic chemotactic factor of anaphylaxis (ECF-A) and histamine have been shown to be important mediators mobilizing eosinophils.

Humoral Component of the Inflammatory Response. Complement System. One of the causes of innate or natural resistance to infection in vertebrates is the complement system. Deficiencies of components of complement can be responsible for severe disorders. Complement is a multimolecular, self-assembling biological system that constitutes the primary humoral mediator of antigen-antibody reactions. Activation of complement may have two distinct biological consequences: (1) the irreversible structural and functional alteration of biological membranes and (2) activation of specialized cell functions for the release of mediators such as histamine from mast cells or the release of lysosomal hydrolases from leukocytes, or the enhancement of phagocytosis and other functions.

In addition to a dozen or more proactivators, activators, inhibitors derived from the complement cascade, and factors unique to an alternate pathway, the complement system consists of 11 proteins that in the classical pathway interact in an organized sequence (Fig. 6).

In spite of its significant biological role, little is known regarding the complement system in the neonate. The third component of complement, C3, can be synthesized in different tissues in the human conceptus beginning as early as 29 days of gestation (113,114). The sites of synthesis for C3 appear to be the fibroblast, the lymphoid cell, and the macrophage (115–117). In adults, there is some evidence that the liver is the major producer of C3 (118). Serum concentration of C3 in the fetus rises almost exponentially from 1.9 mg/100 ml at 5.5 weeks' gestation (113,119) to a range of 52 to 167 mg/100 ml between 28 and 41 weeks. The mean level in cord blood is ±90 mg/100 ml (120), approximately one-half the maternal levels. Studies of C3 phenotypes indicate that C3 is synthesized in utero (120). The concentration of complement in the newborn falls slightly after birth and recovers before the infant is 3 weeks of age. By the age of 6 months, C3 reaches adult levels. Colten et al. (121) have shown that phagocytosis of bacterial products enhances production of complement components. Littman et al. (122) have observed that human peripheral blood mononuclear cells cultured in the presence

BIOACTIVE PRODUCTS OF THE COMPLEMENT SYSTEM GENERATED IN SEQUENCE AND IN BYPASS

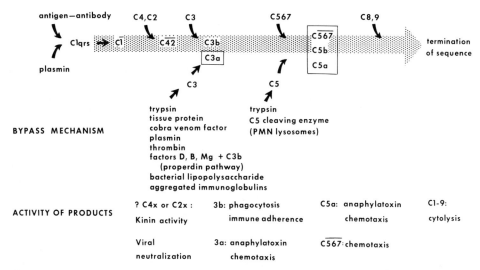

Figure 6. Composite of biologic functions of the complement system and methods by which biologically active products can be generated. From Bellanti, J. A. *Immunology II.* Philadelphia, W. B. Saunders Co., 1978.

of antigen produced hemolytically active second component or complement earlier and in larger amounts than did control cultures of the same cells without antigen. They indicated that the synthesis of C2 came primarily from the adherent cell population and that lymphokines-rich supernatant was able to stimulate more C2 production than supernatants from unstimulated lymphocytes without lymphokines. Thus, it can be deduced that after birth antigen stimulation may play a role in the induction of complement synthesis. Synthesis of C4 by lung and liver has been demonstrated in cells obtained from peritoneal wash in 14-week fetuses (114), and at 18 weeks C4 is detectable in the serum, increasing steadily to levels of about half those in maternal serum at birth (121).

Components C3, C4, and C5 in premature and full-term infants have been found to be deficient when compared with maternal and adult standards. Propp et al. (120) found in cord blood from full-term neonates that C1q, C3, C4, and C5 were slightly higher than 50% of the respective maternal levels. Low levels of properdin, factor B (C3PA), as well as C1, C2, C3, and C4, have also been reported in cord blood (123,124). Interestingly, C1 esterase inhibitor is synthesized in culture by all the tissues that synthesize C3 except blood. At 6.5 weeks of gestation, the serum concentration of the inhibitor was only 20% of normal adult levels; it rose steadily to reach adult levels by 28 weeks. For C1 esterase, it should be noted that the ratio of inhibitor to enzyme activity is higher in the fetus than in the adult. The serum C1 esterase concentration in the infant at birth is only half that of the nonpregnant adult, and C1 esterase inhibitor in term infants is at adult levels. Total hemolytic complement activity against sensitized erythrocytes appears to parallel the development of C3, C4, and C5. At term, it is approximately half that of the mother (124–126). In summary, C1q, C2, C3, C4, C5, factor B (C3PA), properdin level, and total hemolytic complement levels are all lowered in the neonatal period. Most of the biological effects of complement, including opsonization, immune adherence, complement-dependent viral neutralization, generation of anaphylactic and chemotactic factors, and production of cell membrane lesions, require only the first five complement components. Since the fetus can synthesize each of these components in biologically active form within the first trimester of development, but in smaller quantities than the adult, all these immunological functions could be affected to one degree or another by complement levels.

Antibodies. In addition to their direct effect in reacting with antigens, antibodies appear to play a significant role in events mediating inflammatory responses such as phagocytosis, chemotaxis, and the release of mediators. The extent to which the antibodies affect these different functions in the fetus and newborn depends on two main factors: permeability of the placenta to a given antibody (discussed under fetal-maternal relationship) and maturation of the antibody-producing system.

Silverstein et al. (102) have studied the maturation of immunologic capability and lymphoid tissues in the normal fetal lamb in utero (Fig. 7). They have established the sequence of the antibody response to different antigens. Bacteriophage ϕx174 given on day 37 elicited the earliest antibody response, at 41 days of gestation. This is a remarkable observation, since the fetal sheep has little organized lymphoid tissue at this time. At approximately 66 days of gestation the fetus becomes able to respond to the protein ferritin, and not until 125 days of gestation can it respond to egg albumin. Antibodies against *Salmonella typhosa* or BCG appear only after birth. These authors also found that they were unable to induce tolerance until the lamb reached the age at which it was able to recognize the antigen and produce antibody. One can draw an analogy between this phenomenon and the known poor response of human newborn infants to the polysaccharide antigens. We must understand these phenomena in the human if we are to develop adequate immunization techniques and prevent allergic diseases.

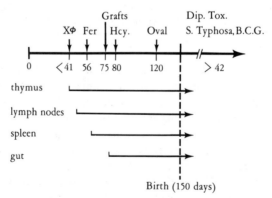

Figure 7. Comparison of immunologic and lymphoid development in the fetal lamb. Numbers on the upper horizontal axis show the earliest times at which antibody responses and graft rejection could be detected. The time at which lymphocytes appear in different tissues is as follows: Xϕ = bacteriophage, Fer = horse ferritin, Hcy. = snail hemocyanin, Oval = hen albumin, Dip. Tox. = diphtheria toxoid. After Silverstein and Prendergast, in Lindahl-Kiessling, K., et al. *Morphological and Functional Aspects of Immunity.* New York, Plenum Press, 1971.

Opsonic Capacity. The opsonic capacity of blood refers to the enhancement of phagocytosis and includes the activities of antibodies, complement, and other not well-defined proteins. In general, IgM appears to have higher opsonic activity. Opsonization has been studied by a number of investigators (82,83,85,88) with somewhat various results. Nevertheless, full-term human newborns, and to a major degree prematures, appear to be relatively deficient in opsonic activity toward a variety of agents. The degree of deficiency varies with different agents. In part, it probably involves antibodies, particularly of the IgM type; this deficiency of antibodies has been claimed and accounts for the predilection for gram-negative infections of the newborn, since IgM antibodies do not traverse the placenta. However, Miller (85) observed that addition of purified IgM to neonatal sera does not enhance opsonization of yeast particles. It has been shown (88) that complement and other heat-labile factors amplify the opsonic activity of IgM to a much greater extent than they amplify IgG opsonic activity. The deficit in opsonic activity derives from deficiencies of complement, as described above (88,127,128), particularly in components C3, C5, and C3PA. In the premature, it has been suggested that lowered levels of IgG may also play a role in the opsonic deficiency (82). Rigorously controlled studies of opsonic capacity of the fetus and newborn are needed in order to decide the usefulness of a potentially harmful treatment such as fresh plasma transfusion in the septicemic neonate.

Specific Immunological Mechanisms

Classically, the lymphoid system develops along two independent pathways leading to morphologically and functionally distinct populations of immune lymphocytes: (1) the B system of humoral or antibody-mediated immunity, which includes the B lymphocyte, and (2) the T system or cell-mediated immunity (CMI) whose principal effector cells are the T lymphocytes and the mononuclear phagocytes. The B lymphocyte is recognized mainly by its easily detectable surface immunoglobulins. The T lymphocyte is recognized for most purposes by its tendency to form nonimmune rosettes with sheep red blood cells (SRBC). The B system responds under antigenic stimulation to give rise to cells actively involved in immunoglobulin production, the plasma cells. The T lymphocytes are considered part of the cell-mediated immune reactions but also participate in nonspecific and humoral reactions. Moreover, there is recent evidence to suggest that the T system functions to enhance or depress B-cell responses. There is a vast range of immunologic reactions in which the T and B lymphocyte systems cooperate so closely that a defect in one cripples or diminishes the reactivity and effectiveness of the other. Moreover, a third cell type that brings about antibody-dependent cell-mediated cytotoxicity (ADCC) reactions has been recently defined. These lymphoid cells, which have also been called "K" or "killer" cells, have not been conclusively identified but appear to be closer to the T-cell lineage than to the B. West et al. (129) have demonstrated that "K" cell activity in adult blood is mainly present in low affinity E-RFC. "K" cells are closely related to the natural killer cells (NK) that are responsible for the natural cytotoxicity (129). We have recently obtained experimental evidence that the "null" fraction from cord blood lymphocytes, which is rich in cells with receptor for the Fc part of IgG and also rich in cells that have human T lymphocyte differentiation antigen (HTLA), is active in ADCC and NK activities (unpublished data and 130). Kaplan has found that lysis of the E^- $HTLA^+$ and E^+ $HTLA^+$ cells in adult peripheral blood lymphocytes abrogates K cell activity (personal communication). This observation supports our hypothesis that the E^- $HTLA^+$ subset is responsible for most of the ADCC activity seen in the "null" fraction isolated from cord blood lymphocytes.

Cell-Mediated Immunity or T-Cell System

This section is concerned primarily with human cell-mediated immunity (CMI). We refer to the T lymphocyte as a cell synonymous with the E rosette–forming cell (E-RFC), which is a lymphocyte that binds three or more sheep red blood cells to its surface. The nature of the receptor responsible for rosette formation is still unknown. Considerable evidence indicates that the E-RFC plays a major role in CMI activity. However, there are other subsets of cells that are partially responsible for some of these CMI mechanisms.

Development of E Rosette–Forming Cells. Table VII shows E-RFC found in 13 fetuses (111). The technique used gave a number of rosettes that later became known as "active" or "early" rosettes, which appear to be much lower than the number of rosettes obtained under optimal conditions. These investigators feel that the number of active rosettes correlates better with cell-mediated immunity than the total number of rosettes (131). Similar experiments done by the same authors, but using fetal calf serum instead of saline, yield higher numbers of E-RFC (Table VIII). Hayward et al., using an improved technique, confirmed these findings (132). Their experiment has to be repeated under optimum conditions in order to be able to draw more valid conclusions. Shown in Table

Table VII. Percentage of Rosette-Forming Cells in the Organs of Human Fetuses Using Lymphocyte/SRBC Ratio 1/8 and Saline as Diluent

Fetus Number	Weeks of Gestation	Thymus	Blood	Spleen	Liver	Bone Marrow
1	11	15	1	N.P.*	0	0.5
2	12	28	N.D.†	0	0	N.D.
3	12	48	0.5	0	0	N.D.
4	13	35	0.5	0	0	N.D.
5	13–14	15	0.5	0.5	0	0
6	13–14	50	0.5	0.5	0	N.D.
7	15	65	N.D.	N.D.	N.D.	3
8	15	47	0.5	0.5	0	N.D.
9	15–16	65	N.D.	N.D.	N.D.	1
10	17	35	2	4	2	0.5
11	18	24	11	11	1	8
12	19	30	N.D.	N.D.	N.D.	N.D.
13	19	30	2.5	2.5	0	N.D.

SOURCE: After D.P. Sites et al. (Reference 111). Development of cellular immunocompetence in man, in Porter, R., and Knight, J. (eds.). *Ontogeny of Acquired Immunity: Ciba Foundation Symposium.* North Holland, Elsevier, Excerpta Medica, 1972, p. 113.

* N.P., not present.

† N.D., not done.

Table VIII. Percentage of Spontaneous Rosette-Forming Cells (RFC) Against Sheep Erythrocytes in 12 Human Fetuses Using FCS as a Diluent

Fetus	Conceptional Age (Weeks)	Thymus FCS (%)	Spleen FCS (%)	Blood FCS (%)	Bone Marrow FCS (%)
1	11	21	NP	ND	0
2	11	NP	NP	0×	0
3	13–14	40×	1	1.5×	ND
4	13–14	ND	ND	3	0
5	14	85	2.5	5	0
6	15	80	ND	ND	0
7	15–16	75	7	ND	ND
8	15–16	71	1×	4	0
9	16	71	2×	3	ND
10	17	57	7	4	0
11	18	34	18	21	4
12	19	32×	6	6	ND

SOURCE: Modified from Wybrant et al., in *Clinical Immunology* 1:408, 1973 (Reference 131).

VIII are the percentages of E rosette–forming cells in the thymus. The data indicate that these cells are present before 11 weeks of gestational age and reach full-term values 1 to 5 weeks later. In peripheral blood, rosette-forming cells are present at or before 11 weeks and reach full-term values after 19 weeks of gestation. In the spleen, the liver, and the bone marrow, these cells are seen at approximately 13 and 17 weeks of gestational age. Percentages of E rosette–forming cells in human newborns have been reported to be similar to (133,134) or lower than percentages in adult peripheral blood (64,135). Bernales et al. (136) observations explain these divergent results. Cord blood lymphocytes separated by a Ficoll-Hypaque method usually contain large numbers of autologous red blood cells. As can be seen in Table IX, these contaminated red blood cells significantly decrease the percentage of rosette-forming cells and may contribute to the lowered levels of rosette formation seen in this age group. Table IX shows clearly that hypotonic shock, which is a common way of getting rid of contaminating red blood cells, also decreases E-RFC. Moreover, because of lymphocytosis observed in cord blood, the

Table IX. Parameters Affecting E Rosette–Forming Capacity of Cord Blood Lymphocytes (CBL)

CBL Used	No.	E Rosette (Mean ± SE) at Various SRBC/CBL Ratios (%)		
		80/1	40/1	8/1
With autologous RBC	3	36.5 ± 4.5	25.8 ± 10.8	3.5 ± 1.8
Pure SRBC	6	63.8 ± 3.0	57.6 ± 4.2	36.3 ± 2.7
After hypotonic shock	6	36.4 ± 4.0	33.8 ± 4.3	19.5 ± 4.7

absolute number of E rosette–forming cells is similar to adult blood. Our observations (136) can also probably explain the lower percentages of early rosettes reported in cord blood as compared with the values seen in adult blood (64).

Developmental Responses to Mitogens

Mitogens are plant extracts or other products that nonspecifically stimulate both T- and B-cell responses. Phytohemagglutinin (PHA) is the mitogen most widely used to evaluate T-cell response. As might be expected, the onset of responses to PHA generally correlates well with the ontogenic appearance of T cells. Fetal thymic lymphocytes acquire PHA responsiveness around 12 to 15 weeks of gestation (35,137–140). Concomitantly, the demarcation of cortex and medulla takes place in the thymus (139), and a rise in peripheral blood lymphocytes occurs (28). From 15 to 18 weeks of gestation, the response to PHA is variable (138) but at times is very high (139).

In a simultaneous study of thymuses, spleens, and bone marrow from 22 fetuses ranging from 16 to 24 weeks of gestational age, it was found that a fourfold increase in tritiated thymidine uptake occurs in the thymus in response to phytohemagglutinin. Fetal spleen responds less uniformly, and liver and bone marrow show mild or no responses (141). A dose-response relationship of PHA responses in fetuses from 5 to 19 weeks old showed responsiveness at an earlier age (111). PHA responsiveness in the thymus was first observed at 10 weeks' gestational age and in spleen and blood 3 to 4 weeks later. Bone marrow and hepatic lymphoid tissues did not respond. It was also observed that cord blood lymphocytes are more sensitive than adult lymphocytes to low concentrations of PHA. The same sequence of appearance of PHA responsiveness in different tissues has been observed by other workers (35,140). These studies indicate the importance of considering dose-response kinetics when interpreting results of PHA stimulation. It is of interest that the beginning of spleen reactivity to PHA appears to correspond with the morphologic differentiation of the cuff surrounding central arterioles in the spleen (thymic-dependent areas) (35).

The response of thymocytes to PHA increases until 18 weeks of gestation. Thereafter, the reactivity declines to adult levels. These relationships appear to correlate with the development of the thymic medulla (44). In general, the responsiveness of fetal organs to PHA is directly correlated with age.

Peripheral blood lymphocytes of full-term newborn infants (62,111,142) and premature infants (142) have been reported to have higher responses to PHA than adult peripheral blood lymphocytes. Other workers have indicated decreased (44,138,143) or similar reactivity to PHA (63,64,144–146). These differences can be best explained by methodological variations in PHA dosage and timing of reading, as well as baseline metabolic activity of cord blood lymphocytes, which is markedly higher than that of adult peripheral blood lymphocytes. How one analyzes the lymphoblastic response is of great importance. Figure 8 shows the curve obtained when a transformation index, the ratio of stimulated to unstimulated culture, is used. It is evident that cord blood lymphocyte responses are lower than adult peripheral lymphocytes. If net counts per minute (CPM) are used (CPM of stimulated cells minus CPM of unstimulated cells) instead of the stimulation index, the resulting conclusions are completely different. Figure 9 shows that cord blood lymphocyte responses to PHA are higher than adult peripheral lymphocytes at lower doses of PHA. At higher doses the responses are very similar. It is also of interest that a fetal plasma factor (143) that suppresses and a monocyte factor

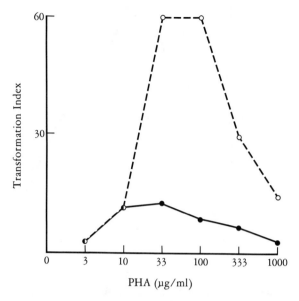

Figure 8. PHA dose-response curve of both cord (●———●) and adult (○ – – – – ○) mononuclear cells when transformation index is used in the calculations:

$$\text{Transformation index} = \frac{\text{CPM of PHA stimulated MNC cultures}}{\text{CPM of unstimulated MNC cultures}}$$

(151) that decreases the response of adult peripheral blood lymphocytes to phytohemagglutinin have been described. The PHA responses of premature infants at their estimated full-term birthday are similar to the responses of adult blood lymphocytes and are reduced when compared with the responses of full-term and premature newborn infants (142,147). This difference might be due to environmental influences.

Response of Fetal Lymphocytes to Allogeneic Cells (Mixed Lymphocyte Culture Reaction)

The mixed lymphocyte culture (MLC) reaction occurs when lymphocytes of two immunologically different individuals are cultured together. In order for the reaction to be studied, proliferation of one set of cells must be first inhibited by treatment with mitomycin C or irradiation. This method is used to detect cell surface antigens. Antigens detected by this assay are known as lymphocyte-defined (LD) antigens. Mixed lymphocyte culture reactions are known to depend on differences encoded by a chromosomal segment called HLA-D, located outside the HLA-B locus on the sixth human chromosome. Although the responsive cell type in the human is not completely known, MLC reactions appear to correlate very closely with cell-mediated immune responsiveness. Seigler et al. (148) have reported the presence of histocompatibility antigens in a fetus of 6 weeks' gestation. MLC responses are first detected in fetal liver as early as 7.5 weeks (149) to 9 weeks (140). The response is earlier than PHA reactivity and precedes MLC reactivity of thymus, which has been noted at various ages ranging from 12 weeks (6,150) or 13 weeks (151) to 16 weeks (152). Analogous observations have been made in combined immunodeficiency patients (153–155). These dissociations between

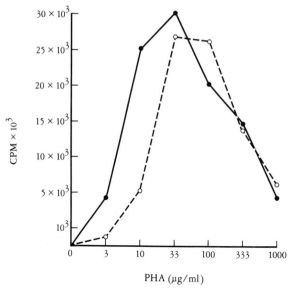

Figure 9. PHA dose-response curve of both cord (●——●) and adult (○----○) mononuclear cells when net counts per minute are used in the calculations:

$$\frac{\text{Net counts}}{\text{per minute}} = \text{CPM of stimulated cultures} - \text{CPM unstimulated}$$

After Carr, M. C., Stites, D. P., Fudenberg, H. H.: Cellular immune aspects of the human fetal-maternal relationship. I. In vitro response of cord blood lymphocytes to phytohemagglutinin. *Cell. Immunol.* 5:21–9, 1972.

MLC reaction and PHA responsiveness are not yet completely understood. However, there is evidence that the human fetal liver probably contains prethymic stem cells (26,140). These observations have been exploited in the initial attempts at immunore-constitutions of six patients with cell-mediated immune deficiencies (27). MLC reactions of the spleen and peripheral blood are seen at 14 to 15 weeks (137).

Cord blood is more active in mixed lymphocyte culture reactions than is adult blood (156,157). The maternal serum appears to provide a compensatory mechanism in the form of a factor that inhibits the MLC as well as the PHA reactions of the newborn infant (158). Fetal cells appear to be as effective as adult lymphocytes in stimulating MLC reactions. Splenic lymphocytes from 13- to 23-week human fetuses are more active than thymocytes from 18- to 23-week fetuses in producing a localized graft-versus-host reaction (GVHR) in the rat kidney capsule (159). These splenic lymphocytes already exhibit GHVR comparable with that of adult lymphocytes. (159).

Cell-Mediated Lympholysis (CML)
It is known that lymphocytes have a natural capacity for spontaneous cytotoxicity (129). They can also be induced to destroy target cells nonspecifically, by either mitogen stimulation or MLC reactions with foreign cells. In the presence of PHA, lymphocytes from the thymus of the 16-week fetus are capable of cytotoxic lysis of xenogeneic cells (150). Earlier ages have not been investigated. Cord blood lymphocytes can also be induced by PHA to exhibit cytotoxicity toward xenogeneic cells (111). The nature of the effector cell is not yet clearly established. Other tissues from 14- to 18-week-old fetuses

vary in their CML capacity induced by phytohemagglutinin. Thymocytes react vigorously to PHA but fail to produce target cell destruction. The opposite effect is observed with bone marrow lymphocytes. The peripheral blood and splenic lymphocytes from the same fetuses showed good proliferative responses to PHA and good cytotoxic capacity. Liver lymphoid cells do not respond in either test. Campbell et al. (160) have reported very low PHA-induced (CML) cytotoxicity against Chang cells. We have observed that cord blood lymphocytes have natural cytotoxicity (NK cells) for myelogenous leukemia cell line K562, as measured in a 4-hr ^{51}Cr release assay (unpublished data). McConnachie et al. (161) have reported that cord blood exhibits extremely low levels of antibody-dependent cellular cytotoxicity (ADCC) against human lymphocytes sensitized with HL-A antibodies. Conversely, Campbell et al. (160), using as a target Chang human liver cells sensitized with anti-Chang antiserum, have found that ADCC activity of cord blood is close to adult values. Using the same system, we had similar preliminary results. Interestingly enough, when we performed natural cytotoxicity and ADCC assays at the same time, they both exhibited parallel results. More recently, Shore et al. (162) found that the ADCC of cord blood against herpes simplex virus type I and II (HSV) infected Chang cells was apparently lower than ADCC activity of adult blood. They found ADCC only if the mother had neutralizing antibodies to HSV. It is worthwhile to stress that absolute numbers of mononuclear cells in cord blood almost doubles the absolute numbers of mononuclear cells in adult peripheral blood. Therefore, any lymphocyte subpopulation that in relative numbers may appear to be lower in cord blood, when compared with adult blood, might not be so in absolute numbers. Using analogous reasoning, Shore et al. (162) concluded that ADCC activity of whole cord blood is similar to the ADCC activity of whole adult blood. At present most evidence supports the suggestion that K and NK are the same cells but that they have two different cytolytic mechanisms. No conclusion as to the maturational state of K and NK cells at birth can be drawn.

Lymphokines

Lymphokines are biologically active factors that can be detected in cell-free supernatants of antigen- or mitogen-stimulated mononuclear cells. Although the cellular source of the great majority of lymphokine activities is still unknown, T lymphocytes have been shown to be the source of some lymphokines such as migration inhibitory factor (MIF). It is by no means clear, however, that T lymphocytes are the only source of lymphokines; production by other cells has in fact been demonstrated. There is evidence to suggest that the monocyte could be a source of some lymphokines (110), particularly those with mitogenic and chemotactic activities. Cord sera have been reported to generate less chemotactic activity for PMN's than do adult sera (106). However, the degree to which these deficiencies reflect the development of complement, lymphokines, or both remains to be demonstrated. Production of lymphocyte-derived chemotactic factor (LDCF) in the absence of stimulation is significantly higher in cord blood lymphocytes than in adult lymphocytes (109). However, phytohemagglutinin brings about only a modest increase of LDCF in cord blood (109); similar effects have been observed for other lymphokines (163). Hahn et al. (164) have reported that cord blood lymphocytes (possibly T cells) produce leukocyte migration inhibition factor (LIF), probably in quantities similar to those produced in adults. In contrast, Handzel (165) has observed that without antigenic stimulation newborns produce only half as much

LIF as adults. Recently, it has been reported that supernatants from cord blood monocytes inhibit normal lymphocyte response to PHA and also inhibit MLC and lymphokine production (110). Eife et al. (163) have shown that lymphotoxin production (LT) is 40% lower in newborns than in adults. The same authors have reported that the dissociation between blast transformation and lymphotoxin production observed in full-term newborns is even more striking in preterm newborns. They also found that the amount of lymphotoxin was correlated with gestational age but not with birthweight.

Interferon is one of the best known lymphokines. It is released by different cells, including lymphocytes, when they are infected with viruses or stimulated by polynucleotides. The main function of these cellular products is to inhibit intracellular viral replication; they also play a role in the recovery phase of viral infection. Fortunately the levels of interferon produced by lymphocytes from fetuses, newborn infants, or adults are no different (166). Nonetheless, the difficulties encountered by children with T-cell deficiencies in coping with viral infections indicate that if interferon is the major factor of recovery, it may be correlated in some way with the operation of cell-mediated immune mechanisms. In conclusion it can be said that developmental analysis of CMI systems strongly suggests that, besides the classical T or E-RFC, there are other subpopulations of lymphocytes responsible for CMI reactions.

Humoral System or B-Cell System and Products

Of all the immunologic systems, the humoral or B-cell system is the best studied. The reason for this is that the B-cell antigen receptors, which are immunoglobulin molecules, are relatively well characterized, unlike those of the CMI system. Moreover, the products—antibody molecules—resulting from recognition of antigens by the B cell have been studied in amazing detail. On the basis of animal and so-called "experiments of nature," several models of B-cell differentiation have been proposed. These models have practical significance for the pediatrician, clinical immunologist, and perinatologist. The most popular model of B-cell development, proposed by Cooper et al. (167), is based primarily on elegant studies performed in the chicken. These studies divide the differentiation pathway into two discontinuous stages. In the first stage (clonal development), differentiation begins in the bursa of Fabricius or other, analogous organs, in the case of the mammal, in the absence of antigen. At this time IgM antibodies are synthesized; most of these are incorporated into the cell membrane. The resultant antibody-bearing cells switch from synthesis of IgM ($C\mu$) to express IgG ($C\gamma$) and later switch from IgG to IgA ($A\alpha$). Investigators suggest that IgE and IgD may arise in a similar fashion, but there is no direct experimental evidence on this point. The second stage of differentiation (clonal selection) is antigen-dependent and comprises all the differentiative events of the humoral immune response. With appropriate cooperation of macrophages and T lymphocytes, the B lymphocytes are stimulated to proliferate; they form memory cells and undergo terminal differentiation to antibody-secreting plasma cells. This model is actually oversimplified and contains many experimental gaps, particularly in the development from stem cells to IgM cells.

In mice, the process of B-cell development is different from that which occurs in the chicken. The switch from IgM to IgG production occurs under the influence of antigen (168–173). The human B-cell system, like that of the chicken, appears to develop early in fetal life under the influence of a microenvironment supposedly free of antigenic stimuli. The first cell to appear (pre-B cell) bears first intracytoplasmic IgM, then surface IgM; cells bearing IgG appear next, followed by cells bearing IgA markers. Since these different cells appear in an orderly fashion from fetus to fetus, Lawton et al. (173) argue that their development does not necessarily depend on contact with antigen. One fact favorable to this model is that cells have been observed to switch from IgM to IgG; this switch occurs, for example, in cultured myeloma cells containing surface-bound IgM and intracytoplasmic IgG. Moreover, patients with infantile types of agammaglobulinemia are deficient in surface IgM (S-IgM) but have normal proportions of pre-B cells that cannot be stimulated to produce surface immunoglobulins (174). Adult percentages of IgA-bearing lymphocytes are present in the 15-week-old fetus; yet adult levels of IgA are not usually seen until puberty, when the thymus is aplastic. To explain this fact, it has been suggested that active IgA synthesis requires some kind of T-cell influence. This has been shown to be the case in some immune deficiencies, in which increased T-cell suppressor activity is responsible for the lack of IgG synthesis (175).

A particularly puzzling problem in the differentiation of B cells from stem cells in mammals is whether a unique lymphoid environment, analogous to the bursa of Fabricius, is required. The bone marrow (176) and the gut-associated lymphoid tissue

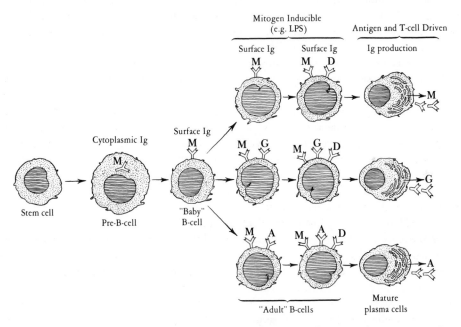

Figure 10. Mammalian B-cell differentiation model. B cells differentiate from a stem cell to a rapidly dividing Pre-B cell lacking functional antibody receptors. These cells initially synthesize cytoplasmic IgM that later become surface IgM ("baby" B cells). These "baby" B cells can be easily made tolerant and are pivotal for further differentiation of immunoglobulin-producing cells. While they continue to express surface IgM, they begin to express one of the surface IgG subclasses or IgA, followed later by the appearance of surface IgD. When these "double" or "triple" cells are triggered by antigen, T-cell help or B-cell mitogens, they become mature plasma cells or memory cells (not illustrated in this figure). The antigen-dependent T-cell driven stage requires the presence of surface IgD that is lost after antigenic stimulation. After Cooper, M. D., et al., in Bellanti, J. A. *Immunology II*. Philadelphia, W. B. Saunders Co., 1978.

(GALT) (177) were originally suggested as the equivalent organ. There is now evidence (173) that GALT is not the bursal equivalent. There are also strong suggestions that bone marrow, although not exclusively (178,179), constitutes one of the equivalents of the bursa. All the evidence (173,179) indicates that the human fetal liver is the first and probably the main organ that plays the role of bursa of Fabricius. Fetal liver occupies the central role in B-cell development, as it probably does in T-cell development. Recently Cooper et al., using newer data particularly related to IgD development, have postulated a more complete model for mammalian B-cell differentiation (Fig. 10) (180). The products secreted by the B cells are covered in the next section.

MATERNAL–FETAL RELATIONSHIPS

One of the most challenging problems in developmental biology is the maternal accept-ance of a fetus bearing foreign, paternal antigens. This maternal-fetal relationship is known to play a prime role in regulating the humoral immunological development of the fetus. Its influence in CMI is only beginning to be studied. In order to explain the acceptance of this allograft transplant by the mother, it has been postulated that (1) the uterus is an immunologically privileged organ, (2) maternal hyporeactivity occurs dur-ing pregnancy, (3) histocompatibility antigens are absent from the fetal-placental unit, or (4) there is a protective barrier between the uterus and the placenta.

Of the hypotheses just enumerated, only the last is supported by evidence convincing enough to explain at least partially the survival of this successful natural tissue graft (181). Relative maternal tolerance during pregnancy has not been considered sufficient to explain by itself a phenomenon of such magnitude. However, recent experimental evidence has revived interest in this hypothesis. Finn et al. (182), using a bidirectional MLC reaction, found tolerance between maternal and fetal lymphocytes. This tolerance appears to require some factor elaborated by fetal cells; it is not seen if the fetal lymphocytes are not viable (one-direction MLC). Rocklin et al. (183) have recently described the absence of a blocking factor in women with chronic abortions; this factor inhibits MIF produced against paternal alloantigens.

The presence of a barrier of fibrinoid material that covers the antigenic determinants of the trophoblast has been definitely proved. By acting as a mechanical barrier, the placenta allows only tiny amounts of formed blood elements to be interchanged between mother and conceptus. However, some antibodies gain access to the fetus very easily and provide protection or, less often, produce deleterious effects. Brambell (184) has extensively studied the transfer of immunoglobulins from mother to conceptus. The Fc fragment is known to play an important role in the transfer, since isolated Fc fragments are passed but Fab fragments are not (185). There are different pathways by which the maternal antibodies are transmitted to the fetus; their relative importance varies from species to species (186) (Table X). In species with large numbers of membranes intervening between the maternal and fetal circulation, the colostrum appears to be the most important route of transfer of antibodies; newborns absorb these antibodies from the gastrointestinal (GI) tract. However, in mammals with fewer placental layers, as is the case in humans, the transplacental transfer of antibodies appears to have assumed greater importance. This by no means detracts from the immunological significance of

Table X. Relationship of Type of Placentation With Character of Maternal-Fetal Transfer of Antibody in Various Species

Animal	Number of Placental Membranes	Relative Importance* of Route	
		Placental	Colostral
Pig	6		
Horse	6	0	+++
Sheep, cow	5	0	+++
Cat, dog	5	+	++
Rat, mouse	4	+	++
Rabbit, guinea pig	3	+++	±
Man, monkey	3	+++	0

SOURCE: Bellanti, J. A. (ed.). *Immunology II.* Philadelphia, W. B. Saunders Co., 1978.

* The relative importance is indicated arbitrarily from 0 (unimportant) to +++ (very important).

breast feeding in humans. For example, the secretory IgA molecules found in breast milk, although not significantly absorbed in the human, have a unique structure that renders them effective in the GI tract and may explain the lowered incidence of enteric and respiratory infections seen in breast-fed infants. In another study (187), GI tract colonization by *E. coli* was found to be significantly diminished in breast-fed as compared with formula-fed infants. This observation could be explained on the basis that lymphocytes reactive to K1 *E. coli* antigen and anti-K1 antibody are present in the milk of women carrying this organism.

The development of serum immunoglobulins during intrauterine and postnatal life is shown schematically in Figure 11. The concentration of immunoglobulin, almost exclusively IgG at birth, may be lower or higher than that of the mother. There are few or no IgA and IgM globulins present in cord blood. The fetus is usually protected in utero from antigenic stimuli and therefore is not called on to synthesize these immunoglobulins actively under normal circumstances. However, if the fetus is challenged in utero as a consequence of immunization, such as immunization of the mother with salmonella (188), or infection (congenital rubella, cytomegalovirus infection, toxoplasmosis), it will respond by producing antibody; the antibody is largely of the IgM variety (189,190). The exclusion of other classes of antibody benefits the fetus in many cases. For example, the exclusion of IgM isohemagglutinins, leukoagglutinins, and the IgE-associated antibodies of allergy prevents major diseases that could be produced by these antibodies. However, it also precludes the passage of other maternal antibodies that would be beneficial to the newborn such as the IgM antibodies, which are important in defense against gram-negative bacterial infection (Table XI); these include the opsonins, agglutinins, and bactericidal antibodies. This lack of transfer may partially explain the increased susceptibility of the newborn to infection with gram-negative organisms such as *Escherichia coli* (191).

The types of antibodies that the fetus obtains by placental transfer vary greatly (Table XI). This variation reflects, in part, the quantity of antibodies in the maternal

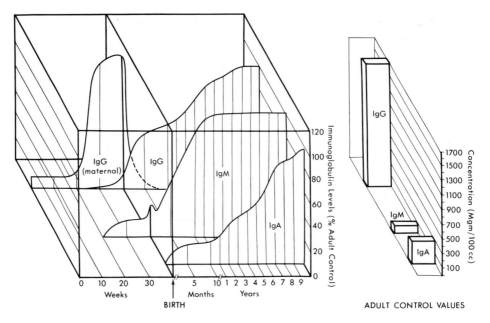

Figure 11. Human postnatal development of serum immunoglobulins. After Alford, C. A., Jr., in Bellanti, J. A. *Immunology II.* Philadelphia, W. B. Saunders Co., 1978.

circulation as well as their molecular structure. For example, low molecular weight IgG antibodies, such as rubeola antibody, which are present in high concentrations in maternal serum, are readily transferred. IgG antibodies, such as those against *Bordetella pertussis,* are present in lower concentrations; they are poorly transferred. Macroglobulin antibodies, such as the Wasserman antibody, are completely excluded. Maternal antibodies that have harmful effects are presented in Table XII. In this framework, we now review the ontogenic development of each individual immunoglobulin.

Table XI. Relationship of Antibody Type With Transplacental Transfer

Good Passive Transfer	Poor Passive Transfer	No Passive Transfer
Diphtheria antitoxin	Hemophilus influenzae	Enteric somatic (0)
Tetanus antitoxin	Bordetella pertussis	antibodies (Salmonella,
Antierythrogenic toxin	Shigella flexneri	Shigella, E. coli)
Antistaphylococcal antibody	Streptococcus MG	Skin-sensitizing antibody
Samonella flagella (H) antibody		Heterophile antibody
Antistreptolysin		Wasserman antibody
All antiviral antibodies		
present in maternal circulation (rubeola,		
rubella, mumps, poliovirus)		
VDRL antibodies		

SOURCE: Bellanti, J. A. (ed.). *Immunology II.* Philadelphia, W. B. Saunders Co., 1978.

Immunoglobulin (Ig) M

Intracellular IgM (pre-B cell) has been seen in the liver of a 7.5-week-old fetus. SIg appears in the liver between 9.5 and 12.5 weeks' gestational age (179). The synthesis of IgM in the human is seen in the spleen at 10.5 weeks of gestation and increases gradually (113). By 11.5 weeks, some IgM is produced by peripheral blood lymphocytes. By approximately 17.5 weeks of gestation, the thymus can also manufacture small amounts of IgM (192). IgM is present in the serum of fetuses earlier than 13 weeks (193). By 15 to 20 weeks of gestation, more than half of the fetuses have detectable levels of serum IgM, some as high as 4 mg%. The level of IgM then increases steadily, and at term the mean concentration is from 13 to 15 mg%. The standard deviation, however, is as great as the mean concentration (193). The serum IgM level reaches adult normal values at about 1 year (194).

Immunoglobulin (Ig) A

Synthesis of this immunoglobulin by the conceptus has not been clearly established. In cases of intrauterine infection, cord serum IgA levels may be higher than normal. Whether this represents synthesis or transplacental transfer is not clear (195,196). IgA molecules do traverse the placenta but at very low rates. The transfer is faster during the first trimester (113), resulting in levels of as much as 10 mg% between 6.5 and 17 weeks of gestation. During the last trimester values range from less than 1 mg% to values below detectable levels (113,193). After birth IgA levels remain low until the third week of life, when they start increasing slowly. Adult levels are reached at about the time of puberty.

Immunoglobulin (Ig) D

The IgD has been found in tissue cultures of fetuses of 11 weeks of gestation (192). Five to eight percent of normal cord blood specimens contain levels of IgD above 2 mg% (197,198). Only 80% of adults have serum levels of IgD above 1 mg%.

Table XII. Maternal Antibodies Which Can Lead to Harmful Effects in the Infant

Maternal Disease	Antibodies	Effect on Newborn
Hyperthyroidism	LATS	Transient hyperthyroidism (exophthalmos)
Idiopathic thrombocytopenia	Platelet antibodies	Transient thrombocytopenia
Isoimmunization (platelets, neutrophils, red blood cells)	Platelet, neutrophil, isohemagglutinins or $Rh_0(D)$ antibodies	Transient thrombocytopenia, neutropenia, anemia
Lupus erythematosus	Autoantibodies to blood elements (LE cell factor, Coombs test, platelet)	Transient LE cell phenomenon, neutropenia, thrombocytopenia, ? congenital heart disease
Myasthenia gravis	Not defined yet	Transient neonatal myasthenia gravis

SOURCE: Modified from Bellanti, J. A. (ed.). *Immunology II.* Philadelphia, W. B. Saunders Co., 1978.

Immunoglobulin (Ig) E

Synthesis of IgE begins at 11 weeks of gestational age, mainly in the liver and lungs (199). This immunoglobulin very slowly crosses the placenta (200) but in minute quantities. The cord blood at term has a level equal to 1% of the mother's level at delivery (201,202). The mean maternal level is 20 to 25 μg/100 ml. At 6 weeks after birth (201,202) the IgE level is 2.5 times that at birth, and at 6 months 10 times the 6-week level (25% of the mean adult level) (200). IgE levels vary widely as a function of genetic factors and environmental stimulation (202).

Immunoglobulin (Ig) G

IgG is present in the serum of the human embryo as early as 4.5 weeks of gestation, with levels remaining at about 5 to 8% of adult values until 15 weeks' gestation (192). The fetal liver and gastrointestinal tract begin IgG production at 11 weeks' gestation, but their contribution is insignificant between 11 and 15 weeks (113). By 18 weeks of gestation, the spleen becomes the principal site of IgG synthesis; this shift in the site of synthesis coincides with a rise of serum IgG values to 10 to 20% of adult values (192). By 26 weeks of gestation, levels reach maternal values (192). Because placental transfer of IgG operates more effectively at relatively low maternal IgG concentrations, the serum level in the infant tends to be higher than that of the mother when maternal concentration is less than 1.6 g/100 ml and lower than that of the mother when the maternal level exceeds 1.6 g/100 ml (203). Immunoglobulins G are mainly passively transferred, and they have a half-life of 20 to 30 days. IgG synthesis takes a significant upturn at 2 weeks to 2 months, then declines rapidly within the first few months of life, and is at its lowest between the second and third months (300 to 600 mg/100 ml, the point at which IgG production equals IgG destruction) (192). During this phase, referred to as physiologic hypogammaglobulinemia, the infant may be susceptible to recurrent infections. During the first few years gamma globulin concentrations increase, mainly because the maturing infant is exposed to antigens in his environment and keeps gaining experience.

There appears to be a sequential development of gamma globulins at different ages: the IgM attains adult concentrations by 1 year of age, the IgG by 5 to 6 years of age, and the IgA by 10 years of age. This pattern of appearance of immunoglobulins recapitulates that which is seen in phylogeny and also appears to parallel the pattern observed after an antigenic exposure during the primary immune response. Morell et al. (204) found that the placental passage of the four subclasses of immunoglobulin G is equally efficient. However, the rate and age of onset of the synthesis for the various subclasses is different. IgG$_3$ rises to considerable levels during the prenatal period and after 3 months reaches adult levels. IgG$_1$ synthesis begins before the third month of postnatal life; concentrations are close to adult levels at 8 months of age. IgG$_2$ and IgG$_4$ production is still far below adult levels at 2 years of age. Exchange transfusion appears to delay the production of the infant's own IgG, an effect that persists for 1 year. Exchange transfusion also delays synthesis of IgA for a short period after birth, whereas it accelerates production of IgM. The mechanism of this effect remains obscure (205).

IMMUNOLOGICAL EVALUATION OF THE NEWBORN INFANT

At this point it seems fair to say that evaluation of the immune system during the prenatal period is by no means an easy task. The evaluator must take into consideration the dynamic, rapidly growing, adaptive, and changing parameters of the immune function in response to a changing internal and external environment. Thus, study of the newborn immune system has to be undertaken with an open mind. Since there are many controversial issues and few known facts, virtually anything that is said can be challenged. In Table XIII are shown some of the major classes of immune deficiencies that can be diagnosed in the newborn period, together with their time of onset and the type of infection that are typically associated with them. However, a detailed history with emphasis on family background, and a careful physical examination, should offer a solid foundation for interpretation of clinical and research laboratory data. Clinical immunology is a relatively young discipline to be speaking in terms of "typical presentation of diseases," particularly in the field of cell-mediated immunity, where with few exceptions the typical is still the atypical. Table XIV presents some suggestions for the clinical evaluation of the newborn. Table XV lists some of the pertinent clinical and historical information that could be useful in the diagnosis of immune deficiency disorders in the newborn period. Although most immunological defects that we see are not usually clinically apparent until postnatal life, it is not unlikely that in certain instances the result of an immunological deficiency may be intrauterine infection with a resultant damaged baby at birth or an aborted conceptus. Zuelzer et al. (206) and others have shown maternal blood–formed elements in fetal circulation. Theoretically, therefore, early passage of immunologically active mononuclear cells from the mother to the fetus could be responsible for graft-versus-host (GVH) reaction. Although direct proof of GVH reactions in the fetus is lacking, several clinical situations suggest that such processes may occur in the newborn and fetus (207). Among these can be cited the report of a XX/XY chimerism in a 12-week-old abortus of a mother who had a number of repeated "spontaneous" abortions (208). A case was reported by Naiman (209) in which, following three exchange transfusions, the infant developed jaundice, aplastic anemia, and marked histiocytosis. This infant also had chimerism, with one line representing donor cells. The striking clinical and histopathological resemblance between GVH reactions and congenital Letterer-Siwe disease (210) and some of the familiar reticuloendothelioses have made some investigators consider the reticuloendothelioses (211) potential examples of GVH reactions.

Evaluation of the Humoral Immune System

Table XVI summarizes the evaluation of the humoral immune system. In general, pure humoral immune deficiency syndromes are not clinically manifested in the prenatal period because of the protective effect of maternal IgG. However, very premature infants, particularly those born at less than 32 weeks' gestation, may have IgG serum levels below 400 mg% (212). Small-for-date infants also have decreased IgG (213), some impairment of specific antibody responses (e.g., to attenuated polio virus), reduction in specific IgA secretory antibody responses (214), and an increased incidence of antibodies to food (215). Another factor to be considered is hypogammaglobulinemia in the mother, which, although rare, would lead to inadequate levels of IgG in the newborn. Other ways to evaluate the humoral immunologic system are described below.

Table XIII. Immune Deficiency Disorders Which Can Be Diagnosed in the Newborn Period

Disorder	Example	Genetics	Time of Onset	Type of Infection
Phagocytic function:				
Quantitative	Neutropenia	Variable	At birth	Virulent bacteria, e.g., staphylococcus
Qualitative	Chronic granulomatous disease	X-linked, autosomal recessive	At birth	Less virulent bacteria, staphylococcus, monilia
Antibody	Agammaglobulinemia Dysgammaglobulinemia	Variable	>6 months, earlier if premature or small for dates	Virulent bacteria
Cell-mediated (delayed hypersensitivity) function	Congenital aplasia of thymus (Di Georges syndrome)	Variable	At birth	Fungal, viral
Combined antibody and cell-mediated function	"Swiss" agammaglobulinemia	Autosomal recessive, X-linked	At birth	Bacterial, viral, fungal, Pneumocystus carinii
Graft vs. host reactions	Spontaneous abortion Fetal transfusion for hemolytic diseases	Nongenetic	At birth; could be later, but no data available	
Combined	Congenital asplenia	Variable	At birth or later	Gram negative
C$_5$ complement deficiency or Leiner disease		Variable	At birth	Gram negative
Variable	Ataxia telangiectasia Wiskott-Aldrich syndrome	Autosomal recessive X-Linked recessive	>6 months >6 months	Fungal, viral

SOURCE: Modified from Bellanti, J. A. (ed.). *Immunology II.* Philadelphia, W. B. Saunders Co., 1978.

Table XIV. Few Remainders for the Clinical Evaluation of Immune System in the Newborn

---

History

Previous newborn deaths in the family; history of immune diseases

Previous isoimmunization in mother (due to pregnancy or transfusions [Rh, ABO], gamma globulin administration)

Previous diseases in the mother (autoimmune diseases, e.g., SLE, thyroiditis, myasthenia gravis, idiopathic thrombocytopenic purpura)

History of medications in mother (quinine, guinidine, Sedormid, Clorpromazine)

History of Infections during pregnancy (rubella, cytomegalic inclusion disease, toxoplasmosis, syphilis, herpes simplex, UTI, vaginal infections, T.B.)

Physical Examination

General appearance (assess degree of activity: hyperactivity, consider hyperthyroidism, passive transfer of LATS; hypoactivity or muscle weakness, consider myasthenia gravis with transfer of antibodies to muscle; purpura, consider thrombocytopenia due to the passive transfer of antibodies to platelets.)

Skin (jaundice in first 24 hr; petechiae are characteristic of isoimmunization, e.g., erythroblastosis fetalis)

Eyes (exophthalmos due to LATS)

Chest (pneumonitis seen in many intrauterine infections)

Cardiovascular (evaluate murmurs for congenital heart disease, e.g., infants of LES mothers)

Abdomen (hepatosplenomegaly: seen in severe erythroblastosis fetalis, also in congenital intrauterine infections and GVH reactions, spleen absence)

Extremities (note deformities and other birth defects)

Neurological (convulsions, weakness)

SOURCE: Bellanti, J. A. (ed.). *Immunology II*. Philadelphia, W. B. Saunders Co., 1978.

Evaluation of the Cell-Mediated Immune System

Table XVII summarizes the evaluation of the cell-mediated immune system of the newborn. Evaluation of the CMI system begins with a total and differential white cell count. Lymphopenia is seen in most of the cell-mediated immune deficiencies, but at times the lymphocyte count may be normal (see Table VI). E$^+$RFC should be quantitated and the total number of T lymphocytes calculated from the WBC value and the percentage of lymphocytes. It should be stressed that E$^+$RFC determinations do not constitute a functional test. Technical details and adequate age-adjusted controls are necessary, since normal numbers for different ages have not yet been established. B-cell determination should be done, using EAC (erythrocyte antibody complement complex) rosettes and by direct immunofluorescence. EAC techniques take advantage of the receptors of B cells for C3b and C3d complement components. The antibody anti-red cell used should be of IgM rather than IgG type to overcome the problem of EA (erythrocyte-antibody complex) rosettes, formed by lymphocytes with receptors for the Fc part of IgG. Fc receptors for IgG are present not only in B cells but also in T and "null" cells. Therefore, apparently normal or augmented numbers of B cells can be detected. The direct immunofluorescence uses antiserum against the B-cell surface immunoglobulins. We prefer to use the Fab$'_2$ fraction of rabbit antihuman immunoglobulins. The use

Table XV. Diagnostic Clues in Suspecting Immune Deficiency Disorders in the Newborn Period

Finding	Comments

Hypocalcemic tetany:
  Absence of thymic shadow
  Moniliasis
	DiGeorge syndrome—diagnosed by DNCB skin testing, in vitro lymphocyte stimulation with phytohemagglutinin, and MLR

History of immune deficiency in other family members	Most immunologic defects genetically determined, and sex-linked most common
Agammaglobulinemia	Quantitative immunoglobulins not useful because of passive transfer of IgG, determination after 2 to 4 months helpful in establishing diagnosis; allotypes helpful
Chronic granulomatous disease	NBT helpful as screening test only because may be nonspecifically elevated; tests of bactericidal function fail to reach normal values in presence of adult sera
Poor growth, splenomegaly, hepatomegaly, diffuse dermatitis, diarrhea	GVH—laboratory findings include anemia, decrease in serum complement, histiocytic infiltration of bone marrow and erythrophagocytosis
Holly Jolly bodies in peripheral smear, absence of spleen, shadow in x-ray	Congenital absence of spleen and other associated malformations
Seborrheic dermatitis	C5 deficiency (Leiner disease)
Chronic diarrhea	Defect in phagocytosis of Baker's yeast particles, secondary to failure of sera to opsonize yeast

of whole rabbit IgG antihuman immunoglobulins, as well as EA complex, can yield misleading results, particularly in cases of severe combined immune deficiency (SCID); this approach can show apparently normal numbers of B cells, which in reality represent Fc receptor-positive cells that have recognized the Fc part of the IgG molecule. If E^+RFC are low, a thymosin induction of E^+RFC will give a good indication, although not definite proof, of the patient's probable response to thymic hormones. If CMI deficiency is suspected before birth, cord blood lymphocytes can be used in thymosin induction of E^+RFC. Normally cord blood contains lymphocytes that can be induced to E^+RFC when incubated with thymosin (130). Absence of this response indicates a probable lack of E^+RFC precursors. A very low initial level of E^+RFC with a brisk thymosin response is more evidence to suggest a probable CMI deficiency syndrome that could respond to thymic hormone. Recently Shore et al. (216) reported a patient with partial CMI deficiency whose bone marrow lymphocytes responded to thymosin only after an "inductive" incubation period in a monolayer culture of epithelial thymic cells. This patient also had a larger than normal thymus, which at biopsy showed a lack of Hassall corpuscles.

Tests of lymphoproliferative responses should be performed, using different concentrations of T-cell mitogens, such as concanavalin A and phytohemagglutinin. Newborn lymphocytes seem to respond better than those of adults at low dosages of mitogens; at higher concentrations they are less responsive than adult lymphocytes

(111). MLC reactions may also be helpful in diagnosing CMI deficiencies. A dissociation of low phytohemagglutinin, with normal MLC, can be seen in some patients with CMI deficiency. On the basis of phylogeny and ontogeny, we may speculate that such a defect originates at a higher level of T-cell differentiation. Lack of MLC responses theoretically suggests a defect occurring earlier in ontogenic development. Determinations of enzymes such as adenine diaminase and nucleoside phosphorylase may help to clarify some of the cases of SCID and orient the clinician toward enzyme replacement therapy.

Radiologic examinations can show bony abnormalities in immune deficiencies with adenosine deaminase (ADA) deficiency, or absence of thymus, which is useful to the diagnostician only when observed in newborns younger than 4 days who have not been previously stressed. A barium swallow may reveal diffuse esophagitis, usually caused by monilia.

Skin testing with fungal, bacterial, and viral antigens for delayed hypersensitivity has not proved useful in the study of the newborn. Skin testing with PHA is claimed to be somewhat more sensitive (217). Contact sensitization to dinitrochlorobenzene (DNCB) offers advantages over intradermal testing (218). DNCB is positive in 90% of normal

Table XVI. Diagnostic Tests for Evaluation of the Humoral Immune Function in Neonates

Test	Comment
Quantitative measurement of immunoglobulins	May reveal elevated IgM or IgA; does not distinguish maternal from fetally produced IgG
B cell mitogen stimulation, e.g.., Pokeweed	As with PHA (routine test) Ig's synthesis determined in supernatant (research tool) or cell stained with intracytoplasmic immunofluorescence techniques
Genetic typing (Gm and Inv.)	Of help in determining origin of circulating immunoglobulins in newborn (not routine test)
IgG subclasses determination	IgG_3 increases in prenatal period and reaches adult levels after 3 months; $IgG_{1,2, and 4}$ close to adult levels many months (years) later
Determination of total number of B cells by EAC or direct immunofluorescence	Does not necessarily correlate with decrease Ig synthesis; helpful to elucidate level of B cell defect
Specific antibody responses de novo sensitization, e.g., salmonella	O antigen induce IgM; H antigen induce IgG
Regional lymph node biopsy after immunization	Helpful for humoral as well as CMI
Coculture of purified B cells from patient with normal T cells	No production of Igs indicates defective Ig production or release
Regional lymph node biopsy after immunization	Helpful for humoral as well as CMI

individuals (218), although Uhr (219) has observed that positive results are less intense and more inconsistent in young infants. If any doubt exists regarding humoral immunity, the last resort is antigenic stimulation with a variety of vaccines, e.g., salmonella or other antigens, followed by a regional lymph node biopsy looking for B- and T-dependent areas. Paired serum specimens taken prior to and after immunization should be studied for specific antibodies. Virus infections sometimes depress CMI, and some of the patients who are referred to us may show anergy because of persistent viral infections. In these cases, sound medical judgment, patience, and repeated studies are necessary. Fetal growth retardation and malnutrition also depress cell-mediated

Table XVII. Diagnostic Tests for Evaluation of Cell-Mediated Immunity in Newborns

WBC and differential	Normal lymphocyte count does not rule out CMI deficiency; low count compatible but not diagnostic
Skin testing with DNCB	Positive result practically rules out CMI deficiency
	Negative or weak result does not confirm diagnosis of CMI deficiency
Immunization with antigens, e.g., diphtheria or tetanus toxoid	Positive in vitro lymphoblastic response to same antigen used for immunization; or MIF release by same Ag compatible with at least partially CMI is present (not routine test)
Determination of absolute number of E$^+$RFC	No functional test but correlates well with CMI status
Coculture of normal lymphocytes, or T lymphocyte, with lymphocytes from suspected patient	Can indicate defective Ig's production due to increase suppressor T-cell activity or decrease in helper T-cell activity
Mitogen stimulation of lymphocytes, e.g., PHA	Optimum, suboptimum as well as over optimum concentrations of PHA should be used
MLR	Could be positive in absence of responses to PHA
Determination of HLTA	Could be helpful in elucidating level of T cell impairment (not routine lab test, may be research tool)
Stimulation of HLTA and E$^+$RFC in PBL or BM	Good response suggests probable response to thymosin treatment (as above)
Thymic hormones determination in blood	Decrease in amount definitely makes diagnosis of thymic insufficiency; if present in normal amount would not necessarily rule out CMI deficiency (as above)
Lymph node biopsy after stimulation with de novo organism	To see if dependent areas are normal
Biopsy of thymus	To be performed in patients with obvious CMI; helps to elucidate different types of CMI deficiencies that could orient new therapeutic measures

Table XVIII. Diagnostic Tests for Polymorphonuclear Function in Newborns

Peripheral blood count and differential	Often of help, count important, Ex/Neutropenia; morphology of cells important, Ex/Chediak—Higashi
Skin window—Rebuck	May give general clue to defect of inflammatory function, particularly ability to marshal leukocytes to site of infection
Phagocytosis	Results vary with assay used; particle being phagocytized critical; assay used must distinguish humoral and cellular components of process
Chemotaxis	Decreased in cellular and humoral activity during neonatal period
Quantitative NBT	Screening test; if normal or high, does not rule out CGD
Bactericidal activity	Measured by direct killing assay; chronic granulomatous disease can be diagnosed during neonatal period
Measurement of specific WBC enzymes	Not done routinely

immune and humoral (213–215,220) responses for several months after birth. Evaluation of the nonspecific immune responses in the newborn is almost limited to testing polymorphonuclear leukocyte function with the Rebuck skin-window technique (Table XVIII), which has not yet been standarized for the newborn. The NBT test may be used as a screening test for chronic granulomatous disease (CGD); the results should be confirmed by bactericidal assay. Lowered numbers of complement components have been described in the prenatal and cord blood, as mentioned above. The extent to which these reflect actual functional abnormalities of complements is uncertain. Phagocytic tests should include evaluation of influences of C3 and C5. Separate evaluation of the complement effects on phagocytosis, chemotaxis, and bactericidal activities must be made. A functional deficiency of C5 activity has been described in Liener disease. Finally, monocyte function, although important, is not usually clinically evaluated because of a lack of adequate methods. Recently Poplack et al. (221) have shown evidence that in humans ADCC activity against red blood cells is dependent only on the monocyte. We hope that this test will prove to be of significance in the evaluation of the monocyte.

CONCLUSION

The neonate is not "immunologically null," it is immunologically nonexperienced and has only a relatively immature immune system. Most of the known immunologic mechanisms develop early in fetal life. At birth some are not fully developed, but maturation proceeds quickly, probably in response to environmental influences. Although the nonspecific defense mechanisms are of vital importance, observations of children with defects of the cell-mediated immune or humoral systems provide definitive proof that the development of specific acquired immune mechanisms is indispensible for survival in normal individuals. Today, as in the early age of immunology, studies of infections can contribute to our understanding of the basic mechanisms of immunity. The question that remains to be answered is what is the difference immunologically between the newborn that develops septicemia and the newborn that does not. Detailed study of pathogenesis and immunity in intrauterine or perinatal infections such as CMV infection, HSV infection, *E. coli* neonatal septicemia, and streptococcus in the newborn will yield a fuller explanation of inexperience and relative immaturity of immune mechanisms in the fetus and newborn infant. Of equal importance is the study of "experiments of nature." Better methods for evaluation of immunological compromise in the newborn are urgently needed. The human neonatal macrophage (monocyte) is the prime candidate for study. Impaired activity of this cell system would explain a number of unusual immune responses observed in the newborn and might provide the basis not only for new therapeutic approaches but for prevention of infectious diseases as well as allergic disorders.

REFERENCES

1. Bellanti, J. A. (ed.): *Immunology II.* Philadelphia, W. B. Saunders Co., 1978.

2. Hildemann, W. H., and Reddy, A. L.: Phylogeny of immune responsiveness: Marine invertebrates. *Federation Proceedings* 32, 1973.

3. Burnet, F. M.: Invertebrate precursors to immune responses, in Cooper, E. L. (ed.): *Contemporary Topics in Immunobiology,* Vol. 4, *Invertebrate Immunology.* New York and London, Plenum Press, 1974, p. 13.

4. Spiegel, M.: The reaggregation of dissociated sponge cells. *Ann. N.Y. Acad. Sci.* 60:1056, 1955.

5. McClay, D. R.: An autoradiographic analysis of the species specificity during sponge cell reaggregation. *Biol. Bull.* 141:319, 1971.

6. Carr, M. C., Stites, D. P., and Fudenberg, H. H.: Dissociation of responses to phytohemagglutinin and adult allogeneic lymphocytes in human foetal lymphoid tissues. *Nature New Biol.* 241:279, 1973.

7. Evans, E. E., Weinheimer, P. F., Acton, R. T., et al.: Induced bactericidal response in a sipunculid worm. *Nature* 222:695, 1969.

8. Evans, E. E., Painter, B., Evans, M. L., et al.: An induced bactericidin in the spiny lobster, *Panulirus argus. Proc. Soc. Exp. Bio. Med.* 128:394, 1968.

9. Weinheimer, P., Acton, R. T., Sawyer, S., et al.: Specificity of the induced bactericidin of the west Indian spiny lobster, *Panulirus argus. J. Bact.* 98:947, 1969.

10. Clem, L. W., and Leslie, G. A.: Phylogeny of immunoglobulin structure and function, in Adinolfi, M. (ed.): *Immunology and Development.* London, Spastics International Medical Publications, 1969, p. 62.

11. Borysenko, M.: Phylogeny of immunity: An overview. *Immunogenetics* 3:305, 1976.

12. Good, R. A., and Papermaster, B. W.: Ontogeny and phylogeny of adaptive immunity. *Adv. Immunol.* 4:1, 1964.

13. Thoenes, G. N., and Hildermann, W. H.: Immunological response of Pacific hagfish: II. Serum antibody production to soluble antigen, in Sterzl, J., and Rika, I. (eds.): *Developmental Aspects of Antibody Formation and Structure,* Vol. II. New York, Academic Press, Inc., 1970.

14. Dreyer, N. B., and King, J. W.: Anaphylaxis in the fish. *J. Immunol.* 60:277, 1948.

15. Ovary, Z.: Reverse passive cutaneous anaphylaxis in the guinea pig with horse, sheep or hen antibodies. *Immunology* 3:19, 1960.

16. Hirata, A., and Campbell, D. H.: Differential anaphylactic susceptibility of chicken and guinea pig intestine. *Proc. Soc. Exp. Biol.* 107:68, 1961.

17. Celada, F., and Ramos, A.: Passive cutaneous anaphylaxis in mice and chickens. *Proc. Soc. Exp. Biol.* 108:129, 1961.

18. Kubo, R. T., and Benedict, A. A.: Passive cutaneous anaphylaxis in chickens. *Proc. Soc. Exp. Biol.* 129:256, 1968.

19. Conway, A. M., van Alten, P. J., and Hirata, A. A.: Passive cutaneous anaphylactic-like reactions in young chicks. *Proc. Soc. Exp. Biol.* 129:694, 1968.

20. Moore, M. A. S., and Owen, J. J. T.: Chromosome marker studies in the irradiated chick embryo. *Nature* 215:1081, 1967.

21. Moore, M. A. S., and Metcalf, D.: Ontogeny of the haemopoietic system: Yolk sac origin of in vivo and in vitro colony forming cells in the developing mouse embryo. *Brit. J. Haemat.* 18:279, 1970.

22. Weiss, L., in Greep, R. O. (ed.): *Histology.* New York, McGraw-Hill, 1966, p. 326.

23. Copenhaver, W. W., in *Textbook of Histology.* Baltimore, Williams and Wilkins, 1964, p. 126.

24. Wintrobe, M. M.: *Clinical Hematology,* 6th ed. Philadelphia, Lea & Febiger, 1967.

25. Thomas, D. B., and Yoffey, J. M.: Human foetal haematopoiesis: II. Hepatic haematopoiesis in the human foetus. *Brit. J. Haemat.* 10:193, 1964.

26. Lowenberg, B.: Fetal liver cell transplantation: Role and nature of the fetal haematopoietic stem cell, thesis. Rotterdam, 1975.

27. Lowenberg, B., Vossen, J. M. J. J., and Dvoren, L. J.: Transplantation of fetal liver cells in the treatment of severe combined immunodeficiency disease. *Blut* 34:181, 1977.

28. Playfair, J. H. L., Wolfendale, M. R., and Kay, H. E. M.: The leukocytes of the peripheral blood in the human foetus. *Brit. J. Haemat.* 9:336, 1963.

29. Gilmour, J. R.: Normal haemopoiesis in intra-uterine and neonatal life. *J. Path. and Bact.* 52:55, 1941.

30. Silverstein, A. M., and Lukes, R. I.: Fetal response to antigenic stimulus: I. Plasma cellular and lymphoid reactions in the human fetus to intrauterine infection. *Lab. Invest.* 11:918, 1962.

31. Wood, C. B. S.: The development of immunity in fetal life and childhood. *J. Roy. Coll. Physcns. Lond.* 6:246, 1972.

32. Rosenberg, M.: Fetal hematopoiesis: Case report. *Blood* 33:66, 1969.

33. Valdes-Dapena, M. A.: *An Atlas of Fetal and Neonatal Histology.* Philadelphia, J. B. Lippincott Co., 1957.

34. Ono, L.: Untersuchungen uber die Entwicklung der menschlichen Milz. *Z. Zeliforsch. Mikr. Anat.* 10:573, 1930.

35. August, C. S., Berkel, A. J., Driscoll, et al.: Onset of lymphocyte function in the human fetus. *Pediatr. Res.* 5:539, 1971.

36. Jones, W. R., Kaye, M. D., and Ing, R. M. Y.: The lymphoid development of the fetal and neonatal appendix. *Biol. Neonate* 20:334, 1972.

37. Yoffey, J. M., and Thomas, D. B.: The development of bone marrow in the human foetus. *J. Anat.* 98:463, 1964.

38. Kalpaktsoglou, P. K., and Emery, J. L.: The effect of birth on the haemopoietic tissue of the human bone marrow. *Brit. J. Haemat.* 11:453, 1965.

39. Gairdner, D., Marks, J., and Roscoe, J. D.: Blood formation in infancy. *Arch. Dis. Childh.* 27:128, 1952.

40. Joppich, G., and Lissens, P.: Knochenmarksuntersuchungen beim lebenden Saugling. *Monatsschr. Kinderheilkd.* 71:382, 1937.

41. Hudson, G.: Bone-marrow volume in the human foetus and newborn. *Brit. J. Haemat.* 11:446, 1965.

42. Arey, L. B.: *Developmental Anatomy.* Philadelphia and London, W. B. Saunders, 1946.

43. Solomon, J. B.: *Foetal and Neonatal Immunology.* New York, American Elsevier Publishing Co., Inc., 1971.

44. Papiernik, M.: Correlation of lymphocyte transformation and morphology in the human fetal thymus. *Blood* 36:470, 1970.

45. Owen, J. J. T., Porter, R. O., Knight, J. (eds.), in *Ontogeny of Acquired Development of Lymphocyte Populations.* Amsterdam, Associated Scientific Publishers, 1972, p. 35.

46. Pinkel, D.: Ultrastructure of human fetal thymus. *Am. J. Dis. Childhood.* 155:222, 1968.

47. Thomas, D. B., and Yoffey, J. M.: Human foetal haemopoiesis: I. The cellular composition of foetal blood. *Brit. J. Haemat.* 8:290, 1962.

48. Thomas, D. B., and Yoffey, J. M.: Developmental changes in the human foetal blood. *J. Physiol.* 157:49, 1961.

49. Dorros, G., Kleiner, G. J., and Romney, S. L.: Fetal leukocyte pattern in premature rupture of amniotic membranes and in normal and abnormal labor. *Amer. J. Obstet. Gynec.* 105:1269, 1969.

50. Xanthou, M.: Leukocyte blood picture in healthy full-term and premature babies during the neonatal period. *Arch. Dis. Childh.* 45:242, 1970.

51. Prindull, G., and Prindull, B.: Leukocyte reserves of newborn infants: I. Observations during exchange transfusions. *Blut* 21:79, 1970.

52. Prindull, G., and Prindull, B.: Leukocyte reserves of newborn infants: II. Restoration of new leukocyte circulating levels after exchange transfusion. *Blut* 21:155, 1970.

53. Moore, M. A. S., and Owen, J. J. T.: Chromosome marker studies on the development of the haemopoietic system in the chick embryo. *Nature* 208:956, 1965.

54. Owen, J. J. T., and Ritter, M. A.: Tissue interaction in the development of thymus lymphocytes. *J. Exp. Med.* 129:431, 1969.

55. Grigoriu, G., Antonescu, M., and Iercan, E.: Evidence for a circulating stem cell: Newly formed erythroblasts found in autologous leukocyte-filled diffusion chambers inserted into bled rabbits. *Blood* 37:187, 1971.

56. Stutman, O., and Good, R. A.: Immunocompetence of embryonic hemopoietic cells after traffic to thymus. *Transplant. Proc.* 3:923, 1971.

57. Yoffey, J. M.: Stem cell role of the lymphocyte-transitional cell (LT) compartment, in *Haemopoietic Stem Cells,* Ciba Foundation Symposium 13 (new series). North Holland, Elsevier—Excerpta Medica—1973, p. 5.

58. Thomas, D. B., Russell, P. M., and Yoffey, J. M.: Pattern of haemopoiesis in the foetal liver. *Nature* 187:876, 1960.

59. Touraine, J. L., Incefy, G. S., Touraine, F. et al.: Differentiation of human bone marrow cells into T-lymphocytes by in vitro incubation with thymic extracts. *Clin. Exp. Immunol.* 17:151, 1974.

60. Incefy, G. S., L'perance, P., and Good, R. A.: In vitro differentiation of human marrow cells into T lymphocytes by thymic extracts using the rosette technique. *Clin. Exp. Immunol.* 19:475, 1975.

61. Kaplan, J., Bernales, R., Inoue, S., et al.: Comparison of E rosette negative and E rosette positive T cell subsets. *Pediat. Res.* 11:488, 1977. Abstract no. 702.

62. Winter, G. C. B., Byles, A. B., and Yoffey, J. M.: Blood lymphocytes in newborn and adult. *Lancet* II:932, 1965.

63. Leikin, S., Mochir-Fatemi, F., and Park, K.: Blast transformation of lymphocytes from newborn infants. *J. Pediatr.* 72:510, 1968.

64. David, R. H., and Galant, S. P.: Nonimmune rosette formation: A measure of the newborn infant's cellular immune response. *J. Pediat.* 87:449, 1975.

65. Pulvertaft, R. J. V., and Pulvertaft, J.: Spontaneous "transformation" of lymphocytes from the umbilical cord vein. *Lancet* II:892, 1966.

66. Faulk, W. P., Wang, A. C., Goodman, J. R., et al.: Immunobiologic parameters unique for the placento-fetal unit. *Pediatr. Res.* 3:499, 1969.

67. Faulk, W. P., Goodman, J. R., Maloney, M. A., et al.: Morphology and nucleoside incorporation of human neonatal lymphocytes. *Cell. Immunol.* 8:166, 1973.

68. Prindull, G., Prindull, B., Arie, R., et al.: Cells in spontaneous DNA synthesis in cord blood of premature and full-term newborn infants. *J. Pediatr.* 86:773, 1975.

69. Yoffey, J. M., Thomas, D. B., Moffatt, D. J., et al.: Nonimmunological functions of the lymphocyte, in Walstenholme, G. E. W., and O'Connor, M. (eds.): *Biological Activity of the Leucocyte.* Ciba Foundation Study Group no. 10, 1961.

70. Bernales, R., and Kaplan, J.: Unpublished observations.

71. Rubini, J. R., Bond, V. P., Keller, S., et al.: DNA synthesis in circulating blood leukocytes labelled in vitro with ³H-thymidine. *J. Lab. Clin. Med.* 58:751, 1961.

72. Warmick, W. J., Good, R. A., and Smith, R. T.: Failure of passive transfer of delayed hypersensitivity in the newborn human infant. *J. Lab. Clin. Med.* 56:139, 1960.

73. Rebuck, J. W., and Crowley, J. H.: A method of studying leukocytic functions in vivo. *Ann. N.Y. Acad. Sci.* 59:757, 1955.

74. Eitzman, D. V., and Smith, R. T.: The nonspecific inflammatory cycle in the neonatal infant. *Am. J. Dis. Child.* 97:326, 1959.

75. Miller, M. E.: Chemotactic function in the human neonate: Humoral and cellular factors. *Pediat. Res.* 5:487, 1971.

76. Maroni, E. S.: Nonspecific immunity in the newborn: Studies on chemotaxis: Deficiency of cellular and humoral components, in Centaro, A., and Carretti, N. (eds.): *Immunology in Obstetrics and Gynaecology,* Proceedings of the First International Congress, New York, 1973.

77. Miller, M. E.: Development maturation of human neutrophil motility and its relationship to membrane deformability, in Bellanti, J. A., and Dayton, D. H. (eds.): *The Phagocytic Cell in Host Resistance.* New York, Raven Press, 1975.

78. Miller, M. E., Oski, F. A., and Harris, M. B.: The lazy-leucocyte syndrome: A new disorder of neutrophil function. *Lancet* 1:665, 1971.

79. Miller, M., Normon, M., Koblenzer, P. J., et al.: A new familial defect of neutrophil movement. *J. Lab. Clin. Med.* 82:1, 1973.

80. Tunicliffe, R.: Observations on anti-infectious power of blood of infants. *J. Infect. Dis.* 7:698, 1910.

81. Gluck, K. L., and Silverman, W. A.: Phagocytosis in premature infants. *Pediatrics* 20:951, 1957.

82. Forman, M. L., and Stiehm, E. R.: Impaired opsonic activity but normal phagocytosis in low-brithweight infants. *N. Engl. J. Med.* 281:926, 1969.

83. McCracken, G. H., and Eichenwald, H. F.: Leukocyte function and the development of opsonic and complement activity in the neonate. *Am. J. Dis. Child.* 121:120, 1971.

84. Matoth, Y.: Phagocytic and ameboid activities of the leukocytes in the newborn infant. *Pediatrics* 9:748, 1952.

85. Miller, M. E.: Phagocytosis in the newborn infant: Humoral and cellular factors. *J. Pediatr.* 74:255, 1969.

86. Gold, F. L., Tuer, W. F., and Steele, R. W.: Neonatal host defenses against K-1 and non K-1 *E. coli. Pediat. Res.* 11:487, 1977. Abstract no. 691.

87. Cocchi, P., and Marianelli, L.: Phagocytosis and intracellular killing of Pseudomonas aeruginosa in premature infants. *Helv. Paediatr. Acta* 22:110, 1967.

88. Dossett, J. H., Williams, R. C., Jr., and Quie, P. G.: Studies on interaction of bacteria, serum factors and polymorphonuclear leukocytes in mothers and newborns. *Pediatrics* 44:49, 1969.

89. Coen, R., Grush, O., and Kauder, E.: Studies of bactericidal activity and metabolism of the leukocyte in full-term neonates. *J. Pediatr.* 75:400, 1969.

90. Cline, M. J.: Metabolism of the circulating leukocyte. *Physiol. Rev.* 45:674, 1965.

91. Brandt, L.: Studies on phagocytic activity of neutrophilic leukocytes. *Scand. J. Haemat. Suppl.* 2:1, 1967.

92. Park, B. H., Holmes, B., and Good, R. A.: Metabolic activities in leukocytes of newborn infants. *J. Pediatr.* 76:237, 1970.

93. Donnell, G. N., Ng, W. G., Hodgman, J. E. et al.: Galactose metabolism in the newborn infant. *Pediatrics* 39:829, 1967.

94. Strauss, G. R., and Seifert, M. S.: Oxidative metabolism in human cord blood neutrophils. *Pediatr. Res.* 11:495, 1977. Abstract 741.

95. Baehner, R. L., Nathan, D. G., and Karnovsky, M. L.: Correction of metabolic deficiencies in the leukocytes of patients with chronic granulomatous disease. *J. Clin. Invest.* 49:865, 1970.

96. Bellanti, J. A., Cantz, B. E., Maybee, D. A., et al.: Defective phagocytosis by newborn leukocytes: A defect similar to that in chronic granulomatous disease? *Pediatr. Res.* (Abstr.) 3:376, 1969.

97. Bellanti, J. A., Cantz, B. E., Yang, M. C., et al.: Biochemical changes in human polymorphonuclear leukocytes during maturation, in Bellanti, J. A., and Dayton, D. H. (eds.): *The Phagocytic Cell in Host Resistance.* New York, Raven Press, 1975.

98. Bellanti, J. A., Cantz, B. E., and Schlegel, R. J.: Accelerated decay of glucose-6-phosphate dehydrogenase activity in chronic granulomatous disease *Pediatr. Res.* 4:405, 1970.

99. Braun, W., and Lasky, L. J.: Antibody formation in newborn mice initiated through adult macrophages (abstract). *Fed. Proc.* 26:642, 1967.

100. Selgrade, M. K., and Osborn, J. E.: Role of macrophages in resistance to murine cytomegalovirus. *Infect. Immun.* 10:383, 1974.

101. Hirsch, M. S., Zisman, B., and Allison, A. C.: Macrophages and age-dependent resistance to herpes simplex virus in mice. *J. Immunol.* 104:1160, 1970.

102. Silverstein, A., Uhr, J., Kramer, K., et al.: Fetal response to antigenic stimulus: II. Antibody production by the fetal lamb. *J. Exp. Med.* 117:799, 1963.

103. Blaese, R. M.: Macrophages and the development of immunocompetence, in Bellanti, J. A., and Dayton, D. H. (eds.): *The Phagocytic Cell in Host Resistance.* New York, Raven Press, 1975, p. 309.

104. Orlowski, J. P., Sieger, L., and Anthony, B. F.: Bactericidal capacity of monocytes of newborn infants. *J. Pediatr.* 89:797, 1976.

105. Kretschmer, R. R., Papierniak, C., Stewardson-Krieger, P., et al.: Quantitative nitroblue tetrazolium reduction by cord blood monocytes (Abstract no. 707) *Pediatr. Res.* 11:489, 1977.

106. Pahwa, S. G., Pahwa, R., Grimes, E., et al.: Cellular and humoral components of monocyte and neutrophil chemotaxis in cord blood. *Pediatr. Res.* 11:677, 1977.

107. Klein, R. B., Rich, K. C., Biberstein, M., et al.: Defective mononuclear and neutrophilic phagocyte chemotaxis in the newborn. *Clin. Res.* 24:180A, 1976.

108. Fischer, T. J., Lkein, R. B., Borut, T. C., et al.: Monocyte chemotaxis in health and disease (Abstr no. 688) *Pediatr. Res.* 11:486, 1977.

109. Kretschmer, R. R., Stewardson, P. B., Papierniak, C. K., et al.: Chemotactic and bactericidal capacities of human newborn monocytes. *J. Immunol.* 117:1303, 1976.

110. Wolf, R. L., Lomnitzer, R., and Rabson, A. R.: An inhibitor of lymphocyte proliferation and lymphokine production released by unstimulated foetal monocytes. *Clin. Exp. Immunol.* 27:464, 1977.

111. Stites, D. P., Wybran, J., Carr, M. C., et al.: Development of cellular immunocompetence in man, in Porter, R., and Knight, J. (eds.): *Ontogeny of Acquired Immunity: Ciba Foundation Symposium.* North Holland Elsevier—Excerpta Medica, 1972, p. 113.

112. Bullock, J. D., Robertson, A. F., Bodenbender, M. T., et al.: Inflammatory response in the neonate re-examined. *Pediatrics* 44:58, 1969.

113. Gitlin, D., and Biasucci, A.: Development of gamma G, gamma A, gamma M, beta 1_c, beta 1α, C'1 esterase inhibitor, ceruloplasmin, transferrin, hemopexin, haptoglobin, fibrinogen, plasminogen, alpha-1-antitrypsin, orosomucoid, beta-lipoprotein, alpha-2-macroglobulin and pre-albumin in the human conceptus. *J. Clin. Invest.* 48:1433, 1969.

114. Adinolfi, M., Gardner, B.,and Wood, C. B.: Ontogenesis of two components of human complement: beta 1E and beta 1C-1A globulins. *Nature* 219:180, 1968.

115. Asofsky, R., and Thorbecke, G. J.: Sites of formation of immune globulins and of a component of C_3: II. Production of immunoelectrophoretically identified serum proteins by humans and monkey tissues in vitro. *J. Exp. Med.* 114:471, 1961.

116. Stecher, U. J., and Thorbecke, G. J.: Sites of synthesis of serum proteins: I. Serum proteins produced by macrophages in vitro. *J. Immunol.* 99:643, 1967.

117. Glade, P. R., and Chessin, L. N.: Synthesis of $\beta 1\chi - \beta 1\alpha$ globulin (C'$_3$) by human lymphoid cells. *Int. Arch. Allergy Appl. Immunol.* 34:181, 1968.

118. Alper, C. A., Johnson, A. M., Birtch, A. G., et al.: Human C'$_3$: Evidence for the liver as the primary site of synthesis. *Science* 163:286, 1969.

119. Adinolfi, M., and Gardner, B.: Synthesis of $\beta 1_e$ and $\beta 1_c$ components of complement in human foetuses. *Acta Paediatr. Scand.* 56:450, 1967.

120. Propp, R. P., and Alper, C. A.: C'3 synthesis in the human fetus and lack of transplacental passage. *Science* 162:672, 1968.

121. Colten, H. R.: Biosynthesis of serum complement. *Prog. Immunol.* 2:183, 1974.

122. Littman, B. H., and Ruddy, S.: Production of the second component of complement by human monocytes: Stimulation by antigen-activated lymphocytes or lymphokines. *J. Exp. Med.* 145:1344, 1977.

123. Kock, F., Schultz, H. E., and Schwick, G.: Komplement faktoren and properdin beim gesunden saugling im ersten lebensjahr. *Klin. Wochenschr.* 36:17, 1958.

124. Feinstein, P. A., and Kaplan, S. R.: The alternative pathway of complement activation in the neonate. *Pediatr. Res.* 9:803, 1975.

125. Natton-Larrier, L., Grimard, L., and Dufour, J.: L'alexine chez le nouveau-né. *Compt. Rend. Soc. Biol.* 125:358, 1937.

126. Coffin, G. S., Hook, W. A., and Murchel, L. H.: Antibacterial substances in placentas and serums of mother and newborn infants. *Proc. Soc. Exp. Biol. Med.* 104:239, 1960.

127. Gitlin, D., Rosen, F. S., and Michael, J. G.: Transient 19S gamma globulin deficiency in the newborn infant, and its significance. *Pediatrics* 31:197, 1963.

128. Michael, J. G., and Rosen, F. S.: Association of "natural" antibodies to gram-negative bacteria with the gamma-1-macroglobulins. *J. Exp. Med.* 118:619, 1963.

129. Kay, D. H., Bonnard, G. D., West, H. W., et al.: A functional comparison of human Fc receptor-bearing lymphocytes active in natural cytotoxicity and antibody-dependent cellular cytotoxicity. *J. Immunol.* 118:2058, 1977.

130. Bernales, R., and Bellanti, J.: E-rosette-forming cells (E RFC) and Tγ cells (suppressor T) precursors in cord blood lymphocytes (CBL): Responsiveness to thymosin fraction V (Presented in APS-SPR Conference). *Pediat. Res.* 12:477, 1978. Abst. no. 683.

131. Wybran, J., Carr, M. C., and Fudenberg, H. H.: Effect of serum on human rosette forming cells in fetuses and adult blood. *Clin. Immunol. Immunopathol.* 1:408, 1973.

132. Hayward, A. R., and Ezer, G.: Development of lymphocyte populations in the human foetal thymus and spleen. *Clin. Exp. Immunol.* 17:169, 1974.

133. Brain, P., Gordon, J., and Willetts, W. A.: Rosette formation by peripheral lymphocytes. *Clin. Exp. Immunol.* 6:681, 1970.

134. Froland, S. S.: Binding of sheep erythrocytes to human lymphocytes: A probable marker of T lymphocyte. *Scand. J. Immunol.* 1:269, 1972.

135. Smith, M. A., Evans, J., and Steel, C. M.: Age related variation in proportion of circulating T cells. *Lancet* 2:922, 1974.

136. Bernales, R., Kaplan, J., and Bellanti, J. A.: Studies of E-rosette-forming capacity of cord blood lymphocytes. *Pediatr. Res.* 11:484, 1977.

137. Carr, M. C., Stites, D. P., and Fudenberg, H. H.: Ontogeny of the human fetus of certain in vitro correlates of cell-mediated immunity. *Pediatr. Res.* 7:362, 1973.

138. Jones, W. R.: In vitro transformation of fetal lymphocytes. *Amer. J. Obstet. Gynec.* 104:586, 1969.

139. Kay, H. E. M., Doe, J., and Hockley, A.: Response of human foetal thymocytes to phytohaemagglutinin (PHA). *Immunology* 18:393, 1970.

140. Miggiano, V. C., Meo, T., Nabholz, M., et al.: Ontogeny of cellular immunocompetence in early human fetuses probed with current and novel in vitro tests, in Centari, A., and Carretti, N. (eds.): *Immunology in Obstetrics and Gynaecology,* Proceedings of the First International Congress, Padera, 7–9 June 1973, New York, American Elsevier Publishing Co., Inc., 1974, p. 156.

141. Pegrum, G. D., Ready, D., and Thompson, E.: The effect of phytohaemagglutinin on human foetal cells grown in culture. *Brit. J. Haematol.* 15:371, 1968.

142. Prindull, G.: An in-vitro quantitative study of phytohaemagglutinin (PHA) induced transformation of lymphocytes from premature newborn infants, from older premature infants, and from full-term newborn infants. *Blut* 23:7, 1971.

143. Ayoub, J., and Kasakura, S.: In vitro response of fetal lymphocytes to PHA, and a plasma factor which suppresses the PHA response of adult lymphocytes. *Clin. Exp. Immunol.* 8:427, 1971.

144. Lindahl-Kiessling, K., and Böök, J. A.: Effects of phytohaemagglutinin on leukocytes. *Lancet* II:591, 1964.

145. Marshall, W. C., Cope, W. A., Soothill, J. F., et al.: In vitro lymphocyte response in some immune deficiency diseases and in intrauterine virus infections. *Proc. Roy. Soc. Med.* 63:351, 1970.

146. Pentycross, C. R.: Lymphocyte transformation in young people. *Clin. Exp. Immunol.* 5:213, 1969.

147. Prindull, G.: Anti-human lymphocyte globulin- (ALG-) sensitive lymphocyte populations in the blood of newborn premature infants, of older premature infants and of full-term newborn infants: A quantitative in vitro study. *Blut* 23:320, 1971.

148. Seigler, H. F., and Metzgar, R. S.: Embryonic development of human transplantation antigens. *Transplantation* 9:478, 1970.

149. Stites, D. P., Carr, M. C., and Fudenberg, H. H.: Ontogeny of cellular immunity in the human fetus: Development of responses to phytohemagglutinin and to allogeneic cells. *Cell. J. Immunol.* 11:257, 1974.

150. Hayward, A. R., and Soothill, J. F.: Reaction to antigen by human foetal thymus lymphocytes, in Porter, R., and Knight, J. (eds.): *Ontogeny of Acquired Immunity: Ciba Foundation Symposium.* North Holland, Elsevier—Excerpta Medica, 1972, p. 261.

151. Pirofsky, B., Davies, G. H., Ramirez-Mateos, J. C., et al.: Cellular immune competence in the human fetus. *Cell. Immunol.* 6:324, 1973.

152. Pegrum, G. D.: Mixed cultures of human foetal and adult cells. *Immunology* 21:159, 1971.

153. Gatti, R. A., Gershanik, J. J., Levkoff, A. H., et al.: DiGeorge syndrome associated with combined immunodeficiency: Dissociation of phytohaemagglutinin and mixed leukocyte culture responses. *J. Pediatr.* 81:920, 1972.

154. Meuwissen, H. J., Bach, F. H., Hong, R., et al.: Lymphocyte studies in congenital thymic dysplasia: The one-way stimulation test. *J. Pediatr.* 72:177, 1968.

155. Seligmann, M., Griscelli, C., Preud'homme, J. L., et al.: A variant of severe combined immunodeficiency with normal in vitro response to allogeneic cells and an increase in circulating B lymphocytes persisting several months after successful bone marrow graft. *Clin. Exp. Immunol.* 17:245, 1974.

156. Lamvik, J. O.: The reactivity of human cord lymphocytes in mixed cell cultures. *Scand. J. Haemat.* 3:325, 1966.

157. Ceppellini, R., Bonnard, G. D., Coppa, F., et al.: Mixed lymphocyte cultures and HL-A antigens. *Transpl. Proc.* 3:58, 1971.

158. Leikin, S.: The immunosuppressive effects of maternal plasma. *Pediatr. Res.* 5:377, 1971.

159. Asantila, T., Sorvari, T., Hirvonen, T., et al.: Xenogeneic reactivity of human fetal lymphocytes. *J. Immunol.* 111:984, 1973.

160. Campbell, A. C., Waller, C., Wood, J., et al.: Lymphocyte subpopulations in the blood of newborn infants. *Clin. Exp. Immunol.* 18:469, 1974.

161. McConnachie, B., Rachelefky, G., Stiehm, E. R., et al.: Antibody-dependent lymphocyte killer function and age. *Pediatrics* 52:795, 1973.

162. Shore, L. S., Milgrom, H., Wood, P. A., et al.: Antibody dependent cellular cytotoxicity to target cells infected with Herpes simplex viruses: Functional adequacy in the neonate. *Pediatrics* 59:22, 1977.

163. Eife, R. F., Eife, G., August, S. C., et al.: Lymphotoxin production and blast cell transformation by cord blood lymphocyte function in newborn infants. *Cell. Immunol.* 14:435, 1974.

164. Hahn, T., Levin, S., and Handzel, Z. T.: Leucocyte migration inhibition factor (LIF) production by lymphocytes of normal children, newborns, and children with immune deficiency. *Clin. Exp. Immunol.* 24:448, 1976.

165. Handzel, Z., Levin, S., Dolfin, Z., et al.: Immune system status in the newborn, European Immunology Congress, 1977, Abstract no. 28, in *Pediatr. Res.* 11:1, 1977.

166. Ray, C. G.: The ontogeny of interferon production by human leukocytes. *J. Pediatr.* 76:94, 1970.

167. Cooper, M. D., Lawton, A. R., and Kincade, P. W.: A two-stage model for development of antibody-producing cells. *Clin. Exp. Immunol.* 11:143, 1972.

168. Herrod, H. G., and Warner, N. L.: Inhibition by anti-chain sera of the cellular transfer of antibody and immunoglobulin synthesis in mice. *J. Immunol.* 108:1712, 1972.

169. Nossal, G. J. V., Szenberg, A., Ada, G. L., et al.: Single cell studies on 19S antibody production. *J. Exp. Med.* 119:485, 1964.

169a. Nossal, G. J. V., Warner, N. L., and Lewis, H.: Incidence of cells simultaneously secreting IgM and IgG antibody to sheep erythrocytes. *Cell. Immunol.* 2:41, 1971.

170. Pierce, C. W., Asofsky, R., and Solliday, S. M.: Immunoglobulin receptors on B lymphocytes: Shifts in immunoglobulin class during immune responses. *Fed. Proc.* 32:41, 1973.

171. Pierce, C. W., Solliday, S. M., and Asofsky, R.: Immune response in vitro: IV. Suppression of primary M, G and A plaque-forming cell response in mouse spleen cell cultures by class-specific antibody to mouse immunoglobulins. *J. Exp. Med.* 135:675, 1972.

172. Press, J. L., and Klinman, N. R.: Monoclonal production of both IgM and IgG antihapten antibody. *J. Exp. Med.* 138:300, 1973.

173. Lawton, A. R., Kincade, P. W., and Cooper, M. D.: Sequential expression of germ line genes in development of immunoglobulin class diversity. *Fed. Proc.* 34:33, 1975.

174. Pearl, E. R., Vogler, L. B., Crist, W. M., et al.: Normal and aberrant B-cell differentiation in bone marrow (Abstr. no. 719). *Pediatr. Res.* 11:491, 1977.

175. Waldmann, T. A., Broder, S., Blaese, R. M., et al.: Role of suppressor T cells in pathogenesis of common variable hypogammaglobulinemia. *Lancet II*:609, 1974.

176. Abdou, N. I., and Abdou, N. L.: Bone marrow: The bursa equivalent in man? *Science* 175:446, 1972.

177. Cooper, M. D., and Lawton, A. R.: The mammalian "Bursa Equivalent": Does lymphoid differentiation along plasma cell lines begin in the gut-associated lymphoepithelial tissues (GALT) of mammals? In Hanna, M. G. (ed.): *Contemporary Topics in Immunobiology.* New York, Plenum Press, 1972, p. 49.

178. Miller, R. G., and Phillips, R. A.: Development of B lymphocytes. *Fed. Proc.* 34:145, 1975.

179. Lawton, A. R., and Cooper, M. D.: Two new stages of antigen-independent B cell development in mice and humans, in Cooper, M. D., and Dayton, D. H. (eds.): *Development of Host Defenses.* Raven Press, New York, 1977, p. 50.

180. Cooper, M. D., and Seligmann, M.: B and T lymphocytes in immunodeficiency and lymphoproliferative diseases, in Loor, F., and Rodants, G. E. (eds.): *B and T Cells in Immune Recognition.* West Sussex, England, John Wiley and Sons, Ltd., 1977.

181. Castro, L. C.: El problema immunologico de la gestacion. *Revista Clinica Espanola* 139:97, 1975.

182. Finn, R., St Hill, C. A., Davis, J. C., et al.: Fetomaternal bidirectional mixed lymphocyte reactions and survival of fetal allograft. *Lancet* II:1200, 1977.

183. Rocklin, R. E., Kitzmiller, J. L., Carpenter, C. B., et al.: Maternal-fetal relation: Absence of an immunologic blocking factor from the serum of women with chronic abortions. *N.E.J.M.* 295:1209, 1976.

184. Brambell, F. W. R.: The transmission of passive immunity from mother to young. *Front. Biol.* 18:102, 1970.

185. Brambell, F. W. R., Hemmings, W. G., Oakley, C. L., et al.: The relative transmission of the fractions of papain hydrolyzed homologous γ globulin from uterine cavity to the foetal circulation in the rabbit. *Proc. Roy. Soc. Ser. B* 151:478, 1960.

186. Vahlquist, B.: Transfer of antibodies from mother to offspring. *Adv. Pediatr.* 10:305, 1958.

187. Beer, E. A., Billingham, R. E., Head, Jr., et al.: Possible influence of maternal-to-perinatal cell transfer on the development of host defenses, in M. D. Cooper and D. H. Dayton (eds.): *Development of Host Defenses.* Raven Press, New York, 1977, p. 266.

188. Bellanti, J. A., and Jackson, A. L.: Characterization of the serum immunoglobulins to the somatic antigen of *S. typhosa* in an infant following intrauterine immunization. *J. Pediatr.* 71:783, 1967.

189. Sever, J. L.: Immunoglobulin determinations for the detection of perinatal infections. *J. Pediatr.* 75:111, 1969.

190. Alford, C. A.: Immunoglobulin determinations in the diagnosis of fetal infection. *Pediatr. Clin. N. Am.* 18:99, 1971.

191. Gotoff, S. P.: Neonatal immunity. *J. Pediatr.* 85:149, 1974.

192. Gittlin, D., and Gittlin, J. D.: Fetal and neonatal development, in Putnam, F. W. (ed.): *The Plasma Proteins Structure and Genetic Control.* Academic Press, 1975.

193. Toivanen, P., Rossi, T., and Hirvonen, T.: Immunoglobulins in human fetal sera at different stages of gestation. *Experientia* 25:527, 1969.

194. Johansson, S. G. O., and Berg, T.: Immunoglobulin levels in healthy children. *Acta Paediat. Scand.* 56:572, 1967.

195. Stiehm, E. R., Ammann, A. J., and Cherry, J. D.: Elevated cord macroglobulins in diagnosis of intrauterine infections. *N.E.J.M.* 275:971, 1966.

196. McFarlane, H., and Udeozo, I. O.: Immunochemical estimation of some proteins in Nigerian paired maternal and fetal blood. *Arch. Dis. Childh.* 43:42, 1968.

197. Evans, H. F., Akpata, S. O., and Glass, L.: Serum immunoglobulin levels in premature and full-term infants. *Amer. J. Clin. Pathol.* 56:416, 1971.

198. Leslie, G. A., and Swate, T. E.: Structure and biologic functions of human IgD: I. The presence of immunoglobulin D in human cord sera. *J. Immunol.* 109:47, 1972.

199. Miller, D. L., Hirvonen, T., and Gitlin, D.: Synthesis of IgE by the human conceptus. *J. Allergy Clin. Immunol.* 52:182, 1973.

200. Miller, D. L., Zapata, R., Hutchinson, D. L., et al.: Maternofetal passage of human IgE in the pregnant monkey, mouse, rat and guinea pig (abstract). *Fed. Proc.* 32:1013, 1973.

201. Berg, T., and Johansson, S. G. O.: Immunoglobulin levels during childhood, with special regard to IgE. *Acta Paediat. Scand.* 58:513, 1969.

202. Bazaral, M., Orgel, H. A., and Hamburger, R. N.: IgE levels in normal infants and mothers and an inheritance hypothesis. *J. Immunol.* 107:794, 1971.

203. Edozien, J. S.: Panel on radioisotope techniques in the study of protein metabolism, in *Radioisotope Techniques in the Study of Protein Metabolism,* Vienna, International Atomic Energy Agency, Tech. Rep. Ser. no. 45, 1965, p. 202.

204. Morrell, A., Skauril, G., Hitzig, W. H., et al.: IgG subclasses: Development of the serum concentrations in "normal" infants and children. *J. Pediatr.* 80:960, 1972.

205. Mantalenaki-Asfi, K., Morphis, L., Nicolopoulos, D., et al.: Influence of exchange transfusion on the development of serum immunoglobulins. *J. Pediatr.* 87:396, 1975.

206. Cohen, F., and Zuelzer, W. W.: Mechanisms of isoimmunization: II. Transplacental passage and postnatal survival of fetal erythrocytes in heterospecific pregnancies. *Blood* 30:796, 1967.

207. Miller, M. E.: Graft-vs-host reactions in man with special reference to thymic dysplasia, in Bergsma, D., and Good, R. A. (eds.): *Immunologic Deficiency Diseases in Man.* Natl. Fnd. March of Dimes, 1968, p. 257.

208. Taylor, A. I., and Polani, P. E.: XX/XY mosaicism in man. *Lancet* 1:1226, 1965.

209. Naiman, J. L., Punnett, H. H., Lischner, H. W., et al.: Possible graft-versus-host reaction after intrauterine transfusion for Rh erythroblastosis fetalis. *N.E.J.M.* 281:697, 1969.

210. Cohen, D. M., Mitchell, C. B., and Alexander, J. W.: Letterer-Siwe disease in a newborn. *Arch. Pathol.* 81:347, 1966.

211. Miller, D. R.: Familial reticuloendotheliosis: Concurrence of disease in five siblings. *Pediatrics* 38:986, 1966.

212. Hobbs, J. R., and Davis, J. A.: Serum gamma-G-globulin levels and gestational age in premature babies. *Lancet* 1:757, 1967.

213. Manerikar, S. S., Malaviya, A. N., Singh, M. B., et al.: Immune status and BCG vaccination in newborns with intra-uterine growth retardation. *Clin. Exp. Immunol.* 26:173, 1976.

214. Sirisinha, S., Suskind, R., Edelman, R., et al.: Secretory and serum IgA in children with protein-calorie malnutrition. *Pediatrics* 55:166, 1975.

215. Chandra, R. H.: Fetal malnutrition and postnatal immunocompetence. *Am. J. Dis. Child.* 129:450, 1975.

216. Shore, A., Dosch, H., Huber, J., et al: In vitro and in vivo definition of a new variant of severe combined immunodeficiency disease (SCID) (Abstr. no. 735). *Pediatr. Res.* 11:494, 1977.

217. Bonforte, R. J., Topilsky, M., Siltzbach, L. E., et al.: Phytohemagglutinin skin test: A possible in vivo measure of cell-mediated immunity. *J. Pediatr.* 81:775, 1972.

218. Catalona, W. J., Taylor, P. T., Rabson, A. S., et al.: A method for dinitrochlorobenzene contact sensitization: A clinicopathological study. *N.E.J.M.* 286:399, 1972.

219. Uhr, J. W., Dancis, J., and Neumann, C. G.: Delayed type hypersensitivity in premature neonatal humans. *Nature* 187:1130, 1960.

220. Ferguson, A. C., Lawlor, G. J., Jr., Neumann, G. G., et al.: Decreased rosette-forming lymphocytes in malnutrition and intrauterine growth retardation. *J. Pediatr.* 85:717, 1974.

221. Poplack, D. G., Bonnard, G. D., Holiman, B. J., et al.: Monocyte-mediated antibody-dependent cellular cytotoxicity: A clinical test of monocyte function. *Blood* 48:809, 1976.

Part 2
SYSTEMIC PROBLEMS IN PERINATAL MEDICINE

11
Fetal Distress

Richard H. Paul, M.D.

Fetal distress, a commonly used obstetrical term, must be a primary focus of concern to those charged with delivering maternal and perinatal care. Attempts to define fetal distress are often confusing, imprecise, and unsubstantiated by the observable outcome. On the other hand, the fact that fetal distress occurs is undeniable, as evidenced by the occurrence of fetal death and the often unexpected delivery of a severely depressed, asphyxiated infant.

In general, the usage of the term *fetal distress* is identified with the events occurring during the labor process. However, chronic disorders during pregnancy are not infrequently associated with "recognizable distress" in the form of antepartum fetal deaths. These problems are most commonly seen in patients with congenital infections, diabetes mellitus, hypertensive disorders, or other medical complications. Neonatal evaluation of infants from complicated pregnancy also suggests that maternal nutritional deprivation, circulatory disorders, and prolonged gestation are chronic distress factors that are associated with intrauterine growth retardation or dysmaturity. Antepartum fetal deaths many times occur without apparent or identifiable maternal disorders. Acute distress that has been objectively documented during labor no doubt contributes to some of these unexplainable antepartum losses. The mechanisms are usually impossible to define, but would include:

1. Acute umbilical cord accidents: entanglement, unrelieved compression, true knot, occult prolapse
2. Excessive uterine activity: spontaneous or induced, possibly related to such factors as unknowing ingestion of an oxytocic agent and coitus

A reality that makes the identification of causative factors difficult or impossible is that fetal death often may occur days or weeks before delivery.

The occurrence of labor imposes a dramatic period of repetitive stress on each fetus. Although deaths prior to labor outnumber those occurring during labor by a factor of about 3 to 1, there is no other comparable time period that contributes as heavily to fetal mortality. The occurrence of intrapartum fetal deaths is generally stated as 2 to 4/1000, and an associated or probable causative factor is found in only about 50% of cases (1).

As one examines the human reproductive outcome, after eliminating the abortion process, it is obvious that the vast majority of newborn infants are judged normal, in excess of 95% of the time. Thus, the unique obstetrical challenge or dilemma is the identification of a relatively small number of fetuses who are at increased risk and the delivery of specialized care that minimizes perinatal mortality and morbidity.

The historical aspect of attempts to evaluate the human fetus have been largely limited to the last 200 years (2). The original observations, not unlike those today, focused on the fetal pulse, heart activity, and meconium passage. Kergaradec in 1822 published what is recognized as a first attempt at fetal evaluation using obstetrical auscultation (3). Auscultation of the fetal heart activity remained the primary method of fetal evaluation until very recent years. Infant and childhood disorders such as cerebral palsy, mental retardation, and dysfunction problems also brought about many retrospective attempts to evaluate intrauterine events as possible contributing factors. Certain general conclusions could be reached from such studies, but many only emphasized that, although suspect, labor and its impact were largely an unobserved and unquantitated process. Questions regarding the role and limitations of auscultation in identifying the distressed fetus were somewhat clarified in the report from a collaborative project (4). With an increased awareness of the limitations in fetal evaluation by auscultation, new techniques have emerged and have been applied in clinical care.

The intrapartum period logically became a major area of investigation because of the known stress factors and the increased frequency of fetal death, which unequivocally demonstrated that a state of fetal distress had occurred. Additional end points were also available that constituted indirect evidence of fetal distress in the observations of severely depressed, asphyxiated newborns.

A primary method of fetal evaluation that emerged in the late 1950s and early 1960s was the continuous recording of fetal heart rate (FHR) and uterine contractions (UC). Another major advance in intrapartum fetal assessment was fetal blood sampling, which was developed in the early 1960s by Saling. These methods provided individualized data on which to make management decisions. The extensive use of these techniques opened new vistas of fetal evaluation and established the foundation on which current concepts of maternal-fetal care are based.

ANTEPARTUM EVALUATION

As previously stated, there is no doubt that fetal distress occurs prior to labor. For convenience, it is helpful to consider these problems as chronically occurring disorders, even though one must concede acute distress may occur. The practical dilemma is the identification of single or multiple acute events over a period of weeks or months, which must, by necessity, remain largely unobserved.

A detailed discussion of antepartum evaluation is beyond the scope of this presentation, but a broad appraisal of current clinical approaches used to identify the distressed fetus before labor includes history and physical examination, biochemical tests, and biophysical evaluations.

History and Physical Examination

The primary screening for a distressed fetus remains largely in the realm of the astute clinical observer, since no practical screening test exists. Once suspect, individual fetal evaluations have proved quite useful in the further definition of the compromised fetus.

Biochemical Tests

Two biochemical methods widely advocated are estriol determinations and human placental lactogen (HPL). The absolute role of these tests is debatable, but many investigators feel that they provide useful data when integrated with the clinical circumstance (5,6). Both testing methods appear to be most useful in selective screening but are plagued by a high incidence of apparently erroneous predictions.

Biophysical Evaluation

The most widely used techniques involve ultrasound, and FHR-UC monitoring.

Ultrasound

Serial ultrasonic measurement provides valuable data demonstrating fetal growth or its absence. The fetus who fails to grow may be logically described as in a distressed state. Relating this observation of chronic distress to factors such as impending demise or the necessity for delivery is clinically difficult. Final decisions usually require additional information from other indicators of fetal well-being, such as estriol measurement or antepartum fetal heart rate testing.

Dynamic ultrasonic approaches are assessing fetal functional status through the study of gross fetal movements and fetal chest wall (breathing) movements. An understanding of these functions may well prove valuable in the determination of fetal well-being (7).

Antepartum FHR Testing (AFHRT)

Attempts to determine fetal well-being using FHR-UC data were explored in preliminary studies in the late 1950s and 1960s (8). More extensive investigation began in the 1970s, based largely on extension of intrapartum observations that certain FHR patterns were associated with fetal compromise (9). Thus, the concept of the contraction stress test (CST) as an indicator of fetal reserve emerged. The rationale of this test was that uterine contractions, which interrupt intervillous blood flow, should provoke FHR patterns of late decelerations in the compromised fetus. The observation of a normal FHR in the presence of uterine contractions of sufficient frequency (3/10 min) was taken as an indicator of adequate fetal reserve. When spontaneous uterine activity was inadequate, oxytocin infusion was given to increase the stress factor and the term *oxytocin challenge test* became the most widely used clinical test of fetal well-being.

The relative role of stress testing (CST, OCT) has become more clearly defined with widespread clinical usage. Problems that are evident include the failure to obtain FHR-UC data and an inability to apply and quantitate the stress factor consistently. As will be pointed out in the intrapartum section, another major problem lies in defining the significance of the positive test (late decelerations) as they relate to available end points that are often remote from the time when the test is performed. The most apparent benefit, as in intrapartum evaluation, appears to be in the observation of a normal FHR, which, at that moment of observation, denotes a normal fetus.

Extensive observations made in Europe and during the process of contraction stress testing have suggested that the FHR is a useful predictor of fetal status even when stress factors are not applied. Thus, much current attention is directed at exploring the concept of nonstress testing (NST) (10,11). The FHR changes, such as accelerations associated with fetal movement (reactive pattern), appear to characterize the normal fetus, whereas observation of a flat, smooth, FHR (nonreactive) is suspect (12). A reactive fetal response appears to be of equal predictive value as a negative CST.

The future individual evaluation of fetal condition will probably include FHR observations, dynamic ultrasonic evaluation of fetal function, and evoked responses to stimuli such as sound, manipulation, and imposed stress factors.

INTRAPARTUM EVALUATION

As previously stated, observation in the intrapartum period, which is of incompassable duration and ends with the emergence of an examinable patient, has given us much of our understanding of human fetal physiology. The development of methods for continuous FHR monitoring supplied data that were more precise and complete than ever before available. Fetal blood sampling permitted direct evaluation of acid-base status and elucidated much of our current understanding of the pathophysiology of FHR patterns (13).

Although clinical factors such as meconium passage, toxemia, and maternal age must be weighed in any comprehensive approach to perinatal care, the ultimate attempt to define the distressed fetus may be currently based on direct observations of data from each individual fetus. The use of continuous FHR-UC monitoring has become commonplace in pregnancies judged to be high risk. This approach has been associated with a decrease in perinatal mortality (14). More specifically, intrapartum fetal deaths are minimized or eliminated by this approach in many institutions (15,16). Likewise, it appears that neonatal condition and survival are enhanced in cases where intrapartum monitoring has been used. Thus, one may reasonably assume that provided with an enhanced awareness of the fetus, fetal distress is, to some degree, recognizable and preventable. These observations have led some to advocate a policy of universal monitoring of all patients during labor (17). This approach seems not unreasonable as one recalls the unexpected fetal losses in normal patients or when fetal distress is encountered during the routine monitoring of the apparently normal patient. On the other hand, risk factors must be weighed: one of the most visible of these appears to be active intervention (cesarean delivery), which in retrospect often appears to have been unnecessary.

With the availability of techniques that assess the fetus, the obstetrical team has accepted the additional responsibility of rendering active intrapartum fetal care. A major dilemma arises when suddenly there is available a continuous flow of data from the fetus that demands interpretation. Likewise, these interpretations must be projected against end points that are equated to some degree with perinatal health. There are enormous problems that arise with such an appraisal, but no practical alternatives exist in the human fetus, who remains largely isolated.

In order to develop a rational, workable clinical approach to fetal distress, one must consider many basic factors. These include the problem that one must attempt to predict the well-being of the fetus from a single biological indicator—the FHR. The prediction of a person's well-being, life or death, even when using multiple testing methods, is perilous, imprecise, and usually approached only with extreme caution. The FHR, which serves as the primary indicator of fetal status, as subsequently discussed in detail, provides direction in patient management, but observed FHR changes are difficult to quantitate (18).

Terms such as late deceleration serve as a descriptive method of communication, and generalized terms such as uteroplacental insufficiency (UPI) denote the associated pathophysiologic mechanisms. Experimental techniques that attempt to define the degree of stress, and associated FHR quantitation necessary to produce a damaged human fetus, are unacceptable. Animal investigation has helpfully served to elucidate some general FHR characteristics associated with demonstrable damage (19). Currently, the approach used in the human to define how bad is bad is based on clinical observations. In such an approach, the tendency is logically chosen that presumably avoids significant fetal distress and prevents any degree of permanent damage.

Labor imposes repetitive stress periods on all fetuses. Uterine contractions repeatedly interrupt uterine blood flow and provoke transient periods of hypoxemia in the fetus. Fetal tolerance or reserve is such that no demonstrable sequelae result from the birth process in the vast majority of circumstances. The other major potential threat to every fetus appears to be the accidental occurrence of umbilical cord occlusion. This mechanism obviously has the potential for asphyxiation, and the perinatal mortality associated with the prolapsed cord is a well-known example.

Other considerations in any discussion of the diagnosis of fetal distress must examine the criteria that, short of death, are confirmatory. Arbitrary values such as a scalp blood pH of 7.20 or less or an Apgar score of less than 7 at 5 min are often subject to question or reflect events which are interposed independently between observations and outcome (20). The most basic dilemma is in the definition of stress and what constitutes a state of distress. Any definition that requires corroboration of the diagnosis fetal distress by demonstration of severe acidemia, newborn asphyxia, or depression is unacceptable in view of the potential risks imposed. Likewise, unwarranted intervention when the fetus is merely reflecting a stress response may impose significant risk to both mother and fetus.

In spite of the confusion surrounding the accurate definition of fetal distress, care must be rendered to the patient. Although the tools used to determine fetal status are imprecise, they provide us with data that, when intelligently used, should enhance patient management. In order to care for the mother and her fetus properly, an attempt is made to develop a clinical approach regarding the recognition and treatment of fetal distress.

As stated in the section on antepartum evaluation, the historical factors and physical examination are fundamental to any rational patient management scheme. Although the primary focus of this presentation is on techniques or tests, the identical data in different patients may indicate quite opposite courses of management, depending on other clinical findings.

Diagnostic Methods

Continuous monitoring of the FHR-UC is the primary method of intrapartum fetal surveillance currently used. The peculiar variations of available monitoring instruments and their limitations must be clearly understood before any patient application. Fetal blood sampling may be intermittently used as a complimentary technique and provides invaluable additional fetal data. Thus, FHR aberrations that are abnormal or confusing can be interpreted in light of their biochemical implication and care enhanced. A detailed discussion of the application of these techniques, their limitations, and classification is beyond the scope of this presentation, and a certain basic understanding must be assumed.

The FHR recording is presently the only continuous method of fetal surveillance. A normal pattern is almost invariably associated with a nonacidemic fetus and normal newborn (21). Aberrations in FHR and pathologic patterns whose pathophysiology is only somewhat understood are the indicators used to diagnose fetal well-being. Although one must clinically assume that late decelerations, as shown in Figure 1, are associated with hypoxemia, the overall judgment regarding such observations and their significance at times remains difficult. Likewise, variable decelerations, as shown in Figure 2, even though denoting a possible lethal potential, are frequently encountered, and yet newborn outcome is seriously compromised only infrequently. At times, FHR changes defy a clear labeling, or, as shown in Figure 3, the potential pathophysiologic mechanism becomes identified only at delivery.

It would seem reasonable to accept the fact that the late decelerations shown in Figure 1 were associated with uteroplacental insufficiency, and, judging from the depressed, acidemic newborn, a diagnosis of fetal distress was justified. In Figure 2, the variable decelerations that became most apparent just prior to delivery were probably the result of umbilical cord compression. Likewise, the patient record presented in Figure 3 could probably be explained through the mechanism of cord compression. In viewing these cases, it becomes apparent that the most dramatic FHR changes were associated with the better newborn state, and the question is raised in the latter cases: Was fetal distress present? Or was this merely a tolerable stress associated with FHR changes that reflected the remarkable cardiovascular adaptations of the fetus? Such questions are largely unanswerable, as is the question: What would the outcome have been in the fetus with six loops of cord around its neck should labor have proceeded?

Assessment of fetal status during labor is primarily based on FHR patterns whose recognition implies a probable pathophysiologic event. Practically, the suspected causes of distress can be divided into two groups: (1) uteroplacental insufficiency and (2) umbilical cord compression through the recognition of late deceleration and variable deceleration. With an understanding of the associated pathophysiology in each of these circumstances, an attempt can be made to identify the precipitating factor and institute proper therapy. Obvious examples would be severe variable decelerations, in which case one would perform a vaginal examination and, on diagnosing a prolapsed cord, commence delivery. Similarly, the observation of late decelerations of FHR in the patient with hypotension, vaginal bleeding, and an abruption would call for prompt therapy, but not necessarily delivery if the pathologic FHR patterns abate.

Clinical Management

Confronted with an abnormal FHR, one can logically assume that some stress factor is responsible. The first step undertaken must be directed at asking: Is the stress factor identifiable? Secondarily, one must ask: (1) Can the stress be altered or removed? and (2) Will this stress reoccur? The most difficult problem is defining the possibility that such a stress may lead to true fetal distress, damage or death. In such cases, supplemental biochemical analysis provides invaluable data, but, in the last analysis, a composite of factors must be considered in arriving at a final clinical decision.

Identifying Stress

When attempting to discover the etiology or the provoking stress associated with an FHR pattern abnormality, one should consider both maternal and fetal factors.

Fetal Factors. The most common fetal problem involves umbilical cord compression or entanglement. Uncommon factors such as fetal anemia are identifiable with FHR changes, the most dramatic of these occurring with rapid hemorrhage from a ruptured vasa previa or fetal-maternal bleed (22).

Maternal Factors. Acute events that alter delivery of oxygen or fetal-maternal exchange at the intervillous site provoke FHR changes as the fetus attempts to adjust. The fetus may become deprived of its oxygen supply in two basic ways: (1) the exchange areas may become disrupted by placental abruption, and (2) oxygen delivery from the mother may be diminished.

The most common factors producing diminished oxygen delivery to the intervillous space are maternal hypotension and excessive uterine activity. In one case, there is a diminished intervillous flow as the result of the lower perfusing pressure, and, in the other, even though pressure is adequate, the vessels are occluded by myometrial contraction. Rarely, maternal hypoxemia secondary to respiratory arrest or severe anemia is causative.

Treatment

Any treatment scheme is largely based on an empiric approach that attempts to identify a probable cause, manipulate maternal factors, and then assess the result in an FHR change.

Variable Deceleration

The approach to cord compression patterns (variable decelerations) is to change the maternal position, thus altering mechanical factors and restoring umbilical circulation.

Late Deceleration

The term *uteroplacental insufficiency,* which is associated with late deceleration, must broadly define whether excessive uterine activity is impeding flow or whether hypotension is the underlying cause. Excessive uterine activity is most often due to oxytocin administration, which abates with discontinuance. Spontaneously occurring activity might logically be treated with uterine relaxant drugs, as these agents become available. When hypotension is encountered, a reason for its occurrence should be sought. Supine hypotension is usually simply corrected by placing the mother on her left side, or with uterine displacement. The hypotensive episode following sympathetic blockade induced by regional anesthesia can be largely prevented with volume expansion and positional therapy. Blood replacement in severe anemia or hypovolemia is necessary. Substances such as vasopressors, which raise the maternal blood pressure, may diminish uterine flow and thus further compromise an already stressed fetus.

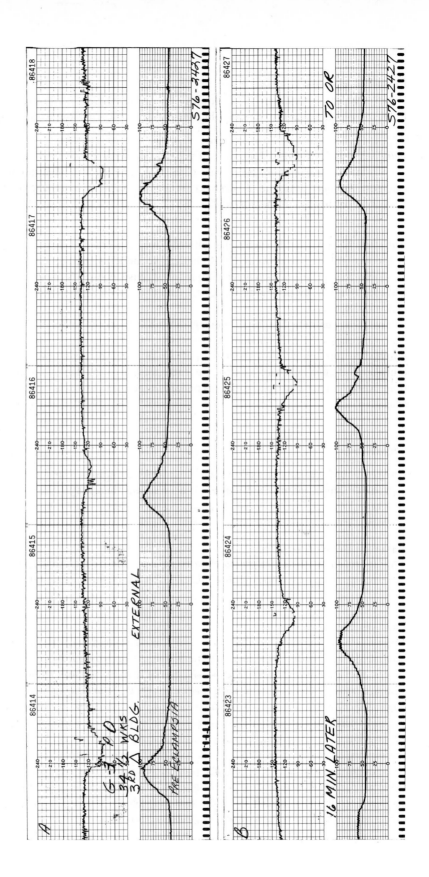

324

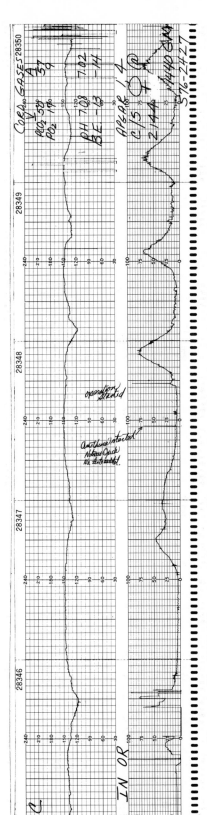

Figure 1. The FHR-UC tracing is from a nulliparous patient at 34 weeks who had mild preeclampsia and vaginal bleeding. Note the smooth baseline FHR in the lower panel (direct method) and repetitive late decelerations. At cesarean delivery the Apgars were 1 and 4, and weight was 1440 g.

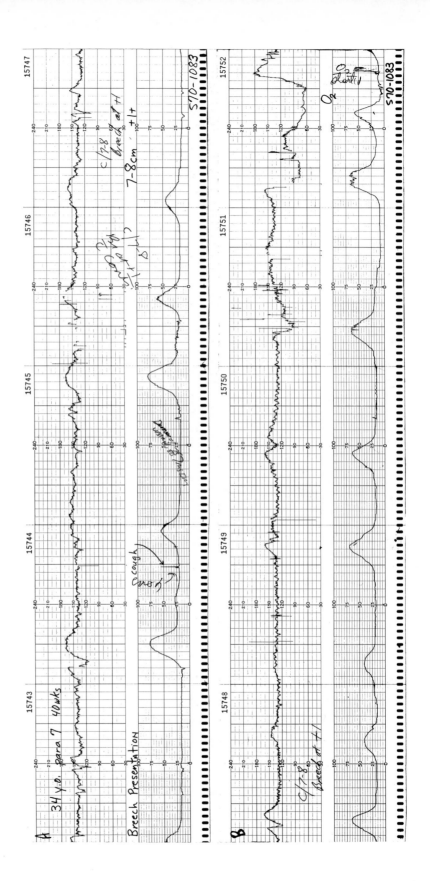

326

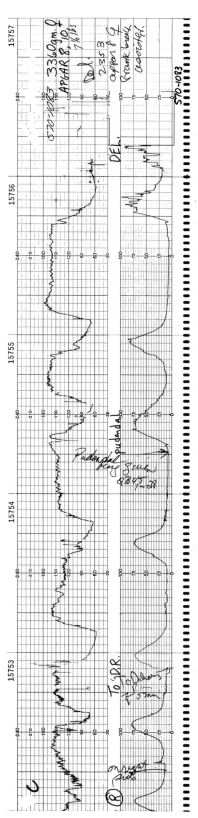

Figure 2. The FHR-UC tracing during labor in a term, nulliparous, breech presentation shows the progressive, rapid development of variable decelerations. In advanced labor (7 to 8 cm) the apparent stress was tolerated, and outcome was good, as noted in the lower right corner. Note the average (normal baseline variability throughout the record.

327

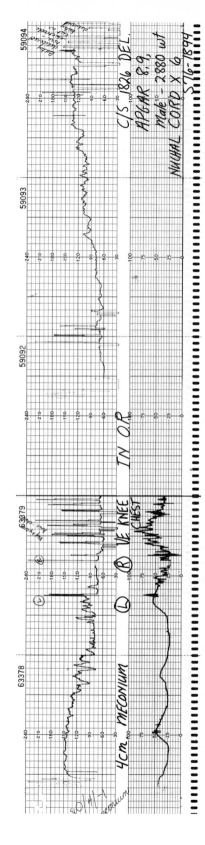

Figure 3. After amniotomy at 4 cm dilatation, a marked FHR fall occurs, and meconium is noted. In view of the persistent bradycardia, delivery by cesarean section was performed. The cord was around the neck six times, and Apgars were 8 and 9.

Maternal oxygen administration causes maternal hyperoxia, which may, to a degree, improve fetal oxygenation. However, fundamental to any attempts designed to relieve fetal distress is the fact that both umbilical and intervillous blood flows must be adequate. Primary therapy must seek to maintain adequate blood flows, and administration of substances such as glucose or bicarbonate to the mother is of questionable value.

Another questionable approach involves maternal administration of therapeutic doses of atropine, which is transferred to the fetus. This drug eliminates the vagal effect, thus modifying the FHR pattern appearance. Although the symptom is relieved, the impact or benefit to the human fetus remains in doubt.

Ongoing Management

As has been pointed out, the FHR serves to bring attention to the stressed fetus. The success of relieving stress is usually identified through the continuum of FHR observation. Thus, when an abnormal pattern reverts to normal, one may assume an improved fetal state. To exemplify this, Figure 4 demonstrates the typical FHR response secondary to the acute stress imposed by a tetanic contraction. As the fetus becomes deprived of oxygen during excessive uterine activity, the FHR falls. As the uterine activity subsides with discontinuance of oxytocin, the FHR rises to a higher level (compensatory tachycardia), and the degree of FHR variability is diminished. Fetal pH sampling at such a time would often reveal pathologic levels (less than 7.20), and yet intervention would be inappropriate with the stress factor removed. The therapy in this case is, first, to recognize a stress—excessive uterine activity—and then discontinue the oxytocin. Most would agree that stress had occurred in such a circumstance, although the long-term significance of such events is unknown. One can practically assume that intervillous flow was interrupted, fetal asphyxia had ensued, and prompt recognition and treatment seems most desirable. In such a circumstance, the poststress FHR abnormality (tachycardia and diminished variability) generally reverts to normal in 10 to 30 min.

Repeated reference has been made regarding FHR variability and its observation. Evaluation of FHR variability is useful clinically and, when present, seemingly reflects an intact central nervous system control of the FHR. Although mathematical machine approaches have been attempted, visual interpretation remains the clinically available tool (23,24).

Ideally the clinical appraisal of fetal well-being can be approached as follows: The FHR patterns are identified, thus providing an indication of possible pathologic mechanisms. The baseline FHR characteristics are evaluated; a decrease in variability and a rise which would reflect probable compensation resulting from an oxygen debt. The reality many times is that the FHR patterns are not so specifically identifiable and that additional factors may also affect FHR characteristics such as maternal drug administration. In such cases, the additional information provided through fetal blood sampling and scalp blood pH is an essential aid in management. In contrast to the acute event shown in Figure 4, a stress state may extend over hours rather than minutes, making recognition more elusive. Thus, many times the stress-distress state must be defined by multiple observations that seek to establish a trend of change in fetal condition. With such an approach, it becomes obvious that there is no magical time limit or standard approach. Each fetus and mother must receive an individualized approach to their care.

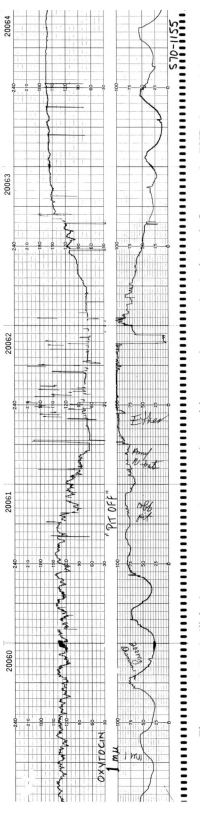

Figure 4. A "typical" fetal response to an acute stress imposed by a tetanic contraction is depicted. Contrast the FHR characteristics before and after the fetal insult.

330

With development of new instrumentation for continuous O_2 or pH, we will better understand the fetal environment. The differentiation of stress from distress remains a dilemma that will become more clearly defined through expanded experience and new approaches.

REFERENCES

1. Quilligan, E. J., and Paul, R. H.: Fetal monitoring: Is it worth it? *Obstet. Gynecol.* 45:96–100, 1975.

2. Gultekin-Zootzmann, B.: The history of monitoring the human fetus. *J. Perinat. Med.* 3:135–144, 1975.

3. Kergaradec, M. D. A. L., de: Mémoire sur l'Auscultation appliquée à l'Etude de la Grossesse ou Recherches sur deux nouveaux signes propres à faire reconnaitre plusieurs circonstances de l'Etat de Gestation; lu à l'Académie royale de médecine, dans sa séance générale du 26 décembre 1821. Paris, 1822.

4. Benson, R. C., Shubeck, F., Deutschberger, J., Weiss, W., and Berendes, H.: Fetal heart rate as a predictor of fetal distress. *Obstet. Gynecol.* 32:259–266, 1968.

5. Spellacy, W. N., Buhi, W. C., and Birk, S. A.: The effectiveness of human placental lactogen measurements as an adjunct in decreasing perinatal deaths. (Results of a retrospective and a randomized controlled prospective study). *Am. J. Obstet. Gynecol.* 121:835–844, 1975.

6. Goebelsmann, U., Freeman, R. K., Mestman, J. H., Nakamura, R. M., and Woodling, B. A.: Estriol in pregnancy: II. Daily urinary estriol assays in the management of the pregnant diabetic woman. *Am. J. Obstet. Gynecol.* 115:795–802, 1973.

7. Martin, C. B., Jr., Manning, F. A., and Platt, L. D.: Assessment of fetal breathing by real time B-scan in the diagnosis of poor fetal growth, submitted for publication.

8. Hon, E. H., and Wohlgemth, R.: The electronic evaluation of fetal heart rate: IV. The effect of maternal exercise. *Am. J. Obstet. Gynecol.* 81:361, 1961.

9. Ray, M., Freeman, R., Pine, S., et al.: Clinical experience with the oxytocin challenge test. *Am. J. Obstet. Gynecol.* 114:1, 1972.

10. Rochard, F., Schifrin, B. S., Goupil, F., Legrand, H., Blottiere, J., and Sureau, C.: Nonstressed fetal heart rate monitoring the the antepartum period. *Am. J. Obstet. Gynecol.* 126:699–706, 1976.

11. Fox, H. E., Steinbrecher, M., and Ripton, B.: Antepartum fetal heart rate and uterine activity studies: I. Preliminary report of accelerations and the oxytocin challenge test. *Am. J. Obstet. Gynecol.* 126:61–69, 1976.

12. Lee, C. Y., Di Loreto, P. C., and Logrand, B.: Fetal activity acceleration determination for the evaluation of fetal reserve. *Obstet. Gynecol.* 48:19–26, 1976.

13. Kubli, F. W., Hon, E. H., Khazin, A. F., and Takemura, H.: Observations on heart rate and pH in the human fetus during labor. *Am. J. Obstet. Gynecol.* 104:1190–1206, 1969.

14. Paul, R. H., Huey, J. R., Jr., and Yaeger, C. F.: Clinical fetal monitoring: Its effect on cesarean section rate and perinatal mortality: Five year trends. *Postgrad. Med.* 61:160–166, 1977.

15. Shenker, L., Post, R. C., and Seiler, J. S.: Routine electronic monitoring of fetal heart rate and uterine activity during labor. *Obstet. Gynecol.* 46:185–189, 1975.

16. Gabert, H. A., and Stenchever, M. A.: Electronic monitoring as a routine practice in an obstetrical service: A progress report. *Am. J. Obstet. Gynecol.* 118:534–537, 1974.

17. Lee, W. K., and Baggish, M. S.: The effect of unselected intrapartum fetal monitoring. *Obstet. Gynecol.* 47:516–520, 1976.

18. Goodlin, R. C.: Fetal cardiovascular responses to distress. *Obstet. Gynecol.* 49:371–381, 1977.

19. Myers, R. E., Mueller-Heubach, E., and Adamsons, K.: Predictability of the state of fetal oxygenation from a quantitative analysis of the components of late deceleration. *Am. J. Obstet. Gynecol.* 115:1083–1094, 1973.

20. Hon, E. H., and Khazin, A. F.: Biochemical studies of the fetus: I. The fetal pH-measuring system. *Obstet. Gynecol.* 33:219–236, 1969.

21. Schifrin, B. S., and Dame, L.: Fetal heart rate patterns: Prediction of Apgar scores. *J.A.M.A.* 219:1322–1325, 1972.

22. Gabbe, S. G., Nelson, L., and Paul, R. H.: Fetal heart response to acute hemorrhage. *Obstet. Gynecol.* 49:247–251, 1977.

23. Paul, R. H., Khazin Suidan, A., Yeh, S., Schifrin, B. S., and Hon, E. H.: Clinical fetal monitoring: VII. The evaluation and significance of intrapartum baseline FHR variability. *Am. J. Obstet. Gynecol.* 123:206–210, 1975.

24. Laros, R. K., Wong, W. S., Heilbron, D. C., Parer, J. T., Shnider, S. M., Naylor, H., and Butler, J.: A comparison of methods for quantitating fetal heart rate variability. *Am. J. Obstet. Gynecol.* 128:381–392, 1977.

12
Newborn and Infant Resuscitation

L. Stanley James, M.D.

The majority of healthy infants breathe spontaneously within a few seconds of being born, even before separation from their mother. Until recently, it was believed that the fetus made breathing movements in utero only under abnormal conditions and that the normal fetus remained entirely in a state of apnea. However, observations on human fetuses in utero have shown that as much as 80% of a 24-hr period is occupied by fetal respiratory movements (1). This period of fetal "breathing" coincides with periods of electrical brain activity usually associated with rapid eye movement (REM) sleep (2). It is possible that fetal breathing permits the fetus a "great deal of practice in utero" for a function so vitally important when the fetus is born.

During fetal breathing there is relatively little displacement of tracheal fluid. Since a considerable quantity of fluid is produced by the fetal lung, there is a net flow of fluid from the lung into the pharynx; some of the fluid is swallowed by the fetus and some of it passes into the amniotic cavity. Fetal respiratory movements appear to be influenced by elevations of $PaCO_2$ and PaO_2; they are also decreased or abolished by analgesic agents and disappear if the fetus becomes hypoxic. Thus, strictly speaking, the first breath is but a continuum of respiratory activity begun in utero. The major change is that respiration becomes continuous and is not interrupted by periods of apnea.

THE FIRST BREATH

Cineradiographic studies have been made of the chest wall as it emerges from the birth canal. The chest wall expansion can draw in between 7 and 42 ml of air to replace fluid squeezed from the air passages during the final stages of delivery and provides an explanation for the cough that occasionally precedes the first inspiratory effort (3). The glossopharyngeal muscles may force down an additional 5 to 10 ml ("frog breathing") (4). Neither of these is essential, however, since uneventful lung expansion occurs in infants delivered by cesarean section or in whom "frog breathing" is prevented by the insertion of a pharyngeal airway.

With the first few inspiratory efforts a gas-liquid interface is formed in the alveolus. This creates surface-tension forces at the gas-liquid interface. The mature lung depends on the surface-active lipoprotein alveolar lining (surfactant) to decrease the surface tension. It has been demonstrated that pressures as high as −70 cm H_2O may be produced to form this initial air-fluid interface in term infants delivered by the vaginal route (3). Much of the air of the first breath remains in the lung as residual volume. However, despite the high negative intrathoracic pressures sometimes observed, it is surprising how often the initial lung expansion appears to require little effort. The first inspiration is usually followed by a cry as the infant expires against a partially closed glottis; this creates a positive intrathoracic pressure of up to 40 cm of water. After the first breaths the lungs are almost completely and evenly expanded, and, within a few minutes, functional residual capacity reaches about three quarters of final aeration.

Little is known about the rate of absorption of the liquid present in the alveoli and air passages at the time of lung expansion. Its low protein content would facilitate rapid absorption as soon as pulmonary blood flow increases, and absorption probably occurs during the first few breaths. Under conditions of severe asphyxia, when pulmonary vascular resistance remains high, removal of fluid could be delayed. This might explain the difficulties encountered in lung expansion under such circumstances. Although the work required for initial lung expansion is undeniably greater than that for quiet breathing, it is not greater than that performed many times a day during vigorous crying.

MAINTENANCE OF BREATHING

A number of excitatory and inhibitory stimuli combine to maintain respiratory acitivity. The excitatory stimuli arise from proprioceptors in the joints, thermal receptors in the skin, and chemoreceptors that respond to hypoxia, hypercarbia, and acidosis (5,6,7). With the occlusion of the umbilical cord there is a widespread sympathetic discharge and a marked increase in the activity of the cervical sympathetic nerves (8). Afferent discharges from the chemoreceptors increase from previously very low levels, blood is shunted from peripheral vascular beds, and cervical vessels dilate (9,10). Finally, cold stimulation appears to play an essential role in the maintenance of rhythmical breathing (11). At the same time inhibitory receptors begin to function. Pulmonary stretch receptors, apparently under vagal control, cause cessation of spontaneous inflation after ventilation of the neonatal lung. Receptors in the upper respiratory passages inhibit respiration in response to fluid in the trachea. Other receptors have been demonstrated in the fetal snout and in the larynx of newly born sheep (12).

FAILURE TO BREATHE

Probably the most common single cause for delay in the onset of breathing is maternal medication producing depression of the respiratory center or the chemoreceptors. However, in most instances, there is a combination of medication plus a more severe degree of asphyxia; the depressant effect of narcotics appears to be potentiated by hypoxia and acidosis. Trauma, as with a rapid molding of the head during a precipitous labor or a difficult aftercoming head in a breech delivery, also appears to contribute, but this effect is difficult to quantitate or to separate from asphyxia, which is usually also present. Added to these factors are the various inhibitory reflexes in the upper airway, (12) particularly in infants who have aspirated meconium or amniotic fluid.

BIRTH ASPHYXIA

During normal labor and delivery there is a reduction of gaseous exchange across the placenta, resulting in a relative degree of hypoxia, hypercarbia, and acidosis (asphyxia). The average value for oxygen saturation is 22%, and, in nearly one quarter of the infants, it is less than 10% (13). Thus, at birth the normal healthy infant has no oxygen reserves. The low oxygen levels are accompanied by varying degrees of hypercapnia and acidosis, the average carbon dioxide pressure being 50 mm Hg; the average pH, 7.28. Although the acid-base status of the developing fetus near term is not known, studies of experimental animals suggest that it is likely to be close to that of the mother (14). Although the oxygen tension of the developing fetus is considerably lower than that of the mother in all the species studied, it can be deduced that the fetus does not suffer from oxygen lack because of its normal acid-base state. This deduction is confirmed by the relatively high cardiac output and the high oxygen consumption of the fetus (15).

Several factors can disturb the normal functional relation between fetal and maternal circulations and cause fetal acidosis. Blood flow through the intervillous space is reduced or may stop during strong uterine contractions; it is also reduced if the mother becomes hypotensive as a result of compression of the inferior vena cava or aorta by the uterus. Maternal hyperventilation leading to alkalosis also appears to lead to a reduction in intervillous flow and to fetal acidosis (16). In addition to these factors, changes in maternal acid-base balance as a result of excessive muscular activity or dehydration during prolonged labor or as a result of respiratory depression from drugs and anesthesia are reflected in the fetus. On the fetal side, cord compression occurs in approximately one-third of all deliveries and probably represents the most common mechanism interfering with transplacental exchange (13).

The composition of cord blood at birth is therefore the result of a disturbance in the functional relationship between mother and fetus during labor and delivery and does not reflect adaptation to a hypoxic environment in utero. This also applies to infants delivered by cesarian section, whether emergency or elective. The posture of the mother, the anesthesia, and the surgical manipulations themselves all probably contribute to disturbances in perfusion of the intervillous space, leading to various degrees of asphyxia.

PHYSIOLOGICAL CHANGES DURING ACUTE ASPHYXIA

During acute asphyxia both blood pressure and heart rate fall, and gasping efforts cease. Following successful resuscitation, both heart rate and blood pressure rise, and gasping resumes. During the initial period of asphyxia there are quite frequent respiratory efforts, followed by a period when respiration stops briefly. This condition is termed primary apnea. Thereafter, for a variable length of time in different species, rhythmic gasping continues until the animal ceases to gasp. The last gasp occurs at about $8\frac{1}{2}$ min in the monkey. After the last gasp nothing restarts gasping except artificial ventilation or, if done soon enough, the rapid correction of blood pH. The reinitiation of gasping requires a variable period of resuscitation, which is directly related to the duration of asphyxia after the last gasp. Observations of severely asphyxiated newborn monkeys indicate that 2 min of resuscitation is required for each minute that has elapsed since the last gasp to reinitiate gasping and 4 min is required before spontaneous breathing is established (17–19). Thus for an infant asphyxiated 3 min after the last gasp, it would require 6 min of resuscitation to initiate gasping and 12 min before spontaneous breathing is established.

The severely asphyxiated infant not only is hypoxic and acidotic but also has profound hypotension and can be considered to be in circulatory collapse.

WHOM TO RESUSCITATE

The Apgar score, which was introduced to facilitate the initial observation and to quantitate the clinical condition of the infant, is a useful guide to the need for resuscitation (20,21). It focuses on five vital signs: heart rate, respiratory effort, muscle tone, reflex irritability, and color, all judged 60 sec after complete delivery of the infant. This particular time interval was chosen, since it coincided with maximal depression in our clinic. These are the five "classic signs" that have been used for many years by anesthesiologists to evaluate a patient's condition during surgery. For each of them, a value of 0, 1, or 2 is given. A score of 0 is given for each of the following: no heart beat, no respiratory effort, no muscle tone, no reflex response to a glancing slap on the soles of the feet, and a blue or pale color. A score of 1 is given for a slow heart beat (less than 100), slow or irregular respiratory effort, some flexion of the extremities, a grimace to a glancing slap on the soles of the feet, and a pink body with blue extremities. Finally, a score of 2 is given for a heart rate over 100, good respiratory effort accompanied by crying, fully flexed limbs, a vigorous cry in response to a slap on the feet, and a completely pink coloration.

The majority of infants are vigorous with a score of 7 to 10, cry or cough within seconds of delivery, and require no resuscitative procedures. Mildly to moderately depressed infants scoring 4 to 6 form the largest group requiring some form of resuscitation. They are pale or blue at 1 min after birth, have not sustained respiration, and may be nearly flaccid. However, their heart rate and reflex irritability are good. Severely depressed infants score 0 to 3. They are pale or cyanotic, apneic, hypotonic, and have a reduced or absent reflex response, and their heart rates are slow or inaudible. Artificial ventilation should be commenced immediately in these infants.

The five signs disappear in a predictable fashion during asphyxiation of the newborn. In vigorous infants who cry lustily as soon as they are born, heart rate, reflex response, and tone are all present to the full extent; the only signs to which the observer has to pay attention are color and respiration. Mildly depressed babies are cyanotic (0 for color), but heart rate and reflex response are usually normal; attention has to be focused primarily on tone and respiration. In severely depressed infants who are pale (0 for color), apneic (0 for respiration), and usually flaccid (0 for tone), attention has to be paid primarily to heart rate and reflex response.

All the signs but reflex response can be seen—respiration from chest movement, tone from flexed or moving extremities, and heart rate from movement of the index finger of the nurse who listens to the heart with a stethoscope. A normal reflex response is present in all vigorous infants. This sign should be tested for in those infants scoring 6 or less and forms part of the resuscitation procedure during the first minute of life. In practice, the heart rate can be slow (under 100) or fast (over 160). In the high score group it is fast, probably in response to catecholamine release due to elevated tension of carbon dioxide and the cold stimulus at birth. In those scoring 6 or less who are not breathing, it is slow either as a result of baroreceptive reflex or myocardial depression.

Initially, the physician may have some difficulty in evaluating the five signs at once. If he makes a mental note of the total clinical picture when 1 min has elapsed, he can then assign a value for each of the clinical signs.

A physician or nurse is soon able to score the infant serially. This has been most useful for record keeping. The busy physician can readily evaluate the infant at 1, 2, 5, and 10 min. If these serial scores are recorded on the infant's chart, his clinical course can be reconstructed readily by the nursery physician, who may not have been present in the delivery room. Thus, the scoring system serves as a rather precise shorthand method describing the recovery rate of an infant whose condition may change rapidly from moment to moment. This is extremely valuable on a busy obstetric service where there may not be time for detailed notation of the changing clinical state.

A further advantage of the scoring system is that it defines the infants at high risk, with regard to both mortality and morbidity. The mortality in low score infants is nearly 15 times that in the high score group, and respiratory distress syndrome occurs significantly more frequently in low score than high score infants.

The time to assign the score is 60 sec after birth. There should be some automatic way to announce the passage of 60 sec. A simple alarm timer should be firmly fixed on the wall and set for 60 sec. When the head and feet of the infant are visible, the timer is started, and when the alarm sounds at 60 sec, the score is assigned.

Experience has demonstrated that the person delivering the infant should not be the one to assign the score. He is usually emotionally involved with the outcome of the delivery and with the family and may not make an impartial decision. It is ideal to have a specially trained observer, whether physician or nurse, but this situation is seldom practical. Until such time as a pediatrically oriented person is routinely present for all deliveries, the anesthesiologist is in a good position to assign the score, particularly if the infant is placed in a bassinet near the head of the delivery table.

RESUSCITATION PROCEDURES

Successful resuscitation of the infant in the delivery room depends on an organized plan coordinating the activites of the obstetrician, anesthesiologist, pediatrician, and delivery room nursing staff. Detailed plans for the management of the asphyxiated infant, including the duties of each member of the team, must be thoroughly understood, and routine procedures should be developed to assure the readiness of equipment and personnel at all times. There must be adequate space set aside in the delivery room to meet the many needs of the infant in distress.

The techniques required to resuscitate a newborn infant are potentially dangerous and when used by unskilled personnel can cause serious injury. Pulmonary resuscitation requires:

1. Establishment and maintenance of the airway
2. Expansion of the lungs
3. Initiation and maintenance of effective ventilation

These goals are most efficiently achieved by endotracheal intubation under direct laryngoscopy with mouth-to-tube or bag-to-tube ventilation. The bag-to-mask or mouth-to-mouth technique is easier to learn and is usually effective when the mask is properly placed and the head and jaw are carefully positioned to ensure an open airway. Mouth-to-mouth resuscitation should be used only if for any reason the other methods are not available. Expansion of the lungs after endotracheal intubation under direct laryngoscopy is the best method, but the resuscitator must maintain his skills through frequent use. Expertise in the use of the laryngoscope and artificial ventilation can best be learned on a cat anesthetized with ketamine.

Following birth, the infant should be held head down to promote drainage of amniotic fluid, blood, and vaginal mucus from the oropharynx. During or at birth, the mouth and throat should be aspirated gently with a suction catheter or ear syringe. To minimize cold stress and a fall in body temperature, dry promptly and place the infant under an infrared heat source.

The moderately depressed infants scoring 4–6 usually respond to relatively simple forms of resuscitation. The airway should be cleared with brief pharyngeal suction, and a small plastic oropharyngeal airway should then be inserted into the mouth and oxygen applied under pressure of 16 to 20 cc of water for 1 to 2 sec. Although this pressure is insufficient to expand the alveoli, some oxygen reaches the respiratory bronchioles. Stimulation of the pulmonary stretch receptors from the positive pressure usually initiates a gasp. If this maneuver produces no response, a brief painful stimulus induced by a quick smack on the soles of the feet may be sufficient to break through depression of the respiratory center and stimulate a cry.

If neither of these procedures has produced a response, it is necessary to intubate the infant and expand the lungs artificially. Intubation is best accomplished with the infant lying supine on a flat surface. A folded towel under the head and slight extension of the neck place him in a position resembling a sniffing posture. The head should be steadied with the right hand and kept in line with the body. The laryngoscope is held in the left hand, and the blade is introduced at the right corner of the mouth and advanced between tongue and palate for about 2 cm. As it is advanced, the blade is swung to the midline. This moves the tongue to the left of the blade. The operator looks along the blade for the rim of the epiglottis. The laryngoscope is gently advanced into the space between the base of the tongue and the epiglottis. Slight elevation of the tip of the blade exposes the glottis as a vertical dark slit bordered posteriorly by pink arytenoid cartilages.

If foreign material such as small blood clots, meconium-stained mucus, or vernix obstructs the larynx, quick brief suction is indicated. When the glottis is seen to be patent, a curved endotracheal tube is introduced at the right corner of the mouth and inserted through the cords until the flange of the tube rests at the glottis. Care must be taken not to intubate the esophagus. The laryngoscope is then withdrawn. Rarely, the glottis is obstructed by a laryngeal web. If this is partial or thin, it may be perforated with a stylet, or the opening may be enlarged with an endotracheal tube. The presence of a thick membrane requires immediate tracheostomy.

If stimuli from these procedures have not initiated a spontaneous gasp, positive pressure should be applied to the endotracheal tube. Brief puffs of air blown through the tube with enough force to cause the lower chest to rise gently usually start spontaneous respiration. If the stomach rises, however, the esophagus has been intubated instead of the trachea, and the position of the tube must be corrected. Pressures between

20 and 35 cm H_2O are necessary to expand the alveoli initially and can be applied safely for 1 to 2 sec. Experience in applying such pressures should be gained by puffing into a spring manometer. Oxygen-enriched gas may be delivered to the infant by placing a tube carrying oxygen in the operator's mouth.

If the endotracheal tube is fitted with appropriate-sized adapters, it can be connected to a rubber bag of oxygen or oxygen-enriched gas mixture or to one of the mechanical devices for applying positive pressure.

Artificial expansion of the lungs can initiate a spontaneous gasp. With the first or second application of positive pressure, the infant usually makes an effort to breathe. The endotracheal tube may be withdrawn after the infant has taken five or six breaths. If at the moment of birth it is clear that the infant is severely depressed from the complete absence of any spontaneous movement, pale color, and complete flaccidity, no time should be lost in establishing ventilation by expanding the lungs after prompt intubation.

CARDIAC MASSAGE

If the blood pressure is unduly low at the beginning of resuscitation, positive pressure ventilation is unlikely to be successful unless cardiac massage is used. Cardiac massage should not be initiated until after the lungs have been well expanded with two or three inflations. If the heartbeat cannot then be heard or if a slow heartbeat has not increased in rate, cardiac massage should be commenced. External manual compression of the heart between the chest wall and vertebral column forces blood into the aorta. Relaxation of pressure allows the heart to fill with venous blood.

The technique consists of intermittent compression of the middle and lower third of the sternum 100 to 200 times per minute with the index and middle fingers. Massage is interrupted every 5 sec to permit two or three inflations of the lung.

ADMINISTRATION OF ALKALI

Currently the most controversial aspect of newborn resuscitation is probably the administration of alkali because of the association found between hypernatremia and intracranial hemorrhage (22). Several lines of evidence have formed the basis for the administration of alkali in the severely asphyxiated infant. It has been shown to reduce the amount of brain damage (23), to reduce the time required to establish spontaneous breathing, and to increase the initial oxygen uptake in asphyxiated newborn monkeys (17). There is a significant decrease in combined cardiac output in fetal lambs in the face of hypoxemia plus acidosis (24). Pulmonary vascular resistance has been shown to vary directly with hydrogen ion concentration (25); a sudden rise in arterial pH improves pulmonary blood flow and increases PaO_2 (26,27). Mortality in the respiratory distress syndrome was reduced with early administration of intravenous glucose and sodium bicarbonate (28), and the early treatment of neonatal acidosis in low birthweight infants was found to be associated with a reduced morbidity rate (29). In addition, the synthesis of lecithin is markedly reduced in the presence of acidosis (30).

However, the demonstration of a significant association of intracranial hemorrhage, hypernatremia, and alkali administration in a retrospective study caused considerable concern (22). Furthermore, in a controlled prospective trial the finding of intracranial hemorrhage in 4 of 26 infants who received alkali by rapid intravenous infusion has raised further doubts about this therapy (31). On the other hand, another retrospective study (32) has failed to confirm the association of alkali therapy and intracranial hemorrhage. In our own clinic the incidence of intracranial hemorrhage was actually higher in those infants who did not receive alkali (33). Examination of the effect of alkali administration in the presence of elevated $PaCO_2$ revealed that a further rise in $PaCO_2$ was transient and bicarbonate appeared to be effective as a base for correcting acidosis (34).

From experimental work there seems little doubt that infusion of hypertonic solutions containing sodium can cause intracranial hemorrhage (35,36) and may in addition also cause hypocalcemia (37). When bicarbonate is administered in a "closed" system, the Pco_2 may rise and pH actually fall (38). Rapid infusion of bicarbonate to newborn puppies with mechanically fixed hypoventilation resulted in a rise in both $PaCO_2$ and osmolality (39).

It is therefore clear that the administration of alkali is not without risk; the risk will outweigh the benefits if alkali is given in too high a concentration, in too great a quantity, and in the presence of severely impaired ventilation. There seems to be little doubt that the adverse effects of alkali have been due to injudicious use, particularly in the presence of impaired CO_2 elimination. Sodium bicarbonate will be ineffective in correcting acidosis if a prompt increase in CO_2 excretion cannot be assured.

With these limitations in mind the beneficial effects of alkali appear to outweigh the risks in the immediate resuscitation of the newborn, provided the lungs can be expanded promptly and pulmonary ventilation established.

In principle, it is advisable initially to correct the metabolic component of the acid-base derangement only by one-half. The most severely asphyxiated infants, that is, those with an arterial pH below 7.0, have a base deficit of 26 mEq/liter or greater. By means of artifical ventilation alone, the base deficit can be reduced by approximately 10 mEq/liter in a matter of 5 to 10 min, provided that good alveolar ventilation is achieved and the infant does not remain in circulatory collapse. This change occurs as a result of bicarbonate shift and should be taken into consideration in calculations for the initial base administration in order to avoid overcorrection. In our own practice we aim first to half-correct this residual metabolic component of the acidosis. Thus, a 3-kg infant receives 7 or 8 mEq of base.

At present we recommend sodium bicarbonate rather than trishydroxyaminomethane, because the latter solution is able to enter the cell and occasionally causes depression of the respiratory center and arrest of breathing. Sodium bicarbonate as it is obtained from the ampule contains nearly 1 mEq/ml (44.7 mEq in 50 ml, 0.9 M solution). This solution has an osmolality of 1400 and a pH of 7.8. The solution is thus very hypertonic. It should be diluted in equal parts with distilled water to reduce its osmolality to 700 and infused at a rate not greater than 2 to 3 ml/min. If the heart rate is slow and irregular, the infusion should be accompanied by intermittent cardiac massage. The alkali may be infused into either the umbilical vein or artery.

The infant's response to alkali administration varies according to the degree of asphyxia, the effectiveness of ventilation, and the responsiveness of the cardiovascular system. It is important, therefore, to have a measurement of his acid-base state as soon as the initial dose of sodium bicarbonate has been given. This can usually be made by 15 min of age. The required amount of sodium bicarbonate for subsequent correction to a pH of 7.3 may then be calculated.

Since most asphyxiated infants have severe hypotension and are in shock, the question arises as to whether volume expansion alone would be a more appropriate therapy. This has been studied during resuscitation of asphyxiated newborn piglets and their recovery. Alkali was found to reduce the time required for establishment of spontaneous respiration. In animals that were asphyxiated to the point of cardiac arrest, the administration of alkali was essential for survival. However, these studies demonstrated that the administration of alkali could be hazardous or even fatal if administered too rapidly in the presence of a severely impaired circulation. Although there is no doubt about the importance of establishing ventilation, oxygenating the blood, and restoring the circulation, the need for volume expanders has not been proved. They should probably not be used unless there is clear evidence of hypovolemia and the blood pressure continues to remain low.

Special Considerations

Depression From Drugs Versus Asphyxia

An infant depressed primarily as a result of maternal analgesic or anesthetics can usually be distinguished by certain clinical signs from one depressed from asphyxia.

The infant depressed from medication has not passed meconium before birth; his skin is cyanotic rather than pale, since he has not received an asphyxial stimulus to cause peripheral vasoconstriction; his heart rate is slow but the pulse strong and full, and the cord is filled with blood, since his cardiovascular system has not been depressed by asphyxia; he is usually not completely hypotonic.

In contrast, the infant depressed primarily as a result of asphyxia is meconium-stained and pale as a result of intense peripheral vasoconstriction; the heart rate is slow and the sounds soft, distant, and occasionally irregular; the umbilical cord is limp and contains little blood.

Delayed Depression From Maternally Administered Analgesia and Anesthesia

Drugs that cross the placenta enter the fetus through the umbilical vein (UV) and the ductus venosus. A variable portion of the UV flow passes through the inferior vena cava through the liver and hepatic veins, and not through the ductus venosus. This places the liver in a strategic position for uptake of drugs, particularly those with a high fat solubility. Over 50% of barbiturates as well as a number of other drugs that have been studied are initially taken up by the liver. From here they can be released slowly over a period of hours. As a result, infants delivered soon after the mother has been given a drug might initially appear vigorous but develop a marked central nervous system depression 2 to 4 hr later. Therefore, when relatively large doses of sedatives or narcotics have been given to the mother and the infant breathes well at birth, he should nevertheless be carefully observed for delayed secondary depression. This may be so severe as to require an exchange transfusion.

Drug Antagonists

Analeptics and drug antagonists are rarely necessary in a modern obstetric practice. If indicated, when depression of the newborn is due to a narcotic, they should never be administered before the lungs have been expanded and the infant oxygenated by artificial ventilation.

Analeptics such as nikethamide serve no useful purpose in resuscitation of the newborn. Although they may shorten primary apnea, they are ineffective in secondary apnea and may cause hypotension and convulsions even if given in the clinically recommended dose.

The morphine antagonist N-allylnormophine has been reported to be of value. The drug should not be given unless the infant's respiratory depression is known to be due to maternal medication, since it augments the depression of asphyxia. Furthermore, the drug should not be given until the lungs have been expanded and the infant oxygenated. The dose is 0.2 mg/kg of body weight. Although crying and restlessness follow administration, this is frequently of brief duration and may be followed by more profound depression.

Toxicity From Local Anesthetics

Rarely local anesthetics may be injected accidentally into the fetus during an attempted caudal anesthesia or paracervical block. The infant is profoundly depressed at birth. However, as soon as he is oxygenated during the course of resuscitation, and the responsiveness of the central nervous system is partially restored, generalized convulsions occur. If the infant convulses after resuscitation, accidental injection to the fetus should be suspected immediately. The presenting part of the infant should be carefully examined for a needle puncture and the convulsion treated promptly with intravenous barbiturates, phenobarbital 15 to 20 mg/kg. It may be necessary to repeat the barbiturate and maintain the infant on a ventilator. As soon as is feasible, a 2 to 3 volume exchange transfusion should be performed.

A generalized convulsion may occur with acute respiratory obstruction or an overdose of analeptic drugs. These should offer no confusion with convulsions resulting from toxicity of local anesthetics, which occur only after the infant has been oxygenated.

Meconium Aspiration

The importance of suctioning meconium from the trachea and bronchi deserves special emphasis. Meconium is passed following an asphyxial episode in utero. If the asphyxial episode is accompanied by prolonged gasping, meconium will be drawn deeply into the lungs. The fetus may recover from this episode with regard to his acid-base state and central nervous system responsiveness but may yet be born with his lungs full of meconium. Such infants may intially be responsive and vigorously attempt to breathe.

If the amniotic fluid is heavily meconium-stained, the mouth and pharynx should be quickly suctioned as soon as the head is delivered and prior to delivery of the rest of the body. As soon as the infant is born, the larynx should then be observed, using a laryngoscope, irrespective of the initial responsiveness. If there is thick meconium at the back of the pharynx, it should be suctioned out under direct vision and the larynx intubated with an endotracheal tube that has a terminal hole (size 12 or 14, French). Suction should then be applied directly to this tube, which is gradually withdrawn while suction is applied. In our unit we use mouth-to-tube suction. Not infrequently, a large piece of meconium, too thick to pass up the endotracheal tube, is observed clinging to the tip of the tube. The trachea should be reintubated immediately and the procedure repeated until only watery mucus is obtained. It appears that the fluid normally produced by the fetal lung continues to form and washes out meconium from the deeper radicals of the lung. If the amniotic fluid is thick and watery and is only stained with meconium and the infant is actively responsive, laryngoscopy and intubation are not indicated. It should be emphasized that thick meconium cannot be removed from the lung through a fine-bore catheter inserted through the lumen of an endotracheal tube. Furthermore, instillation of saline through the endotracheal tube has not been found to be useful but serves only to delay the suctioning procedure.

Inability to Expand the Lungs

Under some circumstances, lung expansion is impossible in spite of proper intubation. There are four conditions in which this occurs: massive aspiration of meconium that cannot be removed by suctioning, intrauterine pneumonia with organization of exudate, large bilateral diaphragmatic hernias with severely hypoplastic lungs, and congenital adenomatous cysts of the lung. Infants with the first two conditions are usually severely depressed at birth. However, those with hypoplastic lungs may be vigorous initially and score as high as 7 at 1 min of age, making strenuous but ineffective respiratory efforts. At present there is no available treatment for this condition. Congenital adenomatous cysts of the lung are usually associated with hydrops fetalis, and the condition is usually fatal.

REFERENCES

1. Boddy, K., Dawes, G. S., and Robinson, J. S.: A 24-hour rhythm in the foetus, in *Foetal and Neonatal Physiology*, Proceedings of the Sir Joseph Barcroft Centenary Symposium. University Press, Cambridge, 1973, p. 63.

2. Dawes, G. S.: Revolutions and cyclical rhythms in prenatal life: Fetal respiratory movements rediscovered. *Pediatrics* 51:965, 1973.

3. Karlberg, P.: Adaptive changes in immediate postnatal period, with particular reference to respiration. *J. Pediat.* 56:585–604, 1960.

4. Bosma, J. F., and Lind, J.: Roentgenologic observations of motions of upper airway associated with establishment of respiration in newborn infant. *Acta Paediat.* 49:18–55, 1960.

5. Parker, H. R., and Purves, M. J.: Some effects of maternal hyperoxia and hypoxia on the blood gas tensions and vascular pressures in the foetal sheep. *Quart. J. Exp. Physiol.* 52:205, 1967.

6. Biscoe, T. J., Purves, M. J., and Sampson, S. R.: Types of nervous activity which may be recorded from the carotid sinus nerve in the sheep foetus. *J. Physiol.* 202:1, 1969.

7. Ponte, J., and Purves, M. J.: Types of afferent nervous activity which may be measured in the vagus nerve of the sheep fetus. *J. Physiol.* 229:51, 1973.

8. Kajikawa, H.: Mode of sympathetic innervation of the cerebral vessels demonstrated by the fluorescent histochemical technique in rats and cats. *Arch. Jap. Chir.* 38:227, 1969.

9. Dawes, G. S., Duncan, S. L. B., Lewis, B. V., Merlet, C. L., Owen-Thomas, J. B., and Reeves, J. T.: Hypoxaemia and aortic chemoreceptor function in foetal lambs. *J. Physiol.* 201:105, 1969.

10. Ponte, J., and Purves, M. J.: The role of the carotid body chemoreceptors and carotid sinus baroreceptors in the control of cerebral blood vessels. *J. Physiol.* 237:315, 1974.

11. Harned, H. S., and Ferreiro, J.: Circulatory effects related to alterations of the ambient environment of the term fetal lamb. *J. Pediat.* 85:120, 1974.

12. Johnson, P., Robinson, J. S., and Salisbury, D.: The onset and control of breathing after birth, in *Foetal and Neonatal Physiology*, Proceedings of the Sir Joseph Barcroft Centenary Symposium. Cambridge, University Press, 1973, p. 67.

13. James, L. S., Weisbrot, J. M., Prince, C. E., Holaday, D. A., and Apgar, V.: Acid-base status of human infants in relation to birth asphyxia and onset of respiration. *J. Pediat.* 52:379–394, 1958.

14. Joelsson, I., Barton, M. D., Daniel, S. S., James, L. S., and Adamsons, K.: A method for prolonged monitoring of physiological function during fetal life. *Am. J. Obstet. Gynec.* 107:445, 1970.

15. Comline, R. S., and Silver, M.: Placental transfer of blood gases, *Br. Med. Bull.* 31:25, 1975.

16. Moya, F., Morishima, H. O., Shnider, S. M., and James, L. S.: Influence of maternal hyperventilation on the newborn infant. *Am. J. Obstet. Gynec.* 91:76, 1965.

17. Adamsons, K., Jr., Behrman, R., Dawes, G. S., James, L. S., and Koford, C.: Resuscitation by positive pressure ventilation and tris-hydroxymethyl-aminomethane of rhesus monkeys asphyxiated at birth. *J. Pediat.* 65:807, 1964.

18. Daniel, S. S., Dawes, G., James, L. S., Ross, B., and Windle, W. F.: Hypothermia and resuscitation of asphyxiated fetal rhesus monkeys. *J. Pediat.* 68:45, 1966.

19. Cockburn, F., Daniel, S. S., Dawes, G. S., James, L. S., Myers, R. E., Nieman, W., Rodriquez de Curet, H., and Ross, B.: The effect of pentobarbital anesthesia on resuscitation and brain damage in fetal rhesus monkeys asphyxiated on delivery. *J. Pediat.* 75:281, 1969.

20. Apgar, V., Holaday, D. A., James, L. S., Weisbrot, I. M., and Berrien, C.: Evaluation of the newborn infant: Second report. *J.A.M.A.* 168:1985, 1958.

21. Apgar, V., and James, L. S.: Further observations on the newborn scoring system. *Amer. J. Dis. Child.* 104:419, 1962.

22. Simmons, M. A., Adcock, E. W., Bard, H., and Battagia, F. C.: Hypernatremia and intracranial hemorrhage in neonates. *New Engl. J. Med.* 291:6–10, 1974.

23. Adamsons, K., Jr., Behrman, R., Dawes, G. S., Dawkins, M. J. R., James, L. S., and Ross, B. B.: The treatment of acidosis with alkali and glucose during asphyxia in foetal rhesus monkeys. *J. Physiol.* 169:679, 1963.

24. Cohn, H. E., Macks, E. J., Heymann, M. A., and Rudolph, A. M.: Cardiovascular responses to hypoxemia and acidemia in fetal lambs. *Am. J. Obstet. Gynecol.* 120:817, 1974.

25. Rudolph, A. M., and Yuan, D.: Response of the pulmonary vasculature to hypoxia and H+ ion concentration changes. *J. Clin. Invest.* 45:399, 1966.

26. Chu, J., Clements, J. A., Cotton, E. K., Klaus, M. H., Sweet, A. Y., and Tooley, W. H.: Neonatal pulmonary ischemia: I. Clinical and physiological studies. *Pediatrics* 40:709, 1967.

27. Russell, G., and Cotton, E. K.: Effects of sodium bicarbonate by rapid injection and of oxygen in high concentration in respiratory distress syndrome of the newborn. *Pediatrics* 41:1063, 1968.

28. Usher, R.: Reduction of mortality from respiratory distress syndrome of prematurity with early administration of intravenous glucose and sodium bicarbonate. *Pediatrics* 32:966, 1963.

29. Hobel, C. J., Oh, W., Hyvarinen, M., Emmanouilides, G., and Erenberg, A.: Early versus late treatment of neonatal acidosis in low birth weight infants: Relation to respiratory distress syndrome. *J. Pediat.* 81:1178–1187, 1972.

30. Merritt, T. A., and Farrell, P. M.: Diminished pulmonary lecithin synthesis in acidosis: Experimental findings related to RDS. *J. Pediat.* 57:32–40, 1976.

31. Bland, R. D., Clarke, T. I., and Harden, L. B.: Rapid infusion of sodium bicarbonate and albumin into high-risk premature infants soon after birth: A controlled, prospective trial. *Am. J. Obstet. Gynecol.* 124:263, 1976.

32. Anderson, J. M., Cockburn, F., Bain, A. D., Forfar, J. O., Turner, T. L., Brown, J. K., and Machin, G. A.: Hyaline membrane disease, alkaline buffer treatment, and cerebral intraventricular haemorrhage. *Lancet* 1:117–119, 1976.

33. Driscoll, J. M., and James, L., unpublished data.

34. Baum, J. D., and Robertson, N. R. C.: Immediate effects of alkaline infusion in infants with respiratory distress syndrome. *J. Pediat.* 87:255, 1975.

35. Finberg, L., Luttrell, C., and Redd. H.: Pathogenesis of lesions in the nervous system in hypernatremic states: II. Experimental studies of gross anatomic changes and alterations of chemical composition of the tissues. *Pediatrics* 33:46, 1959.

36. Luttrell, C. N., Finberg, I., and Drawdy, L. P.: Hemorrhagic encephalopathy induced by hypernatremia: II. Experimental observations on hyperosmolality in cats. *Arch. Neurol.* 1:153, 1959.

37. Finberg, L.: Experimental studies of the mechanisms producing hypocalcemia in hypernatremic states. *J. Clin. Invest.* 36:434, 1957.

38. Ostrea, E. M., Jr., and Odell, G. B.: The influence of bicarbonate administration on blood pH in a "closed system": Clinical implications. *J. Pediat.* 80:671, 1972.

39. Steichen, J. J., and Kleinman, L. I.: Effect of HCO_3 therapy on acid-base homeostasis in newborn dogs with and without ventilatory restriction. *Ped. Res.* 11:543, 1977.

13
Bacterial Infections During Pregnancy

William J. Ledger, M.D.

The topic of intrauterine infection has great significance for obstetricians and neonatologists in the 1970s. A number of medical and social advances in the United States have contributed to a remarkable decline in the perinatal mortality rate in the past 10 years. These include the availability of pregnancy termination in the hospital that eliminates many high-risk pregnancies, a greater obstetrical awareness of high-risk pregnancy with an increasing number of therapeutic decisions for the sake of the fetus, and the development of neonatology as a subspecialty credited with improving survival rates among prematures. The residuum of newborn mortality shows overrepresentation of pregnancies resulting in the delivery of an infant weighing less than 2500 g. There is good evidence that a significant part of fetal and newborn loss in this population of prematures is due to infectious agents, which often cause little or no maternal symptomatology. It is the purpose of this chapter to review diagnostic and therapeutic techniques currently available for the obstetrician that should improve the salvage rates in this high-risk premature population.

Perinatal mortality is not the sole measure of obstetrical performance. Our major emphasis must be on the quality of life that survives. Many infectious agents that are not lethal to the fetus or newborn may cause central nervous system damage with disastrous long-term implications for the survivors. Another goal of this chapter is to focus on the recognition of perinatal infections that could unfavorably influence the future productivity of the survivors.

PATHOPHYSIOLOGY OF PERINATAL INFECTIONS

The fact that mortality and morbidity from infection predominate among newborns weighing less than 2500 g demands a focus on the physiologic events in pregnancies that are terminated prematurely. It is possible that recognizable shortcomings of maternal and fetal host defense mechanisms have contributed to this poor outcome. This area has been largely ignored by obstetricians, for our focus on these problems in the past has been mechanistic. Obstetrical literature is replete with studies that categorize only the length of gestation and the integrity of the membranes as the major variables in the analysis of fetal outcome. There are a number of other observed risk factors that can be

345

identified with currently available technology. Evaluation of these may lead to a better system of recognition of high-risk pregnancies.

There is an association between increased fetal loss and lower socioeconomic status of the mother. This relationship should be acknowledged in every epidemiologic survey that attempts to associate such variables as maternal smoking or vaginal carriage of mycoplasma with increased fetal loss. Few studies have focused specifically on the relationship of poverty to infectious problems in the newborn. The most inclusive evaluation was done by Naeye and Blanc; these investigators found double the rate of perinatal infection among urban poor blacks (1). Of interest was the finding of larger adrenal glands in infected infants, and this led to the speculation that intrauterine infection may be an initiator of premature labor through hyperfunction of the fetal adrenal gland.

Although the reason for the increased rate of perinatal infection in the urban poor is not known, there are a number of observations that may explain this association. Poor urban mothers are likely to have the same demonstrable decrease in the bactericidal and glycolytic activity of leukocytes that has been demonstrated in malnourished adults (2). In addition to the systemic maternal host defense mechanisms, there is evidence of an antibacterial substance present in the amniotic fluid (3). Although this antibacterial activity increases as the patient nears term, there are great individual variations among women, and there is evidence of lower antibacterial levels among poor mothers (4). The evidence of diminished host response to infection is not limited to the mother. In the newborn, black infants have lower serum IgM levels than whites, and half of the perinatal deaths have been reported to occur among infants with the lowest levels of IgM (5).

Cutting across class lines, there is clinical evidence that the fetus' response to a transplacental infection differs from that of the maternal host. It seems clear that antibody formation is different for the fetus and that this difference continues in the newborn period. For example, the fetus exposed to rubella virus early in pregnancy is unable to rid itself of this infective agent, and the newborn infant of such a pregnancy continues to excrete the virus for a long time after delivery. This is a markedly different response to the short-lived period of active virus excretion in the immunologically competent adult.

A major block to both the understanding and prevention of perinatal infections is an unsupported belief in the absolute barrier of intact fetal membranes to intrauterine infection. Most physician thinking about such common problems as premature rupture of the membranes fix the onset of infection with loss of membrane integrity. This truism is not always correct. Infection of the fetus can occur with intact membranes. The organisms may be blood-borne, as documented in a recent case report of a fatal infection with a group A beta hemolytic streptococcus (6). More commonly, the infection may be ascending, occurring across intact membranes, as has been noted by Benirschke (7). Recognition of this possibility should lead to better obstetrical diagnostic techniques, including transabdominal amniocentesis.

TORCH SYNDROME

TORCH is a term coined to categorize a group of microorganisms that cause serious morbidity and occasionally mortality among newborn infants, with little maternal symptomatology. This grouping makes no sense from a microbiologic standpoint, for the pathogens include such dissimilar microorganisms as viruses, bacteria, and protozoa. The justification for the continued use of this acronym lies in the similar clinical findings in the newborn and the serious impact on the reticuloendothelial system and central nervous system of the infants. For the obstetrician, the best understanding of the intricacies of diagnosis, prevention, and treatment will be achieved by discussion of the individual TORCH pathogens.

TOXOPLASMOSIS

Toxoplasma gondii is a protozoan that infects man as an obligatory intracellular parasite. This organism assumes different forms during its life cycle. The trophozoite is seen during the acute phase of infection and invades all types of mammalian cells. This form is easily killed by drying and by maternal antibody. The tissue cysts that develop in the host cells from the trophozoite are resistant to antibody and persist in muscle and the central nervous system. This form is the source of infection in poorly cooked meat consumed by humans, for these cysts are destroyed by temperatures above 50°C. Another form, the oocyst, develops in the intestinal mucosa of the cat family during the acute stage of infection and can be the cause of infection for the susceptible human owner of the acutely infected cat. This animal is thought to be the source of infection for vegetarians and meat eaters who avoid rare meat.

Toxoplasma gondii may result in a wide range of infectious responses. In the adult female, symptomatology associated with an acute infection is usually absent but in a small percentage of cases may be associated with a set of symptoms that resembles mononucleosis. Pregnant patients with "mononucleosis" should have tests performed for toxoplasmosis infection if their heterophile antibody test is normal. In the fetus, there can be intrauterine death or evidence of severe central nervous system or ocular damage. The classic triad of chorioretinitis, hydrocephalus, and intracranial calcification occurs in only a small number of infants (8). Most disturbing is the finding that infected babies that appear grossly normal at birth may develop retinochoroiditis, mental retardation, or seizure disorders in later years. The social costs for the failure to recognize and treat these asymptomatic newborns are enormous.

The pathophysiology of congenital infection has been well investigated. There is controversy about the possibility of fetal infection in a maternal host with a chronic infection, for it is possible this may occasionally occur. Disregarding these infrequent cases, there is a uniform sense that the most common threat to the newborn occurs with the initial acute infection of the mother during pregnancy. Knowing this, a major thrust of obstetrical care must be the early identification of susceptible women and the detection of acute infection during pregnancy. There is a wide range of risk to the fetus, depending on the trimester of maternal acquisition of infection. This is depicted in Figure 1 (9). Transmission of the parasite to the fetus is much more likely to be associated with the third trimester maternal infection than those occurring in the first and second thirds of pregnancy. This risk of infection may be related in part to the observation that placental infection usually precedes fetal infection (see Table I) (9). Additional evidence that supports the importance of the placental lesion are the findings in twin gestations in which one or both of the newborns may have congenital toxoplasmosis (10). The clinical pattern of toxoplasmosis, reflected by the extent and severity of newborn involvement, is similar in monochorial pregnancies, but vast differences in newborn

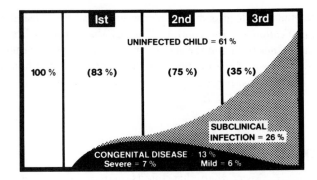

Figure 1. Outcome of pregnancies by trimester in which toxoplasmosis was acquired.

infection occur when there are separate placentas, with the possibility of different degrees of placental involvement. Although the fetus is less likely to be infected with acute maternal infection in the first trimester, the infections that occur then are more likely to have extensive central nervous system involvement at birth (see Fig. 1).

There is a wide range of maternal susceptibility to acute infection with *Toxoplasma gondii*. Adult women in countries in which there is frequent ingestion of raw or poorly cooked meat have a high rate of serologic conversion, usually greater than 75%. In the United States, one study of pregnant women in New York City found evidence of former infection in 1283 out of 4048 (31.7%) pregnant women who were surveyed (11). Within populations with a wide range of susceptible women, there is a small number of women who have an acute infection during pregnancy. In the New York study, there were 6 serologic converters among 2765 susceptible women (11).

The diagnosis of acute *Toxoplasma* infection is dependent on serologic evidence of infection. In the adult, the testing is based on the presence of IgG antibody and can be ascertained by the Sabin-Feldman dye test, a complement fixation test or a hemagglutination inhibition test. To evaluate recent acquisition, an immunofluorescent test for IgM can be performed. Any screening of an adult population will yield a percentage of women without antibody who are susceptible and thus at risk of acquiring infection during the pregnancy.

There is difficulty in the interpretation of the status of women with a low or high initial titer. The low titer should be repeated in 3 weeks to see if there is a significant rise, which would be compatible with recent infection. A high initial titer may occur with a recent or old infection. Recent infections can be correlated with the presence of a high IgM fluorescent antibody titer. In an ideal world, susceptible women could be rescreened late in pregnancy and again at the time of delivery to determine the acquisi-

Table I. Correlation of Toxoplasma Isolations From Placentas and Congenital Toxoplasmosis in the Child

Results	Placenta	Child	Percentage
Positive	40	38	95
Negative	342	5	1.5
Total	382	43	

tion of acute maternal infection. This would pinpoint newborns at risk for infection, who need a complete diagnostic workup. A cost-benefit analysis of such a program has not yet been done. This is important, for studies suggest that asymptomatic infected newborns may benefit from chemotherapy (12). The vagaries of diagnosis of infection in the newborn are detailed in Chapter 14.

The serologic surveillance of pregnant women and newborns is important, for the disease is preventable and treatable. The susceptible pregnant woman with no antibodies at the time of initial screening should be counseled to avoid poorly cooked meats during pregnancy and also intimate contact with a "hunter" cat. The treatment of patients with the many manifestations of toxoplasmosis is currently under study. Experience with chemotherapy is limited to date so that none of the treatment recommendations in this chapter should be considered absolute or binding. There are a number of drugs with laboratory and clinical evidence of effectiveness against *Toxoplasma gondii,* including spiramycin, sulfadiazine, and pyrimethamine. The consequences of adult infection on the adult host are so minimal that chemotherapy for adult symptomatology is not indicated. The justification for chemotherapy should be the elimination of intrauterine infection. Strategies for the use of systemic agents to eliminate this infection may take many forms. There is not likely to be support for first trimester chemotherapy because of concern about potential drug toxicity for the developing fetus, and there will be little enthusiasm for the use of sulfas just prior to delivery. Otherwise, therapy for the pregnant women who has acquired this disease during pregnancy may be recommended. Chapter 14 discusses the pros and cons for the screening of all newborns and the treatment of those with serologic evidence of acquisition of disease during pregnancy.

RUBELLA

The rubella virus was the first recognized viral teratogen. It is of interest that the observation linking this mild or inapparent maternal infection during pregnancy with serious newborn disability was not made in a laboratory devoted to basic research but by a clinically astute observer, in 1941 (13).

Since the first clinical observations by Gregg, repeated investigation in the intervening years has yielded a number of observations about the fetal and newborn manifestations of infection. There is a wide range of newborn risk of infection, influenced greatly by the timing of maternal acquisition of the virus during pregnancy. First trimester infection with "wild" virus can have a serious impact on many rapidly developing organ systems, including the central nervous system, where it causes cataracts, microcephaly, and deafness, and the cardiovascular system, where it causes congenital heart defects. Maternal infection occurring after completion of fetal organogenesis can still have a widespread and long-term impact on the newborn. The 1964 rubella epidemic showed continued long-term replication of virus in the newborns, with persistent shedding of virus for months or years. Some manifestations of fetal viral infection in the newborn may be prolonged hepatosplenomegaly and thrombocytopenia. The persistence of the virus in the newborn after in utero infection may account for the recently observed progessive rubella panencephalitis noted 10 or more years after birth (14,15). Fortunately, there seems to be little impact on the fetus when maternal rubella is acquired during the third trimester.

A number of important laboratory breakthroughs have contributed to our understanding of the impact of rubella in man. The most important was the isolation and identification of the "wild" virus (16,17). This eventually led to modification of the virus so that a live virus vaccine could be developed with the hope of preventing some of the serious newborn problems resulting from maternal acquisitition of "wild" virus during the first two trimesters of pregnancy. Another important advance was the development of serologic testing to determine the susceptibility and, in some cases, the recent acquisition by mothers of "wild" rubella virus during pregnancy. This permits a more scientific evaluation of individual patient risk factors during pregnancy. The absence of maternal antibody indicates susceptibility. Absent or low level of antibody, followed by an acute titer rise of four tubes or more when paired specimens are evaluated in the same laboratory, is strong evidence of acute infection.

The development, licensing, and widespread use of a rubella vaccine has been accompanied by much controversy and many unanswered questions. Very clearly, there was a tremendous variation in national policies toward this vaccine.

In Great Britain, emphasis was placed on immunization of a high-risk population. In the British view, "wild" rubella infection for the child or adult was not associated with sufficient morbidity to justify the widespread use of this vaccine. The population at risk was susceptible women with no antibody to rubella who might become pregnant. The program aimed at identification by serologic testing of susceptible adolescent females and immunization of the population at risk. This public health strategy is not without problems, for a large proportion of the older population develop symptoms of arthritis after immunization.

In the United States, an entirely different approach was used. The decision was made to attempt to achieve complete immunization of a younger population so that "herd" immunity would be gained. This was "safe," for there is evidence that virus could rarely be transmitted from innoculated children to susceptible pregnant women. It was believed that elimination of the pool of susceptible children would remove all risks of future rubella epidemics. This has not been the case. Rubella outbreaks have still been seen in older populations, even though only 15% were susceptible (18). In addition at least one group of investigators has questioned the concept of a pool of susceptible infants being the source of rubella spread among susceptible pregnant women. In a retrospective analysis of congenital rubella, they found no decrease in the frequency of rubella syndrome among women having their first pregnancy (19). This suggests that acquisition of the virus did not always occur because of exposure to infected children within the confines of the household. In addition, other concerns about this immunization program continue to be voiced. There is a real concern about both the peak level of antibodies and duration of immunization. Much lower titers are achieved by rubella immunization than by infection with the "wild" virus. If protection is lost after 6 to 10 years, we would face a whole generation of previously immunized but now susceptible women, instead of the estimated 15% of susceptible adults that existed in the 1960s before the vaccine program was started. It is not known whether the drop in antibody as time intervenes from the immunization will completely protect the fetus when a pregnant woman is exposed to "wild" rubella virus. There have been reports of evident adult infection with "wild" virus, as evidenced by titer rise, after previous immunization programs (20), and these may reflect a loss of immunity. Whether this titer rise was associated with viremia is not known. This information is critical to evaluation of the long-term protection afforded by the vaccine to women who subsequently become pregnant.

Recognition of the shortcomings of the initial immunization program in the United States has resulted in a number of altered strategies by physicians. The primary stimulus has been the recognition that widespread immunization has not eliminated rubella in the community, particularly in susceptible older age groups. The new focus has been on the recognition of susceptible women of childbearing age and selective immunization of this population. Such a program is theoretically simple to carry out. It requires antibody testing to determine susceptibility and the administration of vaccine to the women at risk. The only important proviso is that the woman not be pregnant at the time of vaccine administration or shortly afterward. This is important, for the modified virus used in immunization is "live," and there is evidence that it can cross the placenta and infect the fetus. Unfortunately, the Center for Disease Control Surveillance suggests that many women have received poor medical care. Among 300 women who were pregnant or became pregnant shortly after they received this live virus vaccine, only 61 had prior antibody testing, and 10 out of these women were immune (21). The live vaccine virus has been recovered from products of conception in women who have had a pregnancy termination after inadvertent live virus exposure, and the virus has been recovered from the fetal eye and kidney (22). The identification of susceptible women at delivery and at the time of pregnancy termination followed by administration of vaccine and the use of effective contraception for at least 2 months postpartum seem to be an appropriate strategy for the protection of susceptible women. Another program of vaccine administration to susceptible women, combined with effective contraception, has been reported from Hawaii (23) and among college students (24). In each of these populations, there was a large pool of susceptible women. In all these programs it is important to repeat rubella antibody testing in 2 months to be sure that an antibody response to the vaccine has been achieved. This prolonged interval following vaccine administration is necessary for contraception and evidence of susceptibility. At least one study has shown late sero conversion, 28 days postinnoculation after use of HPV-77, DFS rubella virus vaccine (25).

CYTOMEGALOVIRUS

The cytomegalovirus remains an enigma to practicing obstetricians. The virus is widely disseminated in humans. By serologic testing in the United States, a majority of adult women have been shown to have demonstrable cytomegalovirus antibody, and screening of pregnant women shows excretion of the virus in 2 to 5%. The number of pregnant women with antibody and the number excreting virus far exceed the approximately 1% of newborns with serologic evidence of virus acquisition during pregnancy. The first infection with virus in adults is usually not detected, for it is only infrequently associated with demonstrable clinical disease, except in an immunosuppressed patient. Thus, we have widespread infection with few serious problems for the adult host. In the fetus and newborn, there is serologic evidence that this virus reaches the fetus more than any other known infectious agent (26). Although most of these exposed newborn infants seemingly have no ill effects from intrauterine exposure, the virus can be associated with serious newborn morbidity, including microcephaly and psychomotor retardation. Of great concern is the observation that an apparently normal newborn may show evidence of auditory and mental dysfunction in later years (27). This is a virus with usually undetectable clinical evidence of infection in the mother that can have a serious impact on the newborn.

A major breakthrough in the understanding of intrauterine cytomegalovirus infection is the recognition that transplacental passage of the virus is usually associated with primary maternal infection during pregnancy. This discovery provides a basis for the recognition of susceptible women and for attempts at control of this disease.

Control of cytomegalovirus infection for newborns will depend on techniques of prevention. To date, there have been no reported cases of successful therapy of seriously affected newborns with systemic antiviral medication. Studies are currently being done using antiviral medication in asymptomatic newborns with serologic evidence of acquisition of the virus during pregnancy. For the obstetrician, prevention implies identification of a susceptible female population in the childbearing years. This determination can be accomplished by antibody testing. Means to prevent the maternal viremia of the initial infection might then be used. One technique to reduce the risk of maternal viremia is to screen both maternal recipients of blood during pregnancy and the blood to be administered to them for the presence of cytomegalovirus antibody. This would delineate a population of susceptible women and would indicate units of administered blood that are likely to contain cytomegalovirus particles (28). Of much greater significance as a preventive measure would be the identification of susceptible nonpregnant women and the use of a suitable immunization to provide antibody protection. Clinical trials have been conducted with attenuated live AD-169 strain (29) and Towne 125 strain of human cytomegalovirus (30). The preliminary studies indicate these vaccines elicit an antibody response in susceptible human hosts. Field testing should provide some insight on both the safety and effectiveness of live attenuated cytomegalovirus vaccine in producing long-lasting immunity prior to pregnancy. Future provision of primary care for these susceptible women in the childbearing age groups definitely lies in the province of obstetrical practice.

HERPES

The impact of herpes virus on the fetus and newborn is of a much different magnitude from the other identifiable members of the TORCH complex. The major concern is the immediate prognosis for the fetus, for systemic viral infection may result in neonatal death.

The obstetrical approach to this problem of potential fetal infection is quite different from the other TORCH agents. Adult infection with genital herpes is frequently associated with sufficient symptomatology to result in a visit to a physician, where it can be suspected clinically and diagnosed by appropriate study techniques. Cytologic smears of the lesion may demonstrate multinucleated giant cells. Scrapings of the lesion and viral culture yield positive evidence of the virus within a few days. In addition, serum antibodies to herpes virus can be measured and are indicative of past infections.

A number of observations provide some guidelines for the management of this disease. Although infections due to herpes virus I (usually "cold sores") and herpes II (usually genital) are marked by recurrences at the site of acquisition, maternal antibodies are formed with the initial infection that usually protect against subsequent viremia. Maternal viremia may be the most important factor in transplacental infection, and since antibodies against either herpes virus I or herpes virus II protect against herpes II viremia, a careful history of prior oral or genital herpetic lesions should be obtained in a pregnant woman found to have a genital herpes infection. If there is no prior history, amniocentesis to detect virus is theoretically the best approach. A positive amniotic fluid culture would obviate any consideration for cesarean section at term. To my knowledge to date, there have been no positive amniotic fluid cultures obtained for herpes virus. The major concern for the obstetrician is the fetal acquisition of virus during passage through the birth canal. Although virus can be shed in the genital tract in the absence of gross lesions (31), it appears that a gross genital lesion is associated with sufficient viral shedding to result in the possibility of fetal infection. One obvious approach to the patient with gross genital herpetic lesions is to hasten the evolution and healing of the gross lesions. A popular form of therapy has been the use of heterocycline dyes for photoinactivation of the virus (32). Currently this form of therapy is in disfavor, because of lack of success in a controlled clinical trial (33) and in vitro evidence of oncogenicity (34). To date, no accepted therapy to accelerate local genital healing has gained widespread favor. The current therapeutic regimen includes close observation of the lower genital tract for gross lesion and selection of an appropriate mode of delivery during labor. Intact membranes seem protective, and Amstey and Monif have suggested cesarean section for those women with active genital lesions and membranes ruptured for less than 4 hr, based on the results noted in Table II (35). It should be noted that less than 50% of infants delivered vaginally through an infected birth canal actually become infected after delivery. Although fetal infection is nearly always fatal, there is one observation of a salvage when a systemic antiviral agent was used after newborn lesions appeared (36).

SYPHILIS (TREPONEMA PALLIDUM)

Syphilis properly fits into the general category of the TORCH conditions. The basis of this classification is clinical, not microbiologic, for the causative agent is a spirochete, *Treponema pallidum,* not a virus or protozoan. It is like other TORCH agents in that the mother may be unaware of any recent or past infection and the newborn involvement may take a wide variety of forms. Intrauterine death may occur, or an apparently normal infant can be born who if untreated will develop more widespread manifestations of the disease in later years. Since the disease can be progressive and debilitating, it is important that obstetricians use every tool available to them to detect women with potential intrauterine infection.

The diagnosis of maternal syphilis is of necessity nearly always based on serologic

Table II. Neonatal Outcome in Patients With Genital Herpes Virus Infection Delivered by Cesarean Section

	Number of Deliveries	Normal Infant	Localized Skin Infection	Alive; Severe Defect	Death Due to HV Infection
Membranes ruptured <4 hr	16	16 (1 twin)	0	0	1
Membranes ruptured >4 hr	10	1	1	3	5

SOURCE: Reference 35.

testing. If the patient is seen early in the course of the disease and has a primary lesion, the "chancre," a dark-field examination of exudate from the lesion may reveal spirochetes. Currently, there are no culture techniques available to a clinical laboratory for the isolation of spirochetes, so that diagnosis is dependent on dark-field findings, if there is a lesion, or on serologic changes.

The tests used for the serologic testing for syphilis fall into two categories, nonspecific and specific. The nonspecific tests reflect the detection of nonspecific antibodies (reagins) that are formed to either the lipoidal antigens of the treponema or a lipoidal antigen that results from the reaction of maternal host and treponema. There are many favorable and unfavorable features of nonspecific antibody testing. The positive aspects of the tests are that they are inexpensive and easy to perform in a clinical laboratory because of the reproducible end points of measurements. These nonspecific serologic tests can be used for both screening asymptomatic populations and following the response to antibiotic therapy in patients with syphilis. The disadvantage of the tests is in their lack of specificity. The results may be positive in women without syphilis and may remain positive in women who have had adequate treatment and are free of the spirochete.

The specific serologic tests for syphilis measure antitreponemal antibodies. They have the disadvantages of being expensive and somewhat difficult to perform and evaluate, with some false positive and false negative results (see Table III) (37); and they may remain positive for a long-time. Because of this, the test is not used for screening but is used instead to evaluate asymptomatic women with positive reagin testing. In addition, these tests are not used to follow the response to antibiotics in women with a diagnosis of syphilis. The diagnostic pattern emerges of screening populations with nontreponemal tests, with the utilization of specific treponemal testing for those patients with positive reagin tests.

The treatment of the pregnant woman with serologic evidence of syphilis has the goal of elimination of the spirochete from the fetus with adequate antibiotic therapy. Unfortunately, some of our therapeutic judgments in the past have been based on the false assumption that the spirochete was unable to traverse the placental barrier before the eighteenth week of pregnancy (38). This belief emphasized early detection and treatment of the pregnant woman before the eighteenth week of pregnancy. There is good evidence that the reiterated observation of absence of transplacental passage of the spirochete was based on placental immaturity and inability to demonstrate the pathologic changes of a syphilitic infection, not because of the absence of transplacental passage of

Table III. Reactivity of VDRL, FTA-ABS, and TPI Tests During Various Stages of Syphilis

Category	Number Tested	Percent Reactive		
		FTA-ABS	TPI	VDRL
Primary syphilis	191	85	56	78
Secondary syphilis	270	99	94	97
Late syphilis	117	95	92	77
Latent syphilis	954	95	94	74
Presumably normal	384	1	0	0

spirochetes (39). Clinical antibiotic treatment for fetal syphilis requires the same concern at all points of the pregnancy.

The major clinical determinants for cure seem to be the duration of maternal infection with syphilis plus the ability of the mother to tolerate penicillin therapy. The duration of disease seems important, for this correlates with clinical cure. One study by Schroeter et al. showed remarkably good clinical results in treated patients who had latent syphilis for 1 year or less (40). This type of experience is the basis for the CDC recommendation for treatment of syphilis based on duration. Those having the disease for less than 1 year, i.e., primary, secondary, or latent syphilis of less than 1 year's duration are treated with a smaller total dose of antibiotics than those with evidence of disease for more than 1 year. The penicillin therapy is benzathine penicillin G, 2,400,000 units, or if the patient is allergic to penicillin, erythromycin in any form but the estolate, 2.0 g daily for 15 days (41). This categorization implies a careful physical evaluation of the patient as well as a careful past history. For those women whose infection is of indeterminate length, the CDC recommends treatment as though the disease were of more than 1 year's duration. This includes benzathine penicillin weekly, 2,400,000 units, for three doses, or if the patient is allergic to penicillin, erythromycin, 2.0 g daily, for 30 days (41). A major problem in the treatment of pregnant women with syphilis occurs when the patient is allergic to penicillin. The effectiveness of agents other than penicillin for asymptomatic syphilis of the central nervous system is not known. In addition, the safety of alternative antibiotics for the fetus has not been established, and the level of antibiotics achieved in the fetus with standard maternal dosages is not known. For reasons of safety only erythromycin has been recommended by the CDC. It is known that low levels of erythromycin are achieved in the fetus (42), and congenital syphilis has been found in mothers adequately treated with erythromycin during pregnancy (43); but to my knowledge there have been no reported intrauterine deaths. Any treatment other than penicillin requires special diagnostic and therapeutic considerations for the mother and the newborn. In pregnant women with a history of penicillin allergy and a positive serology and positive FTA-ABS, a diagnostic spinal tap should be done before therapy to be certain that asymptomatic neurosyphilis is not present. In addition, the CDC currently recommends penicillin treatment for all the newborns of the penicillin-allergic mothers who have been treated with erythromycin during pregnancy.

TUBERCULOSIS

Because of remarkable social and medical changes, perinatal infections due to *Mycobacterium tuberculosis* are infrequently seen in the 1970s. There are many reasons for this. The widespread social dislocation and starvation that was associated with the end of World War II made tuberculosis a not uncommon diagnosis among pregnant women. The worldwide elevation in living standards and the introduction of effective chemotherapeutic agents into clinical practice have combined to reduce the incidence of this problem remarkably. Unless the clinician spends time in urban areas of the world with widespread malnutrition and poverty or deals with a large obstetrical population of recent immigrants to the United States, it is unlikely that many women with tuberculosis will be seen. Despite the infrequency of the disease, the pathologic physiology of these cases should be reviewed, for it adds to our understanding of the problem of perinatal infection.

Infections by *Mycobacterium tuberculosis* in the adult may take many forms. Adults who convert their skin test, indicating exposure to the organism, may have a wide variety of response. In the pulmonary tree, the site of initial host-parasite contact, there may be either no radiologic evidence of change, the formation of a Ghon complex, or, in a small minority of patients, widespread progression of the disease to cavity formation. Tubercular infections of other organ systems occasionally are miliary, with a generalized tubercular infection in a critically ill woman, or there can be genital tract involvement with no radiologic evidence of pulmonary tuberculosis (44). Most of the currently seen instances of women whose newborn infants develop tuberculosis probably come from the latter population (45).

In keeping with the diverse human response to this organism, perinatal infections from *Mycobacterium tuberculosis* may take many clinical forms. Transplacental infection during pregnancy can occur. In such instances of blood-borne infection, the primary focus of infection is the fetal or newborn liver (46). In infants under 1 month of age with pulmonary lesions and no evidence of hepatic involvement, it must be assumed that a primary pulmonary infection occurred. This could result from contamination of the respiratory tract during passage through the birth canal or from contact after birth with a contagious member of the household.

The basis of therapy is prevention. Pregnant women, particularly those from lower socioeconomic populations, should be skin-tested. All women with positive skin tests should have adequate roentgenologic examination of the respiratory tract. Recent skin-test convertors should probably be treated in the second and third trimesters with isoniazid as well as a pyridoxine supplement. Pregnant women with an active pulmonary lesion on roentgenologic examination should receive appropriate combination drug chemotherapy. Because of the frequency of reported cases of newborn deafness when streptomycin has been administered during pregnancy, this drug should be avoided if possible (47). The infant of a treated mother requires a workup to determine if chemotherapy or BCG immunization is indicated, for the worst prognosis in tuberculous infants occurs in those under the age of 6 months.

LISTERIA MONOCYTOGENES

Listeria monocytogenes is a bacterial agent that can be associated with fetal or newborn infection. Its significance may be overlooked in some clinical situations. It is a gram-positive aerobic bacillus that can be mistaken for diphtheroids, usually considered a contaminant in most clinical laboratories. There is a wide range of human response to this pathogen. *Listeria monocytogenes* infection may cause no demonstrable symptomatology in humans. It frequently causes mild disease resembling infectious mononucleosis in the adult, and it can be a source of serious infection in an immunosuppressed host. The infection in the fetus and newborn is usually more severe than in a normal adult, but there is a wide variety of clinical manifestations. Infections that occur early in pregnancy may be associated with abortion. Later in pregnancy, the infection may result in a stillbirth or the birth of an acutely ill newborn who dies within a few hours. The major diagnostic problem for the obstetrician is the fact that maternal infection is usually mild or inapparent and may not be detected by the physician, for the mother did not seek medical care.

Infection of the fetus or newborn with *Listeria monocytogenes* may occur in different ways. There may be transplacental infection during pregnancy. This can result from the formation of a placental granuloma and dissemination of the organism to the fetus similar to the mechanism seen with toxoplasmosis. In addition, reported instances of maternal bacteremia with the subsequent delivery of an infected infant provide good documentation of transplacental infection without granuloma formation (48). Further evidence of this transplacental infection is provided by the recovery of *Listeria monocytogenes* from the amniotic fluid of a patient with intact membranes (49). This transplacental mode is evident in the newborns, for they have a generalized miliary infection; but hepatic lesions are particularly frequent and far advanced. The transplacental pathway is not the only route of infection. In some cases, there is evidence that fetal infection occurs because of exposure to infected material in the birth canal during labor (50).

The clinical presentation of infection in the newborn may take many forms. These infections frequently involve premature or low birthweight infants. The onset of symptomatology may be early or late and can progress to mortality. Since antibacterial agents are available that are effective against this organism, the future focus will necessarily be on diagnostic techniques for the early recognition of maternal acquisition of disease or clinical and laboratory signs of newborn infection at birth.

HEPATITIS

Viral infection of the liver (hepatitis) is a serious worldwide problem because of the frequency and severity of the infection. Most practicing physicians are familiar with two main types of hepatitis, but recent studies indicate there may be more than two viruses responsible for the clinical syndrome. Two classic forms of hepatitis have been documented. Type A hepatitis (infectious hepatitis) has a short incubation period and is usually transmitted by contact (fecal-oral route), although parenteral transmission can occur. Type B hepatitis (serum hepatitis) has a longer incubation period and is usually transmitted by the parenteral route, although infection by contact has been documented. The development of specific tests for hepatitis B antigens has expanded our understanding of this disease entity. The continued rapid expansion of knowledge in this area may modify some of the perinatal concepts expressed in this chapter.

The traditional obstetrical concern about hepatitis has been the direct effect on the mother and the pregnancy in which the infection was noted. Varied opinions about maternal morbidity and mortality have been reported in the literature. The American view has been that pregnant women have no different prognosis than similarly aged nonpregnant women (51). In contrast, studies from Saudi Arabia indicate a much worse outlook for the host when hepatitis occurs during pregnancy (52). The critical difference in these two population samples seems to be nutrition, for poorly nourished Middle Eastern women have a much higher mortality rate. For the fetus, the most important consequence of maternal acquisition of hepatitis during pregnancy is an increase in the incidence of premature labor and delivery. In general, the initiation of labor seems to be a response to the systemic effects of the maternal illness and not a direct result of transplacental infection of the fetus with the virus.

The discovery of antigens related to the hepatitis B virus has expanded our understanding of fetal and newborn infection from this virus. Based on diagnostic studies of acquisition of hepatitis B antigen, there is frequent infection of the fetus and newborn with this virus. There is a wide variation in infection rates. Although the transmission of hepatitis B viral antigen can occur to the fetus of seemingly healthy mothers who are HBAg carriers, this is probably less frequent than in women with an acute symptomatic hepatitis B virus infection during pregnancy (53). There also seems to be a variation in fetal risk for viral antigen exposure among women with acute hepatitis during pregnancy. One study demostrated that the highest risk for fetal infection, nearly 50%, resulted from maternal infection occurring from the eighth month of gestation to 2 months postpartum (54). This timing of maternal infection, combined with serologic studies of cord blood, indicates that besides transplacental infection, contamination of the fetus during birth canal passage is also a factor. In addition to the different rates of viral acquisition, there is a wide range of clinical response of the newborn. In most instances, there is no clinical response of the newborn. In most instances, there is no clinical evidence of infection at birth, and evidence of viral infection is detected only by laboratory testing. The persistence of viral antigen in these newborns and the eventual clinical impact of these viruses is not known. There is the possibility of serious newborn outcome because of fetal infection with the virus. There have been reports of the development of serious liver infection in the newborn with progression to death (55).

The current incomplete state of our knowledge of the impact of hepatitis on the fetus and newborn makes it difficult to provide appropriate therapeutic guidelines for the obstetrician. Clearly, prevention should be stressed. Any blood given to a pregnant women should have prior screening for the presence of the hepatitis B antigen. There probably should be limitation of the use of the scalp electrode, unless absolutely necessary, in the fetus of a mother in labor who has had clinical evidence of hepatitis during pregnancy. There is recent evidence, based on limited clinical material, that antibody treatment of the newborn of a mother with hepatitis B virus infection may be effective in preventing neonatal hepatitis B virus infection (56). More observations will be needed to establish the benefits and safety of such a regimen.

GROUP B BETA HEMOLYTIC STREPTOCOCCUS

The recent interest in the group B beta hemolytic streptococcus is not related to any new concern about its pathogenicity for adults. There is evidence that it is a pathogen, for it has been implicated in adult infection. One recent study recorded serious infections in adults due to this organism (57), and a prior publication showed it to be frequently recovered from the bloodstream of obstetric-gynecology patients with bacteremia (58). Most obstetric-gynecologic infections have responded well to antibiotic therapy, although death from adult meningitis has been reported (57). Although the group B beta hemolytic streptococcus was noted to be less susceptible to penicillin in the laboratory than is the group A beta hemolytic streptococcus (57), it is still highly susceptible to antibiotic levels that are easily exceeded in the serum when a standard therapeutic regimen is given. In the adult, this adds up to a picture of an organism causing infection that is easily handled by available therapeutic techniques.

In contrast, fatal newborn infections due to the group B beta hemolytic streptococcus have assumed a major level of importance. In a cooperative multicenter study of neonatal meningitis, there was a dramatic increase in the incidence of group B infections in the early 1970s (59) (see Table IV). Experience at one urban medical center in Dallas, depicted in Figure 2, demonstrates the remarkable emergence of this pathogen as a

Table IV. Etiology of Neonatal Meningitis

	1961–1970 (188) (%)	1971–1973 (131) (%)
Gram negative	71	53
Escherichia coli	43	38
Gram positive	29	47
Group B streptococcus	5	31

major infectious problem in the newborn (60). This is not a unique finding, for it seems to parallel other observations across the United States.

There is a wide range of clinical response of the newborn to infections due to group B streptococcus. A number of clinically distinct syndromes have been noted. Early-onset sepsis is seen in infants with symptoms at birth or within 72 hr of birth (61). In these infants, the clinical and roentgen picture may be difficult to distinguish from respiratory distress syndrome (62). The prognosis is poor, with mortality frequently occurring despite appropriate antibiotics. There is abundant evidence that the source of these organisms is the vagina, with vertical transmission from mother to fetus (63). Late-onset sepsis occurs a week or more after delivery and has a serious prognosis when the

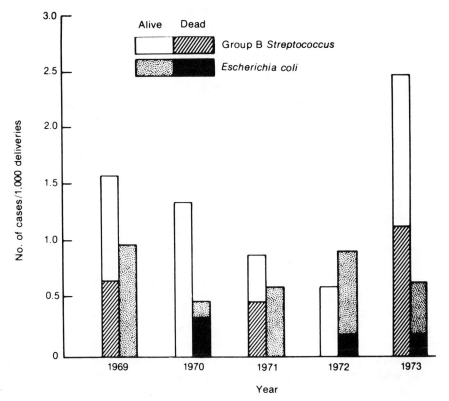

Figure 2. Incidence of infection and of mortality caused by Group B streptococci and *Escherichia coli* at Parkland Memorial Hospital from 1969 to 1973.

mortality rate is considered but does not seem to be as lethal as early-onset problems. There is some evidence that nosocomial transmission of the group B streptococcus can occur in a newborn nursery, and not only from transmission from the maternal vagina (64). In addition to these two well-defined clinical syndromes associated with group B streptococcal infections, a variety of other infections have been noted, including osteo-myelitis and septic arthritis (60). Although most of these infants survived, some had a lethal course. These group B streptococcal infections cause serious problems for the newborn.

To better delineate the epidemiology of these newborn infections, many studies of vaginal colonization during pregnancy have been done. Streptococci can be recovered from the vaginas of asymptomatic pregnant women. The rates can vary from 46/1000 in Denver (61) to 254/1000 in Houston (63). This difference may be related to geographic differences in vaginal colonization, but it more likely reflects the selective antibiotic broth media used in Houston. Maternal carriage of the group B beta hemolytic streptococcus does not seem to be a static phenomenon during pregnancy. One microbiologic evaluation throughout pregnancy found that not all women cultured positive in the first part of pregnancy remained so throughout (65). Another study found a higher incidence of positive vaginal cultures in third trimester sampling (66). In view of the vertical transmission of this organism for mother to fetus, these studies provide an idea of the fetal population pool at risk for infection.

A great dilemma exists in any attempt to formulate measures of control for this serious newborn disease entity. There is a wide gap between the frequency of maternal carriage and the incidence of newborn infection. The ratio of maternal carriage to newborn attack varies from 23/1 in the Denver study (61) to 87.6/1 in Houston (63). This observation suggests that there must be a number of factors that increase the sus-ceptibility of the newborn who becomes infected, as distinguished from the majority of infants who have no clinical evidence of infection.

One clinical approach to this serious problem is an attempt to eliminate maternal vaginal carriage of the group B beta hemolytic streptococcus with prophylactic antibio-tics. One respected pediatric investigator suggested this kind of prophylaxis as a possi-bility (67). Certain aspects of the observed group B beta hemolytic streptococcal data would support this approach. Group B streptococci cause a serious newborn infection that is potentially fatal, despite the use of appropriate antibiotics when clincal sympto-matology is noted. Prophylactic antibiotic therapy in this situation would be directed toward a single organism and one that is quite susceptible to penicillin in the labora-tory. Unfortunately, the results of such an antibiotic strategy have been disappointing. It seems clear that maternal vaginal carriage can be remarkably reduced during and immediately after antibiotic therapy. The Denver group found the organism was eliminated in 13 out of 14 women after penicillin therapy (61). However, this benefit may be short-lived. In an evaluation of a longer follow-up of women treated for 7 days with ampicillin, no striking difference between antibiotic and control groups could be noted (see Table V) (65). These results suggest that vaginal carriage of the group B streptococcus is not a constant finding during pregnancy and that acquisition of the organism may occur from sexual contact with an asymptomatic male carrier. Studies of prophylactic antibiotic therapy for both male and female have not been reported to date, but this added dimension of prophylaxis enforces the sense that this use of antibiotics will not provide the solution to the problem.

Some recent studies indicate that techniques will be available to pinpoint an obstetrical population at high risk for this newborn complication. The most striking

Table V. Colonization of Mothers and Infants With Group B Streptococci

	Treated With Ampicillin		Not Treated	
	Positive	Negative	Positive	Negative
Mothers follow-up, 3 weeks	4	23	14	$<20\,p = <.05$
Mothers at delivery	8	15 (4 unknown)	13	16 N.S. (5 unknown)
Infants at delivery	6	27	10	24 N.S.

study is the report by Baker and Kasper demonstrating the absence of maternal anti-body to type III group B streptococcus in those women whose infants had meningitis due to this organism (69). This is an exciting observation, but is should be noted that in this same study, only 79% of the women with normal neonates had detectable levels of the antibody present. More observations are necessary to see if this lack of maternal antibody is a significant marker for newborn infection. Some clinical observations at the Los Angeles County–University of Southern California (LAC-USC) Medical Center suggest that shortcomings in maternal host defense mechanisms may play a significant role in this overwhelming newborn infectious disease. In those women cultured, whose infant had a group B streptococcal infection, the group B streptococcus was the pre-dominant organism recovered from endocervical culture (69). Problems of newborn infection seem to be related to the dominance of the group B streptococcus in the vaginal flora rather than simply vaginal colonization. There were other suggestive warning signs to the obstetrician. The majority of the infections occur in premature or low birth-weight infants. Nearly one-half of the newborns with group B streptococcal infections had a fetal tachycardia during labor, i.e., a heart rate above 160 per minute for at least 0.5 hr. This frequency was far greater than found in the population at large undergoing monitoring. A number of findings suggest that intrauterine infection with this organism does occur. There is evidence that bacterial infection of the amniotic fluid can occur in the absence of maternal symptomatology. This information, plus the explosive early onset of group B infection in newborns, suggests that in utero infection can occur, in addition to assumed acquisition through passage through a contaminated birth canal.

There are few concrete proposals for prevention and treatment of group B streptococcal infections that can be given to an obstetrician at this time. Mass screening during pregnancy for vaginal carriage of the group B streptococcus and antibiotic prophylaxis for culture-positive women does not seem justified. Patients that fit into a high-risk category because of a premature labor, premature rupture of the membranes, or fetal tachycardia during labor should have endocervical or amniotic fluid cultures. Positive culture results should be transmitted immediately to the neonatologist.

ESCHERICHIA COLI

There are many similarities between serious neonatal infections due to *Escherichia coli* and the group B beta hemolytic streptococcus. *Escherichia coli* infections are frequent problems and rank in frequency with group B beta hemolytic streptococcus as a cause of neonatal meningitis (59). Serious newborn infections with *Escherichia coli* are related to a specific type (70), i.e., those with a K_1 antigen; a similar specificity is seen in type III group B streptococcal infection of the newborn (69). These newborn infections seem to occur in women with an absence of antibody to this specific type of *E. coli* (70), a finding comparable with that reported by Baker and Kasper for the group B streptococcus (69).

There has been little documentation of obstetrical signs in the infants who develop newborn infection due to *Escherichia coli*. Both intrauterine infection and fetal acquisition of the organism during passage through the birth canal are probably involved. Prophylactic antibiotics for the mother have not been recommended, but there is interest in the possibility of developing an immunization program for these antibody-deficient mothers.

REFERENCES

1. Naeye, R. L., and Blanc, W. A.: Relation of poverty and race to antenatal infection. *N.E.J.M.* 283:555, 1970.

2. Selvaraj, R. J., and Bhat, K. S.: Metabolic and bacterial activities of leukocytes in protein calorie malnutrition. *Am. J. Clin. Path.* 25:166, 1974.

3. Schlievert, P., Johnson, W., and Galask, R. P.: Bacterial growth inhibition by amniotic fluid. *Am. J. Obstet. Gynecol.* 125:906, 1976.

4. Galask, R. P., personal communication.

5. Hardy, J. B., McCracken, G. H., Jr., Mellits, E. D., Gilkeson, M. R., and Sever, J. L.: Serum immunoglobulin levels in newborn infants. *J. Pediatr.* 75:1211, 1969.

6. Monif, G. R. G.: Antenatal group A streptococcal infection. *Am. J. Obstet. Gynecol.* 123:213, 1975.

7. Benirschke, K.: Routes and types of infection in the fetus and the newborn. *Amer. J. Dis. Child.* 99:714, 1960.

8. Wolf, A., Cowen, D., and Paige, B. H.: Toxoplasmic encephalomyelitis III. A new case of granulomatous encephalomyelitis due to a protozoan. *Amer. J. Path.* 15:657, 1939.

9. Desmonts, G., and Couvreur, J.: Toxoplasmosis: Epidemiologic and serologic aspects of perinatal infection, in *Infections of the Fetus and the Newborn Infant,* edited by S. Krugman and A. A. Gershon. A. R. Liss Inc., New York, 1975.

10. Couvreur, J., Desmonts, G., and Girre, J. Y.: Congenital toxoplasmosis in twins. *J. Pediatr.* 89:235, 1976.

11. Kimball, A. C., Kean, B. H., and Fuchs, F.: Congenital toxoplasmosis: A prospective study of 4,048 obstetric patients. *Am. J. Obstet. Gynecol.* 111:211, 1971.

12. Alford, C. A., Jr., Stagno, S., and Reynolds, D. W.: Congenital toxoplasmosis: Clinical, laboratory, and therapeutic considerations, with special reference to subclinical disease. *Bull. N.Y. Acad. Med.* 50:160, 1974.

13. Gregg, N. M.: Congenital cataract following German measles in the mother. *J. Ophthalmol. Soc. Aust.* 3:35, 1941.

14. Townsend, J. J., Baringer, J. R., Wolinsky, J. S., Malamud, N., Mednick, J. P., Panitch, H. S., Scitt, R. A. T., Oshiro, L. S., and Cremer, N. F.: Progressive rubella panencephalitis. *N.E.J.M.* 292:990, 1975.

15. Weil, M. I., Habashi, H. H., Cremer, N. F., Oshiro, L. S., Lennette, E. H., and Carnay, L.: Chronic progressive panencephalitis due to rubella virus simulating subacute sclerosing panencephalitis. *N.E.J.M.* 292:994, 1975.

16. Parkman, P. D., Buescher, E. L., and Artenstein, M. D.: Recovery of rubella virus from army recruits. *Proc. Soc. Exp. Biol. Med.* 111:215, 1962.

17. Weller, T. H., and Neva, F. A.: Propagation in tissue culture of cytopathogenic agents from patients with rubella-like illness. *Proc. Soc. Exp. Biol.* 111:225, 1962.

18. Horstmann, D. M., Liebhaber, H., Bouvier, G. R., Rosenberg, D. A., and Halstead, S. B.: Rubella reinfection of vaccinated and naturally immune persons exposed in an epidemic. *N.E.J.M.* 283:771, 1970.

19. Schoenbaum, S. C., Biano, S., and Mack, T.: Epidemiology of congenital rubella syndrome: The role of maternal parity. *J.A.M.A.* 233:151, 1975.

20. Chang, T. W.: Rubella reinfection and intrauterine involvement. *J. Pediatr.* 84:617, 1974.

21. Modlin, J. F., Brandling-Bennett, A. D., Witte, J. J., Campbell, C. C., and Meyers, J. D.: A review of five years experience with rubella vaccine in the United States. *Ped.* 55:20, 1975.

22. Rubella Surveillance, January 1972–July 1973. Center For Disease Control, Public Health Service, Department of Health, Education and Welfare, November 1973.

23. Halstead, E., Halstead, S. B., Jackson, R. S., Char, D., Hale, R., and Pion, R.: Rubella vaccination: Fertility control in a large scale vaccination program for postpubertal women. *Am. J. Obstet. Gynecol.* 121:1089, 1975.

24. Schiff, G. M., Linnemann, C. C., Jr., Shea, L., and Trimble, S.: Rubella surveillance and immunization among college women. *Obstet. Gynecol.* 43:143, 1974.

25. Wilkins, J.: Late sero-conversion following HPV-77, DE5 rubella virus vaccine. *Am. J. Obstet. Gynecol.* 121:998, 1975.

26. Hanshaw, J. B.: Congenital cytomegalovirus infection: A 15 year perspective. *J. Inf. Dis.* 123:555, 1971.

27. Reynolds, D. W., Stagno, S., Stubbs, K. G., Dahle, A. J., Livingston, M. M., Saxon, S. S., and Alford, C. A.: Inapparent congenital cytomegalovirus infection with elevated cord IgM levels. *N.E.J.M.* 290:291, 1974.

28. Monif, G. R. G., Daicoff, G. I., and Florg, L. L.: Blood as a potential vehicle for the cytomegaloviruses. *Am. J. Obstet. Gynecol.* 126:445, 1976.

29. Elck, S. D., and Stern, H.: Development of a vaccine against mental retardation caused by cytomegalovirus infection in utero. *Lancet* 1:1, 1974.

30. Plotkin, S. A., Farguhar, J., and Hornberger, E.: Clinical trials of immunization with the Towne 125 strain of human cytomegalovirus. *J. Inf. Dis.* 134:470, 1976.

31. Bolognese, R. J., Corson, S. L., Fuccillo, D. A., Traub, R., Moder, F., and Sever, J. L.: Herpes virus hominis Type II infections in asymptomatic pregnant women. *Obstet. Gynecol.* 48:507, 1976.

32. Kaufman, R. L., Gardner, H. L., Brown, D., Wallis, C., Rawls, W. E., and Melnick, J. L.: Herpes genitalis treated by photodynamic inactivation of virus. *Am. J. Obstet. Gynecol.* 117:1144, 1973.

33. Myers, M. G., Oxman, M. N., Clark, J. E., and Arndt, K. A.: Failure of neutral-red photodynamic inactivation in recurrent herpes simplex virus infections. *N.E.J.M.* 293:945, 1975.

34. Rapp, F., Li, J. L., Jerkofsky, M.: Transformation of mammalian cells by DNA-containing viruses following photodynamic inactivation. *Virology* 55:339, 1973.

35. Amstey, M. S., and Monif, G. R. G.: Genital herpes virus infection in pregnancy. *Obstet. Gynec.* 44:394, 1974.

36. Amstey, M. S., personal communication.

37. Sparling, P. F.: Diagnosis and treatment of syphilis. *N.E.J.M.* 284:642, 1971.

38. Dippel, A. L.: Relationship of congenital syphilis to abortion and miscarriage and the mechanism of intrauterine protection. *Am. J. Obstet. Gynec.* 47:369, 1944.

39. Harter, C. A., and Benirschke, K.: Fetal syphilis in the first trimester. *Am. J. Obstet. Gynecol.* 124:705, 1976.

40. Schroeter, A. L., Lucas, J. B., Price, E. V., and Falcone, V. H.: Treatment for early syphilis and reactivity of serologic tests. *J.A.M.A.* 221:471, 1972.

41. Center for Disease Control Recommendations for Treatment of Syphilis. 1976.

42. Philipson, A., Sabath, L. D., and Charles, D.: Transplacental passage of erythromycin and clindamycin. *N.E.J.M.* 288:1219, 1973.

43. Fenton, L. J., and Light, I. J.: Congenital syphilis after maternal treatment with erythromycin.

44. Schaefer, G.: Tuberculosis of the female genital tract. *Clin. Obstet. Gynec.* 13:965, 1970.

45. Ramos, A. D., Hibbard, L. T., and Craig, J. R.: Congenital tuberculosis. *Obstet. Gynec.* 43:61, 1974.

46. Davis, S. F., Finley, S. C., and Hare, W. K.: Congenital tuberculosis. *J. Pediatr.* 57:221, 1960.

47. Conway, N., and Birt, B. D.: Streptomycin in pregnancy: Effect on the ear. *Brit. Med. J.* 2:260, 1965.

48. Barber, M., and Okubadejo, O. A.: Maternal and neonatal listeriosis: Report of a case and brief review of listeriosis in man. *Brit. Med. J.* 2:735, 1965.

49. Petrilli, E., and Ledger, W. J., unreported observation.

50. Becroft, D. M. O., Farmer, K., Seddon, R. J., Sowden, R., Stewart, J. H., Vines, A., and Wattie, D. A.: Epidemic listeriosis in the newborn. *Br. Med. J.* 3:747, 1971.

51. Davidson, C. S.: Hepatic disease and pregnancy. *J. Reprod. Med.* 10:107, 1973.

52. Gelpi, A. P.: Fatal hepatitis in Saudi Arabian women. *Amer. J. Gastroenterol.* 53:41, 1970.

53. Muzzur, S., Blumberg, B. S., and Friedlander, J. S.: Silent maternal transmission of Australia antigen. *Nature* 247:41, 1974.

54. Schweitzer, I. L., Wing, A., McPeak, C., and Spears, R. L.: Hepatitis and hepatitis-associated antigen in 56 mother-infant pairs. *J.A.M.A.* 220:1092, 1972.

55. Stokes, J., Jr., Berk, J. E., Malamut, L. L., et al.: The carrier state in viral hepatitis. *J.A.M.A.* 154:1059, 1954.

56. Kohler, P. F., Dubois, R. S., Merrill, D. A., and Bowes, W. A.: Prevention of chronic neonatal hepatitis B virus infection with antibody to the hepatitis B surface antigen. *N.E.J.M.* 291:1378, 1974.

57. Bayer, A. S., Chow, A. W., Anthony, B. F., and Guze, L. B.: Serious infection in adults due to Group B streptococci. *Amer. J. Med.* 61:498, 1976.

58. Ledger, W. J., Norman, M., Gee, C., and Lewis, W.: Bacteremia on an obstetric-gynecologic service. *Am. J. Obstet. Gynecol.* 121:205, 1975.

59. McCracken, G. H., Robbins, J. B., Gotschlich, E., et al.: Escherichiae coli K_1 antigen associated with neonatal meningitis, Read before the 13th Interscience Conference on Antimicrobial Agents and Chemotherapy, Washington, D.C., 1973.

60. Howard, J. B., and McCracken, G. H., Jr.: The spectrum of group B streptococcal infections in infancy. *Am. J. Dis. Child.* 128:815, 1974.

61. Franciosi, R. A., Knostman, J. D., and Zimmerman, R. A.: Group B streptococcal neonatal and infant infections. *J. Pediatr.* 82:707, 1973.

62. Ablow, R. C., Driscoll, S. G., Effmann, E. L., Gross, I., Jolles, C. J., Uauy, R., and Warshaw, J. B.: A comparison of early onset group B streptococcal neonatal infection and the respiratory distress syndrome of the newborn. *N.E.J.M.* 294:65, 1976.

63. Baker, C. J., and Barrett, F. F.: Transmission of group B streptococci among parturient women and their neonates. *J. Pediatr.* 83:919, 1973.

64. Steere, A. C., Aber, R. C., Warford, L. R., Murphy, K. E., Feeley, J. C., Hayes, P. S., Wilkinson, H. W., and Facklam, R. R.: Possible nosocomial transmission of group B streptococci in a newborn nursery. *J. Pediatr.* 87:784, 1975.

65. Hall, R. T., Barnes, W., Krishan, L., Harris, D. J., Rhodes, P. G., Fayez, J., and Miller, G. L.: Antibiotic treatment of parturient women colonized with group B streptococci. *Am. J. Obstet. Gynec.* 124:630, 1976.

66. Baker, C. J., Barrett, F. F., and Yow, M. D.: The influence of advancing gestation on group B streptococcal colonization in pregnant women. *Am. J. Obstet. Gynec.* 122:820, 1975.

67. McCracken, G. H., Jr.: Group B streptococci: the new challenge in neonatal infections. *J. Pediatr.* 82:703, 1973.

68. Baker, C. J., and Kasper, D. L.: Correlation of maternal antibody deficiency with susceptibility to neonatal group B streptococcal infection. *N.E.J.M.* 294:753, 1976.

69. Bobitt, J. R., and Ledger, W. J.: Obstetric observations in eleven cases of neonatal sepsis due to the group B beta hemolytic streptococcus. *Obstet. Gynec.* 47:439, 1976.

70. McCracken, G. H., Sarff, L. D., and Glode, M. P.: Relationship between *Escherichia coli* K_1 capsular polysaccharide antigen and clinical outcome in neonatal meningitis. *Lancet* 2:246, 1974.

14

Perinatal Infections Caused by Rubella, Hepatitis B, Cytomegalovirus, and Herpes Simplex

G. Eric Knox, M.D.
David W. Reynolds, M.D.
Charles Alford, Jr., M.D.

The purpose of this chapter is to summarize methods of diagnosis, implications for the offspring, and clinical management of maternal infections caused by rubella, hepatitis B, cytomegalovirus (CMV), and herpes simplex (HSV). These infections were selected for discussion not only because questions concerning them frequently confront the obstetrician and neonatologist, but because they illustrate a variety of general principles applicable to obstetrical and perinatal viral infectious disease. For example, although symptomatic maternal illness can occur with each of these organisms, in most instances trivial or nonexistent symptomology in the mother commonly causes the infection to be overlooked or ignored. Second, although fetuses acquiring virus as a consequence of active maternal infection may manifest overt disease at or shortly after birth, the asymptomatic and progressive damage occurring in silently infected infants may ultimately represent a public health problem of much greater significance. Finally, these infections illustrate the manner in which most viruses are thought to be transmitted from mother to infant: Rubella can infect a fetus solely by transplacental blood-borne infection; in contrast the overwhelming majority of infants infected with HSV acquire the virus by direct contact at the time of delivery. Fetal and neonatal infections with CMV and hepatitis B can be acquired either transplacentally or by direct contact at or around the time of birth.

Every virus has a unique incubation period, and, therefore, the perinatal expression of maternal infection may vary from a few days (for HSV) to many months (for hepa-

Parts of this work were supported by National Institute of Child Health and Human Development Grants HD01687, HD10699, and HD00413.

titis B). The fact that an infant appears normal at birth and in the early neonatal period does not mean that it has escaped infection in utero or during delivery. Symptomatic or asymptomatic viral illness in the mother demands close communication and cooperation among all members of the perinatal health team in order to achieve a full understanding of the natural history and impact of the disease, including the possibility of remote damage to the infant. Safe and efficacious prevention of infection in the infant will best be achieved through knowledge of the natural history and pathogenesis of the infection.

An exhaustive review of the enormous literature recently acquired on perinatal infection is beyond the scope of this chapter. Therefore, we present a selective summary of the above-mentioned viruses, focusing on general principles and practical considerations involved in prevention and control. The interested reader is referred to recent excellent reviews for additional information and a more comprehensive discussion of viral infections in pregnancy (1–3).

MATERNAL INFECTION: EPIDEMIOLOGY AND CLINICAL EXPRESSION

The approximate percentage of pregnant women in the United States serologically susceptible to primary infection with the viruses under consideration is, for rubella, 10% (4); for cytomegalovirus, 40% (5); for herpes simplex virus, 25% (1,6); for hepatitis B, 84% (7). The major variable influencing serologically defined susceptibility is age, which correlates inversely with susceptibility. Other variables include socioeconomic status, geographic location, sexual activity, housing patterns, and familial living conditions.

Impressive as these figures are, it must also be emphasized that although a clear correlation between immunity and presence of maternal antibody exists for rubella and hepatitis B, recurrent maternal infection and possible fetal involvement with CMV and herpes simplex is not precluded by the presence of circulating maternal antibody, i.e., previous primary infection. Indeed, prospective data indicate that in utero infection with CMV occurs in approximately 3.4% of infants born to mothers known to be seropositive before the beginning of pregnancy (8). In addition, there are reports of mothers who have given birth to more than one infant infected with CMV (9–11). Whether the acquisition of intrauterine CMV infection in the face of circulating maternal antibody represents reactivation of latent virus or reinfection with an antigenically distinct strain of virus remains uncertain, but recent genetic and antigenetic analysis of virus isolated from consecutively infected babies tends to favor the former hypothesis (11). With regard to HSV a similar situation exists. Infection of the neonate can occur as a consequence of recurrent maternal infections as well as during a primary genital infection (12,13).

Although the presence of antibody to hepatitis B usually confers lifelong protection against maternal and fetal infection, asymptomatic chronic carriers of the surface antigen (Australian antigen or HBs Ag positive) can transmit the virus and cause infection of the baby in utero (14–16), at the time of delivery (17–20), or in the immediate newborn period (21,22). Indeed, consecutively infected infants have been born to an asymptomatic carrier of the hepatitis B surface antigen (23). The incidence of perinatal transmission of the hepatitis B virus varies greatly in different parts of the world (24). In the United States, where one woman per thousand is a chronic carrier of hepatitis B, the fetal perinatal transmission occurs in 5% of exposed babies (17).

Thus estimates of the overall incidence of maternal infection are exceedingly difficult because of the clinical and serologic inability to define persistence, chronicity, and recurrence accurately. Nevertheless, several prospective studies have suggested that active maternal infections occur in approximately 14% of all pregnancies, at least in lower socioeconomic groups. By far, the most common is CMV infection, which occurs in about 13% (range 1.3 to 15) of pregnancies (3). The other maternal infections are HSV, 1 to 1.5% (25); rubella, 2 to 4% (epidemic) and 0.17% (interepidemic) (4,26); and hepatitis B, 0.1% (United States asymptomatic carriers) and 0.2% to 2.0% (overt clinical disease) (27). The figures for acute hepatitis B vary from country to country and probably reflect not only the actual incidence of the disease but the efficiency of the public health reporting system as well. Of the four infections, only rubella occurs in well-defined epidemics, with major peaks of activity exceeding the usual incidence by a factor of 20- to 40-fold. Maternal cytomegalovirus and herpes simplex infections are for the most part genital in location and undoubtedly reflect reactivations or reinfections, together with much smaller numbers of primary infections (25,28,29). Their prevalence in any given population depends on socioeconomic status and, in any given individual, on patterns of sexual behavior, at least as regards HSV. The prevalence of asymptomatic carriers of hepatitis B likewise reflects socioeconomic status, particularly as regards living conditions. However, other important risk factors must be taken into consideration. For example, the following situations are associated with an increased incidence of the asymptomatic hepatitis B carrier state: previous or concurrent drug abuse; previous blood transfusions; the presence of a family member with a chronic illness such as leukemia, hemophilia, or lupus erythematosus; the presence of a family member receiving chronic renal dialysis therapy; and, finally, the presence of a family member who has either had symptomatic hepatitis or is discovered to be an asymptomatic carrier of the disease. Careful attention to these factors when taking an obstetrical history may facilitate selective screening of pregnant women for the presence of active infection (circulating hepatis B surface antigen).

Each of these infections is transmitted horizontally within a population primarily by direct contact with the virus at a peripheral site of excretion. Such sites include oropharynx (for all four viruses), urine (for rubella and CMV), genital organs (for HSV and CMV), skin lesions (for HSV), and breast milk (for CMV) (29). During the acute stage or primary infection, blood may also be contagious in each instance. Prolonged viremia is a cardinal feature of hepatitis B and probably CMV as well (1,27,30), and certain persons may thus remain infectious via this source for undetermined periods of time. The usual duration of contagion, with the exception of rubella (1 to 4 weeks), is variable and depends largely on the development of antibody or the carrier state in the case of hepatitis B and on the frequency of recurrences in the case of CMV or HSV. It is noteworthy, however, that the majority of individuals with primary cytomegalovirus infection continue to excrete virus, most prominently in the urine, for many months. Thus, each of these agents, with the exception of rubella, has established an ecological niche within humans that provides for maximal survival potential and long periods of communicability.

With the exception of overt hepatitis, clinically recognizable maternal infection with these organisms is the exception rather than the rule. When compared with the usual "silent" infection with cytomegalovirus, the appearance of primary CMV infection in the form of heterophile negative mononucleosis is an exceedingly rare event. Subclinical rubella occurs at least as often as the clinically apparent infection, which is most often a mild exanthematous disease. The genital lesions of recurrent HSV often go unnoticed because of their location and their largely asymptomatic nature. Primary infections with HSV are more easily recognized because of the fever, adenopathy, and pain involved, but less often appreciated is the fact that virus persists in the genital tract for long periods after the symptoms have subsided (1,31,32). Clinically apparent hepatitis B with jaundice is easily recognized by the clinician, but anicteric hepatitis with its protean manifestations is more often missed. Fever (to 104°) lasting 4 to 5 days, nausea and vomiting, lassitude, anorexia, rashes, or arthralgias are often attributed to other causes or even to pregnancy itself. A heightened awareness of the anicteric forms of hepatitis might lead to additional diagnosis of this disease during pregnancy, with resultant better management of neonates born to infected mothers.

The incidence of fetal infection is a fraction of that occurring in mothers for each infection, and this observation has lead to the concept of the "placental barrier." A precise description of the nature of this "barrier" is not currently possible. Very little information is available regarding maternal, placental, and fetal host defense mechanisms, and especially their ontogeny, which presumably limits the potential for fetal infection following maternal infection. Undoubtedly the so-called protective barrier involves a series of complicated specific events determined by the viral-host interaction at any given stage of gestation. Clearly three hosts are involved: the mother, the placenta and membranes, and the fetus or young infant. It should not be surprising then that even with blood-borne infections the virus may be confined to the mother, infect mother and placenta only, or involve the entire conceptus in a localized or generalized manner. Obviously the fetal outcome of any maternal infection is highly variable and unpredictable.

FETAL AND NEONATAL CONSEQUENCES OF MATERNAL VIRAL INFECTIONS DURING PREGNANCY

Any factor causing disruption of the normal physiology of pregnancy may nonspecifically result in abortion, stillbirth, or premature delivery. Thus, it is not surprising that a maternal viral illness accompanied by high fever, anoxia, dehydration, altered uterine blood flow, or other metabolic derangement can produce the same result in the absence of any direct fetal infection. The occasional coincidence of poor pregnancy outcome and maternal viral illness has fostered the clinical impression that pregnant women are more likely to acquire viral infections and, in addition, have a more severe clinical course than their nonpregnant counterparts. However, careful epidemiological and laboratory studies tend not to substantiate this claim (1,33–35). For the four viruses under consideration, there is little evidence that pregnancy alters incidence of infection or its clinical severity.

Aside from a possible nonspecific disruption of a pregnancy as noted above, the results of a direct fetal infection following hematogenous transplacental spread of virus are diverse. Possible consequences include death and resorption of the embryo, abortion and stillbirth of the fetus, and live birth of a premature or term infant who may or may not be normal (36). Transplacental passage of the viruses under consideration has been established with certainty for hepatitis B, rubella, and cytomegalovirus. Only the latter two agents, however, have been shown capable of producing teratogenic changes and intrauterine growth retardation (1,37). It must be noted, however, that intrauterine growth retardation is an atypical manifestation of congenital CMV infection; well over 90% of infected babies are asymptomatic and appear normal at birth (3). Likewise, establishing any of these agents as a definite cause of embryonic resorption, abortion, or stillbirth is exceedingly difficult, as discussed by Nahmias and Visintine for herpes simplex virus (32). In fact, for HSV, definite proof of transplacental passage leading to fetal death or abortion has only been occasionally suggested (38), and its association with prematurity may simply be secondary to the effects of nonspecific maternal illness. Transplacental passage of the hepatitis B virus has been suggested in the case of babies who become clinically ill sooner after birth than would be expected if the infection were contracted at the time of delivery (19). Transplacental passage has also been inferred for babies who are persistently surface antigen-positive at the time of delivery and whose mothers had clinical hepatitis in the first or second trimester of pregnancy (21,39). Insufficient evidence currently exists to implicate the hepatitis B virus as a cause of abortion or prematurity (except as a secondary result of generalized maternal illness), teratogenic developmental anomalies, or intrauterine growth retardation.

Gestational age of the conceptus at the time of the infection is the single factor most often cited as influencing fetal prognosis and outcome of pregnancy (1,3). As with other factors influencing fetal and neonatal prognosis, the effect of gestational age varies with the infecting agent. In the case of primary maternal rubella, infection of the placenta with transmission to the fetus resulting in major congenital anomalies is generally thought to occur in the first 16 weeks of gestation (3,40,41). Maternal infection after this point in gestation is associated with a mild sensorineural hearing deficit in approximately 5% or less of fetuses thus exposed (42). Even within the first 16 weeks of gestation, the risk to the fetus is sharply defined by the point in pregnancy at which infection occurs. In women contracting the disease within the first 10 weeks of pregnancy, chronic placental infection with fetal infection is common; it has been documented in as many as 85% of pregnancies when clinical maternal rubella occurs before the eighth week of gestation (43). Transmission to the fetus decreases sharply after the tenth week: placental infection also decreases but at a less rapid rate. Thus, for clinical maternal rubella contracted after the tenth week of gestation, isolated chronic placental infection is more common (30%) than fetal infection (5 to 10%) (44). The exact significance of this isolated placental infection is presently unknown, but patterns of disease in newborns parallel intrauterine events (45). Abortion as a result of extensive fetal infection occurs more often with maternal infections in the first 10 weeks of pregnancy; likewise, more surviving infants are born chronically infected, and their disease is usually more severe with a greater tendency for generalized organ system involvement (26). As might be expected, a higher precentage of these infants also have obvious teratogenic defects. After the tenth week, chronic infection of the newborn is less common (26,46). As mentioned previously, it is more often limited to a few organ systems and may well be overlooked for lack of symptoms because the perceptual organs or brain are the major sites of involvement. Although many hypotheses have been put forward to explain the effect of age at infection on fetal outcome, definitive answers are still being sought.

In the case of hepatitis, advanced gestational age increases the fetus' chances of acquiring the maternal infection. The rates of transmission to the fetus are much lower (10%) if the mother acquires clinically apparent hepatitis B in the first or second trimester as opposed to the third trimester or near delivery (50%) (19–21,39). One possible reason for this sequence of events may lie in the relatively long incubation period of hepatitis B (50 to 180 days). It has been postulated that the antibody response following maternal disease confers passive immunity to the fetus as antibody is transferred across the placenta while the virus is still incubating in the fetus (24,39). Regardless of the mechanism involved, the risk of fetal or neonatal acquisition of hepatitis B is higher when clinically apparent maternal disease occurs late as opposed to early in pregnancy.

The effect of fetal age at infection with maternal herpes simplex virus or cytomegalovirus has not been precisely determined. However, since natal acquisition of HSV, whether from a primary or recurrent genital lesion, is a well-defined risk factor for serious neonatal disease, and since there is no definitive proof that HSV is a teratogenic agent or direct cause of abortion, it must be assumed that the clinical situation is analogous to that described for hepatitis B; that is, the poorest outcome occurs following maternal infection late in pregnancy and at the time of delivery. The only statement currently possible about cytomegalovirus is that intrauterine acquisition of CMV (congenital infection) is associated with a worse ultimate outcome than viral acquisition at or near the time of delivery (natal infection). Determining the outcome of subclinical CMV infections, whether acquired in utero, natally, or postnatally, is of continuing paramount importance because of their high incidence. Currently, the intrauterine subclinical infection appears to be more pathogenic because of the tendency to cause sensorineural hearing loss and mental disturbances later in life (47–49). However, at present, follow-up data are inadequate to exclude the possibility that natal and early postnatally acquired CMV cause the same sort of subtle developmental defects already documented for congenital subclinical CMV infections.

Depending on the virus involved, the type of infection (primary or recurrent) occurring in the mother may or may not influence the incidence and severity of fetal infection. For rubella, infections in nonimmune hosts (primary infections) are more dangerous than reinfections (1,3,45). This is probably because of the prolonged blood-borne phase associated with primary infections, as opposed to the local (throat) infections without demonstrable viremia that usually characterize a recurrent infection. Preexisting immunity undoubtedly limits bloodstream spread that occurs with the typical forms of rubella reinfection, thus protecting the placenta from the intensive exposure to which it is subject in primary disease. Whether reinfection of the mother can cause fetal disease and, if so, how often and how virulent are debatable but important questions with regard to current vaccination practices in the United States.

In the case of hepatitis B, it appears that a more severe neonatal outcome may be associated with transmission of virus from mothers who are silent chronic carriers as opposed to mothers who are acutely ill at the time of delivery (23). It must be stressed that the present limited data allow only speculation on this point, but the interesting possibility that the host-immune response to the virus, now thought to be under genetic influence, may in fact turn out to be a powerful determinant of fetal outcome must be considered.

Cytomegalovirus may be transplacentally transmitted to the fetus with either primary (nonimmune) or recurrent (immune) maternal infection (8). Generally the former is thought to be more dangerous for the fetus. However, this assumption is premature, because both types of maternal infection usually cause subclinical congenital infections whose long-term outcomes are not yet adequately defined. In fact, it has yet to be established whether or not a symptomatic congenital infection is exclusively the result of a primary maternal infection.

A number of other factors, mostly theoretical or incompletely defined, have been proposed which may influence fetal outcome following infection in the mother. Among these factors are the genetic constitution of the infected host, the amount of virus to which the fetus is exposed, differences in virulence among different strains of virus, the maternal and fetal immune response, the ability of the placenta to replicate virus at different gestational ages, and the effect of hormonal changes associated with pregnancy on virus replication either in the mother or conceptus. The significance of these and other yet undefined factors as determinants of fetal disease and ultimate outcome needs clarification.

In the case of infections acquired during the course of delivery or the immediate newborn period (HSV, CMV, hepatitis B) maternal infection characterized by persistence or reactivation may prove to be of considerable risk to the baby. In this situation the newborn comes into direct contact with infectious material and may acquire infection with CMV or HSV even in the face of high levels of maternal antibody. Approximately 30% of the infants who are exposed to cytomegalovirus in this manner may become natally infected (1–29). As noted, the ultimate significance of natally acquired CMV infections has not yet been established. Overt disease has not yet been noted in the neonatal period, but a chronic pneumonitis associated with this type of infection has been described in early infancy (50). Such infections are chronic in nature and could conceivably lead to low grade but significant later disease analogous to that described with asymptomatic congenitally acquired infections (47–49). In the case of hepatitis B, the number of infants who become infected following delivery by chronic carriers is much smaller (5% of exposed infants in the United States). However, acquisition of hepatitis B during the perinatal period has been associated with significant progressive liver damage in some infants (20,22,24,39,51). The actual risk that silent maternal excretion of herpes simplex virus poses to a newly born infant has not been established. Given the prevalence of this type of infection in early pregnancy (1 to 2%) (31,32), together with the rarity of neonatal HSV, it must be concluded that either the prevalence of genital infection is decreased near term or, alternatively, that the risk posed for an individual infant is small. However, the low incidence of neonatal infection with HSV stands in marked contrast to the clinical severity and high mortality of the disease produced (52–54).

Clinically apparent disease in the neonate may result from fetal infection with any of the viruses under consideration. The considerable overlap in symptomalogy produced by these diverse agents simply reflects the concept that expression of severe organ dysfunction in the newborn may be independent of its cause through a wide range of etiologies (3). The following signs and symptoms, though nonspecific with respect to the etiologic agent, should suggest the diagnosis of chronic congenital infection: hepatosplenomegaly (single or in combination); jaundice, especially with elevation of direct-reacting bilirubin; hemolytic anemia; petechiae; bleeding tendency with or without reduced platelets; signs of acute central nervous system (CNS) involvement with or without encephalitic changes in the cerebrospinal fluid; signs of chronic CNS disease (microcephaly, cerebral atrophy, or intracranial calcification); pneumonitis; myocarditis; and eye pathology. These findings may be present at birth or develop later in the neonatal or childhood period. Certain findings do lend a degree of specificity to clinical diagnosis. These include, for rubella, signs of patent ductus with or without deformities of the pulmonary isthmus; myocardial infarction pattern on EKG; cataracts, pigmented retina, cloudy cornea, glaucoma; bony radiolucencies (distal and long bones); raised bluish-red skin lesions due to erythrogenic arrest (blueberry muffin syndrome); immunological deficiencies, especially isolated IgA deficiency; and, finally, obvious deafness in early infancy. Findings that add to the specificity of diagnosis for the other infections in the immediate neonatal period include (1) for cytomegalovirus, microcephaly with periventricular calcification and dominance of the central nervous system defects mentioned above under suggestive findings; (2) for herpes simplex virus, keratoconjunctivitis and skin vesicles; (3) for hepatitis B, isolated hepatitis. For expansion on the clinical signs and symptoms the reader is returned to several excellent reviews on the subject (3,55,56).

With the exception of HSV the clinical picture of congenitally infected infants is characterized by a complete lack of signs and symptoms in many of the babies at birth, with variable expression of functional defects appearing in a minority of patients over the next several years of life. Indeed, over 90% of newborns infected with CMV, 50% infected with rubella, and an unknown percentage of babies infected with hepatitis B may appear normal at birth. Hearing, eye, hepatic, or central nervous system disease, even though persistent, most often have no overt manifestations in the newborn and, therefore, can go undetected in early life. However, these disease processes will be expressed as subtle but significant pathology much later (3). Each of the four viruses has the capability of surviving and replicating in the tissues for months or years after in utero or natal infections and causing either silent damage (in chronic active hepatitis and HSV chorioretinitis) (24,32), progressive damage (in CMV pneumonitis and neurosensory hearing loss) (47,50), or sudden symptomatic damage (in late-onset progressive rubella encephalitis). The last example has been documented in four children with clinically stable congenital rubella until the ages of 11 to 14 years (57,58). Excellent clinical care as well as optimal understanding of the morbidity of fetal and perinatal viral infections demands careful diagnosis and serial follow-up of all infants born to infected mothers, with special attention paid to developmental milestones and perceptual abilities. A specific diagnosis, once established, will further aid the physician caring for infected children, since specific long-term problems—hearing for CMV and rubella, visual for rubella and HSV, and liver failure for hepatitis B—may be associated with each viral disease.

Laboratory Diagnosis: Neonates and Infants

Specific viral laboratory diagnosis in the immediate neonatal period is most easily accomplished if several general principles are kept in mind. With the exception of hepatitis B, for which no direct in vitro isolation system currently exists, direct viral isolation is the most definitive diagnostic procedure available. Although virus may be excreted for various periods of time (months to years) after birth, it is imperative that viral isolation be attempted soon after birth for two reasons. First, for diagnostic specificity with regard to intrauterine acquisition, isolation must be attempted early in the neonatal period, since viral excretion after that time may represent natally or postnatally acquired infection carrying a far different prognosis (29,59). Second, as has been demonstrated for rubella, the period of virus shedding is highly variable among individuals, with only 33% of infected infants excreting virus at 4 months and 11% excreting after 8 months (60). When attempting to recover virus, it must be remembered that each virus has a characteristic tissue or body site for optimal viral isolation—for CMV, throat and urine; for rubella, throat; for HSV, the cutaneous lesions, with throat as a secondary site.

A second laboratory technique that can aid in making a specific viral diagnosis is serologic testing. All serologic techniques are based on the fact that specific antibodies are produced following either in utero or natally acquired viral infections. Most of the methods for detection of fetal antibody in cord or neonatal sera are based on the premise that IgM antibody cannot be transferred by the placenta and, therefore, must be produced by the fetus. Such antibody may be useful diagnostically if specific IgM antibody to a particular agent can be demonstrated in cord or neonatal sera (1,3). In addition, general fetal immunologic responses may be used diagnostically as nonspecific screening devices; that is, a demonstration of elevated levels of total IgM in cord sera, as opposed to demonstration of a specific antibody, is taken to indicate excessive intrauterine antigenic stimulation and, in this limited sense, serves as a nonspecific monitor for chronic intrauterine infection (61,62). From a clinical point of view, screening of cord sera for elevated IgM is a useful tool to identify a sizable but unknown percentage of asymptomatic newborns with chronic infections; additionally, an elevated IgM can help select individuals for definitive virologic isolation from among those suspected of having infection by either clinical or epidemiologic criteria. Though IgM is elevated in less than 50% of subclinically infected infants and is thus inefficient as a screening device, it is elevated in the majority of newborns symptomatically infected in utero. Recently, rheumatoid factor has been found to be produced by the fetus in response to intrauterine CMV infections (63). About 38% of subclinically infected infants have rheumatoid factor in their serum at the time of delivery, and another 20% or so develop this substance during the early months of life. At birth none of 155 uninfected infants has yet been found to have rheumatoid factor; consequently this immunologic monitor may also prove to be a useful adjunct in the diagnosis of chronic congenital infection. Like IgM elevations, however, its absence cannot be taken to exclude the presence of subclinical infections, nor is its presence likely to be specific for CMV alone, but rather for infection in general.

The interpretation of neonatal or infant serology based on the ongoing production of specific IgG antibodies is often confusing soon after birth because of the presence of IgG antibodies that are transmitted from the mother to the fetus in infected as well as normal pregnancies (1–3). After delivery, maternal antibodies (IgG) serially decrease with a half-life of 30 days and finally disappear from the sera of uninfected infants at various intervals during the first year of life. In contrast, in infected infants IgG antibody levels comparable with those in maternal sera persist for long periods of time. This fact is useful in the diagnosis of congenital rubella, since demonstration of persistent hemagglutinin inhibiting (HI) antibody during the first year of life is virtually conclusive evidence of intrauterine acquisition. With cytomegalovirus, however, use of serial monitoring for specific antibody is clouded by the fact that the antibody response following infection acquired at or around delivery cannot be easily distinguished from that following intrauterine acquisition with routine procedures like the commonly used complement fixation test. Serologic monitoring for neonatal herpes simplex infection is not practical because of the temporal virulence of the infection in relation to the slower antibody response.

In contrast to CMV, rubella, and HSV, the neonatal diagnosis of asymptomatic hepatitis B is not based on viral isolation or serology and is, therefore, somewhat more complex. As pointed out earlier, an in vitro isolation system for this virus does not exist. In addition, although the presence in serum of specific antibody to the virus is definite evidence of past infection, the time of appearance and magnitude of antibody response is highly variable from individual to individual and, therefore, cannot be generally used to make a diagnosis in the first months of life (64,65). The accepted alternative criterion used to indicate infection with hepatitis B is the appearance in serum of the surface antigen (HBs Ag). However, it must be stressed that the surface antigen may represent complete infectious virions as well as incomplete or noninfectious viral proteins (64); therefore, presence of surface antigen is not a priori evidence of progressive or ongoing infection. In addition, the ability of the surface antigen to cross the placenta, together with the potential for natal acquisition of the virus, renders the presence or absence of surface antigen in cord sera nondiagnostic with regard to current or future infection and prognosis of the infant (24,19). Whether a baby becomes infected after being born to a mother who is either acutely ill or a silent chronic carrier of hepatitis at the time of delivery can only be determined by serial surface antigen determinations and close clinical follow-up, not by the presence or absence of the surface antigen in cord sera.

Diagnosis in the Mother

With the exceptions of clinically recognized rubella, icteric hepatitis B, the heterophile-negative CMV mononucleosis syndrome, and symptomatic genital HSV involvement, these viral illnesses are difficult or impossible to diagnose in the mother on clinical grounds alone. That the majority of women infected during pregnancy with these organisms have no apparent sign of disease, coupled with the fact that recurrent or chronic infections may also lead to significant fetal and neonatal pathology, makes this group of infections one of the most frustrating problems currently faced by the clinician. Nonetheless, therapeutic or preventive measures for current or future pregnancies are obviously predicated on establishing the existence and nature of maternal infection.

Cytomegalovirus

The overwhelming majority of women who are infected with CMV are completely asymptomatic. However, a primary CMV infection should be suspected in a pregnant woman with a heterophile negative mononucleosis syndrome, and diagnosis attempted by complement fixation serology done simultaneously on serum samples collected acutely, and 2, 4, and 8 weeks later. Only one case of CMV mononucleosis has been reported to date in pregnancy (66), and, in this instance, the placenta and fetus were infected with virus. A more realistic estimation of the incidence of primary CMV infections during pregnancy might be obtained if clinicians were to initiate diagnostic studies in women presenting with fever not attributable to other causes. The recovery of CMV from amniotic fluid is theoretically possible, but to date too little experience with this diagnostic procedure has been reported to recommend it for clinical use. It should be emphasized that the intrauterine risk to the fetus associated with recovery of CMV from the cervix or urine in the asymptomatic seropositive pregnant woman has not been established; therefore, counseling recommendations with regard to possible outcomes of pregnancy in this situation are not feasible or appropriate.

Herpes Simplex Virus

Because genital HSV infection is clinically apparent in only about one-third of all cases (31,32,67), case finding might be improved if the clinician were to initiate viral screening on the basis of a history of maternal genital herpes at any time in the past, past history of sexually transmitted disease (1,12,32), genital HSV in contemporary male contacts, and nonspecific signs and symptoms such as pelvic pain and cervical inflammation (discharge). Because the primary risk to an infant is acquisition of infection around the time of birth and because recurrent, as well as primary, disease poses a risk to the infant (32), the most important diagnostic tool available to the clinician is a cytological demonstration or viral isolation of HSV from the cervix. Absolute levels of antibody or changing maternal antibody titers are not helpful in making clinical decisions. It should be emphasized that cytology should only be used as a screening procedure, with viral isolation the definitive procedure on which therapeutic or management decisions are based. A negative cytology in the presence of clinically suspicious lesions should be confirmed by direct culture techniques. In the case of a suspected primary herpetic lesion, isolation of HSV from amniotic fluid or maternal peripheral white blood cells would be confirmatory if positive, but too little clinical experience is available with these procedures to be reassured if virus is not recovered.

Rubella

Proof of symptomatic or asymptomatic primary infection is based on seroconversion, and reinfection is established by a four/fold rise in specific antibody (1,3,45). Difficulty in serologic diagnosis is usually encountered because of inappropriate delay in initiating the necessary serial studies. A history of exposure to rubella or the occurrence of a rubelliform rash in pregnancy demands careful attention and investigation based on the following general principles. The incubation period of this infection may range from 14 to 21 days, and antibody, including hemagglutination inhibition (HI), may appear as early as 14 days after exposure irrespective of clinical illness (3,45). Complement fixation antibodies appear later, peaking 4 weeks to 3 months after exposure (68,69). Therefore, the initial serum specimen should be collected as soon as possible after exposure or illness is reported, and the time of contact with a contagious source established. It must be kept in mind that a contact is potentially infectious up to a week before clinical illness becomes apparent (45). The presence of HI antibody in serum collected within 13 days of the earliest possible exposure date indicates prior immunity, and protection is thought to be complete. A negative result must be followed by a repeat HI determination 35 days after exposure or 14 days after the appearance of the rash. For those women who present 14 or more days after exposure, the initial serum specimen should be followed by a convalescent sample 14 to 21 days later. If seroconversion is found, primary infection has occurred. A four/fold or greater increase in titer could indicate either primary involvement or reinfection. In this case or when stable or rising, but less than four/fold, titers are found, complement fixation or IgM rubella antibody determinations may be performed to establish whether primary infection has occurred as opposed to previous disease or reinfection, respectively. Another helpful procedure in the case of stable antibody titers is to document the presence or absence of rubella in the alleged index case. All the foregoing situations imply absence of maternal illness. Rash or illness occurring after an appropriate incubation period following exposure to a rubella-like illness can be easily documented by a properly timed HI antibody determination (3).

Confusion currently exists with regard to screening of all pregnant women at the first prenatal visit for the presence or absence of rubella antibody. A positive titer in the absence of a history of exposure or rash is sometimes viewed with alarm by the clinician, who intitates serial sampling of the patient and raises the possibility of fetal infection with her. This approach ignores the fact that approximately 85 to 95% of adult women in this country are immune to rubella, that the incidence of interepidemic congenital rubella is 1/1000, and that if serial maternal samples are not run concurrently, the test results may be misleading. If the woman is antibody-negative on the first prenatal visit, she is indeed susceptible to rubella, but serial monitoring for a fortuitous case of rubella reflects wishful thinking. Usually the first serum sample is not drawn until rather late in the first trimester, so that the most critical period for documentation of maternal rubella is therefore overlooked. Indeed, the major purpose of screening all pregnant women for rubella antibodies is for selection of those women who would benefit from rubella vaccination postpartum (see below).

Hepatitis

Specific laboratory diagnosis of hepatitis B infection requires the demonstration of the surface antigen in maternal sera. The presence of antibody to the surface antigen indicates existing immunity to the disease; because of the temporal variability of its appearance following infection, demonstration of seroconversion cannot be used to make a rapid diagnosis. However, antibody testing may be a useful adjunct in establishing a diagnosis of hepatitis B in retrospect. A search for the surface antigen should be a part of any diagnostic workup of pregnant women who present with jaundice as a part of an overt illness. As noted earlier, the variable clinical expression of anicteric hepatitis should alert the clinician to the possibility of hepatitis in all pregnant patients with severe nausea and vomiting, unusual anorexia, fever of undetermined orgin, rashes, or arthalgia and arthritis not easily ascribed to other causes. Because of the low incidence of the asymptomatic carrier state (1/1000), it is probably not reasonable to recommend surface antigen screening as a routine test in prenatal care. However, in mothers who are at special risk for being chronic carriers (see above), determination of their surface antigen status is probably warranted.

Prevention and Control

Rubella

Prevention and control of rubella is unique in that protection is aimed at future fetuses, rather than the current population taking part in control programs (1,70). Moreover, because of the questionable or complete lack of efficacy of either passive immunization or antiviral chemotherapy, control programs in the United States are based on active immunization. The primary goal is to develop a high level of herd immunity among children, who are the major purveyors of rubella virus under natural circumstances. Secondary protection for women of childbearing age is then derived from the presumed decreased circulation of virus in the general population (45). Two major concerns regarding this policy have recently been raised. First, herd immunity as high as 95% has been unable to preclude spread of virus in both open and closed populations (71–73). Second, the attenuated vaccines (HPV-77 and Cendehill) currently in use produce antibody responses that are quantitatively and qualitatively deficient compared with those of natural infection (45–72), with resulting serologic reinfection much more common in the vaccinated than among the naturally infected (71,74,75). Although there has been only one report to date of fetal involvement following reinfection (76), the crucial question regarding fetal risk during reinfection has not been resolved (45). The problems surrounding reinfection are not likely to be solved until a large enough number of females who were initially vaccinated as children or infants reach childbearing age. The antibody status of these children remains under long-term surveillance by the Center for Disease Control; through these and other studies, decisions will be made as to whether or not large segments of the population will require revaccination in time. For those previously vaccinated who are already of childbearing age, the immune status can be determined by serologic assessment. If there is no antibody or the level is low (less than 32) because of a poor initial response, which can be expected to occur in a certain low percentage of people vaccinated, revaccination may be considered. The potential problems of reinfection may be relieved somewhat in the future with the introduction of Plotkin's RA 27-3 vaccine, which confers a broader and more lasting form of immunity than the vaccines in current use (72,77,78).

When vaccinating women of childbearing age, extreme caution must be observed, since vaccine virus can infect the products of conception (79). Though the viral virulence for the fetus of the attenuated strains is unknown, it is prudent to avoid these man-made infections and any potential harmful results. Therefore, pregnancy must be excluded before administering any form of rubella vaccine to women of childbearing age. Contraception is mandatory for 3 months after vaccine administration, since the virus can be transmitted to the products of conception for weeks following inoculation (1). Clearly, the safest time to immunize adult females is the immediate postpartum period, with adequate contraceptive control, when the chances for a subsequent pregnancy are greatly reduced. In any event, serology should be performed before vaccinating any adult female in order to determine that she is susceptible to rubella (seronegative). There is no excuse to vaccinate adult females blindly with the potential hazard at hand, since the great majority are already naturally immune.

In the absence of a perfect preventive control program, the clinician and patient are occasionally forced to deal with a pregnancy complicated by maternal rubella infection. In order to handle the question of therapeutic abortion objectively, the physician must have not only a thorough understanding of the known facts about the pathogenesis of congenital rubella but, more important,deep compassion based on the moral and ethical framework of the family involved. It is clear that the decision rests entirely with the family involved, but the physician must be in a position to advise the family with as much factual knowledge as currently exists. Current abortion laws should have rendered obsolete the practice of using presumed rubella as an excuse for terminating an otherwise unwanted pregnancy.

The therapeutic benefit of gamma globulin following maternal exposure has not been adequately assessed. It clearly is not completely protective, as evidenced by the occurrence of symptomatic fetal infection following its use. At present, it is recommended that this potential preventative be used only in situations where therapeutic abortion is an unacceptable alternative. Large quantities (20 cc) should be given. Even with this approach, protection cannot be assured.

Herpes

At present, there is no completely satisfactory method for preventing neonatal acquisition of HSV. The possible oncogenicity of attenuated live viral vaccines together with the known fact of recurrent genital infections in the face of circulating antibody seems to mitigate against the efficacy and safety of an immunization program in the near future. Although an antiviral agent (adenine arabinoside) has recently been proved effective in the systemic treatment of herpes encephalitis (1), neither this compound nor any other systemic or local treatment regimen has proved of clinical value for the treatment of genital herpes. It has been suggested that pregnant women avoid sexual contact with males with penile herpes, but this suggestion seems to ignore the possibility that the woman herself may be the source from which the male acquired his infection. With intercourse during pregnancy, use of a condom by the male with a known history of recurrent genital herpes is advisable in order to minimize exposure of the female genital tract (32). This suggestion is particularly pertinent in late pregnancy.

Although there are no controlled clinical trials demonstrating the effectiveness of cesarean section in preventing neonatal herpes in infants of mothers with genital HSV infection at the time of delivery (1,32), operative delivery is often the only option available in this situation. In obtaining informed consent for such a procedure, the physician must keep several factors in mind. First, operative delivery may not afford complete protection, and the risk to the infant increases as the time between rupture of membranes and delivery increases (32). Second, the presence of genital virus at or near the time of delivery should be documented. The presence of a primary or recurrent lesion earlier in pregnancy does not mean that virus will necessarily be present near term (31,32,67). Indeed, in primary infections during pregnancy, the virus may be shed from the cervix for as long as 6 weeks to 3 months, but, with recurrent infections, the virus is seldom excreted for more than 10 to 21 days. Therefore, careful virologic monitoring is essential in order to avoid unnecessary operations with attendant maternal mortality and morbidity. In addition, the risk of producing neonatal mortality and morbidity secondary to the elective delivery of a premature infant (80) far exceeds the risk of neonatal herpes. Therefore, careful attention to the lung maturity of the fetus is essential for planning the perinatal management of these infants.

The role of amniocentesis in the care of the pregnant female infected with genital herpes is still questionable. Its use in early pregnancy to detect intrauterine transmission should be avoided, since transplacental transmission of virus during early gestation is very rare and negative results do not exclude the possibility of fetal infection. Use of amniocentesis prior to contemplated cesarean section in later gestation has been suggested (32). If virus is found in the amniotic fluid, it is presumed that the fetus has already been infected; therefore, jeopardizing the mother with an elective operative procedure is not warranted. Once again, however, negative results do not necessarily exclude fetal infection. More important, although positive results should influence the route of delivery (vaginal as opposed to abdominal), the presence of virus in amniotic fluid should not be offered as a reason to delay the timing of delivery, for the infected baby would then be deprived of supportive medical care that could well influence the final outcome of the infection. The outcome of neonatal herpes, though bad, is not irrevocably disastrous, especially with localized varieties limited to involvement of eye, skin, or central nervous system alone. In fact, treatment is available for keratoconjunctivitis (idoxuridine and adenine arabinoside) (1), which otherwise can cause severe visual impairment. Certain of the possible bleeding disorders and secondary effects of the central nervous system damage can be controlled medically for the ultimate benefit of the infant. In other words, the final result of perinatal herpes infections is quite variable and unpredictable. Clearly, decisions concerning whether or not and when to perform a cesarean section in a mother with genital herpes are obviously difficult and require cooperation among the obstetrician, pediatrician, nursery personnel, and virologists. The presence of symptomatic genital lesions at or around the time of delivery is a definite risk factor, particularly so if the infection is primary, because of the higher levels of virus production and persistence. With silent genital herpes fortuitously diagnosed near term by cytology or other means, the actual risk is unknown, because definitive studies have not been done. However, since many cases of neonatal herpes have been documented where the mother has denied any knowledge of genital lesions, one must conclude that virus can be transmitted in absence of apparent lesions. Parenthetically, silent maternal genital HSV infections are much more common than neonatal herpes; consequently, potent inherent protective mechanisms must be operative. Determining what these mechanisms are would greatly facilitate the management of genital herpes in pregnancy and help relieve the present state of agony and frustration.

Cytomegalovirus

Except for the reminder that cytomegalovirus as well as hepatitis B can be transmitted to both mother and newborns via blood transfusion (65,81,82), and the simultaneous caution against the use of transfused blood except where absolutely indicated, there is no prevention or treatment for either maternal or fetal CMV infection. Consideration of abortion with maternal CMV infections must be tempered. Virus can be transmitted with both primary and recurrent maternal infections, but in either event the infection is usually silent in both mother and newborn. The cause of the few virulent fetal infections is unknown. Recognizable maternal disease (CMV mononucleosis) with transmission of virus to the fetus has been documented only once. Recommendations for or against abortion are, therefore, handicapped by the unavailability of a larger experience with this clinical situation. Guidelines with regard to the obstetrical management of an individual pregnant woman silently infected by CMV await definitions of intrauterine transmission and virulence factors, as well as the long-term outcome of silent intrauterine and perinatal infections. One obvious recommendation can be made. Pregnant females, including medical personnel, should avoid close and continuous contact with overtly infected infants or transplant patients, all of whom excrete high levels of virus from throat and urine for long periods.

A vaccination for the prevention of CMV infection has been proposed by many investigators (83–85). Although prevention of CMV is certainly a desirable goal, there are many practical and theoretical disadvantages to the development and testing of a CMV vaccine at this time. Two of the more obvious reasons why caution should be expressed are, first, the question as to the protective effect of naturally acquired antibody; the concept of primary infection as a requisite for passage of infection to the fetus is apparently not an absolute (8). Second, the question arises concerning a possible oncogenic hazard involved in injecting a live virus with in vitro transforming and latency properties into its natural host (86,87). Whether or not the problems involved with vaccine development are resolved or whether primary control of this infection will have to await the development of specific antiviral chemotherapy, control of CMV remains an important research goal for the years ahead.

Hepatitis B

Specific immunity to hepatitis B is afforded by circulating antibody in a manner analogous to that of rubella. Indeed, recent technical advances should lead to the development of a suitable vaccine in the next several years. Development of such a vaccine will eradicate this disease as a threat to mothers and infants. In the meantime, current preventive measures are based on passive immunization, a situation not applicable to CMV, rubella, or HSV. Several studies of individuals at high risk for developing hepatitis B—spouses of infected individuals, renal dialysis personnel, etc.—have demonstrated the efficacy of high titer immune globulin in decreasing both the incidence and severity of subsequent disease (88). Preliminary studies involving a limited number of neonates born to mothers acutely ill or chronically infected with hepatitis B have suggested the efficacy of this preparation in preventing perinatal transmission (89). An important theoretical drawback to this therapeutic approach involves the question of whether prolongation of the carrier state or development of antigen-antibody complex disease may ensue as a result of this treatment (24). Nonetheless, with these reservations in mind, it has been suggested that high titer immune globulin be given to any infant born to a surface antigen-positive mother (acutely ill or chronic carrier). A more definitive recommendation for the use of high titer immune globulin as neonatal prophylaxis or immunotherapy awaits the outcome of further well-controlled studies. In addition, a blanket recommendation may be modified if the interesting preliminary work of O'Kada et al. (90) is borne out in subsequent studies. These workers have suggested that the presence of the 'e' antigen (91) in the serum of surface antigen-positive individuals is a specific marker of perinatal transmission. If this marker is found to be reliable, only infants of 'e' antigen-positive mothers would potentially require passive immunization.

Although it has generally been recommended that a mother who is surface antigen-positive not breast-feed, the specific role of breast feeding as a factor in perinatal transmission of hepatitis B is incompletely defined. Epidemiologic studies have not specifically implicated breast milk in perinatal transmission (22), and surface antigen material has generally been found only infrequently and in low levels in breast milk (92,93). These facts together with the demonstration of Villarejos and his colleagues (94) of the high incidence and duration of surface antigen-positive material in saliva suggests a reexamination of the breast milk recommendation. It may be that the mothering process per se—kissing, fondling, etc.—is more important in early neonatal acquisition of hepatitis B than the isolated act of breast feeding. In the absence of a complete separation of mother and child, it appears that breast feeding may not be so important in the transmission process as previously assumed. It is hoped, however, that passive immunization at present and active immunization in the future will render this question obsolete. As with the control measures cited for the other chronic perinatal viral infections, the ultimate impact of control will be determined by the ability of the clinician to identify correctly, via clinical awareness and a solid epidemiological basis, the mothers at risk in order that the proper type of prophylaxis and treatment can be correctly applied.

REFERENCES

1. Whitley, R., and Alford, C. A.: Chronic intrauterine and perinatal infections caused by rubella, cytomegaloviruses and Herpes simplex virus, in *Antiviral Agents in Man*, edited by G. J. Galosso. Raven Press, New York, in press.

2. Remington, J. S., and Klein, J. O. (eds.): *Infectious Diseases of the Fetus and Newborn Infant*. W. B. Saunders Company, Philadelphia, 1976.

3. Alford, C. A., Stagno, S., and Reynolds, D. W.: Perinatal infections caused by viruses, toxoplasma, and *Treponema pallidum,* in *Clinical Perinatology,* edited by S. Aladjem and A. K. Brown. The C. V. Mosby Co., St. Louis, 1974. pp. 183–204.

4. Sever, J. L., Hardy, J. B., Nelson, K. B., and Gilkeson, M. R.: Rubella in the collaborative perinatal research study. *Am. J. Dis. Child.* 118:123, 1969.

5. Weller, T. H.: The cytomegaloviruses: Ubiquitous agents with protean clinical manifestations. *N. Engl. J. Med.* 285:203, 267, 1971.

6. Nahmias, A. J., and Josey, W. E.: Epidemiology of Herpes simplex Viruses 1 and 2, in *Viral Infections of Humans: Epidemiology and Control,* edited by A. S. Evans. Plenum Publishing Corporation, New York, 1976, pp. 253–271.

7. Maynard, J. E., Bradley, D. W., Hornbeck, C. L., et al.: Preliminary serologic studies of antibody to hepatitis: A virus in populations in the United States. *J. Infect. Dis.* 134:528–530, 1976.

8. Stagno, S., Reynolds, D. W., Huang, E. S., Thames, S., Smith, R. J., and Alford, C. A.: Congenital cytomegalovirus infection: Occurrence in an immune population. *N. Engl. J. Med.* 296:1254–1258, 1977.

9. Embil, J. A., Ozere, R. L., and Haldane, E. V.: Congenital cytomegalovirus infection in two siblings from consecutive pregnancies. *J. Pediatr.* 77:417–421, 1970.

10. Krech, U., Konjajev, Z., and Jung, M.: Congenital cytomegalovirus infection in siblings from consecutive pregnancies. *Helv. Paediatr. Acta* 26:355–57, 1971.

11. Stagno, S., Reynolds, D. W., Lakeman, A., Charamella, L. J., and Alford, C. S.: Congenital cytomegalovirus infection: Consecutive occurrence due to viruses with similar antigenic compositions. *Pediatrics* 52:788–794, 1973.

12. Nahmias, A., and Roizman, B.: Herpes simplex viruses. *N. Engl. J. Med.* 289:667–674, 719–725, 781–789, 1973.

13. Nahmias, A. J., and Visintine, A. M.: Perinatal herpes simplex virus infection, in *Congenital and Perinatal Infection,* edited by J. S. Remington and J. O. Klein. W. B. Saunders, Philadelphia, 1974, pp. 156–196.

14. Stevens, C. E., Beasley, R. P., Tsui, J., and Lee, W. C.: Vertical transmission of hepatitis B antigen in Taiwan. *N. Engl. J. Med.* 292:771–774, 1975.

15. Okada, K., Yamada, T., Mijakawa, Y., and Marjumi, M.: Hepatitis B surface antigen in the serum of infants after delivery from asymptomatic carrier mothers. *J. Pediat.* 87:360–363, 1975.

16. Azia, M. A., Khan, G., Khanum, T., and Siddiqui, A.: Transplacental and postnatal transmission of the hepatitis associated antigen. *J. Infect. Dis.* 127:110–112, 1973.

17. Schweitzer, I. L., Moseley, J. W., Ashcavai, M., et al.,: Factors influencing neonatal infection by hepatitis B virus. *Gastroenterology* 65:227–283, 1973.

18. Skinhog, P., Saremann, H., and Cohen, J.: Hepatitis-associated antigen (HAA) in pregnant women and their newborn infants. *Amer. J. Dis. Child.* 123:380–381, 1972.

19. Schweitzer, I. L., Wing, A., McPeak, C., and Spears, R. L.: Hepatitis and hepatitis-associated antigen in 56 mother-infant pairs. *J.A.M.A.* 220:1092–1095, 1972.

20. Schweitzer, I. L., Dunn, A. E., Peters. R. L., and Spears, R. L.: Viral hepatitis B in neonates and infants. *Amer. J. Med.* 55:762–771, 1973.

21. Cossart, Y. E.: Acquisition of hepatitis B antigen in the newborn period. *Postgrad. Med. J.* 50:334–337, 1974.

22. Merrill, D. A., DuBois, R. S., and Kohler, P. F.: Neonatal onset of the hepatitis-associated antigen carrier state. *N. Engl. J. Med.* 287:1280–1282, 1972.

23. Fawaz, K. A., Grady, G. F., Kaplan, M. M., and Gellis, S. S.: Repetitive maternal-fetal transmission of fatal hepatitis B. *N. Engl. J. Med.* 293:1357–1359, 1975.

24. Crumpacher, C. S.: Hepatitis, in *Infectious Diseases of the Fetus and Newborn Infant,* edited by J. S. Remington and J. O. Klein. W. B. Saunders, Philadelphia, 1976, pp. 492–520.

25. Nahmias, A. J., Josey, W. E., Naib, Z. M., Freeman, M. G., Fernandez, R. J., and Wheeler, J. H.: Perinatal risk associated with maternal genital herpes simplex virus infection. *Am. J. Obstet. Gynecol.* 110:825, 1971.

26. Horstmann, D. M., Banatavala, J. E., Riordan, J. T., Payne, M. D., Whittemore, R., Opton, E. M., and duVe Florey, C.: Maternal rubella and the rubella syndrome in infants. *Am. J. Dis. Child.* 110:408, 1965.

27. McCollum, R. W.: Viral hepatitis, in *Viral Infections of Humans: Epidemiology and Control*, edited by A. S. Evans. Plenum Publishing Corporation, New York, 1976, pp. 235–251.

28. Reynolds, D. W., Stagno, S., Hosty, T. S., Tiller, M., and Alford, C. A., Jr.: Maternal cytomegalovirus excretion and perinatal infection. *N. Engl. J. Med.* 289:1–5, 1973.

29. Montgomery, R., Youngblood, L., and Medearis, D. N.: Recovery of cytomegalovirus from the cervix in pregnancy. *Pediatrics* 49:524, 1972.

30. Langenhuysen, M.: IgM levels, specific IgM antibodies and liver involvement in cytomegalovirus infection: Report of 17 patients. *Scand. J. Infect. Dis.* 4:113–118, 1972.

31. Nahmias, A. J., Josey, W. E., and Naib, Z. M.: Significance of herpes simplex virus infection during pregnancy. *Clin. Obstet. Gynecol.* 15:929–938, 1972.

32. Nahmias, A. J., and Visintine, A. M.: Herpes simplex, in *Infectious Diseases of the Fetus and Newborn Infant*, edited by J. S. Remington and J. O. Klein.. W. B. Saunders, Philadelphia, 1976, pp. 156–190.

33. Adams, R. H., and Combes, B.: Viral hepatitis during pregnancy. *J.A.M.A.* 192:95–99, 1965.

34. Haemmerli, U. P.: Jaundice during pregnancy, in *Diseases of the Liver*, edited by L. Schiff. J. B. Lippincott Co., Philadelphia, 1972, pp. 1023–1036.

35. Horstmann, D. M.: Viral infections, in *Medical Complications During Pregnancy*, edited by B. N. Burrow and T. F. Ferris. W. B. Saunders Co., Philadelphia, 1975, pp. 414–437.

36. Klein, J. O., Remington, J. S., and S. M. Marcy: An introduction to infections of the fetus and newborn infant, in *Infectious Diseases of the Fetus and Newborn Infant*, edited by J. S. Remington and J. O. Klein. W. B. Saunders, Philadelphia, 1976, pp. 1–32.

37. Hanshaw, J. B.: Developmental abnormalities associated with congenital cytomegalovirus infection. *Adv. Teratol.* 4:64–93, 1970.

38. Abrams, C. A.: Isolation of herpes simplex from a mother and aborted foetus. *Ghana Med. J.* 5:41, 1966.

39. Schweitzer, I. L.: Vertical transmission of the hepatitis B surface antigen. *Am. J. Med. Sci.* 270:287–291, 1975.

40. Alford, C. A., Neva, F. A., and Weller, T. H.: Virologic and serologic studies on human products of conception after maternal rubella. *N. Engl. J. Med.* 271:1275, 1964.

41. Alford, C. A., Jr.: Congenital rubella: A review of the virologic and serologic phenomena occurring after maternal rubella in the first trimester. *Southern Med. J.* 59:745, 1966.

42. Hardy, J. B., McCracken, G. H., Gilkeson, M. R., and Sever, J. L.: Adverse fetal outcome following maternal rubella after the first trimester of pregnancy. *J.A.M.A.* 207:2414–2417, 1969.

43. Dudgeon, J. A.: Congenital rubella: Pathogenesis and immunology. *Am. J. Dis. Child.* 118:35, 1969.

44. Alford, C. A., Neva, F. A., and Weller, T. H.: Virologic and serologic studies on human products of conception after maternal rubella. *N. Engl. J. Med.* 271:1275, 1964.

45. Alford, C. A., Jr.: Rubella, in *Infectious Diseases of the Fetus and Newborn Infant*, edited by J. S. Remington and J. O. Klein. W. B. Saunders, Philadelphia, 1976, pp. 71–106.

46. Peckham, G. S.: Clinical and laboratory study of children exposed in utero to maternal rubella. *Arch. Dis. Child.* 47:571, 1972.

47. Alford, C. A., Stagno, S., Reynolds, D. W., Dahle, A., Amos, C., and Saxon, S.: Long-term mental and perceptual defects associated with silent intrauterine infections, in *Intrauterine Asphyxia and the Developing Fetal Brain*, edited by L. Gluck. Year Book Medical Publishers, Inc., Chicago, 1977, pp. 377–393.

48. Hanshaw, J. B., Scheiner, A. P., Moxley, A. W., Gaev, B. A., Abel, V., and Scheiner, B. A.: School failure and deafness after "silent" congenital cytomegalovirus infection. *N. Engl. J. Med.* 925:468–470, 1976.

49. Stagno, S., Reynolds, D. W., Amos, C. S., Dahle, A. J., McCollister, F. P., Mohendra, I., Ermocilla, R., and Alford, C. A.: Auditory and visual defects resulting from symptomatic and subclinical congenital cytomegaloviral and toxoplasma infections. *Pediatrics* 59:669–678, 1977.

50. Whitley, R. J., Brasfield, D., Reynolds, D. W., Stagno, S., Tiller, R. E., and Alford, C. A.: Protracted pneumonitis in young infants associated with perinatally acquired cytomegaloviral infection. *J. Pediatr.* 89:16–22, 1976.

51. Kattamis, C. A., Demetrios, D., and Matsaurotis, N. S.: Australia antigen and neonatal hepatitis syndrome. *Pediatrics* 54:157–164, 1974.

52. Hanshaw, J. B.: Herpesvirus hominis infections in the fetus and newborn. *Am. J. Dis. Child.* 126:546–555, 1973.

53. Miller, D. R., Hanshaw, J. B., O'Leary, D. A., and Hnilicka, J. V.: Fatal disseminated herpes simplex virus infection and hemorrhage in the neonate. *J. Pediatr.* 76:409, 1970.

54. Nahmias, A., Dowdle, W., Josey, W., Naib, Z., Painter, L., and Luce, D.: Newborn infection with *Herpesvirus hominis* types 1 and 2. *J. Pediat.* 75:1194, 1969.

55. Nahmias, A. J.: The TORCH complex. *Hosp. Pract.* 9:65–83, 1974.

56. Alford, C. A., Reynolds, D. W., and Stagno, S.: Current concepts of chronic perinatal infections, in *Modern Perinatal Medicine*, edited by L. Gluck. Year Book Medical Publishers, Inc., Chicago, 1974.

57. Townsend, J. J., Baringer, J. R., Wolinsky, J. S., Malamud, N., et al.: Progressive rubella panencephalitis: Late onset after congenital rubella. *N. Engl. J. Med.* 292:990–993, 1975.

58. Weil, M. L., Itabashi, H. H., Cremer, N. E., Oghiro, L. S., et al.: Chronic progressive panencephalitis due to rubella virus simulating subacute sclerosing panencephalitis. *N. Engl. J. Med.* 292:994–997, 1975.

59. Stagno, S., Reynolds, D. W., Tsiantos, A., Fuccillo, D. A., Long, W., and Alford, C. A.: Comparative serial virologic and serologic studies of symptomatic and sub-clinical congenitally and natally acquired cytomegalovirus infections. *J. Infect. Dis.* 132:568–577, 1975.

60. Cooper, L. Z.: Rubella: A preventable cause of birth defects, in *Intrauterine Infection*, edited by D. Bergsma. New York, The National Foundation, 1968.

61. Alford, C. A.: Immunoglobulin determinations in the diagnosis of fetal infection. *Pediatr. Clin. North Am.* 18:99, 1971.

62. Alford, C. A.: Fetal antibody in the diagnosis of chronic intrauterine infections, in *Prenatal infections*, edited by O. Thalhammer. Stuttgart, Georg Thieme Verlag Kg., 1971.

63. Stagno, S., Volanakis, J. E., Reynolds, D. W., Stroud, R., and Alford, C.A.: Immune complexes in congenital and natal cytomegalovirus infections of man. *J. Clin. Invest.* 60:838–845, 1977.

64. Robinson, W. S., and Lutwich, L. I.: The virus of hepatitis, type B (parts I & II). *N. Engl. J. Med.* 295:1168–1174, 1232–1236, 1976.

65. Krugman, S. and Ward, R.: *Infectious Diseases of Children and Adults*. The C. V. Mosby Co., St. Louis, 1973, pp. 76–95.

66. Davis, L. E., Tweed, G. V., Stewart, J. A., Bernstein, M. T., Miller, G. L., Gravelle, C. R., and Chin, T. D. U.: Cytomegalovirus mononucleosis in a first trimester pregnant female with transmission to the fetus. *Pediatrics* 48:200–206, 1971.

67. Spruance, S. L., Overall, J. C., Jr., Kern, E. R., Krueger, G. G., Pliam, V., and Miller, W.: Natural history of recurrent herpes simplex labialis: Implications for therapy. *N. Engl. J. Med.* 297:69–75, 1977.

68. Horstmann, D. M.: Serologic responses after primary infection and after reinfection with rubella virus, in *Rubella*, edited by H. Friedman and J. E. Prier. Charles C Thomas Publisher, Springfield, Ill., 1973. pp. 84–93.

69. Lennette, E. H., and Schmidt, N. J.: Neutralization, fluorescent antibody and complement fixation tests for rubella, in *Rubella*, edited by H. Friedman and J. E. Prier. Charles C Thomas Publisher, Springfield, Ill., 1973, pp. 18–32.

70. Krugman, S. (ed.): Proceedings of the International Conference on Rubella Immunization. *Am. J. Dis. Child.* 118, 1969.

71. Horstman, D. M., Liebhaber, H., LeBouvier, G. L., Rosenberg, D. A., and Halstead, S. B.: Rubella: Reinfection of vaccinated and naturally immune persons exposed in an epidemic. *N. Engl. J. Med.* 283:771, 1970.

72. Horstmann, D. M.: Rubella: The challenge of its control. *J. Inf. Dis.* 123:640, 1971.

73. Klock, L. E., and Rachelefsky, G. S.: Failure of rubella herd immunity during an epidemic. *N. Engl. J. Med.* 288:69, 1973.

74. Wilkins, J., Leedom, J. M., Portnoy, B., and Salvator, M. A.: Reinfection with rubella virus despite live vaccine-induced immunity. *Am. J. Dis. Child.* 118:275, 1969.

75. Chang, T. W., DesRosiers, S., and Weinstein, L.: Clinical and serologic studies of an outbreak of rubella in a vaccinated population. *N. Engl. J. Med.* 283:246, 1970.

76. Phillips, C. A., Maeck, J. V. S., Rogers, W. A., and Savel, H.: Intrauterine rubella infection following immunization with rubella vaccine. *J.A.M.A.* 213:624, 1970.

77. LeBouvier, G. L., and Plotkin, S. A.: Precipitin responses to rubella vaccine RA 27/3. *J. Inf. Dis.* 123:220, 1971.

78. Liebhaber, H., Ingalls, T. H., LeBouvier, G. L., and Hostmann, D. M.: Vaccination with RA 27/3 rubella vaccine. *Am. J. Dis. Child.* 123:133, 1972.

79. Vaheri, A., Vesikari, T., Oker-blom, N., Seppala, M., Veronelli, J., Robbins, F. C., and Parkman, P. D.: Transmission of attenuated rubella vaccines to the human fetus. *Am. J. Dis. Child.* 110:243, 1969.

80. Goldenberg, R. L., and Nelson, K.: Iatrogenic respiratory distress syndrome: An analysis of obstetric events proceeding delivery of infants who develop respiratory distress syndrome. *Am. J. Obstet. Gynecol.* 123:617–620, 1975.

81. Lang, D. J., and Hanshaw, J. B.: Cytomegalovirus infection and the postperfusion syndrome: Recognition of primary infections in four patients. *N. Engl. J. Med.* 280:1145–49, 1969.

82. Lang, D. J.: The epidemiology of cytomegalovirus infections: Interpretation of recent observations, in *Progress in Clinical and Biological Research,* Vol. 3., *Infections of the Fetus and the Newborn Infant,* edited by S. Krugman and A. A. Gershon. Alan R. Liss, Inc., New York, 1975, pp. 35–45.

83. Just, M., Bürgin-Wolff, A., Emodi, G., and Hernandez, R.: Immunization trials with live attenuated cytomegalovirus Towne 125. *Infection* 3:111–114, 1975.

84. Elek, S. D., and Stern, H.: Development of a vaccine against mental retardation caused by cytomegalovirus infection in utero. *Lancet* 1:1–5, 1974.

85. Plotkin, S. A., Furukawa, T., Zygraich, N., and Huygelen, C.: Candidate cytomegalovirus strain for human vaccination. *Infect. Immun.* 12:521–527, 1975.

86. Albrecht, T., and Rapp, F.: Malignant transformation of hamster embryo fibroblasts following exposure to ultraviolet-irradiated human cytomegalovirus. *Virology* 55:53–61, 1973.

87. St. Jeor, S. C., Albrecht, J. B., Funk, F. D., and Rapp, F.: Stimulation of cellular DNA synthesis by human cytomegalovirus. *J. Virol.* 13:353–362, 1974.

88. Alter, H. J., Barker, L. F., and Holland, P. V.: Hepatitis B immune globulin: Evaluation of clinical trials and rationale for usage. *N. Engl. J. Med.* 293:1093–1094, 1975.

89. Kohler, P. F., Dubois, R. S., Merrill, D. A., et al.: Prevention of chronic neonatal hepatitis B virus infection with antibody to hepatitis B surface antigen. *N. Engl. J. Med.* 291:1378–1380, 1974.

90. Okada, K., Kamiyama, I., Inomata, M., Imai, M., Miyakawa, Y., and Mayumi, Y.: e antigen and anti-e in the serum of asymptomatic carrier mothers as indicators of positive and negative transmission of hepatitis B virus to their infants. *N. Engl. J. Med.* 294:746–749, 1976.

91. Magnius, L. O., and Espmark, J. A.: New specificities in Australia antigen positive sera distinct from the Le Bouvier determinants. *J. Immunology* 107:1017–1021, 1972.

92. Linnemann, C. C., and Goldberg, S.: HB Ag in breast milk. *Lancet* 2:155, 1974.

93. Boxall, E. H., Flewett, T. H., Dane, D. S., et al.: Hepatitis B surface antigen in breast milk. *Lancet* 2:1007–1008, 1974.

94. Villarejos, V. M., Visma, K. A., Gutierrez, A., et al.: Role of saliva, urine, and feces in transmission of type B hepatitis. *N. Engl. J. Med.* 291:1375–1378, 1974.

15
Drugs in Pregnancy

Roy M. Pitkin, M.D.

A particularly prominent feature of medicine during the last quarter century has been the introduction and subsequent widespread usage of drugs of great potency and specificity. New pharmacologic agents have been developed, tested, and incorporated into clinical practice at an ever-increasing rate. Pregnant women share with the general population this increasing exposure to drugs.

Pregnancy represents a unique situation with respect to any environmental influence by virtue of the fact that exposure generally involves, for good or ill, two individuals. Although this concept seems self-evident, full realization of its significance has come only relatively recently, largely as a result of various therapeutic misadventures. Tragic as such occurrences as the thalidomide and diethylstilbestrol experiences have been, some secondary benefit has resulted from the heightened awareness of this fundamental truism among both physicians and patients, underscoring the need for basic research in gestational pharmacology.

Epidemiology of Drug Usage in Pregnancy

A number of surveys have indicated the considerable extent to which populations of pregnant women are exposed to drugs of various types. Selected data from three such studies (1–3) involving the United States, Scotland, and Canada are summarized in Table I. Different methods of data collection were used in these surveys, and this, rather than national differences, probably accounts for apparent variations in usage. The study by Bleyer and colleagues used a medication diary and thus was prospective, as opposed to the questionnaire and hospital record review approaches used in the other two. Therefore, it seems likely that pregnant women, at least in the United States, are exposed to an average of approximately nine drugs throughout gestation, including those given on specific prescription as well as agents of an "over the counter" type. Undoubtedly, many in the latter group are consumed without the physician's knowledge.

The fact that given numbers or types of drugs are taken during pregnancy is not necessarily alarming by itself, for in many instances the indications are sound, and, moreover, agents known to exert adverse effects on mother or fetus or both are relatively few. Nevertheless, such epidemiologic data must be regarded as calling for some concern about the role played by drugs as environmental influences during pregnancy.

Table I. Epidemiology of Drug Usage in Pregnancy (Percentage of Pregnant Women Taking Various Drugs)

	United States (1)	*Scotland (2)*	*Canada (3)*
Vitamins	86	40	
Analgesics	69	63	6
Antacids	60	34	6
Diuretics	30	18	32
Antibiotics	16	15	22
Barbiturates	12	28	12
Mean number of drugs per patient	8.7	3.2	3.3

Aims of Drug Therapy

It is axiomatic in therapeutics that the first step in decision-making regarding treatment involves clear definition and delineation of goals. The process then proceeds through consideration of hoped-for benefits weighed against the risk of potential side effects and complications. In pregnancy, involving as it does two individuals, the entire process becomes greatly complicated because a beneficial effect in one of the partners may or may not be reflected in benefit to the other. If not beneficial, the net result may be at best neutral or at worst actually adverse for the secondary recipient.

By far the most common clinical situation involves that in which the pregnant woman is treated for some condition or state involving herself. In other words, she represents the intended primary beneficiary and the fetus the secondary or passive recipient, the "innocent bystander," as it were. As a general rule it is in the fetus' best interests to have a healthy mother, and things that promote or restore maternal health usually benefit the fetus. For example, pyelonephritis represents a serious condition for the pregnant woman, which, because of its propensity to premature labor as well as hypoxic complications of sepsis, also poses distinct fetal risks. Antibiotic treatment of this primarily maternal disease would thus secondarily benefit the fetus. There are, however, exceptions to the general rule that what is good for the mother is good for the intrauterine patient. In the case of pyelonephritis, treatment with long-acting sulfonamides would probably be ill-advised because of the competitive inhibition of bilirubin binding by these drugs, which, if birth occurs while drugs are present in the fetus, could lead to neonatal jaundice and its complications (4).

Drugs administered during pregnancy, in addition to their potential for adverse fetal effects, may on occasion exert untoward influences on the gravida herself. In such instances, the outcome apparently reflects drug toxicity enhanced by the physiologic adjustments of pregnancy. A classic example is the tetracycline-related liver failure syndrome in which pregnant women appear particularly sensitive to hepatic toxicity of this antibiotic (5).

Although most of drug treatment in pregnancy is directed primarily at the pregnant woman, fetal therapeutics represents an area of recent investigation; the field is still relatively small but certain to grow rapidly in the near future. It had its beginnings in 1943 with the initial report of chemotherapy for fetal syphilis (6)—although strictly speaking, this actually represented combined maternal-fetal therapy—and has continued until the present consideration of glucocorticoid induction of pulmonary surfactant synthesis (7). In general, fetal therapy has been indirect, i.e., maternal administration, but the potential of direct administration by intraamniotic or even intrafetal injection is illustrated by a recent case in which thyroxine was given to a fetus whose mother had inadvertently received a thyroid-ablative dose of radioiodine (8).

PHARMACOLOGY OF GESTATION

Present understanding of gestational pharmacology is beset with many uncertainties and imponderables related to the complex interrelationship among mother, placenta, and fetus. Important determinants of drug effect, such as absorption, distribution, metabolism, and excretion, may be affected in any or all the three components of the gestational unit. Blood reaching the placenta via the uterine arteries contains substances modified qualitatively and quantitatively by maternal metabolism. The placenta transmits agents by various mechanisms and in various amounts and in the process may metabolize them further. Once in the fetus, compounds may exert a variety of influences based on processes characteristic of, and in some instances unique to, developing metabolic systems. These factors are summarized in Figure 1 and discussed below.

Maternal Factors

Pregnancy from the maternal point of view is characterized by a complex set of physiologic adjustments, many of which may potentially influence drug absorption, distribution, and excretion. *Gastrointestinal motility* is inhibited, apparently as an effect of

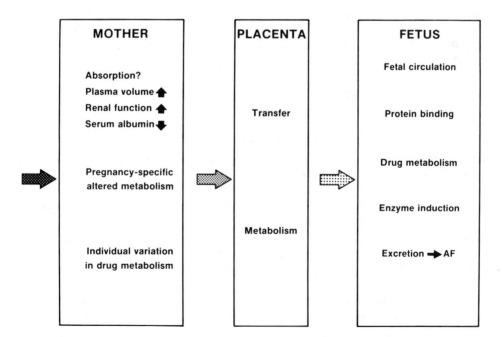

Figure 1. Model of drug distribution in pregnancy. See text description for details.

progesterone. This tends to slow the rate of absorption of orally administered substances, although the extent of gut absorption is if anything enhanced. *Total body water* and *plasma volume* both increase, which can have obvious effects on the volume of distribution of a drug. *Glomerular filtration* increases by as much as 50% during the early weeks of gestation, a phenomenon with readily apparent implications regarding excretion. Characteristic changes in *serum proteins,* especially the physiologic hypoalbuminemia of pregnancy, may influence blood levels of any drug normally bound to protein in vivo.

Although relatively little is known regarding *pregnancy-specific alterations* in maternal drug metabolism, the incomplete evidence available suggests that such influences, presumably resulting from endocrine factors, may be considerable. For example, studies of salicylamide metabolism in parturients indicate that glucuronidation may be inhibited (9). Investigations of the drug-metabolizing ability of the rat liver suggest that pregnancy decreases the capacity of oxidative and reductive pathways but increases that for sulfation reactions (10).

In addition to pregnancy-induced alterations, *individual variation* in drug metabolism may lead to accumulation of metabolites more toxic to the fetus than the parent molecule. For example, recent data indicate that meperidine metabolism follows one of three patterns characteristic for a specific individual and unaffected by pregnancy (11). No cases of newborn depression occurred in patients exhibiting the most common pattern, whereas four out of five depressed infants were born to women with the least common pattern, suggesting that the agent responsible was a metabolite rather than meperidine itself.

Placental Factors

The placenta's most obvious function is that of transferring substances between mother and fetus. The mechanisms involved in *placental transfer* include simple diffusion, facilitated diffusion, active transport, and specialized processes. In *simple diffusion* substances move passively from a region of higher to one of lower concentration in accordance with the Fick principle. Examples of agents crossing the placenta by simple diffusion include water, electrolytes, and respiratory gases. *Facilitated diffusion* refers to a variation in which diffusion occurs at a greater rate than that predicted by physico-chemical characteristics, apparently by use of a carrier system, as in the case of sugars. *Active transport* takes place against an electrochemical gradient and requires energy; amino acids and water-soluble vitamins cross the placenta by this means. *Pinocytosis* is an example of a special process in which large molecules such as proteins are transferred by a process of droplet engulfment.

Most drugs cross biologic membranes by simple diffusion, and this mechanism is the one most commonly involved in their placental transfer as well. As dictated by the Fick equation, the rate and extent of transfer vary directly with the effective concentration gradient and lipid solubility and inversely with molecular size, electrical charge, and thickness of the interposed membrane. However, the implication that placental permeability can be predicted accurately from knowledge of a drug's physicochemical characteristics is deceivingly simplistic. Many other factors are influential in that determination. The nature and extent of *protein binding* is a particularly important consideration, since in general only free or unbound molecules penetrate membranes rapidly whereas bound molecules cross much more slowly if at all. Binding may be specific or nonspecific with respect to a particular drug and may involve plasma or tissue proteins. The importance of protein binding can be illustrated by comparison of two synthetic penicillins, dicloxacillin and methicillin (12). Identical doses produce higher maternal blood levels in the case of dicloxacillin, but maternal-fetal equilibrium is never reached. By contrast, maternal methicillin levels are lower and equilibrate with fetal values by 1 hr after administration. The differences apparently reflect differential degrees of binding to maternal plasma proteins, since dicloxacillin is 95% bound to albumin, compared with 40% for methicillin. Local anesthetic agents represent another example. Bupivacaine is highly bound to plasma protein, and maternal administration results in substantially lower fetal than maternal blood levels of total compound than is the case with less bound compounds such as lidocaine and mepivacaine (13).

Much has been made in the past of an assumed impedimental function of the placenta, a concept embodied in the widely used term "placental barrier." In point of fact, the placenta does not represent much of a barrier at all, at least with respect to drugs. Although it is true that certain drugs, such as heparin and curare, do not cross the placenta in significant degrees and that the placental permeability of others, such as insulin and thyroxine, is quite limited, as a general rule it may be assumed that drugs given to a pregnant woman reach her fetus, usually in "therapeutic" concentrations.

The placenta, in addition to its role as an agent of transfer, represents an active organ in a metabolic sense, and *placental metabolism* is an important consideration in drug disposition during gestation. Studies indicating drug metabolism by the placenta have virtually all been in vitro investigations involving placental slices or homogenates or tissue culture of trophoblast, and their precise meaning in the in vivo situation is uncertain (14). Nevertheless, the capability for a variety of enzymatic reactions seems to exist in the placenta. Catalytic factors for both reduction and hydrolysis have been demonstrated. Conjugation capacity is generally low, with certain exceptions such as glycine conjugation of paraaminobenzoic acid. Oxidative metabolism of drugs seems to be negligible normally, but a response to inducing agents is suggested by observations that the rate of metabolism of benzpyrene is greater in placentas from smoking women.

Placental metabolism, even of limited capacity, has important ramifications with respect to drug effects on the fetus. Such a mechanism may result in metabolites with reduced potency, in which case the net effect might be desirable or undesirable, depending on whether the primary beneficiary of treatment is intended to be mother or fetus. On the other hand, some metabolites formed by the placenta may be more potent than the parent compound, which usually means more toxic and thus posing increased danger to the fetus. The importance of placental metabolism is illustrated by in vitro studies of natural and synthetic glucocorticoids in which cortisol and prednisone were found to be largely converted to inactive 11-keto metabolites, and dexamethasone and betamethasone were essentially unmetabolized (15). Assuming these data are applicable to the situation in vivo, the implication is that cortisol or prednisone would be preferable for maternal treatment, in such conditions as immunologic thrombocytopenic purpura or systemic lupus erythematosus, whereas dexamethasone or betamethasone might be best for specific therapy of the fetus, as for induction of pulmonary surfactant synthesis.

Fetal Factors

Drugs, after having been affected by maternal and placental factors, are carried in umbilical venous blood to the fetus, where they may be subjected to a number of modifying influences. The unique characteristics of the *fetal circulation* represent an important determinant of drug distribution and disposition. A large part of umbilical venous blood flow enters via the ductus venosus, bypassing the liver. Thus, blood levels in the inferior vena cava approximate those of the umbilical vein. Dilution occurs with blood from the superior vena cava and later mixing across the formen ovale and ductus arteriosus, so that aortic levels of a drug are initially half of umbilical values and increase until equilibration is reached.

Approximately 50% of the cardiac output is directed to the placenta, and a significant amount goes to the fetal brain. Blood flow to the lungs and other fetal organs is reduced correspondingly. Thus, equilibration of fetal plasma and tissue levels is reached fairly rapidly in the brain but very slowly in lung and liver. Moreover, the high rate of umbilical arterial flow means that large amounts of drug are returned relatively quickly to the placenta, causing an early decrease in the maternal-fetal concentration gradient, and since most drugs cross the placenta by simple diffusion, a slowing of the transfer rate.

Binding by plasma and tissue proteins of the fetus constitutes an important determinant of drug effect, since greater binding results in lower concentration of free drug but generally longer action, whereas less binding produces higher free levels but shorter duration. Differences between maternal and fetal proteins in binding affinities and capacities have been demonstrated with respect to several drugs, including salicylates, penicillins, and barbiturates, and there is every reason to suspect that this differential effect may apply to both serum and tissue protein binding of many pharmacologic agents. Furthermore, one drug may act as a competitive inhibitor of binding of either another drug or an endogenous substance by displacing the latter from a common binding site, leading to an increased concentration of free substance available for diffusion. For example, sulfonamides compete with bilirubin for binding sites on serum albumin, effectively raising the concentration of free bilirubin. Hyperbilirubinemia does not occur in utero because the free form released by this means diffuses across the placenta to the maternal circulation. With birth, however, the combination of reduced binding capacity due to sulfonamide inhibition, increased bilirubin production, and limited excretory ability may lead to high levels of freely diffusible bilirubin and attendant complications such as kernicterus (4).

Drug metabolism itself in the fetus differs both qualitatively and quantitatively from that in the adult. The fetal liver is generally deficient in smooth endoplasmic reticulum and thus has relatively little drug-metabolizing capacity. Oxidative enzyme and conjugation systems seem to be particularly deficient. Other fetal organs, however, may be capable of substantial metabolic activity, in some instances even greater than that of comparable tissues in the adult, as exemplified by steroid metabolism in the fetal adrenal.

The phenomenon of *enzyme induction,* in which enzyme systems normally deficient during fetal life may be stimulated to premature activity by certain drugs and chemicals, has been recognized for many years. A classic illustration is the induction of glucuronyl transferase activity in hepatic microsomes by pretreatment with phenobarbital, a relationship that has found some degree of successful clinical application in situations in which neonatal hyperbilirubinemia is anticipated. Induction of liver enzymes occurs with a wide variety of drugs, including hypnotics, tranquilizers, analgesics, antihistamines, and ethanol, and indeed Fouts has suggested that drugs that do not modify fetal metabolism are rapidly coming to be regarded as exceptional (16). Moreover, the process tends to be nonspecific in that it typically affects a number of microsomal enzyme systems. Thus, a beneficial effect such as improved bilirubin conjugating ability is likely to be accompanied by induction of other and potentially undesirable metabolic pathways for drugs or endogenous substances. Such pharmacologic manipulation of the normal sequence of developmental metabolism may conceivably exert adverse influences of a long-lasting nature. Thus, fetal enzyme induction by maternal drug administration must be approached with a careful consideration of potential benefits weighed against potential risks.

A final fetal characteristic influencing drug disposition relates to the unique aspects of *fetal excretory activity*. The placenta represents the major fetal organ of excretion, and fetal-maternal transfer seems in general to be governed by the same kinds of constraints as maternal-fetal transfer. However, some differences in rates of bidirectional passage of certain drugs have been described. For example, meperidine in the guinea pig (17) and methylmercury in the rhesus monkey (18) each appear to be transported more slowly from fetus to mother than vice versa. Other than via the placenta, the excretory capacity of the fetus is quite limited. Renal function, especially the tubular secretory mechanism, is relatively poorly developed even by term, and the capacity for biliary excretion is probably even less. Moreover, the amniotic sac represents the repository for fetal urinary excretion as well as transudation across the skin and umbilical cord, and the normal fetal swallowing of amniotic fluid thus effectively recycles excreted products. For whatever reason—differential placental permeability characteristics, impaired or inefficient fetal excretion, or preferential binding by fetal serum or tissues—clearance of drugs by the fetus is generally slower than that of the adult, and fetal tissue and blood levels often are found to persist longer than maternal.

SPECIFIC DRUGS

A listing of all drugs known or suspected of having adverse effects during pregnancy is neither feasible nor advisable. Limitations of space do not permit such a detailed compilation, and even if it were made, today's complete list would be incomplete by tomorrow. There would surely be some additions and perhaps some deletions as well.

The purpose of this section is to survey certain specific drug effects during pregnancy in order to illustrate the different types of adverse actions that may occur. Several excellent reviews of perinatal pharmacology have appeared in recent years (19–21), and the interested reader is referred to these for detailed consideration and documentation. In addition, teratogenicity of drugs is considered in detail in Chapter 16.

Analgesics

Strong analgesics, i.e., *narcotics* and narcoticlike agents, cross the placenta readily and affect the fetus following both acute and chronic administration. Acute administration, typically for pain relief in labor, may cause respiratory depression in the newborn; important determinants include dose, route of administration, timing in relation to delivery, and probably other factors such as maternal metabolic pattern. With modest doses and a healthy fetus, the clinical effect is usually not significant, but large doses or smaller amounts in premature or other types of complicated labor may result in profound neonatal depression.

Chronic narcotic usage results in a state of physiologic dependence in the fetus, just as in the adult. This condition of passive intrauterine addiction becomes manifest by quite typical withdrawal symptoms beginning 24 to 48 hr after birth. The narcotic withdrawal syndrome is particularly serious during the neonatal period, and infants born to known or suspected narcotic addicts require intensive therapy. An additional and particularly intriguing perinatal influence of chronic narcotic abuse is an apparent decreased risk of respiratory distress, presumably due to drug-induced pulmonary surfactant synthesis.

Salicylates represent the prototype of weak analgesics. The ubiquitous aspirin is undoubtedly the most widely consumed of drugs. At one level, the long history of extensive aspirin usage without clear evidence of harm testifies to its safety. However, concern about aspirin ingestion during pregnancy may be raised on several counts. Increased rates of congenital malformation, low birthweight, and perinatal mortality with aspirin usage have all been found in some studies but refuted by others. Laboratory findings indicating interference with blood coagulation—diminished collagen-induced platelet aggregation and factor XII activity—have been noted in newborns in relation to maternal aspirin ingestion during the week or so prior to delivery. Pregnancy appears to be prolonged slightly, with labor delayed an average of a week or two among aspirin users, presumably reflecting inhibition of prostaglandin synthetase. Indeed, indomethacin, a more potent prostaglandin inhibitor than aspirin, has been suggested as therapy for premature labor. Drugs that inhibit prostaglandins, however, should be used with great caution during pregnancy because of the ubiquitous nature of prostaglandins and their role in a variety of fetal homeostatic mechanisms, especially maintenance of patency of the ductus arteriosus. A recent report raises the possibility of an association between maternal indomethacin administration and primary pulmonary hypertension in the newborn.

From a clinical point of view there does not seem to be compelling evidence indicating that aspirin should be categorically proscribed during pregnancy. It seems reasonable, however, to advise heavy or frequent users to reduce their intake. Moreover, in the event of unexplained neonatal bleeding, the possibility of salicylate toxicity should be considered and appropriate diagnostic studies carried out.

Antimicrobials

Sulfonamides, as noted previously, compete with bilirubin for binding sites on serum albumin. Administration within a few days prior to delivery may therefore accentuate neonatal jaundice and could conceivably lead to kernicterus. In the normal-term infant, the margin of safety is probably sufficiently large; however, the infant with potentially impaired bilirubin metabolism because of prematurity or other causes may be a risk for complications of hyperbilirubinemia because of prenatal sulfa administration. Sulfonamides should be avoided during late pregnancy, especially in instances in which jaundice is possible.

Tetracycline has the potential for adverse effects on both mother and fetus. Its maternal toxicity involves the liver, and, though the mechanism is not entirely clear, the combination of high doses of tetracycline and pregnancy has led to fatty infiltration of the liver and even fatal hepatic failure in a number of reported cases. Altered renal function seems to be an important factor in toxicity, since in most instances the indication has been pyelonephritis. The fetal toxicity of tetracycline involves its deposition as a tetracycline-fluorescent complex in the enamel of developing teeth, producing a graying or brownish mottling. Although this dental effect represents only a cosmetic problem, animal experiments suggest that a similar action may occur in growing bone, interfering with osseous development. Thus, from both maternal and fetal standpoints, tetracycline should be regarded as relatively contraindicated in the pregnant woman.

Nitrofurantoins and certain other antimicrobial agents induce hemolysis in the presence of glucose-6-phosphate dehydrogenase (G6PD) deficiency, and hemolytic anemia has been described in fetuses with this metabolic defect exposed to such drugs in utero.

The *penicillin* group of drugs has been used widely in pregnancy and seems to be without specific complication. The amounts reaching the fetus vary from drug to drug, such as the difference in protein binding of methicillin and dicloxicillin discussed earlier, and these characteristics need to be taken into account when selecting therapy for a specific condition. In general, highly bound agents such as dicloxicillin reach the fetus poorly and are thus applicable to treatment of maternal infections, whereas drugs less well bound seem particularly appropriate when fetal sepsis is present. Ampicillin, probably the most popular of penicillins, is only approximately 20% protein bound and yields high levels promptly on the fetal side of the placenta.

Ampicillin and other broad spectrum antibiotics have been noted to produce a fall in maternal estriol levels, apparently as a result of interference with conjugation by gut bacteria affecting the enterohepatic circulation of the hormone. This effect seems to be without clinical consequence, though awareness of it is of obvious importance in interpreting laboratory data.

Chloramphenicol administered to premature newborns has been incriminated in the "gray syndrome," apparently due to deficient excretion by the immature kidney. Use during pregnancy, on the other hand, does not seem to cause this abnormality, because the efficiency of maternal excretory processes prevents accumulation of toxic levels.

Cardiovascular Drugs

Virtually without exception, *vasopressors* tend to diminish uterine blood flow and, depending on whether the primary mode of action involves alpha or beta adrenergic stimulation, may increase uterine contractility as well. Reduced uterine blood flow has certain obvious implications with respect to the fetus, and thus these drugs should generally be avoided in pregnancy. Most disease states causing hypotension in pregnant women involve hypovolemia, for which volume replacement is the obvious therapy.

Blood levels of *digitalis* are significantly lower in pregnant women than in nonpregnant individuals receiving the same dose. Thus, increased dosage during pregnancy may be necessary. The drug crosses the placenta readily, but the fetus exhibits unusual tolerance to digitalis toxicity and there are few if any untoward effects.

The use of *antihypertensive agents* during pregnancy should be approached with considerable caution. Pregnant women, because of their high sympathetic tone, are especially sensitive to alpha adrenergic and ganglionic blockade. Therefore, modest doses may result in marked blood pressure falls. Any significant degree of blood pressure lowering impairs uterine perfusion, with its attendant adverse effects on the fetus. If antihypertensive drugs are to be used during gestation, the specific drug should be selected with careful attention to its cardiovascular effects on the pregnant woman.

For example, hydralazine appears to be among the most useful of drugs, because, in addition to its antihypertensive action, it tends to increase uterine blood flow through positive inotropic, anisotropic and chronotropic effects on the maternal heart.

Propranolol, a beta adrenergic blocker, is being used increasingly for hypertension, cardiac disease, thyrotoxicosis, and dysfunctional labor. Most clinical reports of its use in pregnancy indicate a lack of adverse effects, though questions have been raised about interference with fetal growth. Of possible significance are recent observations that acute administration to sheep increases umbilical vascular resistance and decreases umbilical, but not uterine, blood flow.

Thiazide diuretics have been widely used in attempts at prevention and treatment of toxemia of pregnancy and for alleviation of symptomatic edema. Careful prospective studies have indicated, however, their ineffectiveness in toxemia prophylaxis; their therapeutic use is unwise in view of the contracted plasma volume accompanying this disease. Maternal complications of thiazides include electrolyte imbalance, hyperglycemia, hyperuricemia, and rare cases of acute hemorrhagic pancreatitis. The fetus may be hyponatremic and thrombocytopenic. Although these complications occur relatively infrequently, the fact that thiazides generally offer no therapeutic benefit indicates that they should be used with great caution in the pregnant woman.

Magnesium sulfate, though not strictly speaking a cardiovascular drug, has long been used in treatment of preeclampsia and eclampsia. Magnesium ion crosses the placenta readily, and neonatal elimination of a magnesium load is quite slow. Central nervous system depression and neuromuscular blockade can occur, but the extremely high dosage required is practically never reached if administration is monitored carefully. Some degree of hypocalcemia in mother and newborn occurs regularly with hypermagnesemia, but again untoward consequences are rare. Indeed, the long and widespread use of magnesium sulfate therapy indicates it to be a remarkably safe drug.

Anticonvulsants

Diphenylhydantoin and other anticonvulsant drugs have been the subject of much study because of several suspected adverse effects. Since anticonvulsant drugs tend to be taken in combinations, it is not possible to separate individual drug effects with any degree of certainty. Diphenylhydantoin acts as a metabolic antagonist of folate, and an increased incidence of megaloblastic anemia of pregnancy occurs in women taking this drug. For this reason many authorities advocate routine folate supplementation of such patients. The drug also appears to decrease the concentration of the vitamin K–dependent coagulation factors (factors II, VII, IX, and X) in blood of newborn infants. The question of possible teratogenicity of anticonvulsant drugs has received a great deal of attention. A number of studies have indicated an increased incidence of congenital malformations, particularly cleft lip and palate, saddle nose deformity, and digital hypoplasia. Some type of malformation has been estimated to occur in as many as 30% of women treated with anticonvulsant drugs. The much more common figure, however, is an increase of two- to threefold. Some studies have actually failed to find an increased incidence of congenital malformations.

Assuming that anticonvulsant drugs, particularly diphenylhydantoin, do exert a teratogenic effect, it must be a relatively weak action. Moreover, the mechanism by which it occurs is quite obscure. Although it might be a direct effect of the drug or one of its metabolites, it might also be due to genetic factors, hypoxia during convulsions, or a subclinical folate deficiency induced by the drug. The evidence does not at this time warrant discontinuance of therapy of women with bona fide convulsive disorders. On the other hand, a number of patients take these drugs on relatively vague indications, and such individuals are best advised to discontinue them.

Sex Hormones

Androgens administered chronically during mid- to late pregnancy produce clitoral hypertrophy and fusion of the labioscrotal groove of a female fetus. Though the major problem is cosmetic, the extent of masculinization may at times be severe enough to cause uncertainty in sex assignment at birth. Similar, though less frequent, effects have been reported with progestational therapy, particularly with synthetic *progestins* of the 19-nortestosterone type. For practical purposes there are no indications for androgen treatment of the pregnant woman. Although progestational compounds have been given quite freely in the past for early pregnancy wastage, careful studies fail to indicate any benefit, and their use is not advisable except in unusual instances in which progesterone deficiency can be documented. Under such conditions, natural progesterone is the agent of choice.

Recent reports have raised the question about a possible teratogenic effect of synthetic estrogen-progestin combinations of the *oral contraceptive* type. These agents, typically given shortly after conception to induce withdrawal bleeding as a test for pregnancy, have been associated with a variety of congenital malformations given the acronym VACTERL (V = vertebral, A = anal, C = cardiac, T = tracheal, E = esophageal, R = renal, L = limb reduction). Other studies, however, have failed to demonstrate teratogenicity; so the risk, if present at all, must be very small. Nevertheless, the use of these compounds as pregnancy tests is without merit in view of the wide availability of the more accurate tests for chorionic gonadotropin.

An association between nonsteroidal estrogens, especially *diethylstilbestrol,* administered during early pregnancy and later development of a characteristic variety of abnormalities of the cervix and vagina, has recently been recognized. Careful examination of young women exposed in utero reveals some type of recognizable effect in more than half. The most serious, but fortunately very rare, consequence is a highly malignant clear cell adenocarcinoma of the vagina and cervix. This type of oncogenic effect appearing years after drug exposure during a critical developmental period represents a previously unrecognized complication and has enormous implications. The situation is all the more tragic because the treatment turned out to be ineffective for the various forms of pregnancy complications for which it was used.

Adrenal Hormones

Glucocorticoids have been subjected to close scrutiny because of observations a number of years ago that cortisone treatment of pregnant mice is associated with an increased incidence of cleft palate. Careful analysis of reported data in humans generally indicates a lack of teratogenic action of any natural or synthetic corticosteroids. As discussed previously, certain agents, e.g., betamethasone and dexamethasone, are transferred largely intact. Corticosteroids administered during late pregnancy regularly suppress steroidogenesis in the fetal adrenal, as reflected in substantial falls in maternal estriol levels. This response seems to be without physiologic consequence but can cause confusion if estriol determinations are being used in clinical management. Prolonged adrenal suppression during intrauterine life could conceivably predispose to neonatal adrenal insufficiency, but this complication apparently occurs rarely if at all. A newborn whose mother received prolonged corticosteroids should be observed carefully during the first several days of life, and its later growth and development should be assessed. However, an extensive experience with glucocorticoid treatment during pregnancy, often in high doses and for prolonged periods, indicates that adverse effects on the fetus and newborn are amazingly infrequent. These agents represent the mainstay of treatment for a number of serious illnesses that may complicate pregnancy coincidently, and their use by gravidas should be limited to such situations. Pregnancy per se, however, does not contraindicate necessary treatment of this type.

The possibility of fetal therapy by glucocorticoid administration to women at risk for premature delivery for induction of pulmonary surfactant synthesis is a subject of great current interest and study, as discussed previously. Although preliminary results appear promising in terms of both efficacy and safety, this treatment represents an experimental approach at present, and its use requires rigid adherence to the principles of clinical investigation.

Thyroid and Related Drugs

Thyroxine has limited placental permeability, and its use during pregnancy does not appear to be associated with adverse effects on mother or fetus. *Thiourea drugs,* on the other hand, readily cross the placenta, where they act on the fetal thyroid, after the first trimester, by blocking iodination of tyrosine, just as in the adult thyroid. This can influence the independently functioning thyroid-pituitary axis of the second and third trimester fetus to release excessive amounts of thyroid-stimulating hormone (TSH), leading to development of congenital goiter. Such goiters, which occur in approximately 25% of women treated with propylthiouracil or methimazole, tend to be small and do not obstruct respiration. In most instances, thyroid enlargement regresses spontaneously after birth, and no specific treatment is needed. Some have advocated concomitant administration of thyroxine to "protect" the fetus, but the rationale of such an approach is difficult to reconcile with the known poor placental permeability of thyroid hormones. Others have used the occurrence of congenital goiter to argue for a primary surgical approach to treatment of hyperthyroidism in the pregnant woman. The matter of thyroidectomy versus drugs in hyperthyroidism is controversial, but the majority opinion at present seems to favor the medical approach initially, with surgery reserved for special circumstances such as nodular enlargement, failure of response to drugs, or unacceptable side effects. Relatively minor side effects, such as rash, nausea, and fever, occur in 5 to 10% of patients but usually regress within several weeks. Agranulocytosis, a much more serious complication, occurs in approximately 0.5% of cases, and leukopenia constitutes an absolute contraindication to continued therapy.

At least some cases of hyperthyroidism appear to involve the presence of a 7S immunoglobulin, long-acting thyroid stimulator (LATS), which can cross the placenta and cause a self-limited but potentially serious neonatal thryotoxicosis. Since the biologic half-life of LATS is apparently greater than that of thiourea drugs, the manifestations of neonatal thyrotoxicosis may be masked during the first few days of life by previous maternal therapy, only to become evident at a week or so of age, when the infant typically has been discharged as a normal newborn. Thus, an important caveat is that infants born to thyrotoxic women should be observed carefully for at least the first 2 weeks of life.

Propranolol, a beta adrenergic blocking agent, has recently been advocated for hyperthyroidism and seems particularly valuable in providing rapid control of the thyrotoxic state while awaiting the gradual evolution of thiourea effects. It has also been proposed as the sole agent in long-term management of hyperthyroid gravidas, but this type of usage is more questionable, because the drug affects only peripheral expression without altering the underlying hypermetabolic state.

Iodides ingested chronically and in large quantities during pregnancy have also been associated with congenital goiter, which, in contrast to that observed with thiourea drugs, is often large and obstructive of respiration and may be associated with hypothyroidism. Therefore, prolonged use of iodides, as in expectorant compounds, should be avoided during pregnancy.

Radioactive iodine is concentrated by the fetal thyroid after the twelfth week or so of intrauterine life. In large doses it ablates thyroid function, and even minute amounts may predispose to later development of thyroid carcinoma. Administration during the first trimester does not appear to be associated with any particular adverse effects. Nevertheless, radioiodine should be considered absolutely contraindicated at any time during pregnancy.

Hypoglycemic Agents

Insulin crosses the placenta to a very limited degree. Although concern about a possible teratogenic effect of exogenous insulin might be raised by the well-documented increase in congenital malformation rate among infants of diabetic mothers, there is little to support such a point of view. Moreover, the catastrophic results of failure to control the diabetic state during pregnancy have been demonstrated repeatedly.

Other hypoglycemia agents, especially those of the sulfonylurea group, apparently act by stimulating endogenous insulin production or release, and administration during late gestation increases the risk of neonatal hypoglycemia. *Tolbutamide,* one of the sulfonylureas, is regarded as potentially teratogenic, based on animal experiments and limited human experience. Moreover, diabetics in the childbearing age generally tend to be either insulin-requiring or controlled by diet alone. For all these reasons, oral hypoglycemic agents have no place in obstetric management.

Anticoagulants

Heparin, because of large molecular size and strong electronegative charge, does not cross the placenta, and its use during pregnancy is not apparently associated with any increase in fetal or neonatal complications above that anticipated on the basis of the maternal disease itself. *Coumadin* derivatives, on the other hand, cross the placenta readily and may exert adverse effects in both early and late pregnancy. A teratogenic influence, consisting typically of hypoplasia of the nasal bones and epiphysial stippling seen on long bone x-rays, has been described with coumadin drugs during the first trimester. Occasional instances of fetal or neonatal hemorrhage have been reported with late pregnancy usage, although the risk of this complication may probably be minimized by careful monitoring of the maternal prothrombin time.

Special problems are presented by the gravida needing long-term anticoagulation therapy, such as one with an artifical heart valve. Some authorities recommend changing to heparin during the first trimester, although it should be acknowledged that patients are rarely seen early enough to accomplish this, and again in the last few weeks prior to term. On the other hand, several reports have described quite satisfactory maternal perinatal outcomes in reasonably large series of patients treated with coumadin throughout gestation.

Patients anticoagulated by any means usually tolerate delivery quite well, since normal uterine hemostasis involves the coagulation mechanism to only a minor degree. Incisions of the abdomen and perineum, however, may bleed extensively. If maternal hemorrhage occurs for any reason and treatment becomes necessary, heparinized patients are advantaged because of the ready reversibility of their anticoagulated state by protamine.

Immunosuppressive and Anticancer Drugs

Immunosuppressive drugs are considered teratogenic, but, in view of the growing number of patients treated with them for renal transplants, the effect must be relatively weak or infrequent. Animal experiments indicate that some degree of immunologic disparity between mother and fetus seems in some way necessary for normal fetal growth, which may have a counterpart in the suggestion that immunosuppressed women give birth to small-for-gestational-age infants with greater than expected frequency. Long-term effects of immunosuppression on the developing immune system are generally unknown, but experience thus far has not indicated cause for alarm.

Alkylating agents are also regarded as potentially teratogenic, but again the effect is far from complete. A number of cases have been reported in which women were treated for malignancies throughout pregnancy and normal infants resulted.

Antimetabolites are highly teratogenic. Methotrexate, a metabolic antagonist of folacin, is the most teratogenic drug known in the human and given at an appropriate stage of gestation virtually always causes abortion or congenital malformation.

The indications for these types of drugs all represent serious maternal disease in which pregnancy itself is usually unwise or even frankly contraindicated. The importance of contraception and early pregnancy termination in such situations, although all too obvious, is frequently overlooked.

Psychopharmacologic Agents

Conventional *sedatives* and *hypnotics* such as barbiturates cross the placenta readily because of their relatively low molecular weight and great lipid solubility. The fetal capacity to metabolize them is very limited. Acute administration shortly before birth can result in neonatal respiratory depression, though usually this effect occurs only with large doses. Chronic use by drug addicts has resulted in a few reported cases of a withdrawal syndrome in the newborn. The capacity of these agents to induce hepatic microsomal enzymes has been mentioned previously.

Tranquilizers represent the largest class of drugs prescribed in contemporary American practice, and their use by pregnant women is undoubtedly extensive. The indications are many and varied and include nausea and vomiting of early pregnancy, anesthetic adjuncts during labor, and allaying anxiety at any time. In general, few overt effects of an adverse nature have been recognized. The administration of drugs such as *phenothiazines, meprobamate,* and *chlordiazepoxide* during early pregnancy has been

subjected to particularly close scrutiny, and no clear-cut evidence suggesting teratogenicity has been found. Use in late pregnancy may affect the newborn in some
apparently minor ways. For example, *reserpine* causes lethargy and nasal stuffiness,
and *diazepam* is associated with transient hypotonia and hypothermia. Although careful
study has failed to find an effect on birthweight or perinatal mortality, such effects cannot be dismissed lightly. The situation regarding diazepam, probably the most ubiquitous of these drugs, illustrates the problem. Placental permeability studies indicate that
diazepam and its metabolites tend to accumulate in the fetus, with fetal blood levels
regularly exceeding concomitant maternal values, apparently because of deficient fetal
excretory mechanisms. Highest levels have been found in the fetal heart, which may correlate with the observed diminution of beat-to-beat variability seen on heart rate monitoring. Although no specific adverse influences on fetal outcome have been noted, suggestions that Apgar scores may be lowered or hyperbilirubinemia, hypotonia, and
hypothermia increased must be given some weight, particularly considering the typically
elective or semielective indication for treatment.

Antidepressants are used less frequently than tranquilizers, but usage is still
considerable. A teratogenic effect of *tricyclic antidepressants* was suggested by observations of increased limb reduction defects, though subsequent studies have not been
confirmatory. *Lithium carbonate,* currently enjoying considerable popularity for manic-
depressive illness, may also be teratogenic in view of data from a registry of lithium-
treated pregnancies suggesting an overrepresentation of cardiovascular malformations.
The pregnant woman seems particularly sensitive to lithium toxicity because of her borderline sodium status, and care must be taken to prevent sodium deficiency.

Ethanol

Ethanol, undoubtedly the oldest and most widely used pharmacologic agent, has been
the subject of much recent attention. In addition to its long history of consumption,
ethanol administered intravenously has been advocated for suppression of premature
labor. It crosses the placenta readily and is evenly distributed throughout the water
phase of the fetus. Maternal and fetal blood levels are approximately equal following
maternal administration, but fetal clearance is slower than adult, apparently because of
lower liver levels of alcohol dehydrogenase and greater body water in the fetus. Acute
studies of placental transfer in experimental animals indicate some tendency toward
metabolic acidosis when moderately high blood levels are reached in the fetus. Hepatic
microsomal enzyme induction by ethanol has been mentioned previously.

The current interest in ethanol in pregnancy relates to what has come to be called the
"fetal alcohol syndrome," a complex of physical and developmental characteristics
including a peculiar facial appearance with short palpebral fissures, midfacial hypoplasia, and epicanthic folds (Fig. 2), pre- and postnatal growth retardation, and mental
deficiency. Initially described in children born to chronic alcoholics, it has been suggested recently that effects may occur with more moderate usage. Although ethanol itself
is generally regarded to be the specific cause, the complexity of social and environmental
factors involved precludes firm conclusions about etiology. Indeed, whether it actually
represents a syndrome cannot be stated with certainty. Nevertheless, on the basis of
present knowledge some degree of concern should be expressed, and patients should be
counseled to limit ethanol intake during pregnancy. Complete elimination of alcohol
intake by pregnant women does not seem indicated, nor is it likely to be accomplished.

Another potential adverse effect of ethanol in pregnancy is its influence on maternal

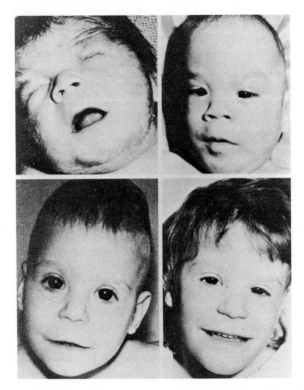

Figure 2. Top: Boy with fetal alcohol syndrome at birth (left) and age 6 months (right). Bottom: Girl with fetal alcohol syndrome at age 16 months (left) and 4 years (right). Note short palpebral fissures, low nasal bridge with short or upturned nose, epicanthic folds, midfacial hypoplasia, and long convex upper lip with narrow vermillion border. Reproduced with permission from Hanson, J. W., Jones, K. L., and Smith, D. W. *J.A.M.A.* 235:458, 1976.

nutritional status. Beer contains 150 kcal per 12-oz bottle and whiskey 125 kcal per 1½-oz serving; so even among moderate drinkers alcohol may represent a significant proportion of total energy intake. Under such circumstances, nutritional status may be modified by displacement of other nutrients from the diet.

GUIDELINES FOR DRUGS IN PREGNANCY

As is readily apparent from this review, a great deal is known regarding pharmacology during gestation, but much more is unknown. During this time, when new information is accumulating at an accelerating pace, an appropriate summation would seem to be the suggestion of guidelines for drug therapy in the pregnant woman:

1. Before giving any drug to a gravida, there should be clear indications and reasonable likelihood of anticipated benefit. An illustrative example is the experience with diethylstilbestrol. In this case the particular tragedy lies in the fact that use of the drug was promulgated without appropriate supporting evidence; moreover, it continued to be used long after therapeutic benefit was disproved.

2. In situations in which a specific drug is clearly indicated for treatment of a maternal life- or health-threatening condition, that agent shoud generally be used. For example, a patient with thyrotoxicosis in pregnancy in whom, by virtue of the nature of her disease, propylthiouracil is the treatment of choice should receive that drug, even though it entails a risk of congenital goiter and possibly even of hypothyroidism.

3. When adequate response is anticipated with either of two agents, the one with the least toxicity or suspicion of toxicity should be selected. For example, necessary anticoagulation during pregnancy is better accomplished with heparin, all other factors being equal, than with coumadin.

4. A general attitude of conservatism is called for with respect to "elective" drugs. The extent of use of psychopharmacologic agents largely reflects efforts to treat social situations pharmacologically. Such therapy is purely elective, as well as being of questionable efficacy, and until a great deal more is known about developmental pharmacology, the potential for subtle and long-term influences dictates a cautious approach. Life is not, after all, a chronic drug deficiency state.

REFERENCES

1. Bleyer, W. A., Au, W. Y., Lang, W. A., and Paiz, L. G.: Studies on the detection of adverse drug reactions in the newborn: I. Fetal exposure to maternal medication. *J.A.M.A.* 213:2046, 1970.

2. Forfar, J. O., and Nelson, M. N.: Epidemiology of drugs taken by pregnant women. *Clin. Pharmacol. Therap.* 14:632, 1973.

3. Shore, M. F.: Drugs can be dangerous during pregnancy and lactation. *Canad. Pharm. J.* 103:358, 1970.

4. Silverman, W. A., Anderson, D. H., Blanc, W. A., and Crozier, D. N.: A difference in mortality rate and incidence of kernicterus among premature infants allotted to two prophylactic antibacterial regimens. *Pediatrics* 18:164, 1956.

5. Whalley, P. J., Adams, R. H., and Combes, B.: Tetracycline toxicity in pregnancy. *J.A.M.A.* 189:357, 1964.

6. Speert, H.: Placental transmission of sulfathiazole and sulfadiazine and its significance for fetal chemotherapy. *Am. J. Obstet. Gynecol.* 45:200, 1943.

7. Liggins, G. C., and Howie, R. N.: A controlled trial of antepartum glucocorticoid therapy for prevention of the respiratory distress syndrome in premature infants. *Pediatrics* 50:515, 1972.

8. VanHerle, A. J., Young, R. T., Fisher, D. A., Uller, R. P., and Brinkman, C. R., III: Intrauterine treatment of a hypothyroid fetus. *J. Clin. Endocrinol. Metab.* 40:474, 1975.

9. Rauramo, L., Pukkinen, M., and Hartiala, K.: Glucuronide formation in parturients. *Ann. Med. Exp. Biol. Fenn.* 41:32, 1963.

10. Rodriguez, H., Catz, C. S., and Yaffe, S. J.: The effect of pregnancy on drug metabolism. *Pediatr. Res.* 6:376, 1972.

11. Morrison, J. C., Whybrew, W. D., Rosser, S. I., Bucovaz, E. T., Wiser, W. L., and Fish, S. A.: Metabolites of meperidine in the fetal and maternal serum. *Am. J. Obstet. Gynecol.* 126:997, 1976.

12. Depp, R., Kind, A. C., Kirby, W. M. M., and Johnson, W. L.: Transplacental passage of methicillin and dicloxacillin into the fetus and amniotic fluid. *Am. J. Obstet. Gynecol.* 107:1054, 1970.

13. Thomas, J., Long, G., Moore, G., and Morgan, D.: Plasma protein binding and placental transfer of bupivacaine. *Clin. Pharmacol. Ther.* 19:426, 1976.

14. Juchau, M. R., and Dyer, D. C.: Pharmacology of the placenta. *Pediat. Clin. N. Am.* 19:65, 1972.

15. Glanford, A. T., and Pearson-Murphy, B. E.: In vitro metabolism of prednisolone, dexamethasone, betamethasone, and cortisol by the human placenta. *Am. J. Obstet. Gynecol.* 127:264, 1977.

16. Fouts, J. R.: Hepatic microsomal drug metabolism in the perinatal period, in *Diagnosis and Treatment of Fetal Disorders,* edited by K. Adamsons. Springer-Verlag, New York, 1968, p. 291.

17. Rosen, M. G., and Bleyer, W. A.: Bidirectional transfer of meperidine across the guinea pig placenta. *Am. J. Obstet. Gynecol.* 101:918, 1968.

18. Reynolds, W. A., and Pitkin, R. M.: Transplacental passage of methylmercury and its uptake by primate fetal tissues. *Proc. Soc. Exp. Biol. Med.* 148:523, 1975.

19. Adamsons, K., and Joelsson, K.: The effects of pharmacologic agents upon the fetus and newborn. *Am. J. Obstet. Gynecol.* 96:437, 1966.

20. Mirkin, B. L.: Developmental pharmacology. *Ann. Rev. Pharmacol.* 10:255, 1970.

21. Yaffe, S. J., and Catz, C. S.: Pharmacology of the perinatal period. *Clin. Obstet. Gynecol.* 14:722, 1971.

16
Teratology

Thomas H. Shepard, M.D.
Ronald J. Lemire, M.D.

Teratology is the science dealing with the causes, mechanisms, and manifestations of developmental deviations of either structural or functional nature (Wilson, 1973); it uses both human and subhuman models to achieve these goals. Approximately 3% of all human newborns have a congenital anomaly requiring medical attention, and approximately one-third of these conditions can be regarded as life-threatening. Close to one-half of the children in hospital wards are there because of prenatally acquired malformations of one kind or another.

Our knowledge of the cause and prevention of these malformations is extremely limited in that approximately 80% are due to unknown causes. About 10% are associated with gene mutations, 5% with chromosomal aberrations, and less than 3% are known to be due to a teratogenic agent. Although there are more than 600 agents known to produce congenital anomalies in experimental animals, less than 25 of these are known to cause defects in the human.

A teratogenic agent may be defined as one that produces, during embryonic or fetal development, a major or minor deviation from normal morphology or function. Chemicals, drugs, physical agents, and viruses as well as certain deficiency states are agents included in this definition.

INFORMATION ON TERATOGENICITY

Information concerning teratogenesis, although widely dispersed throughout most of the biomedical literature, is reviewed in several books. An excellent general discussion of teratology is available in a text written by James Wilson (1973). An annotated catalog by Shepard (1976) of more than 800 agents that are teratogenic in animals and man may prove useful for reference and entry into the literature regarding specific chemical compounds, viruses, and physical agents. Josef Warkany's extensive treatise, *Congenital Malformations* (1971), combines information on teratogenesis in animals with similar anomalies in humans. Several books are available that identify specific malformation syndromes in humans. Included among these are David Smith's book on dysmorphic syndromes (1976) and *Syndromes of the Head and Neck* by Gorlin et al. (1976). McKusick's *Mendelian Inheritance in Man* (1975) includes more than 300 congenital syndromes produced by gene mutations.

PRINCIPLES OF TERATOLOGY

The period of development when exposure to a teratogen occurs controls to a great extent the conceptus' sensitivity to teratogenesis. Damage during the first 14 days (preimplantation and presomite periods) generally produces death of the ovum; if damage occurs during organogenesis (up to 60 gestational days), the embryo is highly sensitive and may undergo major morphological changes. In the fetal period there is less sensitivity to morphologic alterations, but changes in functional capacity such as intellect, reproduction, or aging may occur. In addition, during the latter part of the fetal period, the conceptus becomes sensitive to transplacental carcinogens.

Another principle of teratology is that some species are much more susceptible to teratogenic influences than others. Cortisone, aspirin, and several vitamin deficiencies are highly teratogenic in the rodent, but no evidence has been produced of their teratogenicity in humans. The thalidomide epidemic would not have been prevented by tests in pregnant mice and rats, even though the drug is teratogenic in rabbits, monkeys, and humans. An understanding of pharmacologic, physiologic, and genetic variations that lead to teratogenesis is critically needed if we are to be able to protect the human embryo and fetus from environmental and drug damage.

Most chemicals and drugs when administered in very high doses to pregnant animals produce some fetal toxicity that may be evidenced by fetal growth retardation and immaturity of the skeleton. This does not mean that they are teratogenic or that therapeutic doses in humans produce damage.

MECHANISMS OF TERATOLOGY

The pathogenesis of congenital defects during embryonic and fetal life is possibly as diverse as the causes of pathology in postnatal life. There are many theoretical possibilities, as shown in Figure 1, although little is known because the embryo and fetus are almost inaccessible for direct observation of physiologic and biochemical events. Another problem is that human embryos and fetuses are frequently retained in utero for 4 to 6 weeks following their death; the result is severe autolysis that prevents gross and microscopic studies of the abortus. A second major problem in learning about the pathogenesis of congenital defects is that our knowledge about the genetic control of development is still too small. Even the specific mechanisms of maldevelopment associated with the lack or excess of whole chromosomes are not understood.

It is known that the reaction to injury of embryos is entirely different from the newborn or postnatal individual. A polymorphonuclear response and scar tissue are not found. Instead, following cell necrosis, there is a major macrophage system that cleans up the debris, leaving little trace of the damage that an agent might produce. Although this mechanism has not been thoroughly studied, one model found that embryonic cell death localized to the organs, which were later defective, was produced by a lowering of energy-producing enzyme systems secondary to the agent administered to the rat. In this system the maternal rat is made riboflavin-deficient and given a riboflavin precursor, galactoflavin. Following a major cleanup by macrophages a severe reduction in mesenchyme cells produced absence of digits and very small mandibular sizes.

During embryonic stages there is no hemostatic system; some believe that hemorrhages during this period lead to localized defects. In addition the immune system in the embryo is nonfunctional and viruses that obtain entry grow in an unimpeded manner.

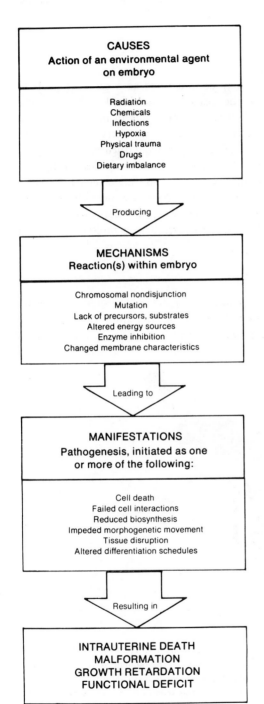

Figure 1. Diagram showing the relationship among cause, mechanism, and manifestation of a teratogenic reaction. Adapted from Wilson, 1973.

405

Other mechanisms of teratogenesis are undergrowth or overgrowth of the embryonic tissue or lack of differentiation.

DETECTION OF TERATOGENS

The existing defenses against teratogenesis may be illustrated as a series of walls or hurdles (Fig. 2). Approximately 2000 new chemicals are introduced each year, thus adding potentially new teratogenic agents. Testing of compounds in pregnant animals represents one defense, which was erected after the devastating effects of thalidomide. The use of chemical structure as a predictor of teratogenicity is theoretically of great promise but to date has limited application. A number of new tests based on in vitro methods are available, but their utility is limited. Our secondary major defenses, which are necessary because of weaknesses in existing screening tests, are those characterized by monitoring: amniocentesis, fetal and newborn monitoring, and surveillance. These various defenses have been described and discussed in detail in a multiauthored text (Shepard et al., 1975).

Testing of Pregnant Animals

The epidemic of limb reduction deformity produced by thalidomide resulted in regulations requiring the testing of new compounds in pregnant laboratory animals. These tests concentrate on the three periods of development: (1) gametogenesis through

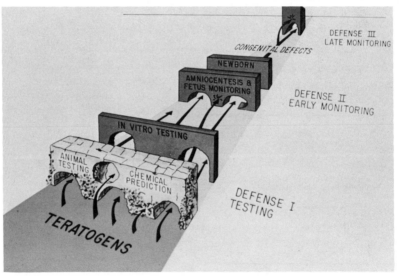

Figure 2. Perspective of our major defenses against teratogenic agents. The first defense is standard testing carried out in pregnant animals. A limited knowledge of the biologic activity of chemical structure contributes. The second wall, which should be in close association with the first, consists of in vitro testing by tissue and organ cultures as well as studies of ova and whole embryo explants. Defense II, or early monitoring of fetus and newborn, is necessary because the first defenses still are inadequate. Late monitoring is illustrated best by the appearance of vaginal carcinomas in young women exposed in utero to diethylstilbestrol. The last defense is manned by the alert medical practitioner. Reproduced through the courtesy of Yearbook Medical Publishers, from Shepard, 1974.

implantation, (2) organogenesis, and (3) late fetal and early postnatal development. Testing that spans two generations and includes all periods is useful as a general screening device.

Pharmacologic principles are important considerations in the choice of test species, as it is advantageous to use an animal model that metabolizes the drug in a fashion similar to man. Variations in absorption rate and transplacental transfer make the choice of species difficult, and dose relationships must be established for the teratogenic zone in each. Usually mice, rats, or rabbits are used to determine the embryotoxic dose and the effects, if any, of the compound at two or three dosage levels that are multiples of the expected human dose. Because of the expense, the long gestation, and the small litter size, tests in subhuman primates usually are reserved for agents either needed during human pregnancy or likely to be taken inadvertently during that time or for testing suspected drugs or chemicals about which a question of safety arises.

In Vitro Tests for Teratogenicity

This second wall of defense against teratogenic agents shows promise but at present has not been fully developed. Tissue and organ culture tests for the study of potential mutagens in in vitro systems are available to deal with a large array of molecular and cellular systems. The techniques of the developmental biologists are especially useful for giving information on the mechanisms of teratogenic action, but to date the in vitro methods have not been used to any degree in testing new drugs.

Whole embryo culturing of rodents has been introduced in the past several years. As these systems allow for direct observation of the embryo, certain previously unavailable physiologic studies may be made. The incorporation of radioactive nutrients or drugs may be measured, and also the effect of certain drugs on embryonic heart rate can be recorded.

In recent years, the exacting nutritional requirements of early ova have been discovered, and this allows for detailed growth and metabolic studies on mammalian eggs. Studies of the effect of drug penetration and teratogenic potential of agents now should be more feasible. In vitro testing is one manner in which early conceptual losses can be evaluated with respect to teratogenic factors. The magnitude and biomedical importance of early conceptual loss in the human has been recognized since the work of Hertig and Rock began in the 1930s. These workers, with the help of volunteer women who were scheduled for hysterectomy, were able to collect many early human specimens, and from these and other observations an estimate of about 60% conceptual loss can be made. Recent studies with material derived from spontaneous abortion have shown that as much as 60% of early human loss is associated with abnormal chromosomal constitution in the embryo. This high-risk group of embryos should be a further source for our understanding of the effect of age and other factors on chromosomal nondisjunction during pre- and postfertilization periods. It is also evident that any condition that might reduce this early loss from the uterus could be expressed as an increase in the number of children born with chromosomal or other defects. For instance, do we know that the routine administration of vitamins to pregnant women does not increase the incidence of defects in their offspring?

Amniocentesis represents the third wall in Figure 2. From 13 to 14 menstrual weeks onward it is possible to obtain 5 to 10 ml of amniotic fluid for analysis in pregnancies where there is a known risk of having an offspring with a serious disorder that can be detected in early development. Chromosome studies of cultured amnion cells can be done to diagnose a fetal chromosome abnormality, and enzyme studies can be done to exclude a homozygous fetus where parents are carriers for some autosomal recessive disorders, e.g., Tay-Sachs disease. Numerous other inherited metabolic defects can be diagnosed by study of cells from amniotic fluid. The sex can also be determined in the fetus of a female carrier for an X-linked recessive disorder such as hemophilia, in which case the male fetus would have a 50% risk of being affected.

Another example of how analysis of amniotic fluid can help detect an anomalous fetus is in pregnancies with open neural tube defects. When anencephaly or meningomyelocele has occurred in a preceding pregnancy, the risk of recurrence of either defect is approximately 5%; this is detected by finding elevated alpha-fetoprotein in the amniotic fluid. If the alpha-fetoprotein is not elevated, anencephaly can be reliably excluded, but only about 90% of the pregnancies with meningomyelocele give positive results. Elective termination of undesired pregnancies is available to parents in such cases. The upper time limit for therapeutic abortion is 18 menstrual weeks, which necessitates that tests on amniotic fluid be performed with expedience and by specialized laboratories.

Monitoring During the Fetal and Newborn Periods

Newborns with congenital defects represent only a small percentage of the total problem of malformations when one takes into account embryonic and fetal loss. One would expect that prenatal losses might be a more dramatic and sensitive index of response to teratogenic agents. Study of abortions during the first trimester should permit an earlier warning system of epidemiologic information up to 6 months before a teratogenic effect could be detected in newborns. Another advantage to the study of spontaneous abortuses is that there is a shorter period from the time of teratogenic exposure to the time of inquiry of the mother. This period may be less than 1 week as compared with the 7- to 8-month time interval involved when a history is obtained from the mother of a newborn.

Continuous recording by time and place and registry of congenital defects observed in the newborn should provide an important warning of teratogenic action by a new chemical or drug. A recent example of the use of newborn monitoring systems occurred following a report from Australia that a tricyclic antidepressant (Imipramine) might cause limb reduction defects. Monitoring groups in Atlanta and Canada, using their existing records, were able to make a rapid, detailed survey of all women who had given birth to children with limb defects. Their negative results in hundreds of women offered strong evidence that if this drug was a human teratogen, at least it was not a highly potent one.

Our current methods of monitoring identify easily recognizable defects but may miss the more subtle anomalies, e.g., changes in intellect secondary to long-term alterations in physiology. More knowledge is needed regarding the possible prenatal drug effects on blood pressure, learning ability, and reproductive function. This form of late monitoring has not been carried out systematically. Most of the significant observations have been reported by alert clinical practitioners. The example of the occurrence of vaginal cancer in adults who were exposed to diethylstilbestrol during the first trimester of fetal life is well known. In this situation, the malignancy probably was initiated by embryonic rests that were retained in the genital tract as a result of the medication.

Prediction of Congenital Defects by Phenotype or Genotype

Some teratologists presume that certain congenital defects are the result of the action of several controlling genes acting in concert with environmental agents. For example, the A/Jax mouse exhibits a higher natural incidence of cleft lip and palate than certain other strains, and this is related to retardation of the process of palatal shelf movement. Other controlling genes for the development of the palate are known to predispose to clefts. Examples such as shortening of the head, changes in mandibular length, or mechanisms that by tongue obstruction might prevent normal closure of the palatal shelf have been studied in inbred animal models. Most of the environmental agents—(aspirin, cortisone)—known to produce clefts are more teratogenic in these inbred strains. This example of multifactorial etiology of teratogenesis is well described by Fraser (1969).

The incidence of cleft lip and palate appears to be about doubled in the offspring of mothers being treated for chronic seizure disorders with diphenylhydantoin. Is this an effect of the drug, or is it possible that these women have a genotype that predisposes to both seizure disorders and clefts? Shapiro et al. (1976) have found an increased incidence of malformation in children fathered by men with chronic seizures. Another example of the importance of finding the teratologically susceptible genotype may be identified by workers in the field of pharmacogenetics. Certainly there must exist small numbers of women who because of molecular changes in their detoxifying enzymes are more vulnerable to the teratogenic action of certain drugs. Mothers with elevated serum levels of phenylalanine secondary to genetically changed amino acid metabolism (phenylketonuria) produce defective brain development in their genetically normal offspring.

Table I. Time Specificity of Action for Human Teratogens

Teratogen	Gestational Age From Fertilization (Days)	Malformation
Rubella virus	0–60	Cataract or heart disease more likely
	0–120+	Deafness
Thalidomide (removed from the market)	21–40	Reduction defects of extremities
Male hormones (Androgens, tumors, progestins)	Before 90	Clitoral hypertrophy and labial fusion
	After 90	Only clitoral hypertrophy
Coumadin anticoagulants	Before 100	Hypoplasia of nose and stippling of epiphyses
Radioiodine therapy	After 65–70	Fetal thyroidectomy
Goitrogens and iodides	After 180	Fetal goiter
Tetracycline	After 120	Dental enamel staining primary teeth
	After 250	Staining of crowns of permanent teeth

Table II. Teratogenicity of Drugs*

Drug	Exposed Infants Studied		Type of Defect	General Comments
	Total	Deformed		
Cancer Chemotherapeutic Agents (Nicholson, 1968; Shepard, 1974):				
Aminopterin and methylaminopterin	41	8	Cranial ossification defect (5), small mandible (5), palate defect (1), hydrocephalus (1)	All potentially teratogenic; first trimester treatment more commonly associated with defects; defects during second and third trimester unknown; often given in combinations and to acutely ill mother; one infant developed leukemia at 9 months of age
Busulfan	30	10	Spontaneous abortion and prematurity (10), cleft palate (1), eye defect (1)	
Chlorambucil	5	1	Absence of ureter and kidney (1)	
Colchicine	16	0		
Cyclophosphamide	4	2	Absence of digits	
Mercaptopurine	26	1	Cleft palate (1), eye defect (1)	
Nitrogen mustard	8	0		
Procarbazine	3	1	Small pelvic kidneys	
Trimethylene melamine	3	0		
Urethan	8	0		
Vinblastine	4	0		
Sedatives:				
Thalidomide	?	10,000	Phocomelia	Rat and mouse fetuses not sensitive; human, monkey, and rabbit sensitive; single dose capable of producing defects in humans
Chlordiazepoxide and meprobamate	2500	See comments	No pattern	One large study found fourfold increase in defects from pregnancies where treatment carried out in first 42 days; another large study could not confirm this

410

Agent	Number	Rate	Defect	Comments
Diazepam	137	See comments	Cleft lip and palate	Two studies found fourfold increase in expected incidence of facial clefts among mothers ingesting this drug during first trimester (Safra and Oakley, 1976)
Androgens: Testosterone, including its ethinyl derivatives	Unknown ? many	50	Masculinization of female genitalia	10–20 mg daily of ethinyl testosterone produces masculinization in about 15% of female fetuses; neither progesterone nor 17-hydroxyprogesterone have produced masculinization
Diethylstilbestrol	Over 500	7–73%	Precancerous adenosis of vagina	Precancerous changes found in 30–73% of offspring exposed before ninth week of gestation but only in 7% exposed after seventeenth week; cancer rate in exposed subjects less than 0.01%, at least by age 22 years
Corticosteroids	688	5	Cleft palate (5)	Little or no teratogenic effect in man
Coumarin anticoagulants	Unknown	9	Small nose, stippled secondary epiphyses, occasional mental retardation, optic atrophy	No case reports have appeared yet in women treated after first trimester
Diphenylhydantoin and trimethadione	Many	? increased	Hypoplasia of terminal digits, nails, cleft palate	A number of large prospective studies have shown no increase in defects; other studies have found small increase in all types of defects; terminal digital hypoplasia may occur in up to 30% of exposed offspring
Radioiodine	Few	5	Athyrotic cretinism	Therapeutic amounts only; diagnostic doses have not caused cretinism; can cause airway obstruction at birth if administered during third trimester; some reports have suggested, but other studies do not confirm, human teratogenicity
Iodides and thioamides	Moderate number	Common	Goiter in newborn	
Oral contraceptives, trace anesthetics, aspirin, lithium, quinine	Many	No increase in pattern		For a balanced discussion on oral contraceptives see Anonymous, 1974

* A more complete referencing of the data is available in Shepard, 1976.

TERATOGENIC AGENTS IN HUMANS

Teratogenic Drugs

With few exceptions drugs have not been a major teratogenic problem in humans. Yet it is a worrisome fact that almost yearly new drugs are moved onto the list of teratogenic agents. Therefore, it may be that in years to come drugs will collectively represent one of the major groups of agents that cause congenital defects in the human population. Table II reviews the present drugs on the list of known teratogens. The cancer chemotherapeutic agents would all seem to be capable of teratogenic action; yet with the exception of aminopterin and busulfan there has been little problem. Because of their mechanism of action as alkylating agents or folic acid antagonists they must be regarded as potentially teratogenic in any woman who is on chemotherapy. Delayed effects of these drugs are also of concern, and therefore for the most part therapeutic abortion should be considered, or at least offered, when one is faced with pregnancy in a woman on chemotherapy.

Among the sedatives, thalidomide, which has now been withdrawn from the market, was the all-time major offender. Numerous malformations were caused by this agent, but the reduction malformations in the extremities were the most dramatic. The thalidomide epidemic permitted for the first time a direct correlation between times of exposures and an arrest in developmental processes. Table I sets forth the relationship between time of exposure and the specific malformation produced. Ear, arm, and leg malformations appeared in that order, depending on when the exposures occurred between the twenty-first and fortieth gestational day. The human model was later duplicated in monkeys, but rat and mice fetuses were not affected by this drug. Numerous analogues of thalidomide also failed to produce comparable defects, and, although the drug was extensively studied, there is still some uncertainty about its real mechanism of action. Other sedatives listed in Table II are presently regarded as having teratogenic potential but are still under investigation.

Androgens and synthetic progestins were definitely found to masculinize female genitalia. The latter drugs were used during the late fifties to prevent threatened abortions. Except for the changes in external genitalia the newborns were entirely normal. An alarming discovery was recently made with respect to diethylstilbestrol: malignant changes were found in the offspring of mothers treated with these drugs during pregnancy. Experience with this drug alone is reason to believe that the teratogenic screening process must continue for a lifetime and that problems arising from intrauterine environmental agents can express themselves at a period long after birth.

Diphenylhydantoin and trimethadione are now regarded as being teratogenic agents but having low teratogenic potential (Hanson and Smith, 1975). Perhaps up to 30% of the offspring of women on these drugs might have minor malformations of their digits and a very small percentage cleft palate.

Infections

Intrauterine viral infections have been a major cause of congenital malformations in humans (see Table III). The virus can reach the fetus by way of the amniotic cavity following a vaginal infection or transplacentally through the bloodstream in the case of maternal viremia. The latter route is suspected to be the more common of the two. In many cases the maternal infection is subclinical, and it is only through postnatal diagnostic procedures that viral infection is confirmed.

Table III. Teratogenic Effects of Maternal Infections

Agent	Gestational Age (Weeks)	Adverse Effects	Diagnostic Tests
Rubella	0–12	Congenital heart disease Microcephaly Microphthalmos Cataracts Deafness Intrauterine growth retardation Thrombocytopenia Chorioretinitis Mental retardation Hepatosplenomegaly	Viral cultures Serology
	12–24	Communication deficits Motor and mental retardation	
Cytomegalovirus	4–28	Microcephaly Chorioretinitis Hepatosplenomegaly Mental retardation Intracranial calcification	Viral cultures Serology
Herpesvirus (Type 2) (Florman et al, 1973)	4–12	Microcephaly Microphthalmia Intracranial calcification	Viral cultures Serology
Toxoplasmosis (Hanshaw, 1970)	8–28	Microcephaly Chorioretinitis Mental retardation Hydrocephaly Hepatosplenomegaly	Sabin-Feldman dye test Serology

Rubella virus was first suspected of being a teratogenic agent in 1941, when an Australian ophthamologist discovered an increased number of cataracts in the offspring of an exposed population. A "rubella syndrome" emerged, consisting of congenital heart disease, microcephaly, microphthalmia, chorioretinitis, cataracts, deafness, and mental retardation. This was later expanded to include intrauterine growth retardation, thrombocytopenia, and hepatosplenomegaly. Later it was appreciated that fetuses acquiring the viremia during the second trimester also have problems in postnatal life. These may consist of communication deficits and motor retardation.

Rubella virus seems to invade sensitive organs directly, where, after multiplication, it produces a cytopathologic effect. This is followed by necrosis and inflammatory response. The central nervous system is one of the primary targets for this virus and one that certainly produces the most drastic sequelae. Degeneration of blood vessels occurs that is associated with the ischemic necrosis of tissue. Vessel walls are found to degenerate, and the layers are replaced by an amorphous granular material. Fibrin and calcium deposits are occasionally present in the subintimal and pericapillary spaces.

The hallmark of damage to the central nervous system is microcephaly, which is present in 70% of cases. This is associated with a decreased number of cells and a retardation of the myelinization process. Subependymal cysts have been described in rubella syndrome as well as in cytomegalovirus infections, which is discussed below.

Cytomegalovirus causes a clinical picture very similar to rubella (Hanshaw, 1970). These children have microcephaly, chorioretinitis, hepatosplenomegaly, mental retardation, intracranial calcification, and frequently seizures. Cytomegalovirus (CMV) is an extremely common infection, with up to 5% of pregnant women having the virus. Several strains exist, and they are closely related to the herpes virus family. Women acquiring the infection during pregnancy frequently have a subclinical infection; the fetus seems most prone to adverse effects during the second and third trimesters. Transplacental transmission of the virus occurs. When CMV gains access to the fetal cells it forms intranuclear cytoplasmic inclusion bodies. Cytomegaly then ensues, and these cells seem to die by a rupture of the cell membrane. Cell counts in the organs concerned reveal an absolute decrease in numbers. After birth periventricular calcifications occur, and microcephaly is common. Deafness, ocular abnormalities, chorioretinitis, microphthalmia, and many other changes in the central nervous system are present in affected patients.

Other viral infections are increasingly of concern, and herpes virus is now considered to be teratogenic. Again there is a predilection for involvement of the nervous system, and findings are similar to those described above for CMV. Toxoplasmosis, a protozoan infection, is also a well-accepted cause of congenital malformations. Microcephaly, chorioretinitis, mental retardation, hydrocephalus, and hepatosplenomegaly are frequently present. With time intracranial calcifications and seizures are found in these patients.

Table IV. Teratogenic Effects of Irradiation in Humans

Source	Dose (Rads)	Gestational Age (Weeks)	Adverse Effects
Atomic Bombs			
Hiroshima	10–19	3–17	Microcephaly Intrauterine growth retardation
	150	3–17	Microcephaly Mental retardation Intrauterine growth retardation
Nagasaki	150	3–17	Microcephaly Mental retardation Intrauterine growth retardation
Therapeutic Pelvic Irradiation	400	2½–4	CNS malformations
	30–250	4–8	Microcephaly Ocular defects Intrauterine growth retardation
	360	4–14	Spontaneous abortion

Table V. Teratogenic Effects of Environmental Agents

Chemical	Adverse Effects	Source
Organic mercury (Murakami, 1972)	Cerebral atrophy Spasticity Mental retardation	Maternal ingestion of contaminated fish, shellfish Fungicide
Alcoholism, chronic (Jones and Smith, 1975)	Microcephaly Mental retardation Congenital heart disease Intrauterine growth retardation	Maternal ingestion
Cigarette smoking	Low birth weight Possible delay in reading (Davie et al, 1972)	Maternal smoking
Organic solvents	Sacral agenesis (?) (Kucera, 1968)	Skin and vapor contact in factories
Polychlorobiphenyls	Intrauterine growth retardation Cola-colored skin Exophthalmos	Maternal ingestion of contaminated cooking oil

Radiation

The teratogenic effects of radiation are well accepted (Brent and Gorson, 1972) (see Table IV). Again the central nervous system is most vulnerable and in fact the only system that seems to be involved in a major way in the human. Irradiation exerts itself by a direct damage of nerves and glial cells and also by an indirect damage secondary to vascular effects. Changes in cell size and shape occur as well as complete destruction. The cell body may be less affected than the axons and dendrites; in the case of glia there may be degeneration.

Microcephaly is the common clinical feature found in humans who have received irradiation in utero. Frequently mental retardation occurs; other abnormalities of the nervous system have been found. When therapeutic pelvic irradiation is given, the doses are usually in the range of several hundred rads. Approximately 25% of the offspring of these gestations have microcephaly. In diagnostic tests where approximately 5 rads have been used, one must consider that chromosomal nondisjunction and perhaps gene mutations can occur. Of additional concern is the suggestion that the incidence of childhood cancer may be increased in the offspring of mothers who have received diagnostic pelvic irradiation. At present the recommendations for judicious use of pelvic x-rays in both pregnant and nonpregnant women seem well advised.

Environmental Agents

Several environmental agents are felt to have some teratogenic potential (see Table V). The problems with organic mercury, which were first delineated at Minamata Bay, Japan, are now well known. Organic mercury had been associated with other focal epidemics and experimentally is a teratogenic agent. The fetal alcohol syndrome is now accepted by most authorities; again the nervous system can be affected. Other agents listed in Table V are less well documented but most certainly qualified for listing.

SUMMARY

The material presented in this chapter summarizes the general field of teratology, giving some of the basic problems and principles as well as outlining our present state of knowledge concerning human teratogens.

Every year new compounds are shown to be teratogenic in animal models, and the mechanisms by which the anomalies arise can now be studied in many cases. Unfortunately, much of this experimental information is not directly applicable to humans. Therefore, relatively few teratogens are known that affect humans. With the high incidence of loss of early embryos, one might expect that a certain percentage of those spontaneous abortions are lost because of anomalies arising from so far unidentified teratogenic influences.

REFERENCES

1. Aksu, O., Mackler, B., Shepard, T. H., and Lemire, R. J.: Studies of mechanisms underlying the development of congenital anomalies in embryos of riboflavin-deficient, galactoflavin-fed rats: II. Role of the terminal electron transport systems. *Teratology* 1:93–102, 1968.

2. Anonymous: Synthetic sex hormones and infants. *Brit. Med. J.* 4:485, 1974.

3. Brent, R. L., and Gorson, R. O.: Radiation exposure in pregnancy. *Current Problems in Radiology* II:3–48, 1972.

4. Davie, R., Butler, N., and Goldstein, H.: *From Birth to Seven: A Report of the National Child Development Study.* London, Longman and the National Children's Bureau, 1972, pp. 175–177.

5. Fraser, F. C., in *Methods for Teratological Studies in Experimental Animals and Man,* edited by Nishimura, H., Miller, J. R., and Yasuda, M. Igaku Shoin Ltd., Tokyo, 1969, pp. 34–49.

6. Gorlin, R. J., Pindborg, J. J., and Cohen, M. M.: *Syndromes of the Head and Neck,* 2nd ed. McGraw-Hill, New York, 1976.

7. Hanshaw, J. B.: Developmental abnormalities associated with congenital cytomegalovirus infection, in Wollam, D. H. M. (ed.): *Advances in Teratology,* Vol. 4. New York, Academic Press, 1970, pp. 62–93.

8. Hanson, J. W., Myrianthopoulos, M. C., Harvey, M. A. S., and Smith, D. W.: Risks to the offspring of women treated with hydantoin anticonvulsants with emphasis on the fetal hydantoin syndrome. *J. Pediatr.* 89:662, 1976.

9. Jones, K. L., and Smith, D. W.: The fetal alcohol syndrome. *Teratology* 12:1, 1975.

10. Kucera, J.: Exposure to fat solvents: A possible cause of sacral agenesis in man. *J. Pediatr.* 72:857, 1968.

11. McKusick, V.: *Mendelian Inheritance in Man,* 4th ed. Johns Hopkins University Press, Baltimore, 1975.

12. Murakami, U.: Organic mercury problem affecting intrauterine life, in Klingberg, M. A. (ed.): *Proceedings of the International Symposium on the Effect of Prolonged Drug Usage on Fetal Development.* New York, Plenum Publishing Corp., 1972, pp. 301–336.

13. Nicholson, H. O.: Cytotoxic drugs in pregnancy. *J. Obstet. Gynec.* 17:316, 1968.

14. Safra, M. J., and Oakley, G. P.: Valium: An oral cleft teratogen? *Cleft Palate J.* 13:198, 1976.

15. Shapiro, S., Hartz, S. C., Siskind, V., et al.: Anticonvulsants and parental epilepsy in the development of birth defects. *Lancet* 1:272, 1976.

16. Shepard, T. H., Lemire, R. J., Aksu, O., and Mackler, B.: Studies of the development of congenital anomalies in embroys of riboflavin-deficient, galactoflavin-fed rats: I. Growth and embryologic pathology. *Teratology* 1:75–92, 1968.

17. Shepard, T. H.: Teratogenic drugs and therapeutic agents, in *Pediatric Therapy,* edited by H. C. Shirkey. C. V. Mosby Co., St. Louis, 1975.

18. Shepard, T. H., Miller, J. R., and Marois, M. (eds.): *Methods for Detection of Environmental Agents That Produce Congenital Defects.* American Elsevier Publishing Co., 1975.

19. Shepard, T. H.: Teratogenicity from drugs: An increasing problem. *Disease-a-Month* June 1974.

20. Shepard, T. H.: *Catalog of Teratogenic Agents,* 2nd ed. Johns Hopkins University Press, Baltimore, 1976.

21. Smith, D. W.: *Recognizable Patterns of Human Malformation,* 2nd ed. W. B. Saunders, Philadelphia, 1976.

22. Warkany, J.: *Congenital Malformations: Notes and Comments.* Year Book Medical Publishers, Chicago, 1971.

23. Wilson, J. G.: *Environment and Birth Defects.* Academic Press, New York, 1973.

17
Clinical Aspects of Twinning

Frank Falkner, M.D., F.R.C.P.
Charles H. Hendricks, M.D.

In primitive societies the occurrence of a multiple birth has always aroused interest out of proportion to the number of such births. The reason for this stems initially from the mysterious nature of twinning and the need for a primitive society to furnish an acceptable explanation for the event and to deal on a practical level with the fate of the infants. Several simplistic explanations for the event have been advanced by primitive societies:

1. Each twin was started by a different father.
2. Twins were fathered by a supernatural being.
3. Intercourse was conducted too recklessly.
4. Something in the woman's diet caused twinning to occur.

Although in many societies twins are welcome and take on somewhat of a supernatural aura, in other societies twins are considered evil or unwelcome (1). In these societies one or both may be killed at birth, especially if they are of opposite sex. In societies where the food supply is precarious, such as in Eskimo civilizations, one child may be permitted to perish through exposure in order that the second child may have enough food to permit a better opportunity for survival.

In modern society our deep preoccupation with the subject of twinning continues among both the lay population and scientific groups. There is a Twin Institute in Rome devoted to the study of twins. International congresses on twin studies are being conducted with increasing frequency. There is an International Twins Club with thousands of members, and in the United States there is a National Organization of Mothers of Twins made up of 9000 members. Scientific organizations find that twinning provides, to some degree, a controlled population for behavioral studies as well as studies dealing with congenital anomalies, epidemiology, cytogenetics, intelligence, and metabolic problems.

CLASSIFICATION OF TWINS

Twins are implanted in the uterus at the same time and thus have the same gestational age, although their birthweights may greatly differ. Both develop as fetuses growing in the same environment and space usually occupied by a single fetus. The placentation is involved in, and related to, prenatal nutrition via a common maternal source. Dizygotic twins are growing in these conditions as siblings, sometimes of different sex, and monozygotic do so with theoretically identical genotypes.

These basic factors play an important role in the subsequent growth and development of each twin and are related to within-pair similarities and differences.

Approximately two-thirds of all twins are dizygotic and one-third monozygotic. Dizygotic twins occur after the independent release of two ova and fertilization of these ova by two separate sperm. Monozygotic twins derive from a single fertilized ovum and division of the embryo at some stage in its development after fertilization.

The blastocysts of each dizygotic twin implant in the tissues of the uterine wall, and two membranes, the chorion and the amnion, surround the fetus. The placentas of these dizygotic twins are separate if the blastocysts implant far apart on the uterine wall but fused if the implantations are close together. If the placentas are fused, there are four membranes separating the twin fetuses: amnion, chorion, chorion, amnion.

In monozygotic twins, the ovum divides, producing a pair derived from a single diploid set of chromosomes. If no abnormalities during replication occur, the twins will be genetically identical. If the division of the ovum occurs before the blastocyst implants, the two blastocysts may implant at different placental sites on the uterine wall. These monozygotic twins will then have separate amniotic and chorionic membranes, just as do all dizygotic twins. And, as in the case of dizygotic twins, the placentas may be separate or fused.

It is more common, however, for the ovum to divide after blastocyte implantation. Such a monozygotic pair has two amnions but only one chorion. An overall estimate of the number of monozygotic twins having dichorial placentation is about 30%, e.g., Benirschke (2), Wilson (3).

Another, and much rarer, type of placentation takes place in monozygotic twins when division occurs in the embryonic disc after amniotic differentiation. This results in the twins' having a single chorion and single amnion. These twins are commonly conjoined and rarely survive. The frequency of monoamniotic twins in all monozygotic twins is approximately 4%.

NATURE OF TWINNING

There is a surprisingly wide variation in the incidence of twinning, as has been known for many years. The occurrence appears to vary according to geography and the ethnic makeup of the population as well as with the factors of maternal age and parity, which are discussed below. The incidence among the white population of the United States has been determined to be 10.1 per 1000 births, and that among the Negro population of the United States is reported at 13.4 per 1000 (4). Data summarized by Nylander (5) indicate that in some African populations the incidence of twin births may be in excess of 40 per 1000, or nearly four times the incidence in the United States. On the other hand, in certain parts of Asia, particularly in Japan, the appearnce is, for unexplained reasons, only about half that observed in the United States.

The monozygotic twinning rates fluctuate within relatively narrow ranges from one population to the other (Fig. 1). The usual monozygotic twinning rate is from 3 to 6 per 1000 maternities. Most of the wide variability in twinning rate appears almost certainly

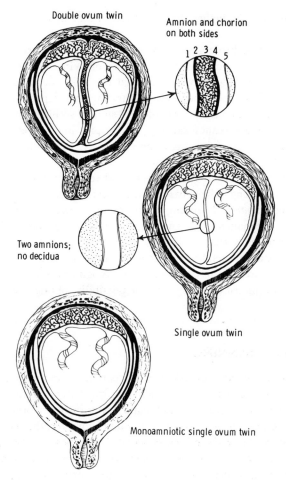

Figure 1. Arrangements of dizygotic and monozygotic twin placentas and membranes. Reproduced with permission from Benson, R. C.: *Handbook of Obstetrics and Gynecology,* 6th ed. Lange, 1977.

to be due to an increase in the number of dizygotic twinnings. A good illustration of this phenomenon is provided by the work of Bulmer (1958), who found in a United States population that the white and Negro monozygotic twinning rates were nearly identical—4.2 and 4.7, respectively—and the dizygotic twinning rates for the same population were 7.1 and 11.1, respectively (6).

In recent years the likelihood of twin and triplet births has been noted to be higher among women who have received ovulogenic drugs. Individual reports of even higher parities have become common to such an extent that the live birth of quintuplets now rates only passing mention in the daily newspapers rather than the headlines that used to be commanded by such an astonishing biological event. Worldwide, virtually every reported case of quintuplets in the last 10 years has been to a woman who received ovulogenic drugs. All twinning among women who receive such drugs is not necessarily due to the use of the drugs. In addition to the normal incidence of twinning in the general population, there is at least some slight evidence that women with polycystic ovarian disease may have a higher than expected rate of twinning after surgical treatment of the ovaries (7).

The overall effect of multiple gestations associated with the use of ovulogenic drugs appears to have little impact on the total incidence of twinning. Any such effect would seem to be well counterbalanced by the fact that the twinning rates in England, Scotland, most Western European countries, Australia, and Japan have been declining progressively for at least the last two decades. A similar secular trend was identified in the United States several decades earlier (8). Despite many speculative attempts to explain these declines in twinning rates, no completely plausible explanation has yet been offered.

The true incidence of twinning can never be determined for certain in any given population, because, among other reasons, the abortion rate in twin pregnancies has never been well documented. Twinning abortions have been demonstrated in tubal as well as intrauterine pregnancies (9). Another reason why the true incidence of twinning is difficult to determine is that a certain number of twins become blighted fetuses attached to the placenta and fetal membranes of an ostensible singleton pregnancy that goes to term (10). Most such cases are not recognized unless all placental and membrane tissue is examined carefully with the possibility of blighted fetus in mind.

INHERITANCE OF TWINNING

The obstetrician is very commonly asked by his patients if twinning is inherited and if "twins skip every other generation." Concerning the latter question, the obstetrician can assure the patient that there is no automatic "skipping every other generation" pattern. Concerning the general question of heritability, however, the issue is not susceptible to a simple answer. From the evidence available, it is possible for the obstetrician to provide a simplistic answer that serves the purpose and provides reasonable information for the patient. Although enormous controversies have arisen on this subject and there continue to be contradictory statements in the literature, the following statements summarize the information currently available quite well (11):

1. The tendency to twinning is not inherited from the father.
2. Any inherited tendency to twinning is almost exclusively among dizygotic pregnancies; thus a woman who has monozygotic twins or who is the relative of monozygotic twins is at no more risk for having twins herself than any other member of the general population. Any heritable tendency to twinning therefore must be confined to dizygotic twinning in maternal inheritance.
3. Women whose mothers have themselves had twins have an increased incidence of twinning, although the precise nature of the inheritance remains to be demonstrated.

Women who have given birth to dizygotic twins have a twofold likelihood as compared with the general population of having additional dizygotic twins in each succeeding pregnancy (12). Among a group of 585 data sets of twins collected by the author, there were three women who each gave birth to three sets of twins. The fact that women giving birth to several sets of twins are usually women of high parity and increasing age means that these individuals have already certain factors that may be enhancing the

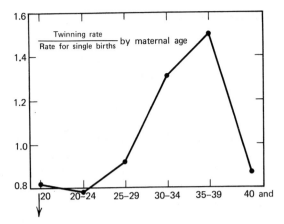

Figure 2. Ratio of twinning to single births by various maternal age groups. From Hendricks. *Obstet. Gynecol.* 27:47, 1966.

further production of multiple pregnancy. Greulich reported the birth of six pairs of fraternal twins to the same parents (13).

MATERNAL AGE AND PARITY

For reasons that are not explained, the twinning rate rises steadily after the age of 20, reaching its maximum some time between age 35 and 39, following which the twinning rate reduces dramatically (Fig. 2). Maternal parity also strongly influences the overall incidence of twinning (Fig. 3). It has now become clear that the effects of increasing maternal age versus those of parity operate independently. The effects of both increasing maternal age and increasing maternal parity appear to be exerted exclusively through altering the incidence of dizygotic twins, the incidence of monozygotic twins remaining relatively constant regardless of age and parity.

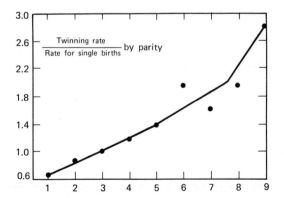

Figure 3. Ratio of twinning to single births at various parities. From Henricks. *Obstet. Gynecol.* 27:47, 1966.

GROWTH PATTERN OF TWINS

From conception until at least 20 weeks' gestation, the weight of a twin conceptus appears to be on average identical with that of a singleton conceptus. Beyond 22 weeks' gestation, however, differences appear, the twin fetus weighing on average less than the singleton fetus. At 38 weeks' gestation, the twin fetus weighs on average only approximately 80% as much as the term singleton fetus—2750 versus 3100 g, respectively (Fig. 4). The disparity between the twin and singleton fetal weights widens beyond 36 weeks of gestation, approaching approximately 20% at term. This may indicate that the mother is incapable of nourishing the average twin fetus as fully as she is the average singleton fetus. This possibility must be entertained despite the fact that in exceptional instances the combined fetal weight of twins may be very high, occasionally totalling more than 20 lb of birthweight.

The problem of raising a twin pregnancy goes beyond the mere challenge of providing nutrient to two growing fetuses. It also involves the problem of intrauterine capacity. As may be seen from Figure 5, the total fetal weight of a twin pregnancy approximates that of a term singleton pregnancy as early as 32.5 weeks' gestation. This means that during a large part of the third trimester the woman carrying twins is coping with carrying an enlarging uterine volume that is progressively more and more in excess of the intrauterine volume reached in term singleton pregnancy. It is widely presumed that the tendency of women carrying twin pregnancy to deliver early may be in response to the

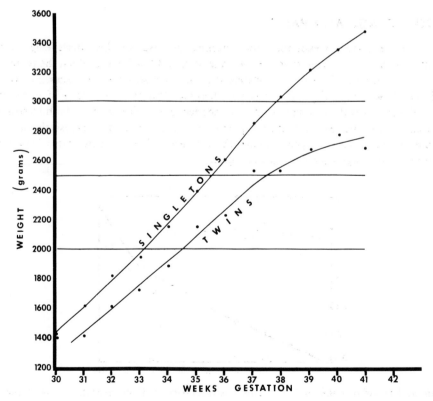

Figure 4. Mean weight of twins and singletons at various weeks of gestation. From Hendricks. *Obstet. Gynecol.* 27:47, 1966.

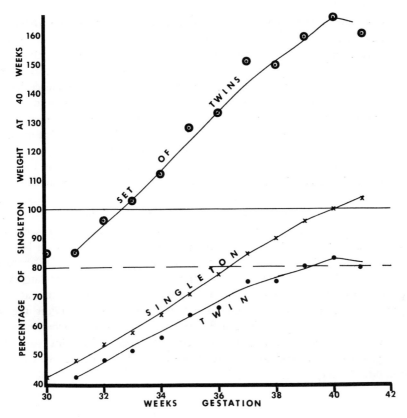

Figure 5. Growth patterns of one twin, singleton, and both twins at various weeks of gestation. From Hendricks. *Obstet. Gynecol.* 27:47, 1966.

two factors of increasing intrauterine volume plus the beginning of intrauterine deprivation of nutrients that may limit the growth of one or both fetuses.

One mechanism occurring in some twin pregnancies that might permit some pregnancies to be carried further toward term without excessive overdistention is the development of intrauterine growth retardation on the part of one fetus. Asymmetric development, to a degree where one fetus weights at least 500 g less than the larger fetus, occurs in only about 15% of twin pregnancies.

VASCULAR ANASTOMOSIS

One important facet of monochorionic placentation is that vascular anastomoses occur between the parts of the placenta supplying each twin. Hence, nutritional and other communications exist via these vascular connections. Indeed, Benirschke and Driscoll (14) found almost all monochorionic placentas to have vascular shunts of some kind, and the transfusion syndrome, where one twin transfuses blood to the other via a placental anastomosis, may occur when an artery-to-vein shunt exists of sufficient magnitude; perhaps one-third of all monochorionic placentas show some degree of the syndrome.

Vascular anastomoses are not found across dichorionic placentas even when these are fused. It must be recorded, however, that although they are not found after birth, blood chimeras have been reported—Benirschke and Driscoll (14)—in twins with dichorionic placentas showing that even if, rarely, there must have been some vascular connection across the dichorionic placentas at some time previously, even if evidence has disappeared by birth. An extremely rare case was also reported by these authors where a small artery-to-artery and vein-to-vein anastomosis was demonstrable in monozygotic twins with dichorionic placentas at birth. The implication thus is still that monozygotic twins with monochorionic placentas should be regarded differently from monozygotic twins with dichorionic placentas—and obviously from dizygotic twins of like sex who always have dichorionic placentas. Since placental "nutrition" presumably has an influence on fetal and early postnatal growth, many substances and agents may be transferred from one twin's placental part to the other's in the case of monozygotic twins with monochorionic placentas. It has been suggested, too, that placental tissue mass supplying each twin, denoting a capacity to supply nutrients, could be regarded subsequently as an indicator of this factor. It was shown—Falkner (15)—that the wet and dry weights of placentas, or placenta parts, were significantly correlated with the corresponding twin's birthweight and that this was so for monozygotic and dizygotic twins with monochorionic or dichorionic placentas. In a series of 92 twins, the within-pair difference in birthweight averaged 326.0 g in monozygotic-monochorionic twins and 227.8 g in monozygotic-dichorionic twins—Falkner (15). This suggests that separated placental parts lead to a greater tendency for monozygotic twins to be more similar in birthweight.

CONGENITAL ANOMALIES AND PERINATAL MORTALITY

The general congenital anomaly rate among twins is variously reported as being two to three times as high as that among singletons. Hendricks (16) reported that among 758 twins the anomaly rate was 10.6% compared with an incidence of 3.3% of all anomalies in the same hospital's population.

The perinatal mortality of twins continues to be distressingly high. Being a twin constitutes a unique biologic burden comprised of an increased incidence of severe congenital anomalies, the threat of premature labor and a high incidence of intrauterine growth retardation, and the threat of traumatic delivery or intrapartum accident. Nearly two-thirds of the perinatal mortalities in Hendricks' series were among infants born prior to 30 weeks' gestation. In those twins born within the time range of 30 to 33 weeks' gestation, the mortality rate was 257 per 1000. In those born in the 34- to 37-week range, the rate was 62.5 per 1000, and among those infants born at 38 or more weeks' gestation the rate was down to 19 per 1000. Each of these rates for the times mentioned is greatly in excess of the perinatal rates for the singleton pregnancies delivered on the service during the same period of time.

The complex relationship among intrauterine growth retardation, perinatal mortality, and congenital malformation is worthy of some examination. Figure 6 bears on this point. Infants were divided into gestational groups of 30 to 35 weeks' gestation and 36 to 40 weeks' gestation, respectively. In each of these chronologic groups the infants were placed into weight categories by standard deviations above or below the mean for the achieved week of gestation, the mean referring at each week of gestation to

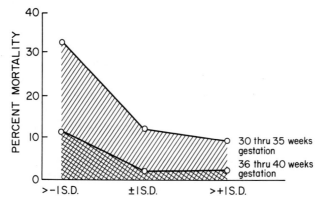

Figure 6. Mortality among premature and term twins in relationship to mean fetal weights. Data from Hendricks (16).

the mean weight of the individual twin rather than to singleton pregnancies. In those infants delivered prematurely within the 30 to 35 week gestation, the perinatal mortality was 32% for those who were more than one standard deviation below the mean but only 8% for those who were more than one standard deviation above the mean. For the more mature 36 to 40 week gestational range, perinatal mortality was 12% for those infants whose birthweight was more than one standard deviation below the mean but only 3% for those who were born at a standard deviation more than one above the mean.

When one examines the relationship between achieved fetal weight at a given number of weeks' gestation and the presence or absence of congenital malformations, a similar pattern emerges (Fig. 7). Once again infants were divided according to gestational groups of 30 to 35 weeks' gestation versus those of 36 to 40 weeks' gestation. In those infants delivered prematurely, congenital anomalies appeared in a startling 27% of those who were more than one standard deviation below the mean weight for twins at the week of gestation when they were born. In individuals whose weight was plus or minus one standard deviation from the mean the anomaly rate was 16%, and among those who had achieved growth to an extent that they were more than one standard deviation

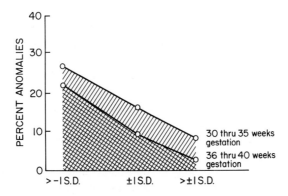

Figure 7. Anomalies among premature and term twins related to mean birth weights. Data from Hendricks (16).

above the mean the anomaly rate was only 8%. Examining the incidence of congenital anomalies among twins born at 36 weeks' or more gestation, one finds that among those who had birthweights more than one standard deviation below the mean the congenital anomaly rate was 21%, those within one standard deviation of the mean had an anomaly rate of 9%, and those who grew to a birthweight more than one standard deviation above the mean had a congenital anomaly rate of only 3%.

This pattern is believed to show that relative intrauterine growth retardation among twins is associated with and possibly causally related to those events which result in perinatal mortality. Each of the factors mentioned above—premature birth, intrauterine growth retardation, congenital anomalies, intrapartum accident, traumatic delivery—appears to play a part in the "formula for reproductive failure" that exists in twin gestation as a threat to the successful completion of parturition.

MANAGEMENT OF TWIN PREGNANCY

It has been commonly stated for many years that only 50 to 75% of twin pregnancies are diagnosed prior to the onset of labor. To the extent that this statement is true, it has significant implications for both the conduct of pregnancy and the conduct of the delivery itself. Without reasonably early diagnosis, the mother of twins may be partially deprived of that intensive prenatal care which helps to optimize the chances for a successful twin pregnancy. Failure to recognize the presence of a second twin until after the delivery of the first may jeopardize the chances of twin B through such mechanisms as the early and possibly injudicious administration of oxytocic preparations after the delivery of twin A, failure to be prepared to deliver twin B, and failure to have arranged in advance for the best available pediatric care.

In a real sense, the management of twin pregnancy starts with the diagnosis. Some clinicians feel that all pregnant women should have ultrasonic scanning in early pregnancy in order inter alia to make a diagnosis of twin pregnancy as early as possible and thus to facilitate the optimum management of the twin pregnancy. Although twin pregnancy has been diagnosed by ultrasonic techniques as early as 5 to 6 weeks by demonstration of two gestational sacs, there are instances where the ultrasonic technique is unreliable and the diagnosis of twins may be missed. Even in the last half of the second trimester, ultrasonic diagnosis is not infallible.

If the physician is going to submit to ultrasonic examination only those pregnancies in whom he observes unusually rapid growth, he ordinarily would not suspect twins much sooner than 16 to 20 weeks' gestation. By that stage of gestation, the ultrasonic scanning techniques have a high degree of accuracy in diagnosing twins.

Those who do not have ultrasonic scanning readily available or who do not elect to use it routinely need to rely on less sophisticated means of making the diagnosis. One often finds that at 16 weeks of gestation the uterine size is already compatible with that which would ordinarily represent a 20-week gestation and at 20 weeks' gestation the fundus is frequently compatible with a 26- to 30-week uterine size.

In theory, it should be possible to diagnose twins by identifying two separate heart rates. In actual practice, it is very difficult to use this "double stethoscope technique" to make a diagnosis. It is only now, with the development of sophisticated electronic monitoring equipment, that methods are being developed to make this diagnostic technique effective. In practice, this approach is of little value because of the development of even better diagnostic methods that permit actual visualization of the twin fetuses in good detail by ultrasonic techniques.

Some, but by no means all, clinicians suspect twin pregnancy if hyperemesis is unusually severe or prolonged. Edema also tends to appear early in the woman pregnant with twins, and in some twin pregnancies there may be excessive weight gain during the first 20 weeks of pregnancy.

The specific management of twin pregnancy is remarkably similar to that required for the optimal management of singleton pregnancy. The mother should report early for prenatal care and have a diagnosis confirmed as soon as possible. Once the diagnosis of twins is confirmed, the patient should be seen at intervals of 2 weeks until the thirtieth week and weekly thereafter.

The dietary intake for a woman with twins should be increased to at least 2400 cal/day with a protein intake of at least 60 g. Maternal weight gain during twin pregnancy most frequently ranges from 30 to 40 lb in those twin pregnancies which progress to term. Supplementary iron should always be provided. Cigarette smoking should be strongly discouraged.

Hydramnios is noted about three times more frequently in twin pregnancy than in singleton pregnancy.

During the latter half of pregnancy there is an increased risk of development of toxemia of pregnancy. Hendricks found the incidence of preeclampsia to be approximately 16% (16). A rare and particularly vicious form of toxemia occurs in twin pregnancy where one twin is a congenital anomaly in the form of a hydatidiform mole and the other and its placenta are raised well into the third trimester. These cases usually progress to eclampsia before the true nature of the pregnancy has been identified (17).

The use of early diagnosis of twin pregnancy plus prolonged rest in bed in the third trimester has been widely advocated by some during the past 20 years. As a matter of fact, in 1939 Hirst (18) proposed maternal bedrest as a means of prolonging multiple pregnancy with a view to reducing neonatal death rate. He suggested that bedrest should last from the thirty-sixth week onward. Since that time, literally dozens of advocates of prenatal bedrest in multiple gestation have gone on record with this recommendation.

No objective studies have yet been done in a strictly controlled series, and there is no prospect that such a study will ever be performed. Most of the advocates of this procedure recommend hospitalization from 32 weeks onward. If one assumes that bedrest is not started until 32 weeks' gestation and does not exert a demonstrably beneficial effect until 33 weeks' gestation, one may gain an idea of what limited advantage is to be anticipated from the thirty-third week onward. Hendricks (16) observed that more than three-fourths of all perinatal losses among a series of 758 twins occurred prior to the thirty-third week of gestation (80 out of a total of 106 perinatal losses); thus any salvage brought about by maternal bedrest presumably would need to be effected from among the remaining one-fourth of losses or those individuals delivering at the thirty-third week and beyond. Here the perinatal loss was 26 out of 646 or 40.2 per 1000. It is certainly possible that part of this perinatal mortality might have been reduced if some of these infants had been carried longer. Demonstrating the truth of such a hypothesis, however, has been very difficult. Jonas (19), in a study of 441 multiple pregnancies cared for between 1954 and 1961, made two important observations: first that "prenatal bedrest in multiple pregnancy does not counteract premature onset of labour before the end of the thirty-second week of gestation. It thus fails to make an impact on immaturity, which is responsible for the bulk of perinatal wastage"; and, second, in multigravid patients, rest initiated at the thirty-third week of gestation may encourage fetal growth. Jonas then concluded, "this may help to overcome prematurity as defined by birthweight, but does not influence perinatal wastage." In 1974 in a smaller American study, Jeffrey, Bowes, and Delaney (20) came to almost the same conclusion. They found that "when gestations of less than thirty weeks are excluded, bedrest does not significantly alter perinatal mortality rate or length of gestation." They did note that bedrest tends to encourage intrauterine growth in twin pregnancies.

In summary, although bedrest initiated after the thirty-second week of gestation may not be expected to have major impact on the huge bulk of twin perinatal mortality, it may possibly serve to improve the overall quality of later twin gestations by enhancing their growth potential.

ASSESSMENT OF FETAL CONDITION

Serial estriol determinations may be useful in certain cases. In general one should anticipate that, because of the total size of the fetal-placental mass, estriol determinations tend to be unusually high as compared with those obtained at a comparable stage in a singleton pregnancy.

Amniocentesis may need to be done for the same reasons as apply in singleton pregnancy. The results obtained from one amniotic sac are by no means automatically translatable to the condition of the other fetus. Special techniques involving the injection of dye into one sac for the performance of amniography have been developed to permit identification of the two sacs. It is not always possible to obtain fluid from both sacs. How vigorous one makes the effort to obtain fluid from the second sac depends on the degree of urgency of obtaining fluid as a diagnostic technique. If one is doing amniocentesis in early midpregnancy to evaluate the alphafetoprotein level, one should not anticipate any correlation whatsoever between the two amniotic fluid cavities. If one is dealing with Rh-sensitized pregnancy, one must be aware that there is a poor correlation between the spectrophotometric absorption profiles (21) of the amniotic fluids from the two sacs, because, for various reasons, there may be substantial differences in fetal condition from one twin to another. If one is performing amniocentesis for the determination of L/S ratio, one may anticipate a fairly good correlation (22), although there may be notable differences in maturation in one twin versus another in certain twin pregnancies.

Fetal growth and development can be graphically documented by ultrasonic techniques. A single such study performed in the second trimester cannot only confirm the presence of twins but can indicate the fetal contours and size. Where subsequent questions arise as to the fetal condition, further ultrasonic scans may provide additional information. This type of study is of both academic and practical interest.

Fetal electronic monitoring is done for the same reasons as for a singleton pregnancy. Simultaneous monitoring of the activity of both fetal hearts requires a fairly high degree of sophistication in instrumentation and interpretation. Oxytocin challenge tests can be carried out, and fetal activity testing is fairly feasible in twin pregnancy. Accurate simultaneous electronic monitoring of fetal cardiac activity during the process of labor can be done, but it requires a much greater degree of expertise than for monitoring singleton labor (23).

PRESENTATION OF TWINS

Guttmacher and Kohl (24) reported on the presentation among 1212 pairs of twins. They found that in 47% of the cases both presented by the vertex. In 37% one was vertex and the other was breech. In 9% both were presenting by the breech, and in the remaining 7% one or both was in a transverse lie. Very similar figures have been reported by others. Approximately 75% of first twins present as vertex (25). Fore-knowledge of the presentation in twin pregnancies is vital information for planning delivery under the safest possible circumstances.

COURSE OF LABOR

Prelabor begins relatively soon in twin pregnancies, probably because of the factor of uterine distention. This in turn leads to an acceleration in cervical effacement and dilatation. Guttmacher (26) also noted an increased likelihood of premature rupture of membranes in twin pregnancy, which occurred in 29% of his cases compared with the singleton rate of 12%.

As already indicated, labor tends to begin prematurely. Under normal conditions the duration of labor may be brief or at least within normal limits, particularly if one is dealing with a vertex presentation of the first infant. Almost paradoxically, a fairly large minority of twin labors develop evidence of uterine dysfunction, presumably due to some combination of the factors of overdistention or abnormal presentation. Because of the enlarged uterine volume, labor is often conducted with contractions of very low or relatively low intrauterine pressure. We have recorded effective labor in twin pregnancies where the average intrauterine pressure developed during labor was only between 30 and 40 mm intensity. After the delivery of the first infant, the intrauterine pressure with contractions tends to become somewhat higher because of the reduced volume about which the same number of myometrical units are contracting.

Postpartum there is some tendency toward uterine atony after any delivery of a large volume of products of conception such as occurs in twins. Manual removal of the placenta and meticulous intrauterine exploration should be done without hesitation after twin delivery per vaginum.

THE SECOND OF TWINS

It has now been established beyond a shadow of a doubt that the birth process, at least in so far as vaginal delivery is concerned, exacts a higher price from the second of twins than from the first. Wyshak and White (27) surveyed the cumulative experience of 28 authors who reported on twin survivorship among 24,194 twin infants. They found the overall perinatal mortality among first-born twins to be 11.14% and that among second-born twins 14.54%. Thus the second twin experienced a perinatal mortality 30.5% in excess of that of the first twin. This large study confirms almost exactly the statement of Guttmacher and Kohl (24) that perinatal loss of the second twin is about 30 per 1000 greater than perinatal loss of the first twin.

To study this problem in detail, Ferguson (28) analyzed birth records of more than 3000 multiple gestation pregnancies reported in Alberta during a time when approximately 140,000 singleton births were occurring. For the singleton births the mortality during the study period was 21.9 per 1000. For the first of twins perinatal mortality was 69.6 per 1000 and for the succeeding infants 115.5 per 1000. Among the most frequently diagnosed causes of fetal loss occurring in other than first babies were hypoxia and intrapartum abruptio placenta; smaller numbers of losses of the second infant were attributed to cord prolapse or to injudicious use of ergonovine maleate after the birth of the first child but before the presence of a twin was recognized.

Ferguson was especially impressed with the problem of intrapartum abruptio placenta where he found that 13 out of the 17 fetal losses in association with placental abruption occurred when the interval between delivery of the first and subsequent babies was in excess of 30 min. An additional three were lost when there was a 15 to 30-min delay and only one from abruptio placenta where there was less than a 15 min delay.

Ferguson's findings reinforce the currently accepted view that if twins are to be delivered vaginally, the second should be delivered no more than 15 min after the first. The presumption is that the second of twins is at particular risk because of the development of severe hypoxia having its onset after the birth of the first twin and also because of potential trauma associated with the delivery itself.

Ware (29), reporting on 207 sets of twins, found that 22.1% of the first-born twins had Apgar scores of 6 or below and 37.6% of second-born twins had Apgars of 6 or below. In a confirmatory study, Ho and Wu (30) found 19.8% of first-born twins had Apgars of 6 or below and 38.3% of second-born infants had Apgar scores of 3 or below.

The moral of the story is reasonably plain. If there are to be twins at all, one must accept the fact that 50% of them will be "the second twin." We must further accept the fact, based on overwhelming evidence, that the second of twins is at substantially greater risk of death than the first twin if delivery is to be done vaginally. To the extent that vaginal delivery continues to be performed for twins, the interval between the birth of the first and second infants should be less than 15 min, and the delivery of the second twin should be conducted as atraumatically as possible.

DELIVERY

There has appeared an increasing tendency to liberalize the use of cesarean section as a means of delivering twins. Assuming that cesarean section can be carried out expeditiously and safely, it appears that the total perinatal mortality among all second twins could be reduced by the magnitude of 30 per 1000 simply by the expedient of performing cesarean section rather than attempting vaginal delivery. Although it appears unlikely that the majority of practitioners at the present time would subscribe to the routine performance of cesarean section for the delivery of all twin pregnancies simply for the well-being of the second twin, there are certainly many instances where a planned or emergency cesarean section might enhance the chances of survivorship of a second twin. Examples of this would be where the second twin was presenting as a breech or transverse lie at the onset of labor. Additional examples might be those situations where there is cord prolapse of the second twin or difficulty in effecting prompt and reasonably atraumatic delivery of the second twin. In those instances, cesarean section delivery for the second of twins might be considered to be justifiable. When the first twin has been delivered vaginally, it is preferable to rupture the membranes of the second sac and to lead the vertex into the pelvis so that delivery may be effected spontaneously or by low forceps. Internal version and extraction of the second of twins is no longer done as freely as it used to be. In rare instances it is not possible to deliver the second twin without undue force: in such cases cesarean section delivery of the second twin is justified.

SPECIAL PROBLEMS ASSOCIATED WITH TWIN DELIVERY

A number of rare but profound problems may be associated with the delivery of twins. No one obstetrician is likely to encounter more than one of the conditions described below during a lifetime of practice. Nevertheless, because of the profound impact these conditions have on the outcome of pregnancy, the physician should be aware of the possibility of these situations and the significance thereof.

Conjoined Twins

Conjoined twins occur only about once in 50,000 deliveries. In this unusual situation where twins are tightly joined together (Fig. 8), safe vaginal delivery is not usually possible at term. Most of these cases tend to be diagnosable before labor or early in labor, either because of some combination of unusual uterine size, uterine contour, asymmetric position of the presenting part in the pelvis, or failure of the presenting part to descend into the pelvis during late pregnancy or early labor. Ultrasonic scanning or X-ray examination confirms the diagnosis. Cesarean section delivery provides both the best opportunity for fetal survivorship and the least danger of damage to the maternal reproductive tract. Unfortunately, conjoined twins may not be easily diagnosed in some instances until labor has been well advanced, because even good X-ray studies do not automatically confirm the diagnosis. This may lead to attempts at vaginal delivery prior to the performance of emergency cesarean section (31,32).

Locked Twins

About once in every 100,000 deliveries there occurs some variety of serious head-to-head entanglement of twin fetuses. Usually the first infant presents by the breech and the second by the vertex, thus producing chin-to-chin locking of the two heads and giving rise to the term of "locked twins." The etiology of locked twins is completely unknown, despite many speculative proposals that have been advanced to explain it. It is not usually diagnosed until part of the first infant has been born and evidence of severe dystocia appears. Ordinarily, interlocking is associated with smaller than normal twin fetuses. In an exceptional case, however, the two locked twins, diagnosed before labor by X-ray, each weighed in excess of 5000 g (33). If the diagnosis should be made before labor is too far advanced, cesarean section is the optimal management. If the fetuses are not too large, it may be possible to deliver both heads together by applying forceps to the head of twin B (34). In some instances decapitation of one fetus is still being used to improve the chances of survivorship of the remaining twin. The overall mortality is reported at 30 to 80%.

Twin Transfusion Syndrome

This is the situation where anastomosis develops between twins in a monozygotic pregnancy and where one twin receives a disproportionate amount of blood from the other (35). Thus the donor twin becomes anemic, and the recipient twin becomes plethoric. The appearance of such twins is striking (Fig. 9). The recipient twin almost always is larger than the donor twin. In one case observed by the author, baby A weighed 2380 g and was born with a hematocrit of 82%, and baby B weighed only 1600 g and had an initial hematocrit of 31%. In general the plethoric infant is subject to the development of cardiac problems, hyperbilirubinemia, and kernicterus. The anemic donor twin may develop hypovolemic shock, and often there is oligohydramnios in his amniotic sac.

Acardius

In this situation one twin only has a heart and thus must sustain the circulatory needs of the second (acardius) twin. In many such cases the cephalic structures are so primi-

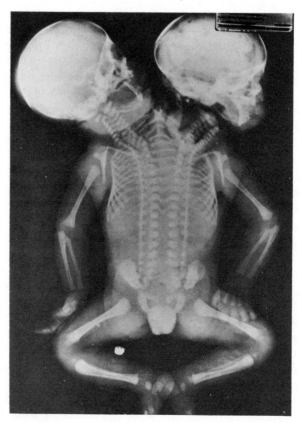

Figure 8. Conjoined twins; term pregnancy. After severe dystocia the diagnosis was confirmed by x-ray. Cesarean section delivery; neonatal death.

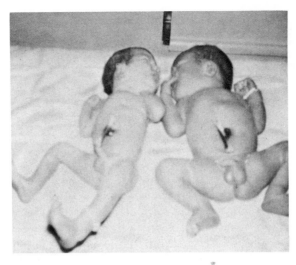

Figure 9. Twin transfusion syndrome (see text). From Morton and Morton. *Obstet. Gynecol.* 26:180, 1965.

tive that the blighted fetus is termed acardius acephalus (Fig. 10) (36). The acardius syndrome represents an extreme form of the twin transfusion syndrome where the circulatory crossover is compounded by a congenital malformation incompatible with extrauterine existence. The acardiac twin is completely dependent on the normal twin for all circulatory support. Only rarely does the presence of acardius result in abnormal labor (37).

PRENATAL AND POSTNATAL GROWTH OF TWINS

Cruise (38) showed that both preterm infants and small-for-date infants grew much faster than full-term infants in the first 9 months and that, given good neonatal care, preterm infants continued catch-up growth and had reached the size of full-term infants by 3 years of age. However, small-for-date infants did not continue to catch up and had not achieved a size equivalent to that of full-term infants by 3 years. Since intrauterine growth retardation, perhaps due to prenatal "fetal malnutrition," is thought to be associated with small-for-date infants, the above example would tend to support this view. However, recently Brandt (39) has demonstrated that two subdivisions of small-for-date infants can exist—those who do catch up and those who do not. The prenatal influences and their evaluation may assume great importance relative to the outcome of growth and development for small-for-date infants.

In fact, it seems to be a comparatively uncommon situation for monozygotic twins to have grossly differing birthweights. Babson and Phillips (40) found in such situations that the twin much smaller at birth does not exhibit sufficient catch-up to achieve the size of his larger twin. Buckler and Robinson (41) however, followed a pair of monozygotic-monochorionic twins, the smaller twin having a birthweight 45% less than that of her larger twin. Rapid catch-up of the smaller twin occurred and continued, and by 10 years both twins were similar in size and mental ability. It is interesting to note that the monochorionic placental part supplying the smaller twin was 87% of the weight of the larger twin's part. The corresponding percentage of the smaller twin's placental

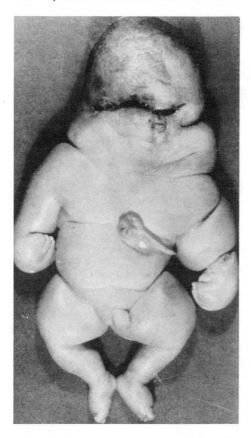

Figure 10. Acardius anceps. Note rudimentry development of head. From Gillim and Hendricks. *Obstet. Gynecol.* 2:647, 1953.

part in a pair of twins whose size difference persisted was 46%, the smaller twin's birthweight being 52% of the larger twin's. This might indicate that placental function, perhaps indicated by placental mass, could be related to differing growth outcome for monozygotic twins or even possibly that there is a "critical level" of size for a placenta or placental part below which growth deficit occurs that may be irreversible. This raises the question of placental size and function as an important factor in prenatal growth for singletons or multiple births. Buckler and Robinson's (41) twin pair also supports the view mentioned earlier that SFDI may be divisible into two subgroups. This pair clearly exhibited sufficient and prolonged catch-up.

Twin growth is studied, in part, in an effort to determine the relative importance of environmental and genetic influences on growth and development.

Standards for growth of twins have been given by Wilson (42,43). When compared with singletons, twins showed a deficit in size at birth that increased with increase of gestational age. Twins born at 33-plus weeks were equal to the thirty-sixth centile for singletons, but at term the twins' average size was below the fifth centile for singletons. Wilson also gave standards for weight, height, and head circumference from birth to 4 years. He compared high and low birthweight pooled groups and found the mean weight gain was similar for the first 2 years. By age 4 years, over 20% of the low birthweight twins were larger than the average for high birthweight twins. After a marked size deficit at birth compared with singletons, there was notable catch-up for 6 months, but only little thereafter. Wilson makes the interesting suggestion that prenatal adipose cell replication may be diminished by the needed nutritional sharing required in a twin pregnancy, since twins nearly caught up with singletons in height by 4 years but remained weight-deficient.

In an effort to examine in more detail some of the general questions raised up to this point, Falkner (44) studied data from a multiple birth cohort in the Collaborative Perinatal Study of the National Institute of Neurological Diseases and Stroke (NINDS)—Niswander and Gordon (45)—and from the Louisville Twin Study—Wilson (43).

In consideration of the influence of chorion condition on monozygotic twins, the Collaborative Study showed, in summary, that physical growth can depend in part on prenatal chorionic condition. Monozygotic-monochorionic pairs become progressively more similar in weight—the difference from 14.4 to 2.9%—between birth and 4 years of age, having at birth notable dissimilarity, and monozygotic-dichorionic pairs maintain in general similar within-pair differences of approximately 10% across the birth-to-4-year period.

Differences at any single age do not emerge until 4 years, and then they are more emphatic for male than female pairs. There appear to be no consistent differences in length, but within-pair differences for head circumference are almost twice as great for monozygotic-monochorionic as for monozygotic-dichorionic twins at birth; such differences are not significant thereafter. This suggests that a monozygotic-monochorionic twin with a deficit at birth exhibits catch-up early in postnatal life.

It appears monozygotic-dichorionic twin pairs are more similar with respect to head circumference than are dizygotic pairs and the difference is significant at each age between birth and 48 months.

It is generally concluded that, although monozygotic twins tend to be more consistently similar in weight, length, and head circumference after birth and up to 48 months of age than are dizygotic twins, there are in addition differences in these growth measures as a function of monochorionic versus dichorionic condition. The chorionic differences are less consistent than the zygosity contrasts, and the data for chorionic differences with respect to length are ambiguous.

In addition, differences between zygosity and chorionic condition changed with development in the case of weight but not for length or head circumference. Monozygotic twins progressively became proportionally more similar to one another, whereas other groups remained the same or showed irregular growth trends. For head circumference, dichorionic pairs were more similar than monochorionic, but only at birth.

In the Louisville Twin Study, birthweight, estimated gestational age, and placental weight were available for the twins. Consequently, it was possible to compare zygosity in the dichorionic condition as well as chorion status in the monozygotic condition for white twin pairs from this sample.

The placental weights were wet weights. Separate placentas posed no problem. When fused, they were divided at the fusion plane. Monochorionic placentas were divided into the respective parts for each twin by cleavage along the vascular equator plane.

The statistical comparisons consisted of a consideration of dichorionic twin pairs on which monozygotic twins were compared with dizygotic pairs. A test was also performed to determine if the differences between these monozygotic and dizygotic twins differed as a function of the sex of the twin pair (only like-sexed pairs were considered). Similarly, among monozygotic twins, monochorionic pairs were compared with dichorionic pairs, and this difference was assessed for possible dependencies on sex. These comparisons were made for the average absolute difference in birthweight within pairs, the average gestational age, and the average absolute difference in within-pair placental weight.

There were no differences in gestational age as a function of zygosity or chorionic condition, nor for the average within-pair absolute difference in placental weight as a function of zygosity or chorionic condition. For birthweight there were no significant differences as a function of zygosity.

The general correlation between actual placenta and birthweight is approximately .36 to .61, and there is no consistent or sizable difference in the level of this relationship as a function of zygosity or chorion. There are no differences in the coefficients of correlation for monozygotic-monochorionic as opposed to monozygotic-dichorionic pairs. Thus, regardless of chorionic condition or zygosity, there is a strong positive relationship between birthweight and placental weight.

In both the Collaborative and the Louisville studies, lack of differences for zygosity are consistent across studies. In the Collaborative Study, zygosity-related differences in weight were not present at birth, though within-pair differences diverged for monozygotic versus dizygotic with development. However, even these developmental contrasts were most pronounced for blacks, and females, whereas the Louisville data are derived from a white sample.

Earlier it was suggested that monozygotic-monochorionic twins were likely to be more different in size than monozygotic-dichorionic twins at birth.

Robson (46) provides some supportive data and also raises some important questions. Her data show 27 monozygotic-dichorionic twins had an average birthweight difference of 261 g, and in the 107 monozygotic-monochorionic twins, the difference was 323 g (20% difference). She points out the need for selection criteria in regard to survival. Among male pairs in which one twin died, the within-pair birthweight differences were 2.2 times greater than in male pairs in which both survived. Among female pairs, no such effect was seen. Along with the need to note the constitution of monozygotic samples—whether there is a higher proportion of monozygotic-dichorionic, for example, than expected—these considerations show the need for care in interpretation of results; they also show that the multifactorial nature of the influences on growth are more complex than has been considered. In the monozygotic-monochorionic condition, for example, it may be necessary to add further factors such as the monozygotic-monochorionic placental status with regard to the shunt-transfusion syndrome. A possible "critical size" factor of placenta, or placenta part, has already been mentioned.

Longitudinal Study

Vandenberg and Falkner (47) used a fitted growth curve for each individual twin and a method of expressing parameters of this curve to summarize the information for that individual in a few numbers. The rate of concordance for growth in height of monozygotic and like-sexed dizygotic twins was very similar for the first few months only. This is not surprising, since it has been shown—e.g., Tanner et al (48)—that the "genetic target" curve is not reached until 2 to 3 years of age, when some prenatal and previous influences on growth have waned. It was found that, at least for height, hereditary influence appears to be of paramount importance only for the deceleration of the growth rate, which takes effect later, and that it is of moderate importance for growth rate, but not significantly important for the initial status.

Wilson (3) supports these general contentions by showing that in his large sample of twins the early strong prenatal influences on growth are gradually neutralized and postnatal growth moves firmly in a direction determined genotypically. Wilson (3) also showed that monozygotic twins were less concordant for birthweight—the chorionic placental factor was not studied—than dizygotic but that this was in some measure due to a few monozygotic pairs who had markedly great within-pair birthweight differences (see earlier in this chapter). However, by 1 year of age, monozygotic twins had become more concordant for size and dizygotic twins had moved further apart, and this trend continued to 4 years. He notes the complex perinatal influences on birth size and the rapid conveyance of each twin onto his own genetic growth curve.

MacMillan and his colleagues (49) found that placental concentration of chorionic somatomammotropin (HCS) and total content of HCS were related to birthweight of twins, the maternal HCS levels being of course common to both twins. This suggests a valid index of placental function. They also found that HCS placental concentration was predictive of length at birth and at 2 years, suggesting that HCS production may represent an influence independent of general placental function. Here is a current example of the need to study the influence of placental nutrition, size, and function on growth pre- and postnatally both in twins and in singletons and to continue study of the human twin as a means to explore other influences on growth.

Zygosity Determination

In deriving information from studies of the human twin, it is usually necessary to be sure of the correct diagnosis of zygosity. Very careful examination of the placenta will diagnose monozygosity if the placenta is monochorionic-diamniotic, or indeed monoamniotic. And it will be helpful in the case of like-sexed twins having a dichorionic placenta. But to be sure of the monozygotic versus dizygotic state, particularly in the latter case, for all practical purposes, it is necessary to blood-type the twins. Wilson (50) in a definitive study described the use of 22 or more antigens in over 700 pairs of twins and showed that there was about a 3% chance that twins concordant for all the major blood groups may be dizygotic, and this chance is even less if parental blood groups are also available.

SUMMARY

The management of twin pregnancy continues to be a challenging part of obstetric practice. The perinatal mortality continues to be excessive. The diagnosis of multiple pregnancy should be confirmed early. Intensive prenatal care should include frequent prenatal visits, excellent nutrition, iron supplementation, and an organized rest pattern. The medical attendant needs to watch for premature labor, premature rupture of the membranes, the development of preeclampsia, and the possibility of polyhydramnios. Delivery should be planned with a special awareness of the problem of the second twin delivery. Anticipation of all the concomitant features of such infants and the associated risks is necessary, and appropriate care must be planned. Special hazards, such as the transfusion syndrome, can be expected and successfully treated. The pediatrician or neonatologist clearly needs to obtain information on the prenatal growth period and placentation of the newly born infants under his care and thus cooperate continually with his obstetric colleagues.

The pediatrician can perform a needed and valuable service by offering explanations and counseling to the parents of multiple-birth infants and by being aware of special parental problems following such a birth.

Although it is clear that interpretation of results from studies of multiple births has to be made with caution, especially since twins are not representative of the general population, more and more information is forthcoming concerning prenatal influences on growth and their multifactorial nature and concerning that often neglected factor of prenatal life, the placenta. It is also clear that much may be learned from multiple births, especially in unraveling influences of nature and nurture on growth and the outcome for the individual infants.

REFERENCES

1. Ford, C. S.: *A Comparative Study of Human Reproduction.* Yale University Publications in Anthropology No. 32, reprinted by Human Relations Area Files Press, 1964.

2. Benirschke, K.: Twin placenta in perinatal mortality. *New York State J. Med.* 289:937, 1973.

3. Wilson, R. S.: Concordance in physical growth for monozygotic and dizygotic twins. *Ann. Human Biol.* 3:1, 1976.

4. Statistical Bulletin of the Metropolitan Life Insurance Company, 1960.

5. MacGillivray, I., Nylander, P. P. S., and Corney, G.: *Human Multiple Reproduction,* Chap. 5. W. B. Saunders Co. Ltd., 1975.

6. Bulmer, M. G.: The numbers of human multiple births. *Annals Human Genetics* 22:158–164, 1958.

7. Stein, I. F., Sr.: Multiple pregnancy following wedge resection in the Stein-Leventhal syndrome. *Internat. J. Fertil.* 9:343–350, 1964.

8. Guttmacher, A. F.: The incidence of multiple births in man and some of the other unipara. *Obstet. Gynec.* 2:22–35, 1953.

9. Arey, L. B.: Two embryologically important specimens of tubal twins. *Surg. Gynec. Obstet.,* 36:407–415, 1923.

10. Bergman, P., Lundin, P., and Malmstrom, T.: Twin pregnancy with early blighted fetus. *Obstet. Gynec.,* 18:348–351, 1961.

11. MacGillivray, I., Nylander, P. P. S., and Corney, G.: *Human Multiple Reproduction,* Chap. 4. W. B. Saunders Co. Ltd., 1975.

12. Hendricks, C. H.: Unpublished data.

13. Greulich, W. W.: The birth of six pairs of fraternal twins to the same parents. *J. Am. Med. Assoc.* 110:559–563, 1938.

14. Benirschke, K. and Driscoll, S. G.: *The Pathology of the Human Placenta.* Berlin, Springer, 1967.

15. Falkner, F.: General considerations in human development, in Falkner, F. (ed.): *Human Development.* Philadelphia and London, W. B. Saunders, 1966, p. 10.

16. Hendricks, C. H.: Twinning in relation to birth weight, mortality and congenital anomalies. *Obstet. Gynec.,* 27:47–53, 1966.

17. Clark, P. B., Gusdon, J. P., and Burt, R. L.: Hydatidiform mole with coexistent fetus: Discussion and review of diagnostic methods. *Obstet. Gynec.,* 35:597–600, 1970.

18. Hirst, J. C.: Maternal and fetal expectations with multiple pregnancy. *Am. J. Obstet. Gynec.* 37:634–643, 1939.

19. Jonas, E. G.: The value of prenatal bed-rest in multiple pregnancy. *J. Obstet. Gynaec. Brit. Cwlth.* 70:461–464, 1963.

20. Jeffrey, R. L., Bowes, W. A., Jr., and Delaney, J. J.: Role of bed rest in twin gestation. *Obstet. Gynec.* 43:822–826, 1974.

21. Beischer, N. A., Pepperell, R. J., and Barrie, J. U.: Twin pregnancy and erythroblastosis. *Obstet. Gynec.* 34:22–29, 1969.

22. Spellacy, W. N., Cruz, A. C., Buhi, W. C., and Birk, S. A.: Amniotic fluid L/S ratio in twin gestation. *Obstet. Gynec.* 50:68–70, 1977.

23. Cetrulo, C. L., Freeman, R. K., and Knuppel, R. A.: Minimizing the risks of twin delivery. *Contemporary Ob/Gyn* 9:47–51, 1977.

24. Guttmacher, A. F., and Kohl, S. G.: The fetus of multiple gestations. *Obstet. Gynec.* 12:528–541, 1958.

25. Portes, L., and Granjon, A.: Les presentations au cours des accouchments genellaires. *Gynécologie et Obstétrique* 45:1459, 1946.

26. Guttmacher, A. F.: Multiple pregnancy: Clinical aspects. *GP* 13:97–102, 1956.

27. Wyshak, G., and White, C.: Birth hazard of the second twin. *J. Am. Med. Assoc.* 186:869–870, 1963.

28. Ferguson, W. F.: Perinatal mortality in multiple gestations. *Obstet. Gynec.* 23:861, 1964.

29. Ware, H. H., III: The second twin. *Am. J. Obstet. Gynec.* 110:865–873, 1971.

30. Ho, S. K., and Wu, P. Y. K.: Perinatal factors and neonatal morbidity in twin pregnancy. *Am. J. Obstet. Gynec.* 122:979–987, 1975.

31. Compton, H. L.: Conjoined twins. *Obstet. Gynec.* 37:27–33, 1971.

32. Lu, T., and Lee, K. H.: Obstetric management of conjoined twins. *J. Obstet. Gynaec. Brit. Cwlth.* 74:757–762, 1967.

33. Costello, J. R.: The interlocking of twins' heads at term. *Med. Ann. D.C.* 34:125, 1965.

34. Khunda, S.: Locked twins. *Obstet. Gynec.* 39:453–459, 1972.

35. Naeye, R. L.: Human intrauterine parabiotic syndrome and its complications. *New Engl. J. Med.* 268:804–809, 1963.

36. Gillim, D. L., and Hendricks, C. H.: Holoacardius: Review of the literature and case report. *Obstet. Gynec.* 2:647–653, 1953.

37. Niles, J. H., and Lowe, E. W.: Holocardius acephalus as a cause of dystocia: Report of a case. *Obstet. Gynec.* 33:541–543, 1969.

38. Cruise, M. O.: A longitudinal study of the growth of low birth weight infants. *Pediatrics* 51:620, 1973.

39. Brandt, I.: Growth dynamics of low birth weight infants with emphasis on the perinatal period, in Falkner, F., and Tanner, J. M. (eds.): *A Treatise on Human Growth: In Three Volumes,* Vol. II. New York, Plenum, in press.

40. Babson, S. G., and Phillips, D. S.: Growth and development of twins dissimilar in size at birth. *New Engl. J. Med.* 289:937, 1973.

41. Buckler, J. M. H., and Robinson, A.: Matched development of a pair of monozygous twins of grossly different size at birth. *Arch. Dis. Childh.* 49:472, 1974.

42. Wilson, R. S.: Twins: Measures of birth size at different gestational ages. *Ann. Human Biol.* 1:57, 1974.

43. Wilson, R. S.: Growth standards for twins from birth to four years. *Ann. Human Biol.* 1:175, 1974.

44. Falkner, F.: Implications for growth in human twins, in Falkner, F., and Tanner, J. M. (eds.): *A Treatise on Human Growth: In Three Volumes,* Vol. I. New York, Plenum, in press.

45. Niswander, K. R., and Gordon, M.: *The NINDS Collaborative Perinatal Study: The Women and Their Pregnancies.* Philadelphia, W. B. Saunders, 1972.

46. Robson, E. B., personal communication on preliminary analysis of Oxford data, 1976.

47. Vandenberg, S. G., and Falkner, F.: Hereditary factors in human growth. *Human Biol.* 37:357, 1966.

48. Tanner, J. M., Healy, M. J. R., Lockhart, R. D., et al.: The prediction of adult body measurements from measurements taken each year from birth to 5 years. *Arch. Dis. Child.* 31:372, 1956.

49. MacMillan, D. R., Brown, A. M., Matheny, A. P., et al.: Relationships between placental concentrations of chorionic somatomammotropin (placental lactogen) and growth: A study using the twin method. *Pediatr. Res.* 7:719, 1973.

50. Wilson, R. S.: Bloodtyping and twin zygosity. *Human Heredity* 20:30, 1970.

Part 3

SPECIFIC DISEASES AFFECTING MOTHER AND CHILD

18

Erythroblastosis
Fetalis

John T. Queenan, M.D.

Erythroblastosis fetalis is an intriguing disease. Symptoms range from slight anemia and mild hyperbilirubinemia in the neonatal period to the extreme of hydrops fetalis with early intrauterine death. The disease process involves a normal fetus who is exposed to a hostile environment. If the disease can be managed successfully, usually the neonate recovers completely.

The development in the 1960s of Rh clinics at several medical centers throughout the United States marked the beginning of modern-day perinatal care. At these centers, perinatal teams were formed that included obstetricians, neonatologists, nurses, blood bank personnel, and hematologists. Their success in managing Rh-disease patients came through cooperative efforts. The team approach to Rh disease served as the prototype for the modern management of high-risk pregnancies.

Rh-IMMUNE PROPHYLAXIS

In 1939, Levine and Stetson (16) noted that a mother who had given birth to a hydropic stillborn developed a transfusion reaction when transfused with her husband's blood. They postulated that erythroblastosis fetalis was caused by an incompatibility between the mother and a fetal red cell antigen inherited from the father. Before that time, erythroblastosis fetalis had been considered a familial disease. No one had suspected that there was an immunologic basis. The next year, Lansteiner and Wiener (14) discovered the Rh antigen, and investigative work on erythroblastosis fetalis was put on a sound scientific basis.

Although maternal immunization can also occur as a result of accidently transfusing an Rh-negative patient with Rh-positive blood, by far the most common cause of immunization is transplacental hemorrhage (TPH). Transplacental hemorrhage can occur during the prenatal course or at delivery. In 1955, Chown (6) reported that transplacental hemorrhage occurred during pregnancy. Subsequently, the development of a simple staining technique for fetal erythrocytes, the Kleihauer-Betke (KB) stain, (13) contributed to our knowledge of the mechanism of Rh immunization. This technique made it easier to quantitate transplacental hemorrhages occurring during the prenatal period and at the time of delivery.

445

Several investigators found that an increasing number of fetal erythrocytes enter the maternal circulation as pregnancy progresses. Furthermore, as pregnancy progresses, an increasing percentage of patients develop these transplacental hemorrhages. At the time of delivery, the number of fetal erythrocytes detected in the maternal circulation increases even more. However, if the fetus is incompatible in the ABO system with the mother, the fetal erythrocytes may be destroyed by the anti-A or anti-B antibodies. Therefore, in the setting of ABO incompatibility, the number of fetal erythrocytes detected in the maternal circulation may be markedly decreased.

By experimental studies, it has been shown that as little as 0.25 ml of Rh-positive cells can immunize a patient to the Rh factor (19). The first exposure to Rh-positive cells causes a primary response. Although an antibody may not yet be detected, this patient clears radioactive chromium-tagged Rh-positive erythrocytes from her circulation at an increased rate. The second exposure causes an anamnestic response with a rapid rise in antibody titer. Two exposures to Rh-positive erythrocytes are not always necessary. If the Rh-negative patient receives a large dose of Rh-positive blood, as in a mismatched transfusion, this may elicit both a primary and secondary response, because there are no antibodies to remove the Rh-positive blood from the maternal circulation. Therefore, this large single exposure to Rh antigen may be sufficient to cause immunization. In many patients, during the course of a pregnancy more than 0.25 ml of blood enters the maternal circulation through the mechanism of transplacental hemorrhage. However, patients may be resistant to becoming immunized because of the high level of steroids in the maternal circulation during pregnancy. The fetal blood may enter the circulation intermittently in minute amounts, and there may not be a sufficient quantity at any one time to cause immunization. In addition, some fetuses are incompatible with the mothers in the ABO blood groups, offering further protection against immunization by transplacental hemorrhage.

SCOPE OF THE PROBLEM

What are the risks of an Rh-negative Caucasian woman mating with a Caucasian male having an Rh-positive child? She stands a 15% chance of mating with a Rh-negative male; in this case all her children would be Rh-negative. There would be no risk of immunization. She stands an 85% chance of mating with a male who is phenotypically Rh-positive. The likelihood of mating with an Rh-positive male can be calculated using the Hardy-Weinberg equation, which expresses the frequency of homozygotes and heterozygotes in a population. Of the phenotypically Rh-positive males, approximately 60% would be heterozygous and 40% would be homozygous for the Rh factor.

If an Rh-negative patient has an Rh-positive partner, the risk of having an Rh-positive infant is approximately 70%. This is because the chance of his being heterozygous is 60%. In this event, half of the offspring would be Rh-positive and half would be Rh-negative. The chance of his being homozygous for the Rh factor is 40%. If he is homozygous, all the offspring would be Rh-positive. Therefore, the overall chance of the offspring being Rh-positive would be 70%. If a genotype indicates the partner is "probable" heterozygous or homozygous, predictions will be even more reliable.

Prior to the advent of Rh-immune prophylaxis, approximately 1% of Caucasian women became immunized to the Rh factor. Since almost 15% of the population was at risk, slightly less than 10% of the at-risk population became immunized.

The Rh-negative patient delivering an Rh-positive infant stands a 1 to 2% chance of becoming immunized with her first pregnancy by the time of delivery (10,5). The incidence of becoming immunized with each subsequent Rh-positive pregnancy increases to 10 to 11% (10). But if only pregnancies in which an Rh-positive fetus is compatible in the ABO blood group with the mother are considered, her chance of becoming immunized is as high as 14 to 17% (3,29).

Rh–IMMUNE PROPHYLAXIS

In the early 1960s, Finn and Clarke in Liverpool (8) and Gorman, Freda, and Pollack in New York City (12) simultaneously but independently embarked on research programs that culminated in the development of Rh-immune prophylaxis. In 1909, Theobald Smith (28) had shown that an antigen capable of stimulating an antibody response would not do so if injected in the presence of an antibody excess. Using the principle of attempting to protect against an antigenic stimulus with an antibody excess, these investigators tested the administration of Rh antibody to protect against the immunizing threat of transplacental hemorrhage.

The New York investigators used prisoner volunteers at Sing Sing. One week after an initial intravenous injection of Rh-positive blood into the volunteers, the investigators injected another 5 ml of Rh-positive blood. At the same time they also injected intramuscularly 5000 μg of Rh-immune globulin. Fifteen other prisoner volunteers were given similar injections of Rh-positive blood but they were given placebo (saline) injections instead of the Rh-immune globulin. At the end of 6 months, 14 out of 15 prisoners injected with the placebo were immunized, but only 1 out of 15 injected with the Rh-immune globulin was immunized. This experiment clearly demonstrated that injection of the antibody could offer protection from the Rh antigenic stimulus.

Over the next 4 years, clinical trials of Rh-immune prophylaxis were conducted. Rh-immune globulin was tested in Rh-negative, unimmunized patients who delivered Rh-positive, ABO-compatible infants. This particular experimental design was selected because of the increased likelihood of ABO compatibility permitting Rh immunization compared with the protective effect of ABO incompatibility. In a collaborative study only 1 out of 1080 (0.1%) patients were immunized when protected with Rh-immune globulin, whereas 51 out of 675 (7.6%) became immunized when no Rh-immune globulin was administered (2). The critical question was what would happen in the subsequent Rh-positive pregnancy. Did the Rh-immune prophylaxis actually confer protection? Of the 145 patients who underwent a subsequent pregnancy, 1 out of 82 (1.2%) of the protected group delivered an Rh-positive infant with erythroblastosis fetalis. In contrast, 7 out of 63 (11.1%) of the control (untreated) group developed erythroblastosis fetalis (2). This impressive record of protection caused worldwide attention, and Rh-immune prophylaxis was initiated in most developed countries.

The problem with this prophylaxis system is that Rh immunization poses a threat every time an Rh-negative patient is exposed to an Rh antigen. In this setting, she must receive Rh-immune prophylaxis with each exposure to the antigen. Even though Rh-immune prophylaxis is administered following her greatest exposure to the Rh antigen, the delivery, the patient still stands a chance of becoming immunized, because exposure can occur with a spontaneous abortion, an induced abortion, amniocentesis, ectopic pregnancy, or even transplacental hemorrhage during a normal pregnancy.

Over the last decade, the use of Rh-immune prophylaxis has markedly decreased the incidence of Rh immunization. The patients who are given Rh-immune prophylaxis within 72 hr postpartum have virtually a 95% assurance that they will not become immunized. If there is a failure, it is generally due to one of four factors:

1. The patient is already immunized, but the antibody levels are so low that the laboratory cannot detect them.
2. There is a large transplacental hemorrhage or a large exposure to fetal erythrocytes at the time of delivery, and the patient does not receive an adequate dose of Rh-immune prophylaxis to achieve an antibody excess.
3. The manufacturer produced Rh-immune globulin less potent than outlined by the standards. This recently occurred with a commercial batch of Rh-immune globulin. Extensive testing revealed that this lot had reduced antibody globulin because of the presence of a protease (20). This particular batch was found to protect against 6 rather than 30 ml of Rh-positive whole blood. A 30-ml transplacental hemorrhage at the time of delivery is very rare, whereas a 3-ml bleed is more common.
4. Finally, the patient is given Rh-immune prophylaxis too late. The original studies showed that Rh-immune globulin is effective if given within 72 hr of the antigenic stimulus. The postpartum patient may be discharged from the hospital before it is discovered that she should have received Rh-immune prophylaxis. By the time the omission is discovered, immunization may have already occurred.

The recent use of Rh-immune globulin with spontaneous abortions and induced abortions will cause a further decrease in the incidence of Rh immunization. The increased use of Rh-immune prophylaxis following amniocentesis in the Rh-negative, unimmunized patient with a partner known to be Rh-positive will eliminate another source of immunization.

Each time an Rh-negative patient is exposed to the Rh antigen, she runs a risk of becoming immunized. Although the risk is small with spontaneous abortion and slightly higher with induced abortion, the consequences of Rh immunization are severe. Therefore, Rh-immune prophylaxis must be considered with each exposure to the Rh antigen. Queenan et al. showed that the risk of the Rh-negative patient's becoming immunized by a spontaneous abortion was 3% (23). This was based on a study of patients who had one or more abortions with curettage as their first obstetrical experience. Because patients having spontaneous abortions usually bleed per vaginum and frequently have embryo-placental circulations that have stopped functioning long before spontaneous expulsion, they are less likely to be exposed to Rh-positive blood. In the instance of the induced abortion, however, the embryo-placental circulation is intact at the time of the suction curettage. If an intraovular injection of an abortifacient is the method of termination, there is a risk from the amniocentesis for instillation of the agent as well as the labor to expel the conceptus. It is, therefore, not surprising that the risk of Rh immunization from an induced abortion is slightly higher (5.5%) than with a spontaneous abortion (24).

Even an ectopic pregnancy can cause Rh immunization. Bergstrom (4) showed that the Rh antigen is present on the fetal erythrocyte as early as 38 days of gestation. Fetal erythrocytes entering the maternal circulation from an ectopic pregnancy at this stage of development or later can immunize a patient.

All three of these obstetrical events require that the patient be protected with Rh-immune prophylaxis. If an appropriate dose is given in time, the protection should be 100% effective.

Recently, Ortho Diagnostics marketed MICRhoGAM. This consists of a 50-µg dose of Rh-immune globulin that should be sufficient to protect against a transplacental hemorrhage from a spontaneous abortion, induced abortion, or an ectopic pregnancy, provided the transplacental hemorrhage does not exceed 4 to 5 ml of fetal erythrocytes. MICRhoGAM does not require a crossmatch and may be given at the time of the spontaneous abortion, passage of the conceptus with an induced abortion, or operation with an ectopic pregnancy. The drug should offer an adequate margin of protection up to 12 weeks' gestation. After that stage a standard dose (300 µg) should be used.

It has been demonstrated that the amniocentesis can cause transplacental hemorrhage. This was shown definitively with Rh-negative patients who were minimally immunized. Following an amniocentesis with recovery of Rh-positive fetal erythrocytes, there was a significant increase in the Rh titer in a number of patients. The patients had an anamnestic response to their Rh immunization (22).

Amniocentesis for genetic diagnosis is usually done at 15 to 17 weeks' gestation. The placenta covers a relatively greater part of the uterine surface at the time, and therefore it is more difficult to avoid piercing the placenta. This situation poses special problems. For example, consider an Ashkenazic Jewish couple who are carriers for Tay-Sachs disease. The woman may undergo one to three pregnancies and genetic amniocenteses prior to carrying a fetus to term who does not have Tay-Sachs disease. If she is Rh-negative and her partner is Rh-positive, it is possible that the genetic amniocenteses and induced abortions for the affected fetuses may cause Rh immunization before this couple has a chance to deliver a genetically normal baby. It is prudent to consider genetic amniocentesis patients as candidates for Rh-immune prophylaxis if the following conditions are met:

1. The mother is Rh-negative, unimmunized.
2. The partner is Rh-positive.
3. There is a reasonable chance that the placenta has been damaged either by virtue of its position or by recovery of Rh-positive fetal erythrocytes determined by Rh typing and by KB stain.

Rh-immune globulin has been successful in reducing the number of patients immunized to the Rh factor. Its protection is quite specific for the Rh antigen. Does it affect the incidence of immunization to other blood group antigens? It is our experience and that of others that there is no change in the incidence of immunization to other antigens like Kell or Duffy.

IRREGULAR ANTIBODIES

Irregular antibodies occur in approximately 1% of pregnant patients (25). They are most commonly encountered in patients who have had blood transfusions, cesarean sections, or induced abortions. They occur in either Rh-positive or Rh-negative patients. The clinical implications of an irregular antibody depend on, first, whether it is an IgG antibody that will cross the placenta and, second, whether the fetus has a corresponding red cell antigen, so that an antigen-antibody reaction will take place, causing erythroblastosis fetalis.

Anti-Kell, anti-Lewis (Le^a and Le^b), anti-c and anti-e immunizations are relatively frequent. With the exception of the anti-Lewis antibody, all these can cause erythroblastosis fetalis and even intrauterine death. Because the Lewis antibody is generally an IgM (saline-reacting) antibody, it does not cross the placenta. Even if it were an IgG antibody and it were capable of crossing the placenta, the antigen is not fixed on the fetal red cells. Therefore, there is no hemolytic disease.

The management of patients with irregular antibodies is essentially the same as for the Rh-immunized patient. The appropriate studies on the father's blood should be done to determine if he has the corresponding antigen. If the father has the antigen, the patient may be managed either by antibody titers or by amniotic fluid analysis, depending on the titer and history.

ABO ERYTHROBLASTOSIS FETALIS

The incidence of ABO erythroblastosis fetalis is approximately 2% of births. It is much more common than Rh erythroblastosis fetalis. Approximately two-thirds of all cases of erythroblastosis fetalis are due to ABO incompatibility. Forty to fifty percent of the cases occur in the first-born infant, in contrast to almost none in the first-born with Rh disease. Unlike Rh erythroblastosis fetalis, the ABO disease does not become more severe with subsequent pregnancies.

ABO erythroblastosis fetalis appears almost exclusively in group A or B infants born to group O women because the anti-A and anti-B produced by group O individuals are predominantly IgG. The IgG antibodies cross the placenta and cause erythroblastosis. ABO erythroblastosis is rarely seen in babies of mothers with A or B blood groups, because the anti-A of group B individuals and the anti-B of group A individuals are predominantly IgM.

The A and B antigens occur commonly in nature. Since they have been demonstrated on gram-negative bacteria that normally inhabit the human gastrointestinal tract, a blood transfusion or pregnancy is not necessary for immunization by A and B antigens. The antigen stimulus from gastrointestinal bacteria produces isoagglutinates in the first 6 months of life in individuals lacking this antigen. The titers of isoagglutinates tend to remain fairly low despite the omnipresence of antigenic stimulation, but they do increase slightly following an ABO pregnancy.

The ABO blood group system is found in all somatic cells in the body with the exception of the nervous system. Eighty percent of these individuals secrete the antigen in soluble form in tears, saliva, urine, and sweat. This represents an enormous antigenic mass that competes with the erythrocyte-bound antigen for any maternal isoagglutinate that enters the fetal circulation. The relatively low affinity of maternal isoagglutinate for fetal A and B antigen probably also contributes to the sparing effect of the hemolytic process.

LABORATORY FINDINGS IN ABO ERYTHROBLASTOSIS

Unlike Rh disease, serologic evaluation of the mother is not helpful. Determining anti-A or anti-B titers does not give a good indication of the severity or the prognosis of ABO erythroblastosis fetalis. Unlike Rh disease, amniocentesis and amniotic fluid analysis are not indicated in ABO disease. Because intrauterine death almost never occurs as a result of this disorder, amniotic fluid analysis is not helpful in evaluating the severity of the disease.

The cord blood direct antiglobulin (Coombs) test is usually positive if done carefully. But, even in excellent laboratories, a negative test or weakly positive test will sometimes be obtained.

The cord blood hemoglobin rarely indicates severe anemia. Usually the hemoglobin is 14 or above. A reticulocyte count may be as high as 25%, indicating significant hemolysis.

The bilirubin level is almost never elevated on the cord blood specimen but tends to rise during the first 24 hr. The maximum levels of bilirubin are obtained on the second or third day of life and thereafter tend to return to normal. The indirect hyperbilirubinemia and reticulocytosis reflect the underlying hemolytic process.

Occasionally, erythroblastosis fetalis exists and it is difficult to detect the causative antibody. In some instances, the ABO system is implicated, and in others the setting exists for ABO erythroblastosis but the actual causative antibody is not detected. Rh disease in the presence of ABO incompatibility occurs but is less frequent than in the setting of ABO compatibility. If the etiology of erythroblastosis is not clear, meticulous laboratory screening of the mother's blood for antibodies and the use of elution techniques on the infant's red blood cells will be helpful in determining which antibody or antibodies are implicated.

NEONATAL CARE OF ABO ERYTHROBLASTOSIS FETALIS

Generally, less than 5% of the affected newborns with ABO erythroblastosis require phototherapy, and only a rare infant requires exchange transfusion. Although ABO erythroblastosis appears milder and is often more insidious than Rh disease, the clinician should realize that it can cause kernicterus, given the tendency to earlier discharge from the hospital. More attention should be paid to jaundice in newborns so that ABO erythroblastosis can be detected and worked up. If a patient were to be discharged on the second or third postpartum day with a significant hemolytic process, the results could be tragic.

CLINICAL MANAGEMENT OF Rh ERYTHROBLASTOSIS

Even though a careful program of administration of Rh-immune prophylaxis following delivery literally decimates the incidence of Rh immunization, there will still be protection failures. Approximately 1 to 2% of Rh-negative patients become immunized during their first pregnancy, prior to the postpartum period when the Rh-immune prophylaxis is generally administered.

During the initial prenatal visit, appropriate blood work should be obtained. The blood group, Rh type, and indirect antiglobulin (Coombs) antibody screening for irregular antibodies should be performed. The blood group is important from the standpoint of ABO incompatibility. The Rh type is extremely important so that the physician will know if follow-up antibody screening is necessary.

If the patient is Rh-negative and unimmunized, she should have repeat antibody screening tests performed at 24 weeks and every 4 weeks thereafter until delivery. This routine pertains to the first pregnancy as well as subsequent pregnancies, even though the patient may have been protected with Rh-immune prophylaxis. The reason for this is obvious. There is always a possibility that there will be an Rh-immune prophylaxis failure or that transplacental hemorrhage during the pregnancy can cause immunization in the antepartum period.

Antibody screening is performed on the initial prenatal visit to detect the presence of irregular antibodies. Queenan et al. found that patients who have had blood transfusions, induced abortions, or cesarean sections have a higher incidence of irregular antibodies (25). If a history of any of these factors is elicited on the initial prenatal visit, antibody screening for irregular antibodies should be performed on the first visit with a follow-up later in pregnancy.

If an antibody is detected, following a schedule of repeat antibody screening at 24 weeks' gestation and every 2 to 4 weeks there-after, the physician can manage the problem properly. Frequently, the initial immunization is determined by detecting a saline-reacting antibody (IgM) that generally does not cross the placenta. Soon thereafter, an albumin-reacting antibody (IgG) appears. Because this antibody is a smaller molecule, it readily crosses the placenta. The IgG antibody causes erythroblastosis fetalis if the fetus has the corresponding antigen.

Once an antibody is detected, it must be identified and an antibody titer obtained. The strength of the antibody is extremely important from the standpoint of prognosis and for determining the clinical management.

MANAGEMENT OF THE IMMUNIZED PATIENT

If an antibody is detected on the initial or subsequent prenatal visit, the setting exists for erythroblastosis fetalis. Since the management and clinical outcome of the first immunized pregnancy are substantially different from a subsequent immunized pregnancy, each is discussed separately in this chapter.

THE FIRST IMMUNIZED PREGNANCY

A first immunized pregnancy is one in which an antibody is not present at the initial prenatal visit but develops during the pregnancy. In this situation, the clinician knows when the antibody first appeared, the strength of the antibody, and approximately how long the fetus has been exposed to this antibody. Because this is quantitative data, the patient, in certain instances, may be managed by monitoring the antibody titer rather than by doing amniocentesis and amniotic fluid analysis.

This consideration has particular import if the placenta is anterior and the amniocentesis poses the risk of piercing the placenta and causing further immunization. The patient with a low antibody titer runs the risk of having her immunization stimulated by transplacental hemorrhage due to the amniocentesis. It has been well established that low antibody titers are generally associated with a favorable pregnancy outcome and almost no risk of intrauterine death (1).

A cautionary note is essential. If the laboratory does not perform a large number of antibody titers and cannot give reliable and reproducible results, then, of course, it is impossible to rely on antibody titers alone. But if the laboratory performs accurate antibody titers and runs the antibody titer in duplicate with the initial serum, the clinician will have excellent information for management of the patient.

From our experience with Rh disease no patients with an antibody titer of 1:16 or less had an intrauterine death. Patients with lower antibody titers generally delivered neonates that did very well clinically, requiring little intervention other than one or two exchange transfusions, a simple transfusion, or phototherapy.

If the antibody titer was 1:32 or higher, there was no way of predicting whether the neonate would have mild, moderate, or severe disease. A *critical antibody titer* for our laboratory was established under which the patient was managed with serial antibody determinations. If the critical antibody titer is reached or surpassed, management would have to be done by amniocentesis and amniotic fluid analysis because the antibody titer no longer correctly reflects the condition of the fetus.

SUBSEQUENT IMMUNIZED PREGNANCY

In the subsequent immunized pregnancy, the antibodies are present at the onset of pregnancy. They can react with Rh-positive fetal erythrocytes even as they are produced in the bone marrow.

In the subsequent immunized pregnancy, the antibody titer and the history are useful to determine when the first amniocentesis should be performed. If the antibody titer is low and the patient has not had a severely affected infant, the initial amniocentesis should be performed at 28 to 29 weeks of gestation. If the antibody titer is high or if the patient has had a history of severe erythroblastosis fetalis, an initial amniocentesis should be performed at 24 weeks' gestation in order to assess the fetus early enough so that an intrauterine transfusion (IUT) can be performed if necessary.

Once the antibody titer is markedly elevated—for instance, 1:512—there is no advantage in following serial antibody titers, because the patient is already fully immunized. Any change, as a falling titer, has absolutely no prognostic value. Furthermore, since the patient is already fully immunized, a rise above 1:512 would not be very significant.

AMNIOTIC FLUID ANALYSIS

The Rh-antibody titer indicates the level of maternal immunization. In the first immunized pregnancy, it may be predictive of the fetal condition and the outcome of the pregnancy. Once a patient is highly immunized or during a subsequent immunized pregnancy, the fetal condition can be completely independent of a high antibody titer. For instance, if her husband is heterozygous, a highly immunized patient with a titer of 1:512 could be carrying an Rh-negative fetus. In this setting, antibody titers are not useful, and amniotic fluid analysis is the only means of determining the fetal condition.

THE AMNIOCENTESIS

In modern obstetrics, the initial amniocentesis should be preceded by an ultrasound scan to visualize the fetus, placenta, and amniotic fluid. In this way, placental trauma

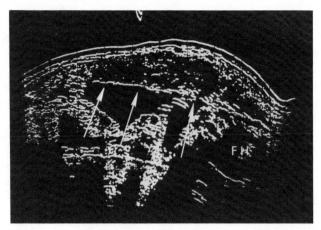

Figure 1. Longitudinal ultrasound scan showing an anteriorly implanted placenta. The arrows point to the chorionic plate. The fetal head (FH) is in the vertex presentation. A sonolucent. pocket of amniotic fluid (AF) is noted posterior to the placenta. From Queenan (21).

can usually be avoided, and the operator does not run the risk of piercing a vital fetal structure. By identifying the sonolucent amniotic fluid, the needle can be directed toward this area so that clear fluid can be obtained. To argue that the ultrasound scan is not necessary overlooks some of the basic principles of management of erythroblastosis fetalis. The major objective is to avoid placental trauma and transplacental hemorrhage when potentially the fetus is already anemic. Furthermore, hemorrhage caused by piercing the placenta may cause additional maternal immunization. The possibility of having unsuspected twins and sampling amniotic fluid from only one sac is another major argument in favor of the ultrasound scan prior to doing an amniocentesis. Figure 1 is a longitudinal scan of an anteriorly implanted placenta. The arrows point to the chorionic plate. Note the sonolucent amniotic fluid beneath the placenta.

The ultrasound scan of the uterus does not have to be repeated for each subsequent amniocentesis. Ideally, it should be done each time because the fetus may change its position considerably, even though the placenta remains stationary. If cost or convenience is a major factor, however, it may be omitted on subsequent amniocenteses.

The amniocentesis is generally done in the areas of the fetal small parts, as shown in Figure 2. If the placenta is located there, the experienced operator may attempt to aspirate amniotic fluid in the area behind the fetal neck (see Fig. 3). The head and neck must be protected with the operator's hand during the insertion of the needle so that no fetal or cord trauma can occur. A third method of performing an amniocentesis is to displace the fetal head upward in the uterus. One hand holds the fetal head up, the other hand inserts the amniocentesis needle suprapubically into the amniotic sac. The objections to this technique are that it is manipulative; there may be a slightly higher incidence of premature rupture of membranes, and the needle must be passed through an area that is difficult to render sterile by a prep.

AMNIOTIC FLUID BILIRUBIN

Once amniotic fluid is obtained, it should be centrifuged immediately to remove any particulate matter. Oxyhemoglobin contamination causes peaks at 412, 540, and 575

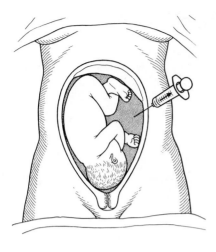

Figure 2. Diagram demonstrating amniocentesis in area of the fetal small parts. From Queenan (21b).

mμ (Fig. 4). The fluid sample must be protected from sunlight, because exposure causes a false low spectrophotometric bilirubin determination.

The amniotic fluid is scanned on a spectrophotometer to determine the bilirubin content. All patients have small amounts of bilirubin in the fluid in early pregnancy. The bilirubin concentration rises until about 22 to 26 weeks' gestation; then it decreases to term. This decrease with increasing gestation is such a constant factor that Mandelbaum (18) reported that it could be used to determine fetal maturity. He showed that the bilirubin content of amniotic fluid generally decreases markedly or disappears as the fetus reaches term (see Fig 5).

The spectrophotometric scan should be done on a continuous recording spectrophotometer. The amniotic fluid is generally scanned from 350 to 750 mμ. If no bilirubin is present, the scan will generally parallel the zero base line with a slightly increased absorbance in the lower wavelengths as seen in Figure 6. When the fluid contains bilirubin, the absorbance starts to increase at 375 mμ, reaching a peak at 450 mμ, and returns to normal at 525 mμ, as shown in Figure 7.

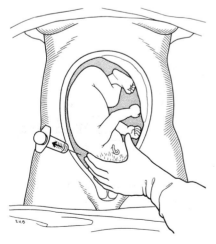

Figure 3. Diagram demonstrating amniocentesis being performed in the area behind the fetal neck. Operator's hand is shielding fetus so that the needle cannot injure it. From Queenan (21b).

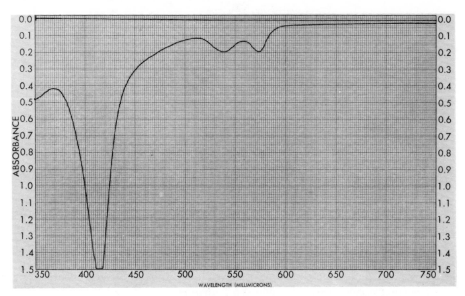

Figure 4. Spectrophotometric scan of amniotic fluid contaminated with blood. Note the peaks at 412, 540, and 575 mμ. This is characteristic of oxyhemoglobin. From Queenan (21).

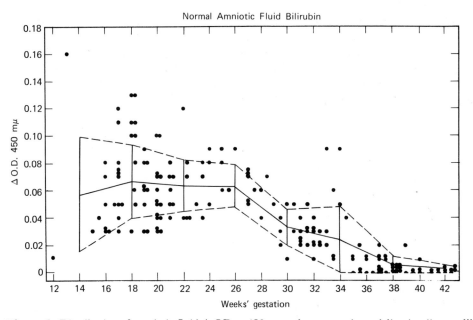

Figure 5. Distribution of amniotic fluid Δ OD at 450 mμ values on patients delivering "normal" infants. The mean values (solid line) and ±1 standard deviation (broken lines) are presented. From Queenan (21a).

456

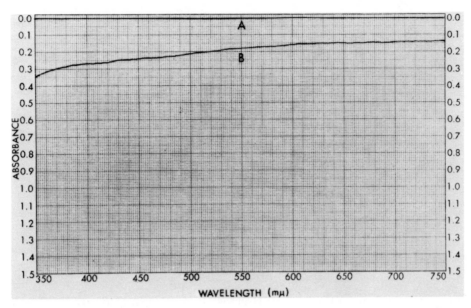

Figure 6. Spectrophotometric scan of amniotic fluid at 34 weeks' gestation (*B*). The infant was Rh-negative. Scan (*A*) is distilled water.

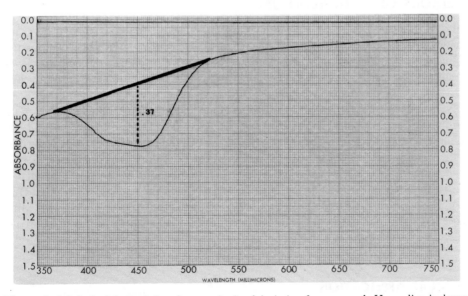

Figure 7. Method of determining the magnitude of deviation from normal. Heavy line is drawn from 375 to 525 mμ. Upright line (interrupted) indicates in absorbance the magnitude of the abnormal scan (0.37). From Queenan (22b).

457

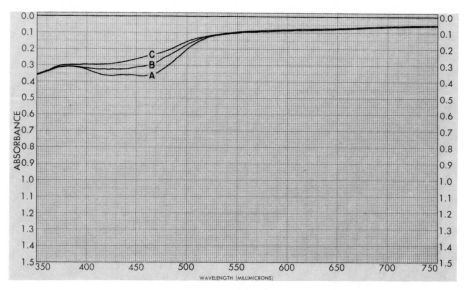

Figure 8. Three spectrophotometric scans of amniotic fluid at 27 (*A*), 32 (*B*), and 35 (*C*) weeks' gestation. Note the decrease in deviation from normal with increasing maturity. From Queenan (21).

Figure 8 shows serial amniotic fluid determinations on a patient at 27, 32 and 35 weeks' gestation. Note that the bilirubin level decreases with increasing gestation.

METHODS OF INTERPRETATION

Liley (17) showed that amniotic fluid bilirubin values placed on a three-zone graph would predict the outcome of pregnancy (Fig. 9). Generally, his method requires two amniotic fluid values on the three-zone graph in order to predict the outcome of the pregnancy. In many instances such a prediction is adequate for clinical purposes. But, occasionally, monitoring the condition of the fetus is necessary.

Numerous other investigators have proposed methods of amniotic fluid analysis in the Rh-immunized pregnancy. At the University of Louisville (21), we studied the fluid bilirubin trend to determine the severity of the disease in the fetus. If the trend of bilirubin is decreasing on serial determinations, the fetus may be Rh-negative, unaffected, or have mild or moderate erythroblastosis (Figs. 10 to 12). If the bilirubin trend is horizontal or rising, the fetus is Rh-positive and may be severely involved or may die in utero (Fig. 13). The amniotic fluid trend is an excellent predictor of the outcome of pregnancy. But, more important, the bilirubin trend monitors the condition of the fetus. It can be used to determine the week-to-week management of the Rh-immunized pregnancy.

CLINICAL APPLICATION

The amniotic fluid bilirubin trend method is based on the principle that serial bilirubin values are extremely reliable in predicting the outcome of pregnancy in the Rh-immunized patient:

1. The initial amniocentesis is performed at 28 or 29 weeks' gestation unless the obstetric history or antibody titer indicates earlier amniotic fluid evaluation.
2. Amniocentesis is repeated at 1- to 3-week intervals, based on the level of amniotic fluid bilirubin.
3. Serial AF bilirubin values are studied to determine the trend.
   a. If the trend is falling, the fetus is safe until scheduled delivery at 38 weeks' gestation (Fig. 14A)
   b. If the trend is rising or horizontal, an intrauterine transfusion is indicated between 25 and 32 weeks (Fig. 14C)
   c. If the trend is rising or horizontal, after 32 weeks' gestation, delivery is indicated (Fig. 14B)

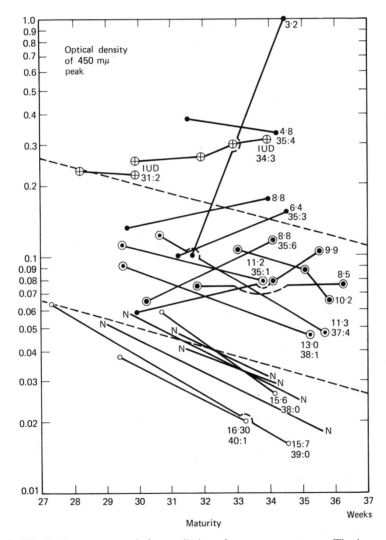

Figure 9. Liley's three-zone graph for prediction of pregnancy outcome. The hemoglobin and weeks' gestation at delivery are recorded. From Liley (16a).

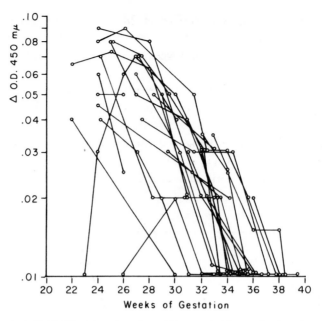

Figure 10. Amniotic fluid bilirubin values from Rh-negative immunized patients delivering Rh-negative (unaffected) infants. Values are recorded as Δ OD. Serial values are connected by lines. From Queenan (21).

4. Amniotic fluid maturity studies and ultrasound are used in conjunction with amniotic fluid bilirubin values to determine the optimal time to deliver.

Amniotic fluid analyses, when properly used, are essentially 100% effective in detecting the fetus that will die in utero. The main source of error is the patient with polyhydramnios. This condition is easy to diagnose clinically. It can cause a false low bilirubin determination, giving a false sense of security while the fetus deteriorates.

Since the various methods of management for the Rh patient are beyond the scope of this chapter, the reader is referred to *Modern Management of the Rh Problem*. (21).

TESTS OF FETAL CONDITION

Amniography

If the patient has an elevated Δ OD at 450 mμ such that the fetus is in danger of dying, additional evaluation of the fetus is necessary. From 25 to 32 weeks of gestation, the clinician may consider performing an intrauterine transfusion, whereas after 32 weeks' gestation, delivery would generally be performed if intrauterine death was imminent.

In order to evaluate the condition of the fetus, an amniogram may be performed (26). An amniocentesis is done, removing amniotic fluid for evaluation. Approximately 10 ml of Hypaque M-75* is injected into the amniotic cavity, rendering the amniotic fluid radioopaque. The patient is allowed to ambulate in order to mix the radioopaque

---

* Sodium and meglumine diatrizoate.

medium; then a roentgenogram of the abdomen is taken to study the various features that indicate the fetal condition. Figure 15 is an amniogram of a hydropic fetus in the breech presentation. Note the massive scalp edema. There is no opacification of the fetal gastrointestinal tract.

Estriols

Twenty-four-hour urinary estriols have been reported to predict fetal deterioration in disorders such as hypertensive disease, renal disease, and diabetes, particularly when there is a vascular component. Unfortunately, they have not been helpful in erythroblastosis fetalis. As a matter of fact, several investigators have been found them to be misleading. Unless there is a pathological condition in addition to the Rh disease, estriol studies are not indicated and only cause additional cost and inconvenience to the patient.

Oxytocin Challenge Test

It is reasonable to assume that the fetus undergoing a severe hemolytic anemia would have a decreased uteroplacental respiratory reserve. One would expect that the severely

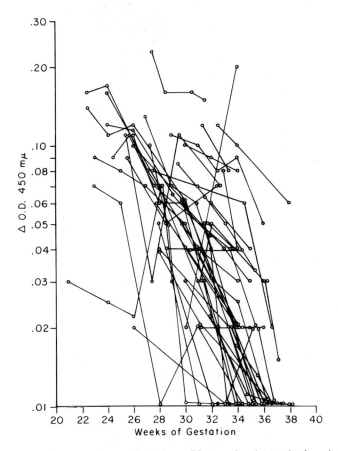

Figure 11. Amniotic fluid bilirubin values from Rh-negative immunized patients delivering infants with mild erythroblastosis fetalis (hgb 14g/100 ml or greater). Values are recorded in Δ OD at 450 mμ. Serial values are connected by lines. From Queenan (21).

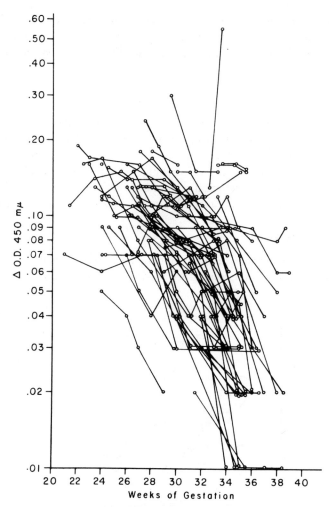

Figure 12. Amniotic fluid bilirubin values from Rh-negative immunized patients delivering infants with moderate erythroblastosis fetalis (hgb from 10 to 14 g/100 ml). Values are recorded as Δ OD. Serial values are connected by lines. From Queenan (21).

anemic fetus would respond with a positive oxytocin challenge test (OCT). At the University of Louisville, five Rh-immunized pregnancies in which the neonate had a cord blood hemoglobin of 5 g or less had negative OCTs just prior to delivery. These studies indicate that the OCT is not helpful in severe Rh disease and furthermore the negative OCT could give a false sense of security.

Fetal Movement

For many years, it has been observed that the fetus that dies because of erythroblastosis fetalis generally has markedly decreased activity prior to dying. The fetus that becomes severely hydropic also has a marked decrease in fetal activity.

The fetal activity may be determined by having the patient count how many times the fetus moves, starting with a certain hour in the morning and waiting to see how long it takes to count 20 movements. The patient may also be instructed to count fetal movements during three 1-hr periods during the day, multiplying her total by a factor to give a 12-hr rate. If there are greater than 10 movements for a 12-hr period, the fetus is in no immediate jeopardy (27).

The fetal activity may also be assessed by real time ultrasound. Generally, the mother perceives movement only when the fetus kicks. By the use of real time ultrasound, additional fetal movement may be observed that the mother does not feel. This fetal movement generally consists of arm and hand movements. The use of this modality has been helpful in ascertaining that the fetus is actively moving. This generally correlates with safety in utero for the next 24 to 48 hr.

Intrauterine Transfusion

If the amniotic fluid analysis indicates that the fetus is deteriorating between 24 and 32 weeks of gestation, an intrauterine transfusion may be indicated. Prior to performing this procedure, an amniogram is done to rule out hydrops fetalis. The likelihood of

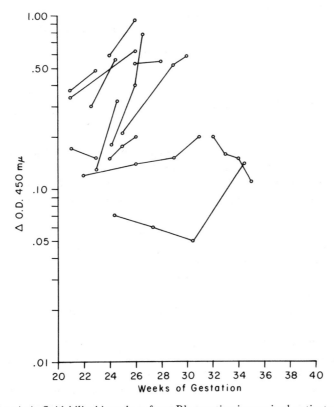

Figure 13. Amniotic fluid bilirubin values from Rh-negative immunized patients whose fetuses died in utero. Values are recorded in Δ OD at 450 mμ. Serial values are connected by lines. From Queenan (21).

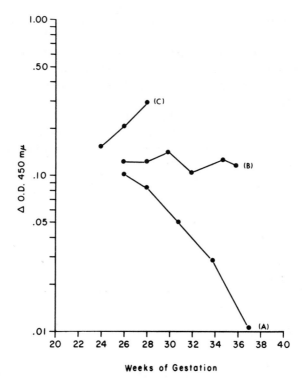

Figure 14. Illustrative examples of the various bilirubin Δ OD trend patterns. (*A*) Decreasing trend, favorable outcome; (*B*) horizontal or rising trend after 32 weeks indicates delivery; (*C*) rising trend prior to 32 weeks may indicate intrauterine transfusion.

salvaging a fetus with severe hydrops fetalis by transfusion is extremely small. Furthermore, injecting blood into the peritoneal cavity has certain inherent dangers if the fetal circulation is markedly compromised or if the fetus dies. Therefore, marked fetal hydrops should not be managed by intrauterine transfusion but by delivery.

The only indication for an intrauterine transfusion is an elevated amniotic fluid bilirubin. If an amniogram reveals that there is no scalp edema and the fetus swallows well, transfusion may be indicated. If history alone is used and an intrauterine transfusion is performed without an elevated amniotic fluid bilirubin, the operator runs the risk of transfusing an Rh-negative fetus. Therefore, an amniotic fluid bilirubin criterion is the only indication for intrauterine transfusion. In the absence of hydrops fetalis, the compromised fetus may receive anywhere from one to four transfusions. The object is to keep the fetus alive while it is maturing enough to survive after delivery.

After successful intrauterine transfusions, the fetus is evaluated for maturity. It is usually delivered at 35 to 36 weeks' gestation. By waiting longer, the clinician runs the risk of unsuspected intrauterine death. Generally, the fetus who has undergone transfusion and completes as much as 35 or 36 weeks' gestation does well after delivery. The number of exchange transfusions in the neonatal period may range from one to eight. However, some neonates do very well with a simple transfusion and as few as one or two exchange transfusions.

Maturity Studies for Delivery

The patient who has intrauterine transfusions for severe erythroblastosis fetalis is generally delivered arbitrarily at 35 or 36 weeks' gestation. The patient who is Rh-immunized but whose disease is not severe enough to require transfusion is delivered at 38 weeks' gestation, or sooner if fetal maturity or fetal deterioration occurs.

If there is any question as to the maturity of the fetus, amniotic fluid maturity studies should be performed prior to delivery. Of course, fetal BPDs would have been obtained earlier in pregnancy with the ultrasound studies prior to amniocentesis. The earlier in pregnancy the BPDs are done, the more accurate they are. This provides strong evidence that the gestational dates are correct.

Since the amniotic fluid analysis for bilirubin is commonly performed in Rh-immunized pregnancies, it is a very simple matter to obtain a lecithin/sphingomyelin ratio and creatinine level when the amniocentesis is being done prior to a planned delivery. In this way, the clinician would never be embarrassed by having delivered an infant early for Rh disease only to find that the hemolytic problem turns out to be mild but the pulmonary immaturity becomes the most critical problem. The management of the Rh-immunized pregnancy is basically a contest to see if the fetus can be kept alive in

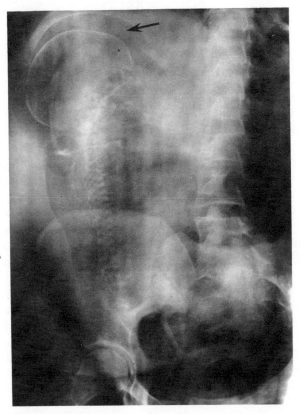

Figure 15. Amniogram of a hydropic fetus in the breech presentation. Note the massive scalp edema (arrow). There is no fetal swallowing.

utero long enough, without becoming extremely compromised hematologically, so that it can be delivered without major problems of prematurity.

Remember, however, that false mature L/S ratios have been reported following intrauterine transfusion (15) and that bloody amniotic fluid may yield falsely lowered L/S ratios (11). Respiratory distress syndrome can develop in an asphyxiated neonate despite a mature L/S ratio. (7).

The Delivery

Most Rh-immunized pregnancies can be delivered by the vaginal route on the scheduled day. Occasionally, it takes 2 days for induction. The first may accomplish softening and effacing of the cervix. The second is for induction and delivery. Obviously, electronic fetal heart rate monitoring must be performed throughout the entire time oxytocin is used. If induction appears to be prolonged or if the fetus is premature or in a precarious condition, cesarean section is the method of delivery. The neonatologist and the blood bank should be alerted well before the delivery so that cooperation can be optimal.

ILLUSTRATIVE CASES

Case History 1

A 25-year-old para 2, gravida 3, living children 1, white, Rh-negative female has a husband who is heterozygous for the Rh factor. The first pregnancy terminated in a full-term spontaneous delivery of a 7-lb male infant. No antibodies were detected during her antepartum course.

At her initial visit for the second pregnancy, it was noted she had an antibody titer of 1:64, by the indirect antiglobulin (Coombs) test. This titer rose to 1:256 at 20 weeks' and 1:512 at 24 weeks' gestation. An amniocentesis at 24 weeks showed a Δ OD of 0.20. A subsequent amniocentesis at 27 weeks' gestation indicated a Δ OD of 0.38. Eleven days later there was no fetal activity. This was prior to the advent of the intrauterine transfusion. At 29 weeks' gestation labor was induced, and a hydropic stillborn infant weighing 3 ½ lb was delivered.

During her most recent pregnancy the patient was seen initially at 6 weeks' gestation. Her antibody titer was 1:256 by the indirect antiglobulin (Coombs) test. She was seen every 4 weeks until 23 weeks' gestation, at which time an amniocentesis was performed. The Δ OD was 0.14. Subsequent amniocenteses revealed the Δ ODs to be 0.12, 0.10, and 0.08 at 26, 28, and 30 weeks' gestation. An amniogram revealed no fetal scalp edema and good fetal swallowing (Fig. 16).

At 33 weeks' gestation the Δ OD was 0.06. The patient was delivered at 36 weeks' gestation after obtaining maturity studies indicating an L/S ratio of 2.4:1 and a creatinine value of 2.1 mg%. The infant weighted 5 lb 3 oz and had a cord blood hemoglobin of 8 g%. The infant underwent three exchange transfusions and two booster transfusions and was discharged home at 3 weeks of age.

Comment

This case shows that a decreasing amniotic fluid bilirubin trend indicates a fetus that will survive. It does not necessarily indicate an Rh-negative or mildly involved fetus but

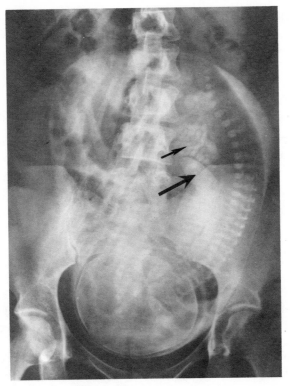

Figure 16. Amniogram of a normal fetus. Contrast material may be seen in the fetal stomach (large arrow) and in the small intestine (small arrow). From Queenan (26).

suggests that the fetus will survive if appropriate management and therapy are administered.

Case History 2

A 25-year-old para 1, gravida 3, living children 1, white, A, Rh-negative female has a husband who is heterozygous for the Rh factor. The first pregnancy was complicated by third trimester bleeding and a diagnosis of partial separation of the placenta. She had a vaginal delivery at 39 week's gestation. The infant was found to be Rh-positive with a negative direct antiglobulin (Coombs) test on the cord blood. The mother received Rh-immune prophylaxis but had no follow-up antibody studies.

The second pregnancy terminated in a spontaneous abortion at 12 weeks' gestation. She had no curettage and received no Rh-immune prophylaxis.

During the third pregnancy she was found to have an antibody titer of 1:32 at her initial office visit. Four weeks later the antibody titer was 1:256. At 24 weeks' gestation an amniocentesis was performed. The Δ OD was 0.12. This was repeated in 4 weeks and found to be 0.11. A repeat antibody titer was 1:512. Serial amniocenteses were done at 31, 34, and 36 weeks' gestation with values of 0.10, 0.09, and 0.12, respectively. At 36 weeks the L/S ratio was 2:1, and the creatinine value was 1.9 mg%. Ultrasound studies indicated that the BPD was consistent with a fetus of 36 weeks' gestation. Labor was induced. The first day was required for softening the cervix. On the second day the induction was continued, and the patient delivered a 5-lb 4-oz male infant with a cord hemoglobin of 9.4 g%. The cord blood bilirubin was 2 mg%. The infant received four exchange transfusions and two booster transfusions and was discharged home at 3.5 weeks of age.

Comment

A horizontal or rising amniotic fluid bilirubin indicates that there is severe erythroblastosis fetalis. If appropriate management is not given, the fetus may die in utero. In this case, the fetus was monitored closely with serial amniotic fluid analysis. The fetus became mature before developing severe deterioration, and delivery could be accomplished. An intrauterine transfusion was not necessary.

Case History 3

A 25-year-old para 2, gravida 3, living children 1, white, A, Rh-negative immunized female has a husband who is heterozygous for the Rh factor. The first pregnancy was uncomplicated, and the patient delivered an Rh-positive 7 ½-lb male infant. Since the delivery occurred before the development of Rh-immune prophylaxis, the patient did not receive protection.

Her second pregancy terminated in a stillborn infant at 23 weeks' gestation. Her antibody titer on her first prenatal visit was 1:256. An amniocentesis at 23 weeks' gestation produced clear, dark-yellow amniotic fluid. The Δ OD was 0.45. There were no fetal movements. Two days later fetal heart tones could not be heard with a Doptone. The patient was observed for coagulation defects. A stillborn infant was delivered following induction of labor with E_2 prostaglandin.

During the latest pregnancy the patient was seen at 6 weeks' gestation; at that time her antibody titer was 1:256. At 24 weeks' gestation the first amniocentesis was performed. The amniotic fluid was clear and pale yellow. The Δ OD was 0.11. On removing the needle a small amount of blood was aspirated. A KB stain showed no fetal erythrocytes. A subsequent amniocentesis was performed at 26 weeks; the amniotic fluid was port wine in color (Fig. 17). Each subsequent amniocentesis revealed port wine amniotic fluid. Fetal activity was excellent. At 30 weeks' gestation, 10 cc of Hypaque 75% was injected into the amniotic cavity, and an amniogram was performed. There was no scalp edema, and there was excellent fetal swallowing. The fetal activity remained excellent throughout the rest of her pregnancy. The amniotic fluid remained port wine in color. One subsequent amniogram was performed at 36 weeks, revealing no scalp edema and excellent fetal swallowing. Labor was induced at 38 weeks' gestation, with the delivery of a 7-lb 4-oz Rh-negative, female infant.

Comment

Occasionally, analysis of amniotic fluid is not possible because of blood or meconium contamination. Other modalities such as amniography, fetal activity, and antibody titers can be helpful in this dilemma.

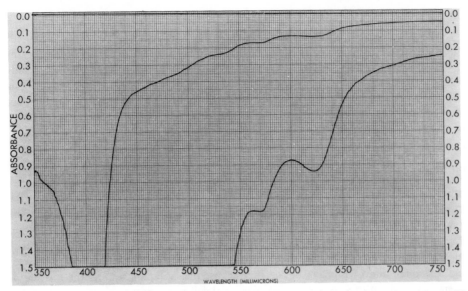

Figure 17. Spectrophotometric scan of amniotic fluid grossly contaminated with blood. The undiluted specimen is off the chart.

Case History 4

This 25-year-old para 2, gravida 4, living children 2, white, A, Rh-negative immunized female has a husband who is heterozygous for the Rh factor. Her first pregnancy ended in an emergency cesarean section for an acute abruptio placenta at 38 weeks' gestation. The infant was born anemic with an Apgar score of 4. After intensive neonatal care, the infant recovered. The patient was given one ampule (300 µg) of Rh-immune globulin. No attempt was made to determine whether a larger transplacental hemorrhage had occurred.

Her second pregnancy terminated in a spontaneous abortion at 8 weeks without a dilatation and curettage. The patient did not receive Rh-immune prophylaxis.

When she was examined for her third pregnancy, she was found to have an anti-Rh titer of 1:128 at 12 weeks' gestation. At 24 weeks her antibody titer was 1:256. An amniocentesis was performed, and the Δ OD was 0.10. At 26, 29, 33, and 37 weeks the Δ OD was 0.08, 0.05, 0.03, and 0.01, respectively. Labor was induced at 38 weeks' gestation, and a 7-lb 6-oz male infant was born with an Apgar score of 9. The cord blood was 0, Rh negative; the direct antiglobulin (Coombs) test was negative.

During her latest pregnancy, she was seen at 8 weeks' gestation, at which time her anti-Rh titer was 1:256. An amniocentesis at 24 weeks was 0.15. Ten days later, the value was 0.22. Because of the rising values, an intrauterine transfusion was performed at 26 weeks' gestation. Eighty ml of fresh, loosely packed, red blood cells were instilled into the fetal peritoneal cavity. Transfusions were repeated at 28 and 31 weeks' gestation, with the instillation of 100 and 120 ml of blood, respectively. Fetal activity was monitored carefully. Although the amniotic fluid bilirubin was evaluated following the third transfusion, it was not interpretable because of the contamination with blood and meconium. An amniogram indicated good fetal swallowing and no scalp edema.

At 35 weeks' gestation a cesarean section was performed. A 5-lb female infant with a cord blood hemoglobin of 8.8 g% and a bilirubin of 2 mg% was delivered. The infant typed O, Rh-negative, with a negative direct antiglobulin (Coombs) test. No fetal erythrocytes were found on KB stain. The infant required minimal resuscitation. The bilirubin began to rise rapidly, and the infant received its first exchange transfusion at 1 hr of age. The infant continued to have rising bilirubins and required a total of six exchanges and one booster transfusion. The infant was discharged from the hospital on the twelfth day of life, to be observed carefully for anemia.

Comment

Amniotic fluid bilirubin determinations are the only indications for an intrauterine transfusion. If the amniotic fluid bilirubin values are evaluated and the trend found to be rising, a transfusion is indicated.

Following an intrauterine transfusion, the monitoring of fetal condition is done by fetal activity and amniography. The amniotic fluid is frequently contaminated with blood and meconium. We have increasingly chosen cesarean section as the method of delivery in this situation because the risk of vaginal delivery is great.

The cord blood specimen typed O, Rh-negative, because all of the cord blood was due to the intrauterine transfusions.

CONCLUSION

Although Rh-immune globulin markedly decreases the incidence of Rh-immunization, this problem still occurs. The incidence of ABO erythroblastosis fetalis will not change. The incidence of erythroblastosis fetalis due to irregular antibodies may increase slightly due to the increased use of blood transfusions. As long as the clinician is alert to detecting the problem, the prognosis will usually be favorable.

REFERENCES

1. Allen, F. H., Diamond, L. K., and Jones, A. R.: Erythroblastosis fetalis: IX. Problems of stillbirth. *N. Engl. J. Med.* 251:453, 1954.

2. Ascari, W. Q., Allen, A. E., Baker, W. J., and Pollack, W.: Rh₀ (D) immune globulin (human). *J.A.M.A.* 205:1, 1968.

3. Ascari, W. Q., Levine, P., and Pollack, W.: Incidence of maternal Rh-immunization by ABO compatible and incompatible pregnancies. *Brit. Med. J.* 1:399, 1969.

4. Bergstrom, H., Nilsson, L. A., Nilsson, L., and Ryttinger, L.: Demonstration of Rh antigens in a 38 day old fetus. *Amer. J. Obstet. Gynecol.* 99:130, 1967.

5. Bowman, J. M.: Current problems in prophylactic treatment of Rh erythroblastosis: An invitational symposium. *J. Reprod. Med.* 6:1, 1971.

6. Chown, B.: The fetus can bleed. *Amer. J. Obstet. Gynecol.* 70:1298, 1955.

7. Donald, I. R., Freeman, R. K., Goebelsman, U., Chan, W. H., and Nakamura, R. M.: Clinical experience with the amniotic fluid lecithin/sphingomyelin ratio. *Amer. J. Obstet. Gynecol.* 115:547, 1973.

8. Finn, R., Clarke, C. A., Donohoe, W. T. A., McConnell, R. B., Sheppard, P. M., Lahane, D., and Kulke, W.: Experimental studies on the prevention of Rh hemolytic disease. *Br. Med. J.* 1:1486, 1961.

9. Freda, V. J.: The Rh problem in obstetrics and a new concept of its management using amniocentesis and spectrophotometric scanning of amniotic fluid. *Amer. J. Obstet. Gynecol.* 93:321, 1965.

10. Freda, V. J., Gorman, J. G., Galen, R. S., and Treacy, N.: The threat of Rh immunization by abortion. *Lancet* 2:147, 1970.

11. Gibbons, J. M., Huntley, T. E., Joachim, E., et al.: Amniotic fluid analysis for fetal maturity: Effect of maternal blood contamination. *Obstet. Gynecol.* 39:631, 1972.

12. Gorman, J. G., Freda, V. J., and Pollack, W.: Intramuscular injection of a new experimental γ_2 globulin preparation containing high levels of anti-Rh antibody as a means of preventing sensitization to Rh. *Proc. 9th Congr. Int. Soc. Hemat.* 2:545, 1962.

13. Kleihauer, E., Braun, H., and Betke, K.: Demonstration von fetalem haemoglobin in den erythrocytes eins blutausstrichs. *Klin. Wschr.* 35:637, 1957.

14. Landsteiner, K., and Wiener, A. S.: Agglutinable factor in human blood recognized by immune sera for rhesus blood. *Proc. Soc. Exper. Biol. (NY)* 43:223, 1940.

15. Lemons, J. A., and Jaffee, R. B.: Amniotic fluid lecithin/sphingomyelin ratio in the diagnosis of hyaline membrane disease. *Amer. J. Obstet. Gynecol.* 115:233, 1973.

16. Levine, P., and Stetson, R. E.: Unusual cases of intra-group agglutination. *J.A.M.A.* 113:126, 1939.

16a. Liley, A. W.: Liquor amnii analysis in management of pregnancy complicated by rhesus sensitization. *Amer. J. Obstet. Gynec.* 82:1359, 1961.

17. Liley, A. W.: Errors in assessment of hemolytic disease from amniotic fluid. *Amer. J. Obstet. Gynecol.* 86:458, 1963.

18. Mandelbaum, B., and Robinson, A. R.: Amniotic fluid pigment in erythroblastosis fetalis. *Obstet. Gynecol.* 28:118, 1966.

19. Mollison, P. L.: Annotation: Suppression of Rh-immunization by passively administered anti-Rh. *Brit. J. Haemat.* 14:1, 1968.

20. Ortho Diagnostics Inc.: News Bulletin. Drug recall information. June 22, 1977.

21. Queenan, J. T.: *Modern Management of the Rh Problem*, 2nd ed. Harper and Row, Hagerstown, Md., 1977.

21a. Queenan, J. T.: Amniotic fluid analysis. *Clin. Obstet. Gynecol.* 14:505, 1971.

21b. Queenan, J. T.: Amniocentesis and transamniotic fetal transfusion for Rh disease. *Clin. Obstet. Gynecol.* 9:491, 1966.

22. Queenan, J. T., and Adams, D. W.: Amniocentesis: A possible immunizing hazard. *Obstet. Gynecol.* 24:530, 1964.

23. Queenan, J. T., Gadow, E. C., and Lopes, A. C.: Role of spontaneous abortion in Rh immunization. *Amer. J. Obstet. Gynecol.* 110:128, 1971.

24. Queenan, J. T., Shah, S., Kubarych, S. F., and Holland, B.: Role of induced abortion in rhesus immunisation. *Lancet* 1:815, 1971.

25. Queenan, J. T., Smith, B. D., Haber, J. M., Jeffrey, J., and Gadow, E. C.: Irregular antibodies in the obstetric patient. *Obstet. Gynecol.* 34:767, 1969.

26. Queenan, J. T., von Gal, H., and Kubarych, S. F.: Amniography for clinical evaluation of erythroblastosis fetalis. *Amer. J. Obstet. Gynecol.* 102:264, 1968.

27. Sadovsky, E., and Polishuk, W. Z.: Fetal movements in utero. *Obstet. Gynecol.* 50:49, 1977.

28. Smith, T.: Active immunity produced by so called balanced or neutral mixtures of diphtheria toxin and antitoxin. *J. Exp. Med.* 11:241, 1909.

29. Woodrow, J. C., and Donohoe, W. T. A.: Rh-immunization by pregnancy: Results of a survey and their relevance to prophylactic therapy. *Brit. Med. J.* 4:139, 1968.

19
Neonatal Management of Erythroblastosis Fetalis

Larry N. Cook, M.D.

More than any other high-risk pregnancy condition, Rh erythroblastosis fetalis requires for its successful management integration of perinatologists and neonatologists. A combined perinatal approach maximizes quality time in utero, thereby reducing the morbidity and mortality associated with severe fetal anemia, iatrogenic prematurity, and postnatal unconjugated hyperbilirubinemia.

It has been predicted that erythroblastosis will become extinct by the 1980s. However, the large pool of immunized women currently in the child-bearing age group and the future generations produced by such phenomena as first-pregnancy immunizations and Rh-immune globulin failures will continue to present sizable numbers of involved fetuses and neonates to care teams in tertiary centers (1).

SEVERITY OF ERYTHROBLASTOSIS FETALIS

Fetal and Neonatal Bilirubin Metabolism

The fetus, like the neonate, generates bilirubin from the catabolism of hemoglobin, 1 g of hemoglobin generating approximately 35 mg of bilirubin. The high maternal to fetal plasma protein gradient facilitates rapid transplacental extraction of unconjugated fetal bilirubin and at the same time suppresses glucuronidation by the fetal liver. Bilirubin so transferred is then conjugated and excreted by the mother (2) (Fig. 1). This mechanism is so efficient that it is uncommon for the neonate to have an elevated cord blood bilirubin level. In severe erythroblastosis, particularly if coupled with placental deterioration, however, unconjugated bilirubin levels as high as 8 mg % can be seen in cord blood (3). Fetuses receiving intrauterine transfusion are often born with high levels of conjugated bilirubin, probably arising from stimulation of fetal glucuronidation coupled with decreased placental permeability to the bilirubin glucuronide (3).

An in-depth discussion of neonatal bilirubin metabolism can be found in many sources (2–4). In simple terms, indirect or unconjugated bilirubin is carried from the

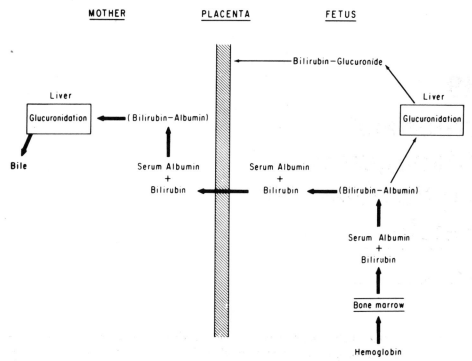

Figure 1. Antepartum excretion of bilirubin. Fetal bilirubin is transferred from fetal serum albumin through the placenta to maternal serum and then is conjugated by the maternal liver with glucuronic acid and excreted into the bile. Fetal glucuronidation is suppressed. The placenta is relatively impermeable to the glucuronide. *From* Dancis, J. Feto-maternal interaction, in Avery, G. B. (ed.): *Neonatology.* Philadelphia, Lippincott, 1975, p. 44, with permission.

reticuloendothelial system bound to albumin and must then undergo hepatic uptake, a process facilitated by acceptor proteins designated Y and Z. In liver microsomes, indirect bilirubin is conjugated with glucuronide or sulfate to direct or conjugated bilirubin. This process is mediated by the enzyme bilirubin glucuronyl transferase. Conjugation having been completed, the liver cell excretes the direct bilirubin into the bowel lumen for subsequent reduction to stercobilinogen or excretion as fecal bilirubin (5) (Fig. 2).

Toxicity of Bilirubin

Conjugated bilirubin is highly water-soluble and, therefore, readily excreted in bowel and urine fluids. Unconjugated or indirect bilirubin, on the other hand, is insoluble in aqueous solution but highly soluble in lipids. Under normal circumstances, unconjugated bilirubin is bound to plasma albumin, a function dependent on the biochemical environment as well as the quality and quantity of albumin. This binding prevents the entrance of free or unbound indirect bilirubin into the lipid-rich central nervous system.

Unconjugated bilirubin is toxic to various tissues. In the central nervous system it causes brain cell staining and necrosis, a pathologic process referred to as kernicterus. There is a particular predilection for the basal ganglia, hippocampus, and subthalamic nucleus (6). The clinical manifestations of CNS bilirubin toxicity are referred to as bilirubin encephalopathy. Affected infants exhibit early symptoms of lethargy, hypotonia, poor feeding, and high-pitched cry. Without intervention there may be progression to convulsions, pathologic posturing, and death.

Surviving infants may have mental retardation, hearing deficits, and choreoathetoid cerebral palsy. Many affected infants, particularly those of low birthweight, have no neonatal symptoms but later in childhood present with hearing deficits, perceptual handicaps, and hyperkinesis.

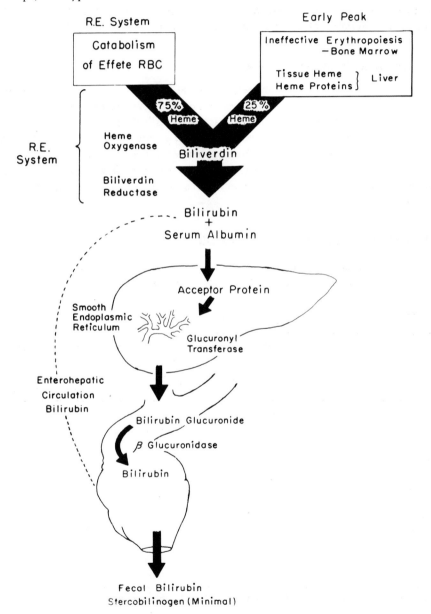

Figure 2. Neonatal bile pigment metabolism. *From* Maisels, M. J. Neonatal jaundice, in Avery, G. B. (ed.): *Neonatology.* Philadelphia, Lippincott, 1975, p. 335, with permission.

The protective binding of unconjugated bilirubin to albumin is limited by the level of serum albumin, an obvious handicap for the hydropic or preterm infant with a low albumin level. Similarly, the binding sites are not exclusive, and bilirubin must compete with nonesterified fatty acids, hematin released during hemolysis, drugs such as sulfas, and probably many unknown agents. Neonatal acidosis exerts a deleterious effect by promoting bilirubin-albumin dissociation.

Certain factors tend to increase the risk of bilirubin toxicity, perhaps by impairing binding or increasing the permeability of the central nervous system (blood-brain barrier) to indirect bilirubin. These factors include prematurity, hypothermia, acidosis, hypoglycemia, hypoxia, (4,6,7) and infection (6) (Tables I and III and Fig. 4).

Spectrum of Erythroblastosis Fetalis

In approximately 9% of Caucasion pregnancies an Rh-negative woman carries an Rh-positive fetus. Only 1 in 15 pregnancies at risk, however, results in a neonate with clinical disease (9). Fifty percent of these infants require either no treatment or treatment of mild to moderate hyperbilirubinemia with phototherapy alone. Of the remaining 50%, 25 to 30% are live-born with variable anemia but with the potential for severe hyperbilirubinemia in the absence of aggressive intervention. The remaining 20 to 25%, if not treated with an early delivery or intrauterine transfusion, become hydropic before the fortieth week (10).

Pathophysiology of Erythroblastosis Fetalis

Maternal IgG crosses the placenta and causes intravascular hemolysis and splenic sequestration of fetal erythrocytes. This results in anemia, the severity of which depends

Table I. Factors Influencing the Risk of Kernicterus

	Reduced Albumin-Binding Capacity	Competition for Binding Sites	Increased Cell Susceptibility to Bilirubin Toxicity
Prematurity	+	−	?
Hemolysis	−	+	?
Asphyxia	+	−	+
Acidosis	+	−	?
↑ NEFA	−	+	−
Cold stress	−	+	−
Starvation	−	+	−
Hypoalbuminemia	+	−	+
Hypoglycemia	−	+	?
Infection	+	−	?
Drugs	−	+	−
Male sex	−	−	?

SOURCE: From Brown, A. K. *Original Article Series* 6;22, 1970, with permission.

+ has an effect

− has no effect

? unknown

on the balance between red blood cell destruction and production. Even surviving cells may be metabolically compromised by the surface attachment of the antibody. Anemia is the main component of fetal morbidity, and extreme anemia leads to hydrops fetalis. The maternal-placental unit prevents bilirubin toxicity to the fetus.

For the neonate, the pathophysiology involves variable anemia, postnatal hyperbilirubinemia, and a variable degree of prematurity with its associated problems—hyaline membrane disease and other pathophysiologic events such as hepatic coagulopathy, hypoglycemia, congestive heart failure, and necrotizing enterocolitis.

Preparation for the Birth of a Severely Involved Neonate

The neonatal care team should be aware of the pregnancy complicated by Rh incompatibility and should make risk-benefit decisions of early delivery versus intrauterine transfusions in accordance with the expertise of the particular center. Preparation begins with the mutual decision that delivery should take place.

Prenatal Consultation
In advance of the delivery, the neonatologist should meet with the parents to present, in a calm and reassuring fashion, the potential problems to be encountered, the mechanics of dealing with these problems—i.e., assisted ventilation, exchange transfusion—and realistic expectations for the outcome for the neonate.

Preparation of the Newborn Intensive Care Unit
In the case of a planned delivery, the unit should be appropriately alerted to assure the availability of an isolette, proper equipment, and personnel.

Blood Products
The availability of blood products, in advance of the delivery, is mandatory. In our institution, O-negative frozen red cells, reconstituted in fresh AB plasma, are cross-matched against the mother for subsequent use in the neonate. In anticipation of a severely involved neonate, a unit of packed red blood cells, two units of whole blood, and several units of platelets are available at the time of delivery.

Attendance at Delivery
A neonatal care team consisting of a staff neonatologist, neonatal fellow, resident, critical care nurse, and respiratory therapist should be present at the delivery.

Resuscitation and Cardiopulmonary Stabilization
On delivery, the infant is placed in a radiant warmer, toweled dry, the upper airway suctioned, and adequate cardiopulmonary status established by whatever means are necessary, including intubation and assisted ventilation. The delivery room physical assessment, with reference to the severity of Rh disease, is performed and the cord blood laboratory evaluation requested and coordinated.

Delivery Room Assessment

Presence or Absence of Hydrops
Profound anemia, cardiac decompensation, generalized edema, particularly of the face and scalp, ascites, and pleural effusions with respiratory distress characterize hydrops

fetalis and should prompt immediate transfer to the critical care facility after cardiopulmonary stabilization.

Assessment of Cardiopulmonary Status

As with any neonate, Apgar scores should be recorded. Suctioning of the airway, drying to prevent evaporative heat loss, and specific treatment for asphyxia, pleural effusions, compromising ascites, or prematurity with early hyaline membrane disease should be initiated. Because of the underlying handicap of decreased red cell mass and the role of acidosis and hypoxia in facilitating bilirubin-albumin dissociation and increased permeability of blood-brain barrier to bilirubin, resuscitation should be prompt and efficient.

Assessment of Gestational Age

In prehydropic and hydropic infants as well as those receiving intrauterine transfusion, birthweight is not a reliable indicator of gestational age. Using the physical and neurologic parameters of Lubchenco (13), a gestational age should be assigned, since this affects care decisions, such as the critical level of bilirubin for exchange transfusion, and indicates the likelihood of complications, such as hyaline membrane disease and hypoglycemia.

Pallor and Color

Pallor correlates with the magnitude of anemia, the quantitator of severity of fetal disease. Only extreme anemia is recognizable, and most infants with mild to moderate anemia have normal color.

Jaundice

Because of placental clearance of bilirubin, most infants are not icteric at birth. In severe disease with cord bilirubin levels of 6 mg % or higher, early facial icterus can be detected by blanching the skin of the forehead or tip of the nose. The presence of icterus at birth is an indication of severe hemolytic disease.

Hepatosplenomegaly

In an effort to compensate for the antibody-mediated destruction of red cells, the fetus reverts to a more primitive form of erythropoiesis, the production of red blood cells in the liver and spleen—extramedullary hematopoiesis. A massive enlargement of these viscera often occurs. Because of the predisposition to rupture, palpation of the spleen should be done gently. Generally, the more severe the disease, the larger the liver and spleen.

Purpura

In association with severe erythroblastosis, thrombocytopenia is often seen with purpura visible shortly after birth or bruisability at sites of manipulation. The etiology of the thrombocytopenia is unknown, but it is probably secondary to marrow displacement of megakaryocytes by red blood cell precursors.

Congenital Malformation

No data are available to support an increased incidence of congenital malformations in erythroblastotic infants; however, as with all neonates an examination to exclude complicating congenital malformations is indicated.

Delivery Room Laboratory Assessment

Cord blood studies provide little more than the confirmation of Rh incompatability and base line hemoglobin and bilirubin values on which further treatment—phototherapy or exchange transfusion—will depend. In the baby with severe disease, the cord blood studies provide the basis for a logical sequence of care. Lab slips should be made out in advance, the laboratory placed on standby, and a runner should be in attendance at delivery to carry the specimen to the lab and bring blood to the critical care unit in time to meet the baby.

The important parameters in cord blood include:

Type/Rh/Coombs—Direct and Indirect

Under normal circumstances, the presence of anti-Rh globulin is confirmed by a positive direct and indirect Coombs test. In situations of severe sensitization, it is possible for the fetal red cells to be so completely covered with antibody as to give a negative direct Coombs test and even a false negative result for Rh typing (3). Similarly in the case of multiple intrauterine transfusions, the baby may type Rh-negative because of almost complete replacement of its own cells with donor erythrocytes.

Hemoglobin

The hemoglobin concentration is the most accurate index of the severity of fetal disease. In severe disease, however, borderline normal hemoglobin can be found when bone marrow and extramedullary hematopoiesis have effectively compensated for severe hemolysis. Near-normal hemoglobin values do not ensure against severe hemolysis and malignant indirect hyperbilirubinemia requiring multiple exchange transfusions. In hydropic infants, hemoglobin concentrations of 3 to 6 g % may be seen, and normal values may be seen in neonates undergoing successful intrauterine transfusion (14). The role of the cord hemoglobin in determining the initial treatment is discussed under "Treatment."

Reticulocyte Count and Nucleated Red Blood Cell Count

These are measurements of the efforts of the hemotopoietic system to compensate for destruction of red blood cells. Reticulocyte counts as high as 30 to 40% and nucleated red blood cell counts as high as 100 NRBC/100 WBC can be seen in severe disease (3). Generally, the more severe the disease, the higher these values.

Platelet Count

For reasons previously discussed, severe disease often is associated with platelet counts as low as 20,000 to 30,000 (3). Hepatic extramedullary hematopoiesis often interferes with the ability to synthesize vitamin K–dependent clotting factors. Coupled with potential hypoxic capillary damage seen in extreme anemia, the potential for a hemorrhagic diathesis is great, and prophylaxis is required.

Bilirubin—Direct and Indirect

The majority of erythroblastotic neonates do not have significant cord blood bilirubin elevations; however, in severe disease, levels of 4.5 to 6.0 mg % and occasionally as high as 8 mg % are seen (3). These levels are important in deciding whether to use immediate or delayed exchange transfusion (see "Treatment"). In neonates receiving intrauterine transfusions, it is not uncommon to see significantly elevated levels of direct bilirubin (4).

Total Protein

Levels of cord total protein decrease with decreasing gestational age (15). Severe hypoproteinemia occurs with hydrops fetalis. Knowledge of the total protein level, particularly albumin concentration, is essential in evaluating tolerance to indirect hyperbilirubinemia.

Glucose

Hyperinsulinism due to beta cell hyperplasia of the pancreas is seen in association with severe erythroblastosis fetalis (16). The mechanism of hyperinsulinism is speculated to be the inactivation of circulating fetal insulin by the products of fetal red cell destruction (17). A base line glucose concentration facilitates appropriate prophylaxis against hypoglycemia in an erythroblastotic neonate.

Respiratory Gas Concentration

Abnormalities are often seen in hydropic infants with severe anemia, cardiac decompensation, and respiratory embarrassment from extravascular fluid collections—ascites and pleural effusions. In asphyxiated infants or the premature infant with hyaline membrane disease, cord blood gases or blood obtained in the delivery room by arterial puncture allow for early correction of acidosis and hypoxia.

Hemoglobin Electrophoresis

In babies receiving intrauterine transfusion, it is our custom to send cord blood for hemoglobin electrophoresis. The percentage of adult hemoglobin is a measure of the efficiency of uptake of transfused blood as well as an indirect quantitation of the number of surviving fetal cells available for hemolysis.

Treatment of the Neonate with Erythroblastosis Fetalis

An approach to the treatment of erythroblastosis fetalis must take into consideration the severity of the disease, the presence of complicating factors, and the many treatment modalities available (Fig. 3).

Treatment of the Mildly Involved Neonate

Fifty percent of erythroblastotic neonates fall into this category. A severe fetal or neonatal hemolytic process is not present. These babies are born usually at term with normal cord hemoglobins and bilirubins and a positive Coombs test. Postnatally they experience an insignificant drop in hemoglobin concentration and mild hyperbilirubinemia. They can be monitored at frequent intervals with the institution of phototherapy on rate-of-rise criteria or when critical peak bilirubin levels are reached. Prophylactic phototherapy from birth coupled with careful laboratory monitoring is also acceptable management.

These babies are susceptible to the latent anemia of erythroblastosis fetalis. This is a consequence of the physiologic anemia associated with bone marrow arrest that occurs in all neonates and the slow hemolysis secondary to the persistence of anti-D (Rh) globulin, which has a 28-day half-life (9). These infants should be followed with serial hemoglobins for 6 weeks after discharge with transfusions as necessary for significant anemia.

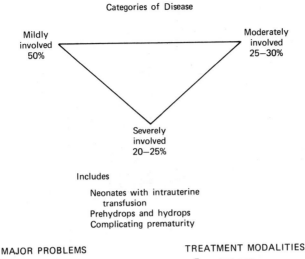

Figure 3. Treatment of erythroblastosis fetalis.

Treatment of the Moderately Involved Neonate

This group of infants constitutes 25% of erythroblastotic neonates. Most represent scheduled deliveries at 38 weeks of gestation and by definition do not have intrauterine transfusions, hydrops, or significant prematurity. They have a variable but not compromising cord blood hemoglobin, usually in the range of 10 to 12 g %, strongly positive Coombs tests, high reticulocyte counts, and borderline cord bilirubin concentrations in the 4 to 5 mg % range. As a rule postnatal hyperbilirubinemia is severe.

Infants in this group must be considered for immediate exchange transfusion. Precise criteria for exchange transfusion vary from center to center (5,6,18). Figure 4 and Tables II and III demonstrate some of the many protocols for immediate exchange, delayed exchange, and repeat exchange transfusion.

There is general agreement that if the cord blood hemoglobin concentration is less than 12 g % or if the cord bilirubin is greater than 5 mg %, an immediate exchange transfusion is indicated (5,6,18). It must be appreciated that the first exchange transfusion has as its goal the removal of sensitized erythrocytes (85% removed in the first double-volume exchange) and achieves as an additional benefit the establishment of a more favorable hemoglobin concentration. The removal of a moderate amount of bilirubin occurs. Repeat exchange transfusions are for the purpose of bilirubin removal and control.

In situations where an immediate exchange transfusion is not clearly indicated—hemoglobin 12 to 14 g % and bilirubin 4 to 5 mg %—vigorous phototherapy should be instituted, and, there should be careful lab surveillance of hemoglobin and bilirubin concentrations, with determinations made every 4 hr. The rate-of-rise criteria of Diamond (Fig. 5) are generally accepted with appropriate modification for the

Table II. Need for Exchange Transfusion in Infants With a Positive Coombs Test

	Observe	Consider Exchange	Do Exchange
At birth:			
History of previous offspring	No need for exchange transfusion	Exchange transfusion necessary for kernicterus	Death or near death from erythroblastosis
Maternal Rh antibody titer	<1:64	>1:64	
Clinical situation	Apparently normal	Induced or spontaneous delivery of premature infant	Jaundice, fetal hydrops
Cord hemoglobin	>14 g/100 ml	12–14 g/100 ml	<12 g/100 ml
Cord bilirubin	<4 mg/100 ml	4–5 mg/100 ml	>5 mg/100 ml
After birth:			
Capillary blood hemoglobin	>12g/100 ml	<12 g/100 ml	<12 g/100 ml and falling in first 24 hr
Serum bilirubin	<18 mg/100 ml	18–20 mg/ml	20 mg/100 ml in first 48 hr or 22 mg/100 ml on two successive determinations at 6- to 8-hour intervals after 48 hr Clinical signs suggesting kernicterus at any time or any bilirubin level

SOURCE: From McKay, R. J. *Pediatrics* 33:763, 1964.

Table III. Indications for Exchange Transfusion at the Albert Einstein College of Medicine*

Birthweight (*g*)	*<1250*	*1250 to 1499*	*1500 to 1999*	*2000 to 2499*	*2400 and Up*
Uncomplicated course	13+	15	17	18	20
Complicated course†	10	13	15	17	18

SOURCE: From Lee, K., Gartner, L. M., Eidelman, A. I., and Ezhuthachan, S. Unconjugated hyperbilirubinemia in very low birth weight infants, in *Symposium on the Tiny Baby: Clinics in Perinatology,* Dweck, H. S. (ed.). Philadelphia, W. B. Saunders Co., 1977, pp. 305–320, with permission.

* Total serum bilirubin concentrations, mg per dl.

† Complicated course includes Apgar score 3 or less at 5 minutes; Pao_2 less than 40 mm Hg for over 1 hr; pH 7.15 or less for over 1 hr; rectal temperature 35°C or less; serum albumin content 2.5 g/dl or less; signs of the central nervous system deterioration; proved sepsis or meningitis; evidence of hemolytic anemia; or birthweight of 1000 g or less.

presence of mitigating factors. As a rule, as soon as it is established that a critical level will in time be reached, the exchange transfusion should be performed. In a tertiary care center, where these procedures are done frequently, the morbidity and mortality are minimal. The risk-benefit ratio clearly favors the procedure. Undue delay allows for large tissue accumulations of bilirubin, resulting in rapid rebound as postexchange bili-·rubin equilibrates from the tissues back into the vascular space, a phenomenon usually necessitating additional exchanges. A mounting body of data indicates that the duration of time spent at a critical bilirubin concentration is more significant in bilirubin toxicity than the peak bilirubin concentration (19).

Repeat exchange transfusions are done in recognition of the rebound phenomenon and to avoid reaching the critical bilirubin level in a particular baby, modifying factors having been taken into consideration. Generally, a steady exchange transfusion over 60 to 75 min results in maximum bilirubin removal. The rebound value at 4 hr after the exchange transfusion approximates two-thirds of the immediate preexchange value. Albumin priming—administration of 1 g/kg of salt-poor albumin to the baby 1 hr prior to the exchange or the addition of albumin to the bag of exchange transfusion blood—is recommended to increase the efficiency of bilirubin removal (10).

Phototherapy is used to decrease the number and frequency of additional exchange transfusions. A discussion of phototherapy physiology as well as theoretical and real side effects can be obtained in many standard reference texts (5,6).

This moderately affected group of babies is similarly susceptible to the latent anemia referred to in the mildly affected group.

Treatment of the Severely Involved Neonate

This group of neonates presents the greatest challenge to the neonatologist. It includes the neonates who have received single or multiple intrauterine transfusions and also includes those with hydrops fetalis or bordering on that state (prehydrops). Prematurity

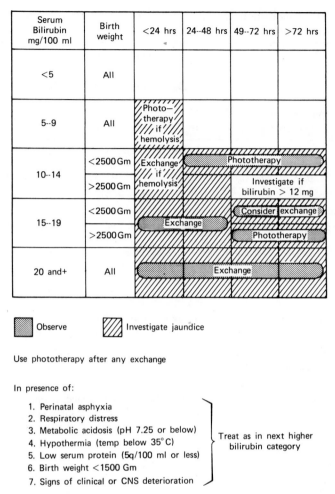

Serum Bilirubin mg/100 ml	Birth weight	<24 hrs	24–48 hrs	49–72 hrs	>72 hrs
<5	All				
5–9	All	Photo— therapy if hemolysis			
10–14	<2500 Gm	Exchange if hemolysis	Phototherapy		
	>2500 Gm			Investigate if bilirubin > 12 mg	
15–19	<2500 Gm	Exchange		Consider exchange	
	>2500 Gm			Phototherapy	
20 and+	All	Exchange			

▨ Observe   ▧ Investigate jaundice

Use phototherapy after any exchange

In presence of:

1. Perinatal asphyxia
2. Respiratory distress
3. Metabolic acidosis (pH 7.25 or below)
4. Hypothermia (temp below 35°C)
5. Low serum protein (5g/100 ml or less)
6. Birth weight <1500 Gm
7. Signs of clinical or CNS deterioration

} Treat as in next higher bilirubin category

Figure 4. From Maisels, M. J., Neonatal jaundice, in Avery, G. B. (ed.): *Neonatology.* Philadelphia, Lippincott, 1975, p. 335, with permission.

with its associated problems, chiefly respiratory immaturity, is an inevitable consequence of scheduled early delivery. The high incidence of associated problems and complications requires very sophisticated monitoring, diagnostic, and treatment procedures. These infants are usually quite ill from the moment of birth. After delivery room assessment and stabilization, they are transferred to the critical care area. Most neonates in this group are placed immediately on life support with endotracheal assisted ventilation or external positive airway pressure, i.e., CPAP. It is our practice to insert both umbilical artery and umbilical vein catheters immediately. The arterial line is connected to a blood pressure transducer, and arterial respiratory gases are monitored frequently. The venous line is connected to a CVP monitor. Either line can be used for infusion or administration of drug or for exchange transfusion. By the time the catheters are placed, the stat lab work and blood for exchange should be available. Additional lab studies include Dextrostix, coagulogram (PT, PTT, fibrinogen), and repeat blood gases.

Prophylaxis against hypoglycemia is achieved with an infusion of 10% dextrose in water. All infants receive 1 to 2 mg of intravenous vitamin K (Aquamephyton). Acidosis is treated with adjustments in assisted ventilation or the slow careful infusion of one-half strength sodium bicarbonate. An admission chest and abdominal radiograph is obtained to evaluate catheter placement, heart size, and the presence of effusions, i.e., pleural and peritoneal. At this point, in hydropic infants, emergency paracentesis or thoracentesis is often necessary to relieve respiratory embarrassment.

The immediate problem for these infants is an overwhelming anemia, often as extreme as 3 g % in the hydropic infant. In a hydropic infant digitalization and diureses with lasix are begun immediately. In all babies in this group, except some born after intrauterine transfusion who have excellent hemoglobins, a packed cell, limited volume,

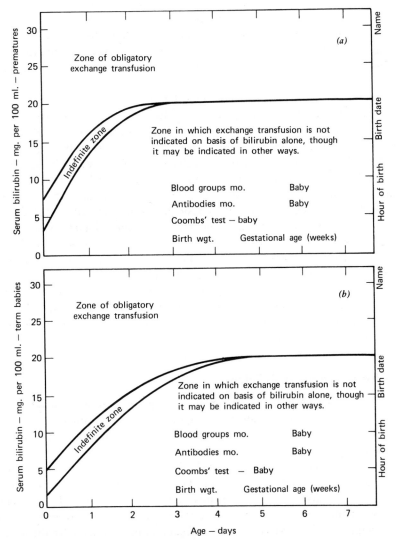

Figure 5. Bilirubin charts for term and premature newborns. (Courtesy of Dr. Louis K. Diamond and the Blood Grouping Laboratory, Boston.)

usually isovolumetric exchange transfusion is done with considerable speed to achieve a hemoglobin concentration of at least 12 g %.

In the hydropic infant, massive intravascular overloading may occur because of the protein infusion contained in the packed cells. Vigorous diuresis, increases in positive airway pressure to combat pulmonary edema, and monitoring of MAP and CVP are critical at this time.

Having accomplished the packed red blood cell exchange transfusion, an hour or so can be taken for stabilization of acid-base status and other parameters. As soon as the newborn is stable, a double-volume whole blood exchange transfusion (in our institution using O-negative frozen red blood cells reconstituted in fresh AB plasma) is done to remove sensitized erythrocytes. Platelet counts that are low or marginal are further reduced by the washout phenomenon of the exchange transfusion, and our usual custom is to conclude the first exchange transfusion with the infusion of a unit of platelets.

The double-volume exchange transfusion having been completed, the neonate is placed under phototherapy and monitored closely until the absolute bilirubin value or the rate of rise justifies an additional exchange transfusion. As a rule, multiple exchange transfusions, as many as twelve in our experience, may be required for neonates in this group.

These infants must be carefully monitored for the problems associated with severe erythroblastosis fetalis and extreme prematurity: hypoglycemia, congestive heart failure, thrombocytopenia and hepatic coagulopathy, hypocalcemia, electrolyte disturbance, hyaline membrane disease, intracranial hemorrhage, and splenic rupture.

A particularly catastrophic occurrence in this group of infants is the vascular bowel catastrophe known as necrotizing enterocolitis (10). Undoubtedly, bowel hypoperfusion secondary to anemia, bowel hypoxia, variable vascular dynamics brought about by multiple exchange transfusions as well as basic prematurity are all related (20–22). We tend to be very conservative in initiating feedings in these infants, since necrotizing enterocolitis is seldom seen without the presence of substrate (milk) in the bowel (20). Usually these infants are kept on 1 to 2 weeks of parenteral nutrition following the last exchange transfusion; then feedings are carefully initiated.

Obviously, the degree of instrumentation that these neonates are subjected to provides multiple opportunities for nosocomial infection. Although it is not our custom to use prophylactic antibiotics in these children, we maintain continuous surveillance for infection and treat when indicated.

Outlook for Erythroblastosis Fetalis

As in all aspects of neonatal care, our goal is not merely survival but intact survival. For infants in the mild and moderate categories, with appropriate management the prognosis for growth and development differs little from that of control populations without the disease.

The true measure of our efforts is seen in the outcome of the most severe neonates, i.e., those receiving intrauterine transfusion. Here risk factors like extreme prematurity, hyaline membrane disease, severe anemia, and maximum hyperbilirubinemia are greatest. Bowman, reporting on 87 intrauterine transfusion survivors with extended follow-up, found that 74 were completely normal and in the remainder the incidence of mental retardation, cerebral palsy, and major handicaps is very limited (10). Data from our own institution (23) and several others are in agreement (24,25).

Clearly the extraordinary efforts expended on these infants have not only resulted in minimizing mortality but also achieved minimum morbidity with excellent quality of life in the survivors.

REFERENCES

1. Naiman, J. L.: Current management of hemolytic disease of the newborn infant. *J. Peds.* 80:1049–1059, 1972.

2. Davies, J.: Feto-maternal interaction, in Avery, G. B. (ed.): *Neonatology.* Philadelphia, Lippincott, 1975, pp. 44–45.

3. Oski, F. A., and Naiman, J. L.: Erythroblastosis fetalis, in *Hematologic Problems in the Newborn.* Philadelphia, W. B. Saunders, 1972, pp. 176–236.

4. Maisels, M. J.: Bilirubin: On understanding and influencing its metabolism in the newborn infant. *Pediat. Clin. North Am.* 19:447, 1972.

5. Maisels, M. J.: Neonatal jaundice, in Avery, G. B. (ed.): *Neonatology.* Philadelphia, Lippincott, 1975, pp. 335–377.

6. Lee, K., Gartner, L. M., Eidelman, A. F., and Ezhuthachan, S.: Unconjugated hyperbilirubinemia in very low birth weight infants, in *Symposium on The Tiny Baby: Clinics in Perinatology,* Dweck, H. S. (ed.). Philadelphia, W. B. Saunders, 1977, pp. 305–320.

7. Brown, A. K.: Variations in the management of neonatal hyperbilirubinemia: Impact on our understanding of fetal and neonatal physiology, in Bergsma, E. (ed.): *Bilirubin Metabolism in the Newborn: Birth Defects: Original Article Series,* 6:22, 1970.

8. Odell, G. B.: Studies in kernicterus: I. The protein binding of bilirubin. *J. Clin. Invest.* 38:823, 1959.

9. Oski, F. A.: Hematologic problems, in Avery, G. B. (ed.): *Neonatology.* Philadelphia, Lippincott, 1975, pp. 379–422.

10. Bowman, J. M.: Rh erythroblastosis fetalis 1975, in *Current Problems in Pediatric Hematology,* Oski, F. A., Jaffe, E. R., and Miescher, P. A. (eds.). New York, Grune & Stratton, Inc., 1975, pp. 29–48.

11. Abrahamov, A., and Diamond, L. K.: Erythrocyte glycolysis in erythroblastotic newborns. *Am. J. Dis. Child.* 99:202, 1960.

12. Schrier, S. L., Moore, L. D., and Chiapella, A. P.: Inhibition of human erythrocyte membrane mediated ATP synthesis by anti-D antibody. *Am. J. Med. Sci.* 256:340, 1968.

13. Lubchenko, L. O.: Assessment of gestational age and development at birth. *Pediat. Clin. North Am.* 17:129, 1970.

14. Queenan, J. T.: Intrauterine transfusion, in *Modern Management of the Rh Problem,* Queenan, J. T (ed.): New York, Harper and Row, 1977, pp. 149–190.

15. Andrews, B. F.: Amniotic fluid studies to determine maturity, in *Ped. Clin. North Am.: The Small-for Date Infant,* Andrews, B. F. (ed.). Philadelphia, W. B. Saunders Co., 1970, pp. 49–67.

16. Barrett, C. T., and Oliver, T. K., Jr.: Hypoglycemia and hyperinsulinism with erythroblastosis fetalis. *New Eng. J. Med.* 278:1260, 1968.

17. Steinke, J., Gries, F. A., and Driscoll, S. G.: In vitro studies of insulin inactivation with reference to erythroblastosis fetalis. *Blood* 30:359, 1967.

18. McKay, R. J.: Current status of exchange transfusion in newborn infants. *Pediatrics* 32:763, 1964.

19. Odell, G. B., Storey, G. N. B., and Rosenberg, L. A.: Studies in kernicterus: III. The saturation of serum proteins with bilirubin during neonatal life and its relationship to brain damage at five years. *J. Peds.* 76:12, 1970.

20. Barlow, B., Santulli, T. V., Heird, W. C., Pitt, J., Blanc, W. A., and Schullinger, J. N.: An experimental study of acute neonatal enterocolitis: The importance of breast milk. *J. Ped. Surg.* 9:587–594, 1974.

21. Frantz, I. D., L'Heureux, P., Engle, R. R., and Hunt, C. E.: Necrotizing enterocolitis. *J. Peds.* 86:259–263, 1975.

22. Suntulli, T. V., Schullinger, J. N., Heird, W. C., Gongaware, R. D., Wigger J., Barlow, B., Blanc, W. A., and Berdon, W. E.: Acute necrotizing enterocolitis in infancy: A review of 64 cases. *Pediatrics* 55:376–387, 1975.

23. Franco, S., and Andrews, B. F.: Reduction of cerebral palsy by neonatal intensive care, in *The Newborn: Pediatric Clin. North Am.* 24, B. F. Andrews (ed.). Philadelphia, W. B. Saunders Co., 1977.

24. Gregg, G. S., and Hutchinson, D. L.: Developmental characteristics of infants surviving fetal transfusion. *J.A.M.A.* 209:1059, 1969.

25. Phibbs, R. H., Harvin, D., Jones, G., Talbot, C., Cohen, M., Crowther, D., and Tooley, W. H.: Development of children who had received intrauterine transfusions. *Pediatrics* 47:689, 1971.

20
Thyroid and Parathyroid Diseases in Pregnancy

Jorge H. Mestman, M.D.

Disease of the thyroid gland is one of the most common medical problems found during pregnancy. In addition to the well-known changes in thyroid function tests that occur in pregnancy, signs and symptoms occurring normally in pregnancy may mimic the clinical picture found in disorders of the thyroid gland. An understanding of the relationship between mother and fetus is helpful when therapy for thyroid disorders is under consideration. Recent advances in our knowledge of thyroid metabolism in the fetus and the newborn have helped in the diagnosis of thyroid disorders early in life.

THYROID PHYSIOLOGY IN NORMAL PREGNANCY

The thyroid gland enlarges during pregnancy, but prevalence figures for thyroid enlargement vary with geographical area and also with the clinical criteria used to define goiter (1). The greater incidence of goiter among pregnant women in Scotland as compared with pregnant women in Iceland has been attributed to the high iodine intake in the latter (2,3).

The reason for this enlargement of the thyroid gland is unclear, although alterations in iodine metabolism and the production of placental thyroid stimulators may be involved. Human chorionic gonadotropin (hCG) has thyroid-stimulating activity; whether this hormone plays a role in thyroid enlargement is a matter of speculation at this time (4).

It is a well-known fact that during pregnancy there is an increase in total serum thyroxine (T_4) and total serum triiodothyronine (T_3). Since the work of Doweling et al. (5) it is known that this increase in serum thyroid hormones is caused by increases in thyroxine-binding globulin (TBG) due to an increase in estrogen production. In spite of this increase in total serum thyroxine, the amount of free hormone levels remains the same.

Ingested dietary iodine is reduced to iodide in the gastrointestinal tract. In the thyroid gland it is oxidized and bound to tyrosine. Mono- and diiodotyrosine combine to form the iodothyronines thyroxine (T_4) and triiodothyronine (T_3). Under the influence

489

of thyroid-stimulating hormone (TSH), T_4 and T_3 are released into the circulation, where they become bound to serum proteins (TBG, thyroxine-binding prealbumin, and albumin).

About 60% of thyroxine is bound to thyroxine-binding globulin, 30% to thyroxine-binding prealbumin (TBPA), and the rest to albumin. Serum TBG doubles between 8 and 12 weeks of pregnancy and rises progressively until term (6–8). Levels return to normal during the 6 weeks after delivery.

Changes in the concentration of thyroxine-binding prealbumin (TBPA) have been measured during pregnancy, and they show only a slight decrease. The normal binding capacity of TBG ranges from 19 to 30 μg per 10 ml and doubles during pregnancy. In spite of the elevation in serum thyroxine in the course of pregnancy, the concentration of the metabolically active or free hormone is not significantly different from that in nonpregnant women (9,10). However, slightly increased (11) or decreased values (8) have been reported. The free or unbound fraction exerts its physiological action by binding to nuclear receptors in the cell, initiating new protein synthesis.

The metabolism of thyroxine in pregnancy is altered because of the increase in TBG (5). This increase in thyroxine-binding capacity produces a decrease in the fractional rate of thyroxine turnover, which is about 10% of the total body pool of T_4 per day in nonpregnant subjects. However, the absolute rate of thyroid hormone degradation is unchanged because of the increase in total serum thyroxine concentration. Dowling et al. (12) found that net T_4 turnover and thyroid hormone requirements were unchanged during normal human pregnancy.

Serum triiodothyronine (T_3) is secreted by the thyroid gland. However, most of the circulating T_3 is derived from peripheral conversion of circulating serum thyroxine (T_4) (13,14). Triiodothyronine has weaker affinity for TBG; therefore its volume of distribution is greater, and the turnover is more rapid. It has been calculated that 40% of circulating T_4 is converted into T_3.

Thyroglobulin is the storage form of the thyroid hormone in the thyroid gland. After stimulation by TSH, T_4 and T_3 are released into the circulation. TSH exerts its effects by binding to a specific receptor on the thyroid cell membrane; binding of TSH activates the intracellular enzyme adenyl cyclase, which converts ATP to cyclic AMP. Cyclic AMP then initiates a series of biochemical events that ultimately results in stimulation of thyroid hormone production (15). The secretion of TSH is stimulated by TRH (thyrotropin releasing hormone), which is produced by the hypothalamus. The feedback control of TSH secretion appears to operate at both the pituitary and hypothalamic levels. A decrease in thyroid hormone levels results in enhanced TSH secretion, and elevated concentrations of thyroid hormone suppress TSH secretion.

The effect of TRH has been investigated in normal persons and in pathological situations. Administration of TRH intravenously in doses of 100 to 500 μg produces an increase in serum TSH levels; the peak occurs 15 to 30 min after administration of the releasing hormone (16).

The effect in pregnancy was studied by several groups. Although Burrow found an exaggerated TSH response in patients 16 to 20 weeks pregnant but not in patients 6 to 12 weeks pregnant (17), Kannan et al. (18) found a normal increase in TSH responsiveness to TRH.

Whether plasma TSH levels are normal or elevated in pregnancy has not been resolved yet. Plasma TSH has been reported to be elevated early in pregnancy, returning to normal in the second half of gestation (9). However, significant elevations throughout pregnancy and even in the early puerperium have also been reported (18). Early reports of elevated serum TSH (19) might have represented cross-reactivity with hCG. Although slightly elevated, serum TSH values are within the normal limits as compared with nonpregnant women.

A group of patients with trophoblastic tumors have been reported in whom thyroid function tests were abnormally high. Some of these patients presented with hyperthyroid symptoms and signs (20). It appears that human chorionic gonadotropin (hCG) has thyrotropic activity. Although it is a very weak thyrotropin, the very high concentration achieved in patients with trophoblastic disease can cause significant thyroid stimulation and eventual hyperthyroidism. Hershman et al. (21) have calculated that hCG is only 1/4000 as potent as pituitary TSH on a molecular basis.

Normal full-term placentas also contain various amounts of a thyroid stimulator with a molecular size and structure similar to that of human TSH. This human chorionic thyrotropin (hCT) does not cross-react with human TSH but does so with bovine TSH. Highly purified hCT has a potency that is about 10 to 20% of that of human pituitary TSH. The role of placental thyrotropin in the regulation of thyroid function is unknown and only a matter of speculation at present (21). Serum concentration of hCT is low, its physiological role is not known.

THYROID FUNCTION TESTS IN PREGNANCY

In the past few years the development of new techniques for the direct quantitation of hormones in blood have improved the diagnosis of thyroid diseases. Tests of thyroid hormones may be divided into two groups: (1) those which measure the levels of circulating thyroid hormone and (2) tests for circulating thyroid hormone binding proteins.

Several methods are available for the direct determination of serum thyroxine (T_4). Tests like the protein-bound iodine (PBI), the butanol-extractable iodine (BEI), and thyroxine quantitation by column methods have been superseded by new techniques. These new techniques are specific for the measurement of circulating T_4 levels. Radioimmunoassay techniques or the competitive protein-binding displacement assay are the most commonly used at present. These methods have the advantage of not being influenced by inorganic iodine or organic nonthyroxine iodine contamination. Measurement of serum thyroxine by the radioimmunoassay technique offers an advantage over competitive protein-binding displacement assay (CPB) in that it involves no extractions and requires very small amounts of serum. Serum thyroxine measured by this technique includes total serum T_4, the part that is bound to thyroxine-binding globulin and the minute amount that is free. As mentioned before, in situations in which there is an increase in TBG—estrogen administration, pregnancy, or contraceptive pills—there is an increase in the total amount of serum T_4. However, in these circumstances, patients maintain a normal free thyroxine level. As discussed below, in order to interpret the free thyroxine level, a determination of serum T_4 along with an evaluation of the amount of TBG should be made.

Serum triiodothyronine (T_3) is the other thyroid hormone with biological activity. The total amount of T_3 may be measured by radioimmunoassay technique. The concentration of circulating T_3 is quite low relative to that of T_4 (1/100), because the affinity of the binding proteins in human serum is much less for T_4 than for T_3. Normal values in nonpregnant patients have been reported between 70 and 200 ng/100 ml.

This value may vary slightly from laboratory to laboratory, depending on the method used. Since serum triiodothyronine is bound to protein in serum, adjustments must be made in patients with alterations in the amount of circulating TBG. In pregnancy the normal values increase about 50%; therefore normal values up to 300 ng % are considered normal in pregnancy (22,23). The main value of T_3 determinations is in the diagnosis of hyperthyroidism. Cases have been described in which hyperthyroidism is associated with an elevation of circulating T_3 but not of T_4, a condition called T_3 thyrotoxicosis (24).

As mentioned before, it is the free hormone rather than the total thyroid hormone that is the best index of the euthyroid state and presumably is the feedback regulator of hypothalamic-pituitary regulation. When there is an increase in serum TBG concentration, there is both a transient increase in thyroid hormone production and a transient decrease in metabolic clearance until a new steady state is achieved at which absolute free hormone concentration is within the normal range. Therefore, direct measurement of free hormone concentration would identify patients with thyroid dysfunction. However, this method of direct measurement is too costly and complex for routine use. Instead, the total hormone levels are evaluated in the context of TBG concentration or the so-called TBG assessment (25).

Several methods are available to assess serum TBG. Direct measurement of TBG is not yet in general use. Resin uptake tests are more practical and available, and they give an indirect evaluation of the amount of circulating TBG. The resin T_3 uptake (RT_3U) reflects unbound TBG binding sites in the patient's serum. The test assesses the distribution of a tracer amount of radioactive T_3 between the patient's unoccupied TBG binding sites and a T_3-binding exchange resin added to the serum. The result is reported as a percentage of the amount of radioactive T_3 taken up by the resin. In pregnancy or situations in which the serum TBG is elevated, more unoccupied binding sites are available, and, therefore, the T_3 uptake by the resin is decreased. When the serum TBG is reduced, the unbound binding sites are also reduced, and the resin T_3 uptake (RT_3U) is increased (26) (Fig. 1). (Alterations in serum TBG concentration are summarized in Table I.)

Resin T_3 uptake is not a thyroid test. It is of value only when used in conjunction with the serum T_4 for calculation of the "free thyroxine index" (27) or "adjusted total thyroxine" value (28). The index correlates very well with the actual amount of free thyroxine in serum (29). In order to calculate the free thyroxine index or adjusted total thyroxine, the normal values for T_4 and resin R_3 uptake for a given laboratory have to be known. The formula used is as follows:

$$T_4 \times \frac{RT_3U}{\text{Mean } RT_3U \text{ normal value}} = \text{free thyroxine index}$$

The normal value for the free thyroxine index is the same as the normal value for serum T_4. Therefore, if the index is low, it will be consistent with hypothyroidism, and if it is elevated, hyperthyroidism can be ruled out (26).

Serum free thyroxine can be estimated directly by a dialysis method (30). However, this method is not used for routine clinical purposes, since the calculation of the free thyroxine index gives the same information. A decrease in free thyroxine with progression of pregnancy was reported by Auruskin et al. (8). At the same time there was a decrease in serum free triiodothyronine. These changes are not clearly under-

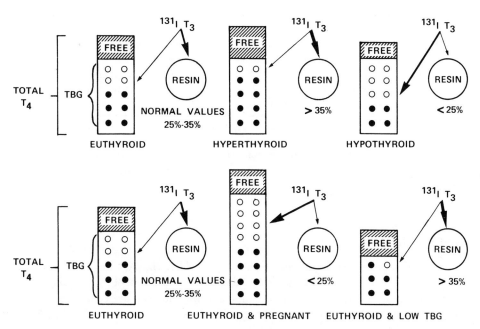

Figure 1. Interpretation of Resin T_3 Uptake (RT_3U) in euthyroid, hyperthyroid, and hypothyroid patients, and in situations of thyroxine binding globulin (TBG) abnormalities.

stood, since the same authors could demonstrate no concomitant changes in serum TSH levels.

SERUM TSH CONCENTRATION

Measurement of serum TSH concentration is the most sensitive test available for detection of thyroid gland hypofunction. Serum TSH concentration is increased in patients with hypothyroidism of thyroidal origin. During pregnancy an increase in serum TSH indicates primary thyroid deficiency. Serum TSH may be elevated as an early manifestation of thyroid failure at a time when the patient is clinically euthyroid and the serum T_4 is in the normal range. The question whether to treat or not to treat patients with so-called decreased thyroid reserve has not yet been resolved. It is the author's opinion that, particularly in pregnancy, patients with elevated serum TSH in spite of normal serum thyroxine concentration should be treated with thyroid replacement therapy. This is discussed in more detail in the section on hypothyroidism in pregnancy.

The association of a normal or undetectable serum TSH concentration with clear-cut hypothyroidism is diagnostic of secondary hypothyroidism of hypothalamic or pituitary origin (31).

Table I. Alterations in Thyroxine-Binding Globulin (TBG) Concentration

Increase	Decrease
Pregnancy	Androgens
Estrogen therapy	Anabolic steroids
Acute intermittent porphyria	Acromegaly
Infectious hepatitis	Nephrotic syndrome
Genetically determined	Genetically determined
Chronic perphenazine administration	

Values for TSH concentration are normal in the serum of pregnant women despite the fact that the normal placenta produces the thyroid-stimulating peptide, human chorionic thyrotropin (hCT).

MISCELLANEOUS TESTS

Other indirect tests like basal metabolic rate (BMR), the Achilles reflex time, and serum cholesterol concentration are of no value in the evaluation of thyroid disorders.

Determination of thyroid uptake of iodine and thyroid scan are contraindicated during pregnancy. Studies done in early pregnancy show an elevated uptake of radioactive iodine by the thyroid (32,33). The reason for this elevation is not clear, although an increase in renal clearance of iodide and increase in thyrotropin activity, which have been postulated to be present in early pregnancy, have been implicated.

THYROID ANTIBODIES

The determination of thyroid antibodies is of value in the diagnosis of Hashimoto thyroiditis. Of the different types of thyroid autoantibodies, the antithyroglobulin antibodies and the antimicrosomal are the most commonly used. The autoantibodies are immunogloblulins and they are organ-specific. The presence of antibodies appears to correlate with the histological presence of focal thyroiditis. High titers of antibodies are also seen in some patients with Graves disease or primary thyroprivic hypothyroidism. Although antibodies to thyroidal antigens are known to cross the placenta freely in man, a cause-effect relationship between such transmission and thyroid disease has not been clearly established (34).

PLACENTAL TRANSFER OF HORMONES AND DRUGS

Transplacental passage of thyroid hormones (Table II) does occur, but the magnitude and direction of this transfer remain uncertain. Recent studies in pregnant rhesus monkeys by Azukizawa et al. (35) showed that TRH can transverse the placenta from mother to fetus. The placenta is not permeable to pituitary TSH. Studies of T_4 and T_3

transfer from the mother to the fetus near term have suggested that such transfer occurs but is minimal. It appears that T_3 is transferred at a faster rate than thyroxine (36–39).

Placental transfer of long-acting thyroid stimulator (LATS) is known to occur in cases of neonatal thyrotoxicosis (40). Long-acting thyroid stimulator is an immunoglobulin G (IgG) that is found in some patients with Graves disease; its role as the etiological agent in Graves disease has been questioned. Its presence in the serum of neonates with thyrotoxicosis has been reported by several authors (41–43). Recently, cases of neonatal hyperthyroidism caused by another immunoglobulin G that seems to stimulate only the human thyroid have been reported (44,45). This LATS protector (LATS-P) initially reported by Adams and Kennedy (46) is present in most patients with Graves disease, and it has been suggested to be the thyroid stimulator responsible for the hyperthyroidism of Graves disease. LATS protector was detected in cord blood in infants born of thyrotoxic mothers (44,45).

Iodine crosses the placental barrier and may cause goiter or hypothyroidism in the fetus. Short-term treatment with iodine for preparation for subtotal thyroidectomy does not appear to affect the fetus. Thiourea compounds cross the placental barrier (47–49), and several cases of fetal goiter have been reported (49–51).

GOITER IN PREGNANCY

The thyroid gland enlarges during pregnancy, although the incidence of goiter depends on the geographical area and the clinical criteria used to define a goiter. Incidence of goiter does not appear to be increased in areas of high iodine intake such as Iceland (3). In Scotland, 70% of pregnant women had goiter in comparison with 38% of women who were nonpregnant (3). The reason for this enlargement of the thyroid gland is not very well known at the present time. Studies by Aboul-Khair et al. (52) have shown an elevation of iodide renal clearance beginning early in pregnancy. This early rise in the renal clearance of iodine may decrease plasma inorganic iodine concentration, and, as a consequence, there is a diminished amount of iodine available for the synthesis of thyroid hormone. However, Dworkin et al. (53) found no significant difference in iodine balance between pregnant and nonpregnant women in the United States. Autopsy studies of the thyroid gland during pregnancy have shown only slight thyroid hyperplasia (54). It has been suggested that an early increase in serum TSH in pregnancy due to the depression of free thyroxine concentration secondary to TBG increase may

Table II. Placental Transport of Thyroid Hormones and Drugs

Do Cross	Do Not Cross
TRH	Thyroxine
LATS	Triiodothyronine
LATS-protector	TSH
Propylthiouracil	
Methimazole	
Iodide	

account for the etiology of this simple goiter of pregnancy (55). The role of placental thyrotropins as a goiterogenic stimulus has been also mentioned (55).

Regardless of the etiologic factors, the thyroid gland may be slightly enlarged in pregnancy, and no specific treatment is indicated. On physical examination the gland may be visible, easily palpable, diffuse, painless, and soft to palpation. Furthermore, thyroid tests, including free thyroxine index and serum TSH, should be within normal limits. If the thyroid gland, on examination, is definitely enlarged, irregular in shape, with nodules, and of altered consistency, this enlargement is not related to pregnancy and constitutes nontoxic goiter, assuming thyroid tests are within normal limits.

Simple or nontoxic goiter may be defined as any thyroid enlargement that is not associated with thyrotoxicosis or hypothyroidism and does not result from an inflammatory or neoplastic process (56). Diffuse or multinodular goiter has been reported to occur more commonly during adolescence and pregnancy. The clinical features depend on the local effect of the goiter. Sometimes displacement or compression of the esophagus or trachea may occur, leading to dysphagia, a choking sensation, and inspiratory stridor. Occasionally, acute pain may develop in a goiter because of hemorrhage into a nodule.

The evolution of nontoxic goiter from its initial diffuse form to its late multinodule stage is similar to the natural history of goiters in endemic areas. In some patients, thyroid antibodies may be elevated, indicating that some of these goiters are related to chronic lymphocytic thyroiditis or Hashimoto disease. Some patients may develop hypothyroidism and others Graves disease. For these reasons patients with nontoxic goiters should be followed at regular intervals.

If detected during pregnancy, a determination of free thyroxine index and a serum TSH should be performed to evaluate the function of this goiter. If the patient is clinically and chemically euthyroid, suppressive therapy with thyroxine hormone is the treatment of choice. Levo-thyroxine in a dose 150 to 200 μg daily produces the maximum state of thyroid suppression in most patients. Complete regression of diffuse goiters has been reported only in 30 to 50% of patients after long-term treatment. And, multinodular goiters do not respond so well as diffuse goiters. Suppression therapy may prevent further growth of the goiter rather than cause reversion of the goiter. Surgery is rarely indicated in pregnancy and should be performed only in the exceptional case of obstructive symptoms.

CHRONIC THYROIDITIS

Chronic thyroiditis is one of the causes of goiter and hypothyroidism. It is an autoimmune disease and is four times more common in women than in men. The diagnosis is confirmed by the clinical findings, the histological changes, and the findings of high titers of thyroid autoantibodies in serum. The histological changes consist of a combination of diffuse lymphocytic infiltration, obliteration of thyroid follicles, and fibrosis.

The clinical picture is characterized by the presence of a goiter that is firm in consistency and moves freely when the patient swallows. There is a diffuse enlargement of the thyroid gland, but often one lobe is larger than the other. The natural course of the goiter is to remain unchanged or enlarge gradually over many years if left untreated. Most patients develop hypothyroidism over several years. However, some cases may present with symptoms of mild thyrotoxicosis, particularly in the early phase of the disease. The association of Hashimoto thyroiditis with other autoimmune diseases has been reported, particularly pernicious anemia, rheumatoid arthritis, and systemic lupus erythematosus.

Maternal thyroid antibodies have been reported to cross the placenta, and simultaneous occurrence of thyroid antibodies in both mother and newborn has been reported in some cases of cretinism (57). However, a relationship between these antibodies and thyroid diseases in the newborn has not been established. Beierwaltes was unable to document maternal transmission of thyroid antibodies in man (58). Blizzard and coworkers postulated the transplacental transfer of an unidentified thyrocytotoxic factor in addition to thyroid antibodies to account for the familial occurrence of congenital hypothyroidism (57). Transient hypothyroidism in the neonatal period with presence of antibodies was demonstrated in all six offspring of one member of a family with autoimmune thyroid disease. In these cases, the babies were born with chemical evidence of hypothyroidism, but the tests reverted to normal at a later time (34). The authors postulated that a factor with cytosuppressive effect on thyroid tissue may cross the placenta from the mother and produce a transient suppression of the fetal thyroid. However, studies done by Thier et al. (59) failed to demonstrate such a factor.

A remission of hypothyroidism in pregnancy in a patient with chronic thyroiditis was reported by Nelson and Palmer (60). Their patient had high titers of thyroid antibodies that decreased during pregnancy. In addition, the elevated serum TSH returned to normal during pregnancy, and the goiter remitted. Following an uneventful pregnancy and a normal delivery, the patient became hypothyroid 6 weeks postpartum with an enlargement of the thyroid gland. The infant was euthyroid, with no goiter, and had a negative titer for thyroid antibodies.

Transient hypothyroidism in the postpartum period was reported recently in patients with autoimmune thyroiditis (61,62). The syndrome is characterized by high incidence of previous goiter, thyroid enlargement at 1 to 4 months postpartum, hypothyroidism at 3 to 5 months postpartum, return to euthyroidism 5 to 10 months postpartum, positive titers of antithyroid microsomal hemagglutination antibodies, and decrease in size but persistence of goiter. Thyroid function tests return to the normal range concomitantly with the decrease in goiter size at 6 to 9 months after delivery. A decrease in thyroid autoantibody titer in pregnancy and an increase after delivery were reported in three patients with chronic thyroiditis (63). It has been postulated that these changes in thyroid function during pregnancy and in the postpartum period in patients with chronic thyroiditis are due to changes in immune response during pregnancy or after delivery. Postpartum relapses or aggravation have been reported in patients with rheumatoid arthritis, systemic lupus erythematosus, and idiopathic thrombocytopenic purpura. Changes in thyroid antibody titers during and after pregnancy have been reported in patients with chronic lymphocytic thyroiditis (63,64).

An association between high titers of thyroid antibodies and Down syndrome occurring in the offspring was reported by Fialkow (65).

Treatment of chronic thyroiditis consists of thyroid hormone replacement. Treatment is indicated in patients in whom the diagnosis of chronic thyroiditis is made. Replacement doses of 1-thyroxine in amounts of 150 to 200 μg/day are indicated. Surgery is justified only if pressure symptoms or an excessively large gland does not respond to a trial with thyroid hormone replacement.

SOLITARY NODULE OF THE THYROID IN PREGNANCY

One of the most controversial subjects among endocrinologists is the management of patients with a single nodule of the thyroid gland. The question of carcinoma is unresolved until a pathological diagnosis is made. The incidence of malignancy in these nodules varies, according to different series, between 5 and 40% (66,67). From the clinical point of view, it is very difficult to establish the diagnosis unless metastasis or local extension becomes evident. There are a group of findings that may favor a diagnosis of malignancy. The younger the patient, the greater the likelihood that the nodular thyroid harbors a malignancy. A history of radiation to the head, neck, or chest during childhood suggests the likelihood of carcinoma, as does a history of recent painless growth or a nodule of very firm or stony, hard consistency. Late manifestations of the disease are fixation, vocal cord paralysis, or extension to regional lymph nodes.

Histologically papillary carcinoma is most common in young people. An occasional case of pregnancy in a patient with medullary thyroid carcinoma has been reported in the literature (73).

Routine laboratory tests are normal, including the serum T_4 and T_3. Recently, it has been suggested that determination of serum thyroglobulin may provide a potential tumor marker, but it is not specific, since it has been found elevated in patients with Graves disease and Hashimoto thyroiditis (68).

In nonpregnant patients, a cold or hypofunctioning nodule on scintiscan is an additional criterion for malignancy. Obviously this test cannot be performed in pregnancy. Recently, the use of ultrasound techniques has helped in differentiating a cystic from a solid lesion; the presence of a cystic lesion favors a nonmalignant outcome (69).

Needle biopsy appears to be regaining popularity, but its use in pregnancy has not been described (70).

Therefore, during pregnancy the presence of a solitary thyroid nodule presents a diagnostic problem because of the limitations in our diagnostic possibilities. In the presence of a solitary nodule on palpation, and in a euthyroid patient, thyroid suppression therapy with L-thyroxine 0.2 mg daily for the remainder of pregnancy is a sound approach, since it is widely accepted treatment even in nonpregnant patients for a few months. Surgery during pregnancy should be carried out only if there is any evidence of enlargement of the tumor during suppressive therapy or if there is any evidence of local metastasis.

Subsequent pregnancies in patients with thyroid carcinoma do not appear to have an adverse effect on the course of the malignancy (71,72).

HYPOTHYROIDISM AND PREGNANCY

Hypothyroidism is rarely associated with pregnancy (74). Early studies by Goldsmith et al. (75) indicated that 70% of myxedematous women were anovulatory. Studies by Mann and coworkers (76) suggested that 3% of pregnant patients had hypothyroxinemia. At the time of the studies serum butanol-extractable iodine (BEI) was measured. The results suggested that inadequately treated mothers had children with lower IQ than children whose mothers had received proper treatment. As stated by Burrow (77), there was no good clinical evidence to suggest that these patients were truly hypothyroid. Very few of the patients were studied after delivery in order to define their thyroid status. The reason for these findings is not very clear, since it is known that the fetal thyroid functions autonomously of the maternal system and the placental transfer of thyroid hormones is minimal. As suggested by Fisher (78), if maternal hypothyroidism affects the fetus, it must do so by altering placental function or compromising fetal substrate supply in some other way.

Montoro et al. (78a) reported 11 pregnancies in 9 women who were profoundly hypothyroid but nevertheless were able to conceive and sustain their pregnancies. Ten children were born alive; there was 1 intrauterine death at 29 weeks which occurred in the only patient who developed preeclampsia. There were no neonatal deaths and only 1 infant with congenital abnormalities (Down's syndrome), but the mother was 41 years old.

Hypothyroidism may be due to pituitary or hypothalamic disease or an intrinsic disorder of the thyroid gland (primary hypothyroidism). The former is very uncommon, particularly in pregnancy. Therefore, in this chapter we discuss only primary hypothyroidism. This is a disease that is more common in women than in men and occurs most often between the ages of 40 and 60. In many patients, primary hypothyroidism is the end stage of chronic thyroiditis. In these cases, thyroid antibodies are present, and the thyroid gland may not be enlarged to palpation. In the so-called goitrous hypothyroidism there is an impaired ability of the thyroid gland to synthesize thyroid hormones. This leads to hypersecretion of TSH, which in turn produces goiter. Finally, hypothyroidism is frequently seen in patients following total or subtotal thyroidectomy or radioiodine treatment for Graves disease.

The onset of hypothyroidism is usually so insidious that the classic clinical manifestations may take months or years to appear. Early symptoms of hypothyroidism are variable and nonspecific. Tiredness, lethargy, and weakness are very common. Sensitivity to cold may be an early manifestation. Menorrhagia or anovulatory cycles with infertility has been reported. Women frequently complain of hair loss, brittle nails, and dry skin. Weight gain often occurs. The voice may become husky, and periorbital puffiness may become evident, particularly in the early morning hours. Stiffness and aching of muscles are sometimes misdiagnosed as rheumatoid arthritis. Muscle cramps could be an early manifestation of this disease (56).

Routine thyroid tests like a serum T_4 and a free thyroxine index may be low or in the low-normal range. The diagnosis is confirmed by an elevation of serum TSH. TSH determination appears to be, at the present time, the most sensitive and specific test for the diagnosis of primary hypothyroidism. Unfortunately, early reports of patients with mild hypothyroidism in pregnancy did not have the confirmatory evidence of an elevation in TSH, since this test was not available then.

The development of TSH radioimmunoassays has allowed the more precise recognition of minor degrees of thyroid failure. Subclinical hypothyroidism has been defined as an entity in which the level of thyroid hormones is normal or slightly reduced but there is an elevation in serum TSH. Studies of the effect of subclinical hypothyroidism in pregnancy and fetal development have yet to be undertaken. In recent years we have seen several cases with minimum symptoms of hypothyroidism in which the serum TSH was elevated in the presence of low-normal or normal thyroid indices. One such case presented with carpal tunnel syndrome as the only complaint. Until more information is available, full thyroid replacement dosage is justified in asymptomatic pregnant mothers in whom mild elevation of serum TSH is found (55). Replacement therapy can be achieved using thyroxine in a total dose from 0.2 to 0.3 mg/day. Serum T_4 and TSH should be followed, but it must be kept in mind that serum TSH may require up to 8 weeks to return to base line values following initiation of therapy (79).

Patients with goiter, family history of thyroid disease, past history of thyroidectomy, or radioactive therapy should be screened for hypothyroidism. If the serum TSH is elevated, thyroid replacement therapy is indicated.

HYPERTHYROIDISM AND PREGNANCY

The incidence of hyperthyroidism in pregnancy ranges from 0.02 to 3.7%, with an average of about 0.2% (80,81) as compared with 0.4% in the general hospital population (82). In most patients, hyperthyroidism is diagnosed during pregnancy with symptoms dating months and sometimes years before the patients became pregnant (83). There is no convincing evidence that fertility is impaired in hyperthyroidism, although menstrual function is usually disturbed. However, in most patients ovulation occurs (56). Since the symptoms of hyperthyroidism in most pregnant women are mild to moderate, it appears that fertility in severe thyrotoxicosis might be impaired and only those patients with a mild form of the disease are able to conceive.

Hyperthyroidism during pregnancy imposes no unusual risk for the mother, although the incidence of toxemia has been reported by Javert to be higher (84), and thyroid storm, although unusual, has been reported (85). Early reports of fetal wastage indicated that the incidence was as high as 45% in those patients in whom the disease was not controlled by either medical or surgical treatment (86). On the other hand, when hyperthyroidism is well controlled, fetal wastage ranged from values comparable with those for pregnancy in normal individuals to values as high as 24% (87–93). Recent reports indicate a low perinatal mortality in those patients treated with either surgery or antithyroid drug therapy (83,94–97).

Graves disease is the most common cause of thyrotoxicosis in pregnancy; multinodular goiter and toxic nodular goiter (Plummer disease) are relatively infrequent during the third and fourth decade and thus constitute relatively less common causes of thyrotoxicosis during pregnancy. Other causes of hyperthyroidism in pregnancy, although uncommon, include subacute thyroiditis and thyrotoxicosis factitia. Subacute thyroiditis, also known as granulomatous giant cell or de Quervain's thyroiditis, is an acute process of the thyroid gland, possibly of viral etiology. Women are far more frequently affected than men, and the maximum incidence is in the fourth and fifth decades. In the author's experience, the disease is uncommon in pregnancy, representing no more than 2% of all cases of hyperthyroidism in pregnancy. The characteristic feature of this disease is a gradual or sudden onset of pain in the region of the thyroid gland with radiation to the ear, the jaw, or the occiput (56); on palpation the thyroid gland is slightly or moderately enlarged, firm, and tender, one lobe being generally more severely affected than the other. These physical findings may change in a few days during the course of the disease. Low-grade fever, lassitude, malaise, nervousness, and palpitations are frequent complaints. Thyroid tests are in the hyperthyroid range or slightly elevated; the thyroid ^{131}I uptake is very low (contraindicated in pregnancy). The clinical course is characterized by an initial stage of hyperthyroidism, followed by a hypothyroidlike phase and recovery over a period of weeks or months in most cases (98).

Treatment with analgesics in mild cases and corticosteroids in most severely affected patients is almost invariably effective. Prednisone in doses of 30 to 60 mg relieves the symptoms in a few days; then the amount of medication may be decreased and usually can be discontinued after 3 to 6 weeks of therapy (99).

Thyrotoxicosis factitia is due to ingestion, usually chronic, of excessive quantities of thyroid hormones. Generally the patient denies that she is taking thyroid hormones. The thyroid gland is not enlarged, and in nonpregnant patients a low thyroid ^{131}I uptake is characteristic.

The clinical diagnosis of hyperthyroidism in pregnancy may be very difficult, since many of the symptoms of the disease occur in normal pregnancy. It is not unusual, during gestation, to complain of excessive warmth and nervousness. Mild tachycardia, hyperdynamic circulation, and slight enlargement of the thyroid gland and tremor are not uncommon in normal pregnancy. The presence of persistent tachycardia, weight loss or failure to gain weight despite a good appetite, and eye signs such as lid lag, lid retraction, and exophthalmos are very suggestive of thyrotoxicosis. It has to be kept in mind that, with the most liberal use of thyroid tests, earlier diagnosis is possible at the time when the clinical symptoms are few and of moderate severity. Normal pulse rate, absence of goiter, and weight gain have been observed more frequently nowadays in patients with hyperthyroidism (Table III).

The diagnosis is sustained by an elevation of the free thyroxine index calculated from the values of serum T_4 and RT_3U. In hyperthyroid pregnant patients the RT_3U value may be within the normal limits for nonpregnant patients, but such a value is definitely elevated for pregnancy. In those patients with borderline values a serum T_3RIA determination is helpful. Values over 300 ng % are definitely abnormal and consistent with a diagnosis of hyperthyroidism. With the use of the free T_4 index and the T_3RIA, one is able to make the proper diagnosis in most cases. In those patients in whom no definite diagnosis can be made, follow-up without treatment is indicated. Suppression tests with triiodothyronine (Cytomel) are not very useful in pregnancy, because complete suppression is difficult to achieve in the presence of elevated TBG. The TRH stimulation test has not yet been evaluated for use in pregnancy (100,101).

Hyperthyroidism in pregnancy does not seem to carry any special threat to the mother; it is generally accepted that hyperthyroidism is ameliorated by pregnancy (83,102–104). The risk for the infant of the untreated mother is premature delivery with an increased incidence in neonatal mortality and morbidity (83). The treatment of choice for thyrotoxicosis in pregnancy is antithyroid drug therapy, using the minimum amount of drug to maintain the patient clinically and chemically euthyroid

Table III. Common Symptoms and Signs of Hyperthyroidism

Nervousness	Tachycardia
Palpitations	Goiter
Heat intolerance	Eye signs
Weakness	Plummer's nail (onycholysis)
Weight loss	Hyperkinetic reflexes
Excessive perspiration	Bruit over thyroid
Fatigability	Tremor
Diarrhea	Skin changes

(77,83,94,105,106). Subtotal thyroidectomy, although recommended by some (107–109), should be reserved for patients with large goiters and pressure symptoms, those who have allergies to all the usual antithyroid drugs, and perhaps those who, for geographical reasons find it difficult to attend a hospital for careful control of the thyroid state during pregnancy (110).

Thiourea compounds—propylthiouracil and methimazole—are the antithyroid drugs used in this country. These drugs block the synthesis of thyroid hormones by inhibiting the oxidation and organic binding of thyroid iodide thus inhibiting the formation of monoiodotyrosine (MIT) and diiodotyrosine (DIT). They also inhibit the coupling of MIT and DIT to form T_3 and T_4 (Fig. 2). The response to antithyroid therapy occurs after a latent period of 3 to 6 weeks, because these agents do not effect the release of thyroid hormones. Therefore the reduction in the supply of hormone to the tissues must await depletion of glandular hormone stores (56). The amount of drug to be given depends on the severity of the thyrotoxicosis and size of the goiter.

Propylthiouracil (PTU) and methimazole (Tapazole) have been used interchangeably without evidence that one or the other has definite therapeutic advantages (111). Both may be given in a twice-a-day dosage, but, from a theoretical standpoint, it has been suggested in the past to use them every 6 to 8 hr. The usual standing dose is 200 mg of PTU or 20 mg of Tapazole twice a day. In severe cases 300 mg of PTU twice a day or 30 mg of Tapazole twice a day may be used. Most patients show signs of improvement by 2 to 4 weeks after initiation of treatment. The best clinical signs in this regard are an increase in weight and amelioration of the tachycardia. Along with the clinical improvement a fall in the free thyroxine index is observed. After 3 to 4 weeks of treatment, the

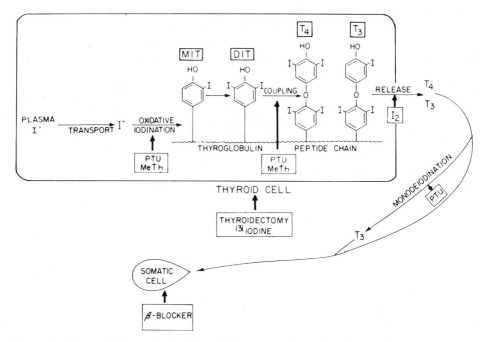

Figure 2. Scheme for biosynthesis of thyroid hormone and the site of action of antithyroid treatments. From Hershman, J. M., in *Gynecologic Endocrinology,* ed. by J. R. Givens. Year Book Medical Publishers, 1977, p. 256.

amount of antithyroid drug should be decreased by half and further reduced after the patient becomes euthyroid, using the minimum amount of antithyroid medication to maintain the mother at the euthyroid level. Maintenance may be achieved using 10 mg of Tapazole or 100 mg of PTU daily. If the mother has responded promptly to the treatment, it is possible and advisable to discontinue the drug by 30 to 34 weeks of gestation, particularly if treatment was given for at least 12 weeks. Recent evidence in nonpregnant patients appears to indicate that a large number will have a remission after 3 months of antithyroid drug therapy; patients with a small goiter and recent onset of symptoms are the ones most likely to respond to this short therapeutic regimen (112). If thyrotoxicosis recurs when the dosage is reduced, the initial dose should be given again.

If after 6 weeks of therapy there is no improvement, which is very unlikely, the antithyroid medication should be given every 6 or 8 hr. It is our experience that those patients showing no clinical response are those with poor compliance.

Adverse reactions to antithyroid drugs occur in a small percentage of patients (Table IV). The most serious adverse reaction is agranulocytosis, which occurs in about 0.1 to 0.4% of patients. Agranulocytosis occurs within the first few weeks or months of treatment; sore throat and fever are the first manifestations, and every patient should be instructed to discontinue the drug and notify the physician immediately if these symptoms develop. If the diagnosis is confirmed, complete isolation and the use of glucocorticoids and antibiotics should be instituted at once. If the diagnosis of agranulocytosis is made early, recovery occurs. Thereafter, the patient should never be given the same drug, but the alternative drug may be given a cautious trial. Since granulocytopenia is frequent in untreated thyrotoxicosis, a white cell count should be made before antithyroid drug therapy is started in every patient.

Of the less severe reactions, skin rash is the most common and occurs in about 4 to 7% of patients. The incidence of this reaction appears to be slightly greater with methimazole than with PTU. Any reaction to these drugs is an indication for withdrawal and the use of an alternative agent.

Treatment with antithyroid drugs was reported in 1951 by Astwood et al. (88). Nineteen patients completed 22 pregnancies with only 3 premature infants. Mestman et al. (83) had 1 fetal death in a group of 18 viable pregnancies. Mytaba and Burrow (97) reported their experience of 21 women during 26 pregnancies; there were 2 abortions and 2 stillbirth, the latter occurring at 21 and 26 weeks of gestation. Five children had congenital defects—developmental retardation, scalp defects, hypospadia, imperforate anus, and aortic atresia—4 of the infants were born with goiter, and 3 of these had neonatal thyrotoxicosis. However, not all mothers had frequent serum thyroxine determinations; therefore, the relationship of drug therapy, maternal hypothyroidism, and control of the disease to the outcome of these pregnancies cannot be inferred.

The incidence of congenital malformations does not appear to be increased in thyrotoxicosis patients regardless of the type of treatment given. Both methimazole and propylthiouracil cross the placenta (47–49) and may cause fetal complications, including hypothyroidism and goiter (49–51). Burrow (51), in a retrospective study of 41 pregnancies in 30 patients who had received antithyroid medications during pregnancy, found 5 infants born with a goiter; however, other factors, including maternal hypothyroidism, iodine therapy, and familial thyroid disease could not be excluded as cause of the goiter. The incidence of goiter or hypothyroidism in infants is indeed very low. However, it is advisable to avoid hypothyroidism in the mother. In order to achieve

Table IV. Toxic Reactions to Thiomide

Agranulocytosis*
Skin rash†
Fever†
Arthralgias
Neuritis
Hepatitis (cholestasis)
Alopecia
Thrombocytopenia

* More serious, but uncommon.
† More common.

this goal, the mother should be seen every 2 to 3 weeks, and blood tests should be done at each visit. As soon as the thyroid tests return to normal, the amount of antithyroid medication should be reduced. In order to prevent neonatal goiter, a combination of thyroid-antithyroid therapy was suggested by Fraser and Wilkinson (113), Asper and London (114), and Herbst and Selenkow (115). This approach has been used successfully in several reported series (91,115,116). At the time these studies were conducted, it was thought that thyroid medication given to the mother would cross the placenta. However, present evidence indicates that thyroid hormones do not cross the placenta in significant amounts (36–39). Furthermore, studies in animals (117) and humans (118) have shown failure of triiodothyronine administration in preventing hypothyroidism in the newborn in mothers treated with antithyroid drugs.

When antithyroid therapy is compared with antithyroid-thyroid treatment (83), the perinatal mortality and the incidence of goiter and hypothyroidism in the newborn appear to be the same. In order to achieve similar serum PBI values at the end of pregnancy, the group on antithyroid-thyroid therapy received a mean dose of methimazole of 26.3 mg daily as compared with 7.0 mg in the group given antithyroid drugs alone (83). The addition of thyroid hormone to the antithyroid drug regimen in pregnancy may lead to neglect of the important principle of minimizing drug dosage and is not recommended (83,119,120).

The most important question that currently cannot be answered concerns the possibility that infants born of mothers treated for hyperthyroidism might have lower intelligence quotients than they would have had if the mothers had no thyroid abnormality. Data presented by Burrow et al. (121) did not suggest that propylthiouracil therapy during pregnancy had an adverse effect on subsequent growth and development of a child, but, as it was pointed out by the authors, the number of children was too small to make any definite conclusions.

There are a few reported cases of scalp defects (aplasia cutis) in the offspring of mothers treated with methimazole (97,122). We have had no opportunity to see such complications in any of our patients; on the basis of this inconclusive data, it was suggested that PTU may be preferable in the therapy for thyrotoxicosis during pregnancy (97).

If surgery is to be performed, it should be done before the third trimester of pregnancy. As mentioned above, the indications for subtotal thyroidectomy during gestation are few. To us, perhaps the only "indication" is a hypersensitivity reaction to both antithyroid medications. Patients undergoing surgery should be clinically euthyroid at the time of surgery. Emslander et al. (109) prepared their patients with Lugol solution for 10 to 14 days before surgery; other authors recommended the use of antithyroid drugs and iodine solution (89,93,108). The use of large doses of iodides in pregnancy is contraindicated, since large goiters and hypothyroidism have been reported in newborns. The use of small doses of iodides (5 minims three times a day of Lugol solution yields approximately 46 mg of iodine) for 10 to 14 days appears to be safe (55). Propanolol has been used in a few patients in preparation for thyroidectomy in pregnancy (123). The authors reported four pregnant patients with thyrotoxicosis who were prepared with doses of propanolol from 320 to 800 mg a day. The patients were treated for 5 to 10 days before surgery without any ill effects on the infants. The major advantage of propanolol is the rapidity with which the patient can be prepared for surgery. The medication should be restarted after surgery, in order to prevent recurrences of hyperthyroidism and the possibility of thyroid storm. Propanolol has been proposed as the sole mode of therapy in the treatment of hyperthyroidism in pregnancy (124). The safety of propanolol in pregnancy has not been established. The use of propanolol has been linked with intrauterine growth retardation, intrapartum asphyxia, neonatal bradycardia, and neonatal hypoglycemia (125–127). It is our opinion that, at the present time, there is no indication for the use of propanolol as the only medication for the treatment of thyrotoxicosis.

Many years ago it was suggested that small amounts of iodide be added to antithyroid drug therapy in the last 4 weeks of gestation (102,128). It was reasoned that antithyroid medication could be stopped, decreasing the risk of neonatal hypothyroidism, but it is now known that iodides do cross the placenta and in excessive dosage may produce fetal goiter and hypothyroidism. Therefore, this form of treatment is not recommended (55).

Thyroid storm is an unusual complication of thyrotoxicosis in pregnancy. It is precipitated by infection, ketoacidosis, or surgery in a previously undiagnosed or poorly controlled patient. It is characterized by fever of over 103°F, tachycardia, nausea, vomiting, and abnormalities in the central nervous system, including tremor, delirium, or stupor. Therapy in the intensive care unit includes (1) intravenous fluid; (2) propanolol 40 mg orally every 6 hr or if the patient is unable to take oral medications, 1 or 2 mg given slowly intravenously until the pulse rate is around or below 100 per minute; (3) 1 g of intravenous sodium iodide to block the secretion of thyroid hormone; (4) 300 mg of PTU every 6 hr; (5) induction of hypothermia; and (6) hydrocortisone 100 to 300 mg in the first 24 hr. The most common cause of death is tachyarrhythmia and high output failure. In spite of the treatment above the mortality may run as high as 20%.

After delivery the patient should be followed at regular intervals, since recurrence of thyrotoxicosis is not uncommon in the next 6 to 12 weeks postpartum. It is recommended that the patient be seen 2 weeks postpartum and the thyroid tests repeated. Patients on antithyroid therapy should not breast-feed their babies, since the drugs are secreted in breast milk.

Postpartum thyrotoxicosis has been recently reported in five patients with painless thyroiditis. Conservative treatment with propanolol is advised, since this is a self-limited disease and return to normal thyroid function is the rule. Since many of these patients present with biopsy findings consistent with chronic thyroiditis and high antibody titers, the risk of developing permanent hypothyroidism later in life should be kept in mind (129). Aquino et al. (130) described four cases of Graves disease whose hyperthyroidism, following antithyroid therapy, was in remission at the time of conception. During pregnancy the patients remained euthyroid without therapy. At 1 to 3 months following delivery hyperthyroidism recurred, but all four patients returned spontaneously to the normal range at 4 to 6 months after delivery. The titers of serum antithyroid microsomal antibodies that had decreased during pregnancy increased at the time of the thyrotoxicosis. The authors suggested that immunological changes after delivery may account for this transient phenomenon. It is similar to the transient hypothyroidism in the postpartum period reported by the same group (61) in patients with autoimmune thyroiditis.

One of the most controversial subjects is the treatment of the hyperthyroid woman wishing to become pregnant in the near future. Medical management may produce a remission in less than 40% of patients, and since antithyroid drug therapy may produce side effects in the infant, therapy with radioactive iodine or surgery should definitely be considered; both treatments are acceptable and proven to be very effective. It is the author's opinion that, because of the theoretical possibilities of genetic defects following 131 iodine therapy, subtotal thyroidectomy is the treatment of choice.

HYDATIDIFORM MOLE AND HYPERTHYROIDISM

Clinical symptoms of hyperthyroidism have been reported in patients with trophoblastic disease, with resolution occurring a few days after delivery of the mole (131,132). Galton et al. (134) and Kock et al. (133) reported several cases of increased thyroid function in patients with molar pregnancy but without clinical evidence of hyperthyroidism. The thyroid gland is generally not enlarged or only slightly increased in size. Several cases of severe hyperthyroidism with congestive heart failure have been reported (135). Higgins et al. (136) studied 14 women with hydatidiform mole, 6 of whom had moderately severe hyperthyroidism easily detected clinically, 3 had mild hyperthyroid symptoms, 4 were euthyroid by all criteria, and 1 was biochemically hyperthyroid but clinically euthyroid. None of the patients had exophthalmos, but 2 had thyrotoxic myopathy. Nagataki et al. (137) reported 15 patients with molar pregnancy, and, although none of them was clinically thyrotoxic, thyroxine levels were elevated in 13 patients. Therefore, it appears that most patients with trophoblastic disease are clinically euthyroid in spite of laboratory findings of hyperthyroxinemia.

Galton et al. (134) found high levels of thyrotropin in serum from 13 patients with hydatidiform mole; this activity could not be detected after evacuation of the mole. This thyroid stimulator originates in the molar tissue and differs biologically and immunologically from pituitary thyroid-stimulating hormone (TSH), the chorionic TSH (cTSH) of normal placenta, and thyroid-stimulating immunoglobulins. Studies carried out by Hershman (138,139) and Nisula and Ketelslegers (140) indicate that this thyroid stimulator is indeed hCG (human chorionic gonadotropin). On a molecular basis it was calculated that hCG contained approximately 1/4000 the thyrotropic activity of pituitary TSH. They postulated that in conditions of grossly elevated serum hCG levels, such as hydatidiform mole, the thyrotropic activity could be sufficient to produce hyperthyroidism (138). The association of hyperthyroidism and hydatidiform mole must be suspected particularly when serum levels of hCG exceed 300 IU/ml (136). Miyai et al. (141) studied the response to TRH in 12 patients with trophoblastic disease of whom 4 had hydatidiform mole. In those patients with abnormally elevated serum free thyroxine and free triiodothyronine, serum TSH was undetectable and did not respond to the administration of TRH. After treatment the TSH response to TRH became positive. The authors speculated that, in some patients with trophoblastic disease, the trophoblastic tissue produces an abnormal thyroid stimulator that stimulates the thyroid gland, and, in turn, excess T_4 and T_3 suppresses TSH secretion from the pituitary gland by a negative feedback mechanism. The reason for the absence of clear thyrotoxicosis despite marked elevations in serum T_4 and T_3 is not known; a low serum T_3/T_4 ratio as a possible explanation was suggested by Nagataki et al. (137).

Treatment consists of prompt removal of the molar tissue. The use of intravenous sodium iodide caused a significant preoperative fall in serum T_3 levels (136). Propanolol (40 mg every 6 hr) and intravenous fluids along with 1 g of sodium iodide administered intravenously are the treatment of choice. The hyperthyroidism has been shown to remit after successful treatment of the trophoblastic tumor.

MATERNAL INGESTION OF IODINE

Congenital goiter caused by maternal ingestion of iodine has been known for many years. In 1940, Parmelee (142) reported three cases of newborn infants with goiters. In each case the mother had taken iodine-containing preparations throughout pregnancy. Similar cases of sporadic goiters have been reported since then (143–146). The thyroid of the fetus may become very large, and pressure on the trachea may interfere with respiration (147). Carswell et al. (145) reported eight cases of congenital goiter and hypothyroidism, and two of these babies were mentally retarded. The source of iodine was medications taken by the mothers because of respiratory problems. The goiter in the newborn usually disappears with or without thyroid replacement therapy. It is advisable to avoid use of long-term iodine during pregnancy.

IODINE DEFICIENCY

Iodine deficiency is the primary factor causing endemic goiter and, in many parts of the world, endemic cretinism, a disease that sometimes is associated with hypothyroidism (148). Endemic cretinism is characterized by multiple neurological defects, including deaf mutism, cerebral diplegia, squint, and mental deficiency. The administration of intramuscular iodized oil to women before conception prevents the development of endemic cretinism (149). In one instance, the withdrawal of a rich source of dietary iodine precipitated a local epidemic of the disease. Iodine deficiency is strongly implicated in the pathogenesis of the syndrome, and it exerts its effect before birth or even, possibly, before conception (150). Fierro-Benitez et al. (151) studied the incidence of endemic cretinism and goiter in eight rural villages in the Andean provinces. The prevalence of endemic cretinism is clearly associated with the prevalence of endemic goiter. However, there was no evidence of overt hypothyroidism. Pharoah et al. (152) studied a group of pregnant women in an isolated area of New Guinea where iodine deficiency is very common. Their results appear to indicate that iodine deficiency causes fetal loss late in pregnancy or death postnatally in contrast to the infertility or repeated abortion of myxedema. Furthermore, the syndrome of endemic cretinism is peculiar to iodine deficiency.

RADIOACTIVE IODINE GIVEN IN PREGNANCY

The amount of radiation that the mother receives during a radioactive iodine uptake is insignificant in terms of exposure of the thyroid gland. When a dose of 10 μCi is given for the purpose of determining iodine uptake, the approximate radiation absorbed by the thyroid is 10 rads (77). If a patient receives 10 mCi; of ^{131}I (for treatment of hyperthyroidism), she would receive 5.1 rads of total body radiation (153). The mean gonadal dose is 0.45 rads/mCi (153,154). Whether this radiation dose is sufficient to cause genetic defects is not clear. However, chromosome abnormalities have been reported in the white cells of patients receiving treatment for thyrotoxicosis (155). In the case of the pregnant patient treated with radioactive iodine, it is known that a higher percentage of the dose per gram is concentrated in the fetal thyroid. Several cases of hypothyroidism have been reported in the offspring of mothers receiving therapeutic doses of 131 iodine for hyperthyroidism or cancer (156–161).

If the mother has received radioactive iodine, and is subsequently found to have been pregnant at the time of treatment, nothing further needs to be done (77). Even if therapeutic doses of 131 iodine were given for the treatment of hyperthyroidism, most authorities do not advise therapeutic abortion if the dose was given in the first trimester (162). However, a case can be made for termination of pregnancy because of the possibility of significant radiation effect to the fetus (77). In a recent survey, Stoffer and Hamburger (162) reported 237 cases of mothers who had received inadvertent radioiodine therapy for hyperthyroidism during the first trimester; 116 physicians were involved. Therapeutic abortions were advised for 55 patients by 22 physicians. From the 182 remaining pregnancies there were 2 spontaneous abortions, 2 stillbirths, 1 neonate with biliary atresia, and 1 with respiratory distress. This complication rate was no greater than might be expected in a similar number of random pregnancies. There were three documented cases of hypothyroidism in the infants, two of them with evidence of mental deficiency. From this survey the authors concluded that no therapeutic abortion should be advised in mothers that inadvertently received 131 iodine therapy early in the first trimester. They stressed the fact that a pregnancy test should be performed routinely on all women in the childbearing age group prior to the administration of therapeutic doses of 131 iodine.

If the mother has received radioactive iodine therapy in the second half of pregnancy, the possibility of hypothyroidism in the newborn is very high. Since thyroid medication given to the mother does not cross the placenta in significant amounts, intramniotic administration of thyroxine in order to prevent hypothyroidism in the fetus has recently been reported (163,164). In both experimental cases the infants developed normally. The authors suggest that this modality of treatment may help to minimize irreversible mental retardation in known high-risk infants.

LITHIUM, THYROID FUNCTION, AND PREGNANCY

Since the introduction of lithium carbonate for the treatment of various psychiatric disorders, a number of reports have appeared describing the development of thyroid enlargement or symptomatic hypothyroidism in patients receiving this drug (165–167). Studies of the effect of lithium on the hypothalamic-pituitary-thyroid function tests have shown that in some patients there is an increase in thyroid ^{131}I uptake, a decrease in 'um thyroxine, an increase in serum TSH, and an exaggerated TSH response to avenous thyrotropin releasing hormone (TRH). In some cases, though basal TSH are normal, there is an exaggerated TRH response. Schou et al. (165) described ant with a large goiter that remitted after a few months, born from a mother that 'eloped a goiter during lithium therapy. High levels of serum TSH were detected 'born from a mother treated with lithium during pregnancy; there was no the infant's thyroid tests returned to normal a week after delivery. In this her was treated for lithium intoxication at the eighth month of gestation. 'ne and TSH concentrations were normal in the mother, and a 6-month ' baby disclosed no nervous system disturbance (168).

IYROID REPLACEMENT THERAPY DURING PREGNANCY

in daily practice is the pregnant woman already on thyroid hor-
times without a proved thyroid disorder. In order to evaluate
y-thyroid function in patients on thyroid replacement therapy, it is
discontinue the drugs for at least 5 weeks (169). However, since
represent a risk to continuation of the pregnancy, it is our
hyroid replacement therapy during pregnancy, adjusting the dose
function tests. A serum TSH determination helps in deciding if
ough medication, and the determination of a free thyroxine index
the patient is taking excessive amounts of hormone. In most
e with thyroxine of 0.2 mg daily is needed to keep the patient
euthyroid (170).

C   JM METABOLISM IN PREGNANCY

Calcium plays a key role in many fundamental biologic processes. In spite of variations in intake and excretion, the concentration of calcium in cellular and extracellular fluids remains constant. This is due mainly to the effect of parathyroid hormone, vitamin D, and calcitonin.

The average adult human body contains approximately 1000 to 1200 g of calcium, of which approximately 1 g exists in the extracellular fluids. The rest is in the bone in the form of hydroxyapatite crystals. The normal adult ingests between 600 to 1000 mg of calcium daily. The calcium is absorbed primarily in the duodenum and upper jejunum. In addition to the calcium ingested in the diet, some 600 mg is added to the intestinal contents in the various intestinal secretions. Of this total of 1600 mg, about 40 to 50% is reabsorbed and the rest appears in the feces. The calcium that is absorbed enters the extracellular pool and is being exchanged constantly with that in the intracellular fluid, the glomerular filtrate and the bone. In addition, the calcium is filtrated through the kidney, but almost all of it is absorbed and only a small amount (about 100 mg) appears in the urine each day (171).

The calcium in plasma exists in three forms: ionized, ultrafiltrable, and protein-bound. Of the total calcium, about 46% is protein-bound, primarily to serum albumin, 48% is ionized and the remainder exists as ultrafiltrable complexes, chiefly citrate and phosphate. The ionized calcium concentration is the one that regulates a variety of biological processes. This is a very important concept since changes in plasma protein concentrations may lead to changes in total plasma calcium without a change in calcium ion concentration. This is particularly true in pregnancy since normally there is a decrease in serum protein concentration. Since the measurement of ionized calcium concentration is not easily carried out, the changes in total plasma calcium should be interpreted in the light of the above observation.

In addition to calcium, inorganic phosphate and magnesium are important elements in the regulation of mineral metabolism. The adult human body contains 500 to 600 g of phosphate, 85% of which is in the skeleton. In contrast to calcium, the concentration of plasma phosphate varies with age, diet and hormonal status. In the human adult, the range of values is 2.5 to 4.3 mg/100 ml.

More than 70% of ingested phosphate is absorbed from the intestinal tract. Vitamin D appears to have an active function in the absorption of the phosphate, independent of its effect on calcium absorption. The major excretory route for phosphate is the kidney. Normally about 600 mg is excreted in 24 hr.

Plasma magnesium concentration is between 1.3 and 2.0 mEq/liter in the human adult. Although very little is known about the factors involved in magnesium homeostasis, there is increasing evidence that one of these factors is parathyroid hormone.

Daily calcium requirements in pregnancy have been estimated by the National Research Council to be about 1200 mg/day, which is an increment of 400 mg above the nonpregnant daily requirement. This amount of calcium is easily provided by ingesting a quart of milk a day. For mothers unable to drink milk, 800 mg of calcium may be obtained in 100 g of cheese. In subjects with milk intolerance due to intestinal lactase deficiency, the calcium requirements have to be given in form of calcium salts. This increase in calcium intake is needed, since earlier studies have shown that the skeleton of newborn human infants contains 25 g of calcium (172). This was thought to be compensated by an accumulation of approximately 30 g that occur during pregnancy (173). Heaney and Skillman (174) studied 15 normal pregnant women, using a stable isotope of calcium, [48]calcium, for mineral balance and kinetic studies. They confirm that nitrogen, calcium, and phosphorus retention are associated with fetal development. In addition, they show a 20% increase in miscible calcium pool by term and a doubling of both pool turnover and bone mineral accretion rates, rising progressively with duration of pregnancy. They suggest that these changes represent maternal adjustment in advance, since 80% of fetal calcium is acquired during the last trimester of pregnancy. According to this study, pregnancy does not produce a net loss of calcium. In order to explain the mechanism for this, they postulated that an increase in growth hormone–like activity (human chorionic somatomammotropin (HCS) is responsible for the elevation in intestinal calcium absorption, urinary calcium secretion, and skeletal remodeling. At the same time, high estrogen levels decrease bone reabsorption and in turn produce an increase in parathyroid hormone (PTH) secretion; this in turn enhances calcium absorption and antagonizes the hypercalciuric effect of HCS. Heany and Skillman postulate that, with progression of gestation, parathyroid levels rise and as a result bone reabsorption rises and urinary calcium falls. As we will see later, increases in serum PTH levels in pregnancy have been reported (175).

Total serum calcium falls during pregnancy. This decline begins shortly after conception and is progressive until the middle of the third trimester, after which there is a slight rise (176,177). Serum phosphorus declines until approximately 30 weeks, at which time a drop of 6% from nonpregnant levels has occurred. Serum phosphorus then rises, to nearly nonpregnant levels by term. The most likely explanation of the decline in serum calcium in pregnancy is the fall in serum proteins. However, some reports have indicated a slight decrease in ionized calcium levels during pregnancy (178,179). Serum calcium appears to be actively transported from the mother to the fetus. At term the plasma total ultrafiltrable calcium and ionized calcium levels in the fetus exceed those in the mother. The placental transfer of isotopic calcium has been demonstrated in a number of species (180). However, there is a considerable species variation in the placental transfer of calcium. In the sheep, transfer of calcium occurs only from mother to fetus. In the monkey, bidirectional placental exchange occurs (180).

Parathyroid Hormone

Chemically, the parathyroid hormone is a single polypeptide chain of 84 amino acid residues. A fragment of this hormone, consisting of 33 amino acids at the N-terminal region of the molecule, is sufficient for the peptide to exert its characteristic biologic effect. A large parathyroid hormone (prohormone) with a molecular weight of 11,500 has been found. This proparathyroid hormone is converted in the gland to a molecule of 9500 for storage and secretion. The 9500-molecular-weight hormone is secreted as such, but in the periphery it appears to be converted to the 7500- and 4500-molecular-weight fragments (171,181,182). Most of the immunoreactive parathyroid peptides present in the peripheral circulation have been shown to have a molecular weight of approximately 7500 and to be biologically inactive. The major factor controlling parathyroid hormone secretion is the plasma level of ionized calcium.

The major function of PTH appears to be regulation of the rate of activation of bone metabolic units and the maintenance of plasma calcium concentration.

The major target organs for PTH action are kidney and bone. Parathyroid hormone also acts on the intestine, but here its effect may be indirect, achieved by controlling the renal synthesis of $1,25(OH)_2D_3$.

The most imprtant effects of PTH can be summarized as follows:

1. Increasing plasma calcium concentration and decreasing plasma phosphate concentration
2. Increasing excretion of phosphate and hydroxyproline in the kidney and decreasing excretion of calcium
3. Increasing the rate of skeletal remodeling and the net rate of bone reabsorption
4. Increasing the extent of osteocytic osteolysis in bone and increasing the number of both osteoclasts and osteoblasts on bone surfaces
5. Increasing the rate of conversion of $25(OH)D_3$ to $1,25(OH)_2D_3$ in renal tissue
6. Activating adenyl cyclase in the cells of its target tissues
7. Increasing the gastrointestinal absorption of calcium

Changes in parathyroid hormone levels in pregnancy have been reported by Cushard et al. (175). These authors reported a decrease in midpregnancy and a significant increase thereafter. The mean values of PTH doubled from the nonpregnant levels in the last 6 weeks of pregnancy. This increase in PTH was not correlated with changes in serum calcium and could be due to the increased calcium demands by the fetus in the last part of gestation. These changes appear to be specific for the pregnant state, for they revert to the prepregnancy levels soon after delivery regardless of whether lactation occurs. High values of PTH at the time of delivery were reported by Samaan and coworkers (183). It has been suggested that maternal parathyroid hormone facilitates the transport of calcium from mother to fetus (184).

Vitamin D

In the last few years it has been realized that, in order for vitamin D_3 (cholecalciferol) to be active, it must be metabolically altered (Fig. 3). It is known now that vitamin D_3 is metabolized in the liver to $25(OH)D_3$ and it is further converted in the kidney to $1,25(OH)_2D_3$. It has been shown that the latter is the metabolically active form. Nephrectomized vitamin D–deficient animals do not show intestinal calcium transfer response or bone calcium mobilization response to physiological doses of vitamin D_3 (cholecalciferol) or $25(OH)D_3$ (185). The concentration of $1,25(OH)_2D_3$ in blood is related to the serum calcium concentration; hypocalcemia stimulates the production of $1,25(OH)_2D_3$, and it was shown that PTH regulates its synthesis (186, 187). In the presence of elevated serum calcium, the kidney produces another metabolite, $24,25(OH)_2D_3$, instead of $1,25(OH)_2D_3$. The former metabolite is much less active than $1,25(OH)_2D_3$ (185).

The function of vitamin D is to maintain normal plasma calcium and phosphate. It accomplishes this by stimulating intestinal calcium absorption, activating phosphate transport in the small intestine, and mobilizing calcium from previously formed bones. The last processes also require parathyroid hormone.

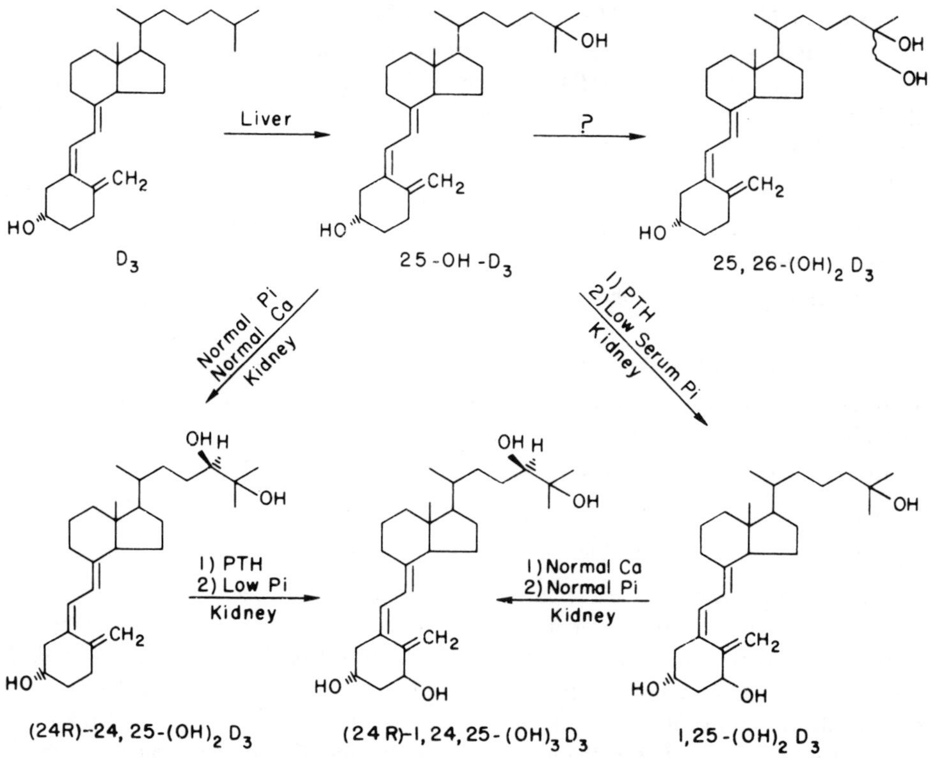

Figure 3. Vitamin D metabolism. From De Luca (185).

Levels of serum $25(OH)D_3$, the first step in the metabolism of vitamin D and the major circulating metabolite, were reported in pregnant women by Hillman and Haddad (188). The concentration was higher in summer than in winter months, but no seasonal difference in serum calcium was noted. They also concluded that regardless of race, ultraviolet exposure was the major determinant of maternal $25(OH)D_3$ in their patients in St. Louis. Turton et al. reported a decrease in plasma $25(OH)D_3$ in 33% of the group of pregnant women studied in South London. The reason for this change is unknown, but the authors proposed an enhanced maternal metabolism or increased utilization of vitamin D by the fetus (189). In other reports, neonatal rickets occurred in a group of mothers with low serum $25(OH)D_3$ and with evidence of osteomalacia (190–192). Rosen et al. (193) have postulated an association of low serum $25(OH)D_3$ and early neonatal hypocalcemia. Placental transfer of 25-hydroxyvitamin D $(25(OH)D_3)$ was suggested by the positive correlation between the higher concentration of total $25(OH)D_3$ in maternal serum and the lower concentration in cord serum (193,194). Vitamin D and its metabolites appear to be bound in serum to a protein (vitamin D–binding protein or DBP) (195–197); their concentration increases during pregnancy, whereas in cord serum a lower concentration is found (197). The free rather than the total concentration of steroids is the important factor in the placental transfer of steroids. The authors found a highly significant positive correlation between maternal and cord serum concentration of total and free $25(OH)D_3$. They suggested that, in view of the low circulating stores of $25(OH)D_3$ at birth, a vitamin D supplementation either during pregnancy or during early life could be used (197).

The daily vitamin D requirement in pregnancy is the same as in nonpregnant patients, 400 IU a day. It has been suggested that excessive amounts of vitamin D taken during pregnancy may be responsible for the syndrome of infantile hypercalcemia. However, this suggestion has not been confirmed (198,199).

Serum 25-hydroxyvitamin D $(25(OH)D_3)$ was measured by Fairney et al. (200) in a group of mothers who were breast-feeding and in a similar group who were not. Values were obtained during the first 3 days after delivery and at 4 to 6 weeks. The values were higher in the breast-feeding group, which suggested to the authors that no supplementary vitamin D is indicated during lactation.

CALCITONIN

Calcitonin is a small polypeptide hormone secreted by the thyroid gland and involved in calcium metabolism. It consists of a single sequence of 32 amino acid residues and has a molecular weight of 3000. The source of the hormone is specialized C cells, or parafollicular cells, that exist as small groups in the thyroid tissue. The only known physiologically important regulator of the rate of calcitonin secretion is the concentration of calcium ion in plasma. An increase in the serum calcium produces a secretion of calcitonin, which keeps the calcium within normal limits. Calcitonin appears to act on the bone, regulating the rate of skeletal remodeling and inhibiting bone reabsorption (201).

Calcitonin is produced in excessive amounts in patients with medullary carcinoma of the thyroid (171,202).

Calcitonin has been measured in pregnancy at the time of delivery by Samaan et al. (203). The mean calcitonin value in maternal peripheral blood was significantly higher than in normal nonpregnant subjects. The value in umbilical arterial blood was significantly higher than in umbilical venous blood. Serum calcitonin was found to be high early in life and to diminish with age. The suggestion was made that calcitonin may be of physiological significance in bone formation during intrauterine life and childhood. The difference between arterial umbilical blood and umbilical venous blood suggests that calcitonin is produced by the fetus and not by the placenta. It is possible that high levels of serum calcitonin in the newborn infant might be important in producing the hypocalcemia commonly seen in the first days of life.

PRIMARY HYPERPARATHYROIDISM

Primary hyperparathyroidism is a clinical condition caused by excessive secretion of parathyroid hormone due to a primary disease of the parathyroid glands. The incidence varies in different series. With automated laboratory facilities and routine analysis of serum calcium for all patients regardless of symptoms, the incidence of hyperparathyroidism has been reported to be as high as 1 per 1000 (204–206). It is more common among women than men. Women of childbearing age account for 20 to 25% of the cases reported (206,207). However, no more than 70 cases of hyperparathyroidism in pregnancy have been described in the English literature.

In nonpregnant patients, single adenomas account for 80% of the cases reported. These tumors are histologically of the chief cell type. More than one adenoma has been reported in 3% of the cases. Parathyroid carcinoma is a rare entity. Primary hyperplasia accounts for 15% of cases of primary hyperparathyroidism. In pregnancy, most cases have been due to single adenoma, and two cases of chief cell hyperplasia have been reported (208,227).

Patients with primary hyperparathyroidism may present with renal lithiasis, with bone disease, or without symptoms; the diagnosis is made by serendipity. The mode of presentation is shown in Table V. Recent reviews have emphasized many other symptoms that in the past were unrecognized, particularly weakness and fatigability,

Table V. Mode of Presentation of Hyperparathyroidism (%)

Renal stones	40
Osteitis fibrosa	10
Gastrointestinal symptoms	15
Hypertension	10
Pancreatitis	4
Psychiatric disorders	3
Myopathy	
Weakness	
Fatigability	
Weight loss	
Arthralgias	15
Pancreatitis	
Hyperparathyroid crisis	
Neonatal hypocalcemia in the patient's infant	
Serendipity	?

anemia, weight loss, psychiatric disturbances, gastrointestinal symptoms, and hypertension (209–211).

On physical examination, signs due specifically to hypercalcemia are few. Arterial hypertension has been reported in about 5 to 10% with primary hyperparathyroidism. Corneal calcification—thin linear aggregation, of coarsely granular appearance, on the lateral aspects of the cornea—is seen in 20% of patients with hyperparathyroidism. However, this sign is not specific and is present in patients with chronic hypercalcemia of any etiology. Parathyroid adenomas are rarely palpable. When palpable, it usually turns out to be a thyroid nodule. It is interesting that, in three cases of hyperparathyroidism in pregnancy, the nodules felt on physical examination were due to parathyroid adenomas (212–214).

Renal stones are the form of presentation in about 40% of patients with primary hyperparathyroidism. The incidence of primary hyperparathyroidism in patients with renal stones, however, is less than 5%. The stones contain calcium phosphate more often than oxalate and are radio-opaque. Less common disturbances are nephrocalcinosis, inability to concentrate the urine with symptoms of polyuria and nocturia. Renal function tests are normal in most patients with renal stones unless nephrocalcinosis or bilateral renal stones with urinary obstruction or infection are present.

Bone disease (osteitis fibrosa cystica) used to be a very common presentation of patients with primary hyperparathyroidism. The disease produces aches and pains, simulating rheumatism or myositis. At a later stage, severe bone pain and tenderness occur, sometimes with spontaneous fracture and deformities. In 1946, Norris reported the incidence of osteoitis fibrosa in patients with hyperparathyroidism to be 90% (215). However, recent surveys have shown a much lower incidence (205–206). The most characteristic radiological signs of bone disease are subperiosteal bone reabsorption in the metacarpals and phalanges of the fingers. These bone changes produce no symptoms. The serum alkaline phosphatase is usually elevated when these radiological changes are present. Advanced bone disease is characterized by single or multiple cystic lesions, granular appearance of the skull ("ground glass"), and generalized osteoporosis.

Hypercalcemic crisis is a medical emergency. It presents with marked weakness, mental deterioration, severe nausea and vomiting, progressive uremia, coma, and death within a short period. Dehydration is often an important contributory factor in the development of the crisis in patients with hypercalcemia.

Hyperparathyroidism in Pregnancy

The occurrence of hyperparathyroidism in pregnancy is a rare event. It was described for the first time by Friederischen in 1939 (216). He described a case of neonatal tetany due to hypocalcemia. The mother had hypercalcemia, renal calcification, and bone changes of hyperparathyroidism. In 1962, Ludwig (212) reviewed the literature and found 15 patients that displayed symptoms and signs of hyperparathyroidism during pregnancy and described two cases of his own. Only rarely was hyperparathyroidism recognized and diagnosed during gestation, and in most cases it was suspected only when the infant displayed tetany. Tetany appeared in many infants only when they were given cow's milk, which has a higher content of phosphorus. The fetal mortality in the cases reviewed by Ludwig was 50%. The diagnosis of hyperparathyroidism in pregnancy appeared certain in only 10 patients. Of the 20 pregnancies in these 10 patients, there were 4 stillbirths, 1 neonatal death, 4 premature infants with tetany, 7 normal infants at time of birth, and 1 spontaneous abortion. Therefore, perinatal mortality was 30% and prematurity was 20%. Of the 5 cases of neonatal hypocalcemia, 4 were premature babies. These mothers had not had treatment during pregnancy with the exception of the case reported by Petit and Clark (213), in which an adenoma was removed successfully during pregnancy. The infant developed no hypocalcemia at birth.

In 1972, Johnstone et al. (208) reported three cases of their own and reviewed 39 viable pregnancies in 35 patients with primary hyperparathyroidism. The perinatal mortality was 25% and there was a 50% incidence of neonatal tetany. The authors stated properly that patients described in the literature had a more severe form of hyperparathyroidism than is usually seen today. When screening tests are used more frequently, more asymptomatic cases are going to be discovered. Indeed, in the cases reviewed by Johnstone and coworkers, the incidence of renal stones and nephrocalcinosis was almost 80%. This incidence is much higher than the one reported in recent surveys in nonpregnant patients (205,206,209). Delmonico et al. (217) have reviewed 13 cases of proved hyperparathyroidism in pregnancy since the report by Ludwig in 1962 (212). The incidence of renal calculi in these patients was about 50%, the incidence of neonatal tetany was 50%, but the perinatal mortality was 1 case out of 12 viable pregnancies. In contrast to the early report by Ludwig, there were no stillbirths and most of the babies were born at full term. Although neonatal tetany is common in premature babies, the incidence in the full-term neonate is about 2%. Several cases of prolonged neonatal parathyroid suppression in infants of mothers with hyperparathyroidism have been reported (218,219).

Severe nausea and vomiting in the first trimester of pregnancy have been reported to be a common problem in patients with hyperparathyroidism (220).

Delmonico et al. (217) reported a case of secondary hyperparathyroidism following renal transplantation. Surgery was performed in the sixth month of pregnancy because of persistent hypercalcemia. At surgery, 3¾ hyperplastic glands were removed, and the histological diagnosis was chief cell hyperplasia. This case is very provocative; it suggests that, with the long-term increase in the population of female patients who have been successfully treated by renal transplantation, more cases of secondary hyperparathyroidism in pregnancy may be seen in the future (221,222).

Hypercalcemic crisis has been reported in two patients during pregnancy (223,224). Intensive treatment with fluid and furosemide (225) has improved the outcome for these patients.

Confirmation of the diagnosis of hyperparathyroidism is based on the demonstration of persistent hypercalcemia. The other causes of hypercalcemia must be considered and ruled out (Table VI).

Normal serum calcium values have been reported to be between 9 and 11 mg% in nonpregnant patients. Several factors modify the concentration of serum calcium, mainly the concentration of serum proteins in plasma. In pregnancy, there is a gradual decrease in serum calcium in the course of gestation. This decrease appears to be due to changes in serum albumin, although recent reports suggest there is a slight decrease in ionized serum calcium as well (178,179). Borderline or marginal hypercalcemia has been reported in 20 to 30% of nonpregnant patients with proved hyperparathyroidism (205,206). A persistent serum calcium in pregnancy of 10 mg% or above should be considered very suggestive of hypercalcemia, and other tests such as ionized serum calcium, serum phosphorus, and serum PTH determination may be helpful to confirm the

Table VI. Causes of Hypercalcemia

Primary Hyperparathyroidism
Carcinoma with bone metastasis
Vitamin D intoxication
Sarcoidosis
Thiazide diuretics
Milk-alkali syndrome
Multiple myeloma
Ectopic PTH production
Thyrotoxicosis
Acute adrenal insufficiency

diagnosis. Serum phosphorus determinations are abnormal in only 50% of patients with primary hyperparathyroidism (226). In pregnancy, serum phosphorus falls slightly from nonpregnant levels until approximately 30 weeks of gestation and then rises to nearly nonpregnant levels. Therefore, a serum phosphorus value below 2.5 mg% should be considered abnormal in pregnancy. Measurement of ionized serum calcium would be ideal, since there is only a slight decrease during pregnancy.

Parathyroid hormone assays are helpful in the diagnosis of hyperparathyroidism. As mentioned before, parathyroid hormone levels have been reported to increase during pregnancy, particularly after 32 weeks' gestation (175). Because of the normal feedback mechanism, it is expected that patients with hyperparathyroidism will have an inappropriate serum parathyroid hormone level in the presence of hypercalcemia. In the two cases reported with parathyroid hormone assays in pregnancy these values were definitely elevated in the presence of hypercalcemia (227,228). Therefore, the use of serum PTH would be of value in the evaluation of patients with hypercalcemia during pregnancy, since the other causes of hypercalcemia are associated with low or normal serum PTH values.

Eight cases of primary hyperparathyroidism treated during pregnancy have been reported, and in all but one of them (227) a single adenoma was found. In the patient reported by Gaeke et al. (227), surgery was performed during the seventeenth gestational week; four abnormal parathyroid glands were identified (chief cell hyperplasia), and partial parathyroidectomy was done. The mother delivered a normocalcemic baby. In most of these cases surgery was done in the first or second trimester of gestation; the exception is the case reported by Dorey and Gell (228), in which surgery was done at 36 weeks' gestation. Of these eight cases, there was only one fetal loss, of a 700 g premature baby (214). There was no case of neonatal hypocalcemia in the other seven cases. In the only case of secondary hyperparathyroidism reported by Delmonico et al. (217), the infant developed symptomatic hypocalcemia, requiring supplemental calcium gluconate. As mentioned before, this patient underwent surgery in the sixth month of her pregnancy.

In view of the data above, it seems appropriate to consider surgical treatment for symptomatic maternal hyperparathyroidism during pregnancy. Most patients treated during pregnancy have had marked elevations in the serum calcium. Of the eight cases reviewed by Johnstone et al. (208), more than 90% had serum calcium values greater than 12 mg%. Whether patients with minimal elevations of serum calcium and no evidence of complications such as renal calcinosis should be treated during pregnancy is not known at the present time. Whether the infants of these mothers would have an increase in perinatal mortality is uncertain. The maternal mortality and morbidity appears to be comparable with that of nonpregnant patients. Surgery is the only definite treatment yet devised for primary hyperparathyroidism. Following surgery, hypocalcemia follows in many patients, but it is of short duration and very mild, requiring no treatment. In patients with bone disease, hypocalcemia may be profound, and aggressive treatment is needed (229).

Tingling in the lips and fingers are common hypocalcemic symptoms on the day following surgery. Daily serum calcium determinination should be ordered, since the fall in calcium may occur a few days after surgery. In patients with minimal symptoms, a high calcium diet—four glasses of milk daily—is the only requirement. In patients with more severe symptoms, such as mental confusion, Trousseau signs and tetany, calcium gluconate—20 ml of the 10% solution—should be given slowly intravenously two or three times a day. Patients with bone disease should be treated with calcium supplement from the day of surgery, since these are the patients that will develop severe hypocalcemia. Vitamin D may be used, but it is very slow in taking effect. Recently, Montoro et al. (229a) reported 2 cases of hyperparathyroidism treated with oral phosphate because surgery was contraindicated. In both mothers the serum calcium returned to normal limits and the newborns developed no hypocalcemia.

HYPOPARATHYROIDISM

By far the most common cause of hypoparathyroidism is damage to or removal of the parathyroid glands in the course of an operation on the thyroid gland (230). Idiopathic hypoparathyroidism is a much less common cause of the disease; it occurs in children, and about twice as many females as males are affected. Less than 150 cases of idiopathic hypoparathyroidism have been reported in the literature. Other causes are much less common. A recent review proposed a new classification based on physiological principles (231).

The incidence of hypoparathyroidism following thyroid surgery has been estimated to be between 0.2 and 3.5%. In many cases the hypocalcemia in the immediate postoperative period is only transitory.

Idiopathic hypoparathyroidism has been associated with other endocrine diseases such as hypothyroidism, Addison disease, and ovarian failure. Antibodies against these endocrine tissues have been reported (232).

Several cases have been reported of idiopathic hypoparathyroidism occurring in the mother and her children (233,234). Transient hypoparathyroidism in the newborn infant has been reported many times in hyperparathyroid mothers. Unexplained hypocalcemia in the infant is an indication for serum calcium determination in the mother.

The diagnosis of hypoparathyroidism is based on previous history, particularly of thyroid surgery, and on clinical, radiological, and laboratory information. The symptoms of hypoparathyroidism are due to low concentration of serum calcium. Hypocalcemia is manifested by numbness and tingling in the fingers, toes, and around the lips, and if this is severe, it may produce carpopedal spasms, laryngeal stridor, dyspnea, and cyanosis. The patient may have convulsions. Mental abnormalities may occur in hypoparathyroidism with symptoms of irritability, emotional lability, impairment of memory, depression, etc. On physical examination, papilledema and cataracts may be seen. Some patients may present with ectopic calcification in the basal ganglia and subcutaneous tissue. In patients with idiopathic hypoparathyroidism changes in the teeth, skin, nails, and hair are very common.

Two signs may reveal latent tetany. The Chvostek sign, which is a twitch of the facial muscles, notably those of the upper lip when a sharp tap is given over the facial nerve in front of the ear. This test is not specific for hypocalcemia, since it has been described in 10% of normal adults. The Trousseau sign is the induction of carpopedal spasm by reducing the circulation in the arm with the blood pressure cuff. The constriction should be maintained above the systolic blood pressure for 2 min before the test is considered to be negative.

The electroencephalogram may be abnormal, with changes typical of idiopathic epilepsy.

The diagnosis is confirmed by low serum calcium and high serum phosphate levels. The plasma alkaline phosphatase level usually is normal or slightly low. The differential diagnosis of hypocalcemia includes rickets and osteomalacia and hypomagnesemia. In rickets and osteomalacia, the serum phosphate level is low, and the alkaline phosphatase level is increased. There is also a characteristic radiographic appearance of the bones. Hypomagnesemia may be due to chronic diarrhea, abuse of diuretics, or chronic alcoholism.

Although hypoparathyroidism in pregnancy appears to be uncommon, it is interesting to know that, in 1942, Anderson and Musselman (235) reviewed the literature on pregnancy and tetany and collected 240 cases. Twenty-six of these cases were due to postthyroid surgery; there were 145 cases of the so-called idiopathic type. It is likely that, in some of these cases, tetany was not due to hypoparathyroidism. Before specific therapy was available, fetal and maternal mortality was so high that therapeutic abortion was routinely recommended. With the availability of vitamin D and the use of calcium supplementation, the prognosis was much better, and the babies revealed no unusual abnormalities.

Graham et al. (236) reported several cases of hypoparathyroidism that were well controlled during pregnancy with vitamin D; there were no problems with the newborn infants. However, if the mother is not treated properly, hypoparathyroidism with hypocalcemia may be deleterious to the newborn. Several of the cases of hyperparathyroidism in the newborn were reported in untreated or poorly controlled hypoparathyroid mothers. Aceto et al. (237) reported a case of idiopathic hypoparathyroidism in a pregnant women who did not receive the proper amount of vitamin D during her pregnancy; the infant had radiological changes of hyperparathyroidism during intrauterine life. Later they reported another infant from the same mother without evidence of bone disease in spite of hypocalcemia in the mother during gestation (234). Landing and Kamoshita (238) reported a pair of twins born prematurely of a hypoparathyroid mother. Both infants had marked parathyroid hyperplasia and typical bone changes of hyperparathyroidism. These changes reverted to normal in 4 to 9 months. Bronsky et al. (239) reported two cases of intrauterine hyperparathyroidism secondary to maternal hypoparathyroidism. They suggested the passage of parathyroid hormone from fetus to mother, since the symptoms of hypocalcemia in the mother remitted during pregnancy.

An unusual case of hypocalcemia and tetany brought about by the use of magnesium sulfate was reported in a pregnant woman with toxemia (240).

Treatment of hypoparathyroidism in pregnancy does not differ from the nonpregnant state (236,241). Vitamin D requirements do not seem to increase during pregnancy; the recommended dietary allowance is 400 IU/day for both pregnant and nonpregnant individuals. Therefore, the patient should continue with the same amount of vitamin D that she was taking before pregnancy, an amount that usually ranges from 50,000 to 150,000 IU/day. She should also take the normal calcium supplementation for pregnancy, about 1.2 g/day. As an alternative to vitamin D, dihydrotachysterol can be given in doses from 0.1 to 0.5 mg daily. The major problem in the treatment of hypoparathyroidism is that recurrent episodes of hyper- and hypocalcemia are common even in conscientious patients (242). The therapeutically effective and the toxic doses of vitamin D are often close to each other. In addition, because vitamin D acts slowly, it is difficult to anticipate therapeutic activity. Furthermore, because of the prolonged storage of vitamin D in the body, when hypercalcemia develops, it may persist for months (243). For this reason, serum calcium should be checked at frequent intervals in order to maintain the serum calcium concentration at approximately 9 mg/100 ml. In patients who do not respond to vitamin D administration, hypomagnesemia should be ruled out. Magnesium supplementation has been reported to improve the management of such patients (244).

Hypercalcemia during treatment with vitamin D should be treated promptly with discontinuation of vitamin D and calcium, hydration, and, if needed, corticosteroid therapy in the form of Prednisone (from 20 to 60 mg/day). The most common symptoms of vitamin D intoxication are nausea, constipation, fatigue, headaches, and, in more severe cases, vomiting and dehydration.

In the postpartum period serum calcium determination should be performed in hypoparathyroid patients, since postpartum hypercalcemia has been reported by Wright et al. (245). A similar case has been seen by us (246). In these patients hypercalcemia developed postpartum in spite of good hydration and taking the same amount of vitamin D and calcium during pregnancy. There is no explantation for this phenomenon, and it is suggested that careful monitoring of serum calcium be done in the postpartum period (245).

Since the doses of vitamin D required to achieve normal calcemia in patients with hypoparathyroidism are large and variable and the effects are slow in onset, new synthetic metabolites of vitamin D_3 have recently been used in the treatment of this condition. Preliminary reports appear to indicate advantages with the use of these new metabolites (247,248).

Lactation in mothers taking vitamin D is perhaps not indicated, since a metabolite of vitamin D, 25-hydroxyvitamin D_3 has been detected in breast in high content in a mother taking 50,000 units of vitamin D daily for the treatment of hypoparathyroidism (249).

OSTEOMALACIA IN PREGNANCY

The term osteomalacia was applied originally to the distinct clinical syndrome consisting of severe bone pain, skeletal deformity, depressed serum calcium × phosphorous ion product, and wide osteoid borders in bone—all associated with vitamin D deficiency (250). The term is now used for patients with some clinical features of the disease.

In the United States, the disease is due to malabsorption syndromes, particularly idiopathic sprue. It has been reported in 15% of patients following gastrectomy and in patients with Fanconi syndrome. Recently, several reports have indicated an increased incidence of osteomalacia in patients on anticonvulsive drugs (251–253).

An increase in osteomalacia has been observed in Great Britain among the Asian immigrant population (254), and this was observed, too, in pregnant women and newborns (191,192). Watney et al. (190) described an increase in subclinical hypocalcemia on the sixth day of life in full-term infants, especially during the winter months in babies of Asian parents. It appears that lack of contact with direct sunlight is the major reason for hypovitaminosis D. Ford et al. (191) described two cases of neo-natal rickets in the offspring of Asian immigrant mothers suffering from osteomalacia.

The diagnosis of osteomalacia is based on clinical, radiological, and laboratory find-ings. Bone pain and proximal muscle weakness are typical. Wide osteoid borders are characteristic on biopsy. Pseudo-fractures are seen on radiological examination of the ribs, pelvis, or long bones.

Low serum calcium, low serum phosphate, and elevation in serum alkaline phos-phatase are typically seen. In addition, the calcium in the urine is low.

Treatment is directed toward the underlying disease and the use of vitamin D. The amount of vitamin D varies, but in patients with a malabsorption syndrome, up to 50,000 units a day may be required. New metabolites of vitamin D have been recently reported to be very effective therapy; this has been discussed previously (247,248).

ACKNOWLEDGMENT

The author is indebted to Mrs. S. Rodriguez for her secretarial assistance.

REFERENCES

1. Tunbridge, W. M. G., and Hall, R.: Thyroid function in pregnancy. *Clinics Obst. Gynec.* 2:381–393, 1975.

2. Crooks, J., Aboul-Khair, S. A., Turnbull, A. C., and Hytten, F.: The incidence of goitre during preg-nancy. *Lancet* 2:334–336, 1964.

3. Crooks, J., Tullock, M. I., Turnbull, A. C., Davidsson, D., Skulason, T., and Snaedal, G.: Compara-tive incidence of goitre in pregnancy in Iceland and Scotland. *Lancet* 2:625–627, 1967.

4. Hershman, J. M., Kenimer, J. G., Higgins, J. P., and Patillo, R. A.: Placental thyrotropin, in *Perinatal Thyroid Physiology and Disease,* edited by Fisher, D. A., and Burrow, G. N. Raven Press, 1974, p. 11.

5. Dowling, J. T., Freinkel, N., and Ingbar, S. H.: The effect of estrogens upon the peripheral metabolism of thyroxine. *J. Clin. Invest.* 39:1119, 1960.

6. Dowling, J. T., Freinkel, N., and Ingbar, S. H.: Thyroxine-binding by sera of pregnant women, newborn infants and women with spontaneous abortion. *J. Clin. Invest.* 35:1263, 1956.

7. Rastogi, G. K., Sawhney, R. C., Sinha, M. K., Thomas, Z., and Devi, P. K.: Serum and urinary levels of thyroid hormones in normal pregnancy. *Obst. Gynec.* 44:176–180, 1974.

8. Auruskin, T. W., Mitsuma, T., Shenkman, L., Sau, K., and Hollander, C. S.: Measurements of free and total serum T3 and T4 in pregnant subjects and in neonates. *Am. J. Med. Science* 271:309–315, 1976.

9. Malkasian, G. D., and Mayberry, W. E.: Serum total and free thyroxine and thyrotropin in normal and pregnant women, neonates and women receiving progestogens. *Am. J. Obst. Gynec.* 108:1234–1238, 1970.

10. Soume, J. A., Niejadlick, D. G., Cottrell, S., et al.: Comparison of thyroid function in each trimester of pregnancy with the use of triiodothyronine uptake, thyroxine iodine, free thyroxine and free thyroxine index. *Am. J. Obst. Gynec.* 116:905–910, 1973.

11. Oppenheimer, S. H., Squef, R., Surks, M. I., et al.: Binding of thyroxine of serum proteins evaluated by equilibrium dialysis and electrophoretic techniques: Alterations in non-thyroidal illness. *J. Clin. Invest.* 42:1769, 1963.

12. Dowling, J. T., Appleton, W. G., and Nicoloff, J. T.: Thyroxine turnover during human pregnancy. *J. Clin. Endoc. Metab.* 27:1749, 1967.

13. Braverman, L. E., Ingbar, S. H., and Sterling, K.: Conversion of thyroxine (T4) to triiodothyronine (T3) in athyreotic human subjects. *J. Clin. Invest.* 49:855, 1970.

14. Surks, M. I., Schadlow, A. R., Stock, J. M., and Oppenheimer, J. H.: Determination of iodothyronine absorption and conversion of L-thyroxine (T4) to L-triiodothyronine (T3) using turnover rate techniques. *J. Clin. Invest.* 52:805, 1973.

15. Carlson, H. E., and Hershman, J. M.: The hypothalamic-pituitary-thyroid axis. *Med. Clin. N.A.* 59:1045–1053, 1975.

16. Haigler, E. D., Jr., Pittman, J. A., Jr., Hershman, J. H., and Baugh, C. M.: Direct evaluation of pituitary thyrotropin reserve utilizing synthetic thyrotropin releasing hormone. *J. Clin. Endoc. Metab.* 33:573, 1971.

17. Burrow, G. N.: Thyroid and parathyroid function in pregnancy, in *Endocrinology of Pregnancy,* 2nd ed., edited by Fuchs, F., and Klopper, A. Harper and Row, Publishers, 1977, pp. 246–270.

18. Kannan, V., Sinha, M. K., Devi, P. K., and Rastogi, G. K.: Plasma thyrotropin and its response to thyrotropin-releasing hormone in normal pregnancy. *Obst. Gynec.* 42:547–549, 1973.

19. Hennen, G., Pierce, J. G., and Freychet, P.: Human chorionic thyrotropin. *J. Clin. Endoc. Metab.* 29:581, 1969.

20. Higgins, H. P., Hershamn, J. M., Kenimer, J. G., Patillo, R. A., Bayley, A., and Walfish, P.: The thyrotoxicosis of hydatidiform mole. *Ann. Int. Med.* 83:307, 1975.

21. Hershman, J. M., and Starnes: Extraction and characteristics of a thyrotropic material from the human placenta. *J. Clin. Invest.* 48:923, 1969.

22. Hotelling, D. R., and Sherwood, L. M.: The effects of pregnancy on circulating triiodothyronine. *J. Clin. Endoc. Metab.* 33:383, 1971.

23. Larsen, P. R.: Triiodothyronine: Review of recent studies of its physiology and pathophysiology in man. *Metabolism* 21:1073, 1972.

24. Sterling, K., Refetoff, S., and Selenkow, H. A.: T3 thyrotoxicosis: thyrotoxicosis due to elevated serum triiodothyronine levels. *J.A.M.A.* 213:571, 1970.

25. Larsen, P. R.: Tests of thyroid function. *Med. Clinics N.A.* 59:1063, 1975.

26. Mestman, J. H.: A practical approach to thyroid function tests. *Contem. OB/GYN* 9:28, 1977.

27. Clark, F., and Horn, D. B.: Assessment of thyroid function by the combined use of the serum protein bound iodine and resin uptake of 131I-triiodothyronine. *J. Clin. Endoc. Metab.* 25:35, 1965.

28. Stein, R. B., and Price, L.: Evaluation of adjusted total thyroxine (free thyroxine index) as a measure of thyroid function. *J. Clin. Endoc. Metab.* 34:225, 1972.

29. Hamada, S. Nakagawa, J., Mori, T., and Torizuka, K.: Re-evaluation of thyroxine binding and free thyroxine in human serum by paper electrophoresis and equilibrium dialysis, and a new free thyroxine index. *J. Clin. Endoc. Metab.* 31:166, 1970.

30. Sterling, K., and Brenner, M.: Free thyroxine in human serum: Simplified measurement with the aid of magnesium precipitation. *J. Clin. Invest.* 45:153, 1966.

31. Hershman, J. M., and Pittman, J. A.: Utility of the radioimmunoassay of serum thyrotropin in man. *Ann. Int. Med.* 74:481, 1971.

32. Pochin, E. E.: The iodine uptake of the human thyroid throughout the menstrual cycle and pregnancy. *Clinical Science* 2:441–445, 1952.

33. Halman, K. E.: The radioiodine uptake of the human thyroid in pregnancy. *Clinical Science* 17:281–290, 1958.

34. Goldsmith, R. E., McAdams, A. J., Larsen, P. R., Mackenzie, M., and Hess, E. V.: Familial autoimmune disease and thyroiditis: Maternal-fetal relationship and the role of generalized autoimmunity. *J. Clin. Endoc.* 39:265, 1973.

35. Azukizawa, M. Murata, Y., Ikenoue, T., et al.: Effect of thyrotropin-releasing hormone on secretion of thyrotropin, prolactin, thyroxine, and triiodothyronine in pregnancy and fetal rhesus monkeys. *J. Clin. Endoc. Metab.* 43:1020, 1976.

36. Grumbach, M. M., and Werner, S. C.: Transfer of thyroid hormone across the human placenta at term. *J. Clin. Endoc.* 16:1392, 1956.

37. Raiti, S., Holzman, G. B., Scott, R. L., and Blizzard, R. M.: Evidence for the placental transfer of triiodothyronine in human beings. *N.E.J.M.* 277:456, 1967.

38. Dussault, J., Row, V. V., Lickrish, G., and Volpe, R.: Studies of triiodothyronine concentration in maternal and cord blood: Transfer of triiodothyronine across the human placenta. *J. Clin. Endoc.* 29:595, 1969.

39. Abuid, J., Stinson, D. A., and Larsen, P. R.: Serum triiodothyronine and thyroxine in the neonate and the acute increases in these hormones following delivery. *J. Clin. Invest.* 52:1195, 1973.

40. McKenzie, J. M.: Neonatal Graves' disease. *J. Clin. Endoc.* 24:660, 1964.

41. Sunshine, P., Kusamoto, H., and Kriss, J. P.: Survival time of circulating long-acting thyroid stimulator in neonatal thyrotoxicosis: Implication for diagnosis and therapy of the disorder. *Pediatrics* 36:869, 1965.

42. Farrehi, C., Mitchell, M., and Fawcett, D.: Heart failure in congenital thyrotoxicosis. *Pediatrics* 37:460–466, 1966.

43. Green, W. L.: Humoral and genetic factors in thyrotoxic Graves' disease and neonatal thyrotoxicosis. *J.A.M.A.* 235:1449–1450, 1976.

44. Nutt, J., Clark, F., Welch, R. G., and Hall, R.: Neonatal hyperthyroidism and long-acting thyroid stimulator protector. *Brit. Med. J.* 4:695, 1974.

45. Dirmikis, S. M., and Munro, D. S.: Placental transmission of thyroid-stimulating immunoglobulins. *Brit. Med. J.* 2:665, 1975.

46. Adams, D. D., and Kennedy, T. H.: Occurrence in thyrotoxicosis of a gamma globulin which protects LATS from neutralization by an extract of thyroid gland. *J. Clin. Endoc. Metab.* 27:173, 1967.

47. Aaron, H. H., Schneierson, S. J., and Siegel, E.: Goiter in newborn infant due to mother's ingestion of propylthiouracil. *J.A.M.A.* 159:848, 1955.

48. Freiesleben, R., and Kverulf-Jensen, K.: Effect of thiouracil derivatives on fetuses and infants. *J. Clin. Endoc. Metab.* 7:47, 1947.

49. Elphinstone, N.: Thiouracil in pregnancy: Its effects on fetuses. *Lancet* 1:1281, 1953.

50. Branch, L. K., and Tuthill, S. W.: Goiters in twins resulting from propylthiouracil given during pregnancy. *Ann. Int. Med.* 46:145, 1957.

51. Burrow, G. N.: Neonatal goiter after maternal propylthiouracil therapy. *J. Clin. Endoc. Metab.* 25:403, 1965.

52. Aboul-Khair, S. A., Crooks, J., Turnbull, A. C., and Hytten, F. E.: The physiological changes in thyroid function during pregnancy. *Clinical Science* 27:195–207, 1964.

53. Dworkin, H. J., Jacquez, J. A., and Beierwaltes, W. H.: Relationship of iodine ingestion to iodine excretion in pregnancy. *J. Clin. Endoc. Metab.* 26:1328, 1966.

54. Stoffer, R. P., Joeneke, I. A., Chesky, V. E., and Hellwig, C. A.: The thyroid in pregnancy. *Am. J. Obst. Gynec.* 74:300–308, 1974.

55. Innerfield, R., and Hollanger, C. S.: Thyroidal complications of pregnancy. *Med. Clinic N.A.* 61:67–87, 1977.

56. Ingbar, S. H., and Woeber, K. A.: The thyroid gland, in *Textbook of Endocrinology*, ed. by R. Williams. W. B. Saunders Co., 1974, p. 212.

57. Blizzard, R. M., Chandler, R. W., Landing, B. H., Pettit, M. D., and West, C. D.: Maternal autoimmunization to thyroid as a probable cause of athyrotic cretinism. *N.E.J.M.* 263:327, 1960.

58. Beirwaltes, M. H., Dodson, V. N., and Wheeler, A. H.: Thyroid autoantibodies in the families of cretins. *J. Clin. Endoc. Metab.* 19:179, 1969.

59. Thier, S. O., Black, P., Williams, H. C., and Robbins, J.: Chronic lymphocytic thyroiditis: Report of a kindred with viral, immunological and chemical studies. *J. Clin. Endoc. Metab.* 25:65, 1965.

60. Nelson, J. C., and Palmer, F. J.: A remission of goitrous hypothyroidism during pregnancy. *J. Clin. Endoc. Metab.* 40:383–385, 1975.

61. Amini, N., Miyai, K., Onishi, T., et al.: Transient hypothyroidism after delivery in autoimmune thyroiditis. *J. Clin. Endoc. Metab.* 42:296, 1976.

62. Amino, N., Miyai, K., Kuro, R., et al.: Transient postpartum hypothyroidism: Fourteen cases with autoimmune thyroiditis. *Ann. Int. Med.* 87:155–159, 1977.

63. St. Hill, C., Finn, R., and Denye, V.: Depression of cellular immunity in pregnancy due to a serum factor. *Brit. Med. J.* 3:513, 1973.

64. Parker, R. H., and Beirwaltes, W. H.: Thyroid antibodies during pregnancy and in the newborn. *J. Clin. Endoc. Metab.* 21:792, 1961.

65. Fialkow, P. J.: Autoimmunity and chromosomal aberrations. *Am. J. Human Genetics* 18:93, 1966.

66. Shimaoka, K., Badillo, J., et al.: Clinical differentiation between thyroid cancer and benign goiter. *J.A.M.A.* 181:179, 1962.

67. Silverberg, S. G., and Vidone, R. A.: Adenoma and carcinoma of the thyroid. *Cancer* 19:1053, 1966.

68. Schneider, A. B., Favus, M. J., Stachura, M. E., et al.: Plasma thyroglobulin in detecting thyroid carcinoma after childhood head and neck irradiation. *Ann. Intern. Med.* 86:29–34, 1977.

69. Gershengorn, M. C., McClung, M. R., Chu, E. W., et al.: Fine-needle aspiration cytology in the preoperative diagnosis of thyroid nodules. *Ann. Intern. Med.* 87:265–269, 1977.

70. Walfish, P. G., Hazani, E., Strawbridge, H. T. G., et al.: Combined ultrasound and needle aspiration cytology in the assessment and management of hypofunctioning thyroid nodule. *Ann. Intern. Med.* 87:270–274, 1977.

71. Rosvoll, R. V., and Winship, T.: Thyroid carcinoma and pregnancy. *Surgery Gynec. Obst.* 121:1030–1042, 1965.

72. Hill, C. S., Jr., Clark, R. L., and Wolf, M.: The effect of subsequent pregnancy on patients with thyroid carcinoma. *Surgery Gynec. Obst.* 122:1219, 1966.

73. Gillstrap, L. C., III, Brekken, A. L., and Harris, R. E.: Sipple syndrome and pregnancy. *J.A.M.A.* 235:1136, 1976.

74. Echt, C. R., and Doss, J. F.: Myxedema in pregnancy *Obst. Gynec.* 22:615, 1963.

75. Goldsmith, R. E., Sturgis, S. H., Herman, J., and Stansbury, J. B.: The menstrual pattern in thyroid disease. *J. Clin. Endoc. Metab.,* 12:846, 1952.

76. Mann, E. B., Holden, R. H., and Jones, W. S.: Thyroid function in human pregnancy: VII. Development and retardation of 4-year old progeny of euthyroid and hypothyroxinemic women. *Am. J. Obst. Gynec.* 109:12, 1971.

77. Burrow, G. N.: *The Thyroid Gland in Pregnancy.* W. B. Saunders Company, 1972.

78. Fisher, D.: Thyroid physiology in the fetus and newborn, in *Current Concepts and Approaches to Perinatal Thyroid Disease in Diabetes and Other Endocrine Diseases During Pregnancy and in the Newborn,* ed. by M. I. New and R. A. Fine. Alan R. Liss, Inc., New York, 1976, p. 221.

78a. Montoro, M., Frazier, D., Collea, J. V., and Mestman, J. H.: Hypothyroidism and pregnancy. Report of 11 pregnancies in 9 women and review of the literature (in preparation).

79. Maeda, M., Kuzuya, N., Masuyama, Y., et al.: Changes in serum triiodothyronine, thyroxine, and thyrotropin during treatment with thyroxine in severe primary hypothyroidism. *J. Clin. Endoc. Metab.,* 43:10, 1976.

80. Mussey, R. D., Haines, S. F., and Ward, E.: Hyperthyroidism and pregnancy. *Am. J. Obst. Gynec.* 55:609–619, 1948.

81. Jondahl, W. H., Banner, E. A., and Howell, L. P.: Management of pregnancy complicated by toxic goiter: Report of case. *Proc. Staff Meet. Mayo Clin.* 24:358–361, 1949.

82. Fursyfer, J., Kurland, L. T., McConahey, W. M., and Elveback, L. R.: Graves' disease in Olmstead County, Minnesota, 1935 through 1967. *Mayo Clin. Proc.* 45:636–644, 1970.

83. Mestman, J. H., Manning, P. R., and Hodgman, J.: Hyperthyroidism and pregnancy. *Arch. Int. Med.* 134:434, 1974.

84. Javert, C. T.: Hyperthyroidism in pregnancy. *Am. J. Obst. Gynec.* 39:954–963, 1940.

85. Hoffenberg, G. R., Louw, J. H., and Voss, T. J.: Thyroidectomy under hypothermia in a pregnant patient with thyroid crisis. *Lancet* 2:687–689, 1961.

86. Gardiner-Hill, H.: Pregnancy complicating simple goiter and Graves' disease. *Lancet* 1:120–124, 1929.

87. Asper, S. P., Jr., and London, F.: Thyrotoxicosis and pregnancy. *Trans. Am. Clin. Climatol. Assoc.* 72:110–118, 1960.

88. Astwood, E. B.: The use of antithyroid drugs during pregnancy. *J. Clin. Endoc. Metab.* 11:1045–1056, 1951.

89. Bell, G. O., and Hall, J.: Hyperthyroidism in pregnancy. *Med. Clinics N.A.* 44:363–367, 1960.

90. Hawe, P.: The management of thyrotoxicosis during pregnancy. *Br. J. Surg.* 52:731–734, 1965.

91. Herbst, A. L., and Selenkow, H. A.: Hyperthyroidism during pregnancy. *N.E.J.M.* 273:627–633, 1965.

92. Bokat, M. A.: Treatment of hyperthyroidism during pregnancy, in Astwood, E. B., Cassidy, C. E. (eds.): *Clinical Endocrinology,* New York, Grune and Stratton Inc., 1968, vol. 2, pp. 236–243.

93. Becker, W. F., and Sudduth, P. G.: Hyperthyroidism and pregnancy. *Ann. Surg.* 149:867–874, 1959.

94. Ayromlooi, J., Zervoudakis, I., and Sadaghat, A.: Thyrotoxicosis in pregnancy. *Am. J. Obst. Gynec.* 117:818–823, 1973.

95. Worley, R. J., and Crosby, W. M.: Hyperthyroidism during pregnancy. *Am. J. Obst. Gynec.* 119:150–155, 1974.

96. Goluboff, L. G., Sisson, J. C., and Hamburger, J. I.: Hyperthyroidism associated with pregnancy. *Obst. Gynec.* 44:107–116, 1974.

97. Mujtaba, Q., and Burrow, G. N.: Treatment of hyperthyroidism in pregnancy with propylthiouracil and methimazole. *Obst. Gynec.* 46:282–286, 1975.

98. Lebacq, G., Therasse, G., Schmidt, A., Delannoy, A., and Destailleurs, C.: Subacute thyroiditis: Eleven cases with histological confirmation and thyrotropin response to thyrotropin releasing hormone. *Acta Endocrinologica* 81:707–715, 1976.

99. Volpe, R.: Thyroiditis: Current views of pathogenesis. *Med. Clinics N.A.* 59:1163–1175, 1975.

100. Ormston, B. J., Garry, R., Cryer, R. J., Besser, G. M., and Hall, R.: Thyrotrophin-releasing hormone as a thyroid function test. *Lancet* 2:10–14, 1971.

101. Franco, P. S., Hershman, J. M., Haigler, E. D., Jr., and Pittman, J. A., Jr.: Response to thyrotropin-releasing hormone compared with thyroid suppression tests in euthyroid Graves' disease. *Metabolism* 22:1357, 1973.

102. Piper, J., and Rosen, J.: Management of hyperthyroidism during pregnancy. *Acta Med. Scand.* 150:215, 1954.

103. Prout, T. E.: Thyroid disease in pregnancy. *Am. J. Obst. Gynec.* 122:669, 1975.

104. Werner, S. C.: Hyperthyroidism in the pregnant woman and the neonate. *J. Clin. Endoc. Metab.* 67:1637–1654, 1967.

105. Komins, J. T., Snyder, P. J., and Schwartz, R. H.: Hyperthyroidism and pregnancy. *Obstet. Gynec. Surgery* 30:527, 1975.

106. Selenkow, H. A., Birnbaum, M. O., and Hollander, C. S.: Thyroid function and dysfunction during pregnancy. *Clin. Obstet. Gynec.* 16:66, 1973.

107. Hawe, P.: The management of thyrotoxicosis during pregnancy. *Brit. J. Surg.* 52:731, 1965.

108. Talbert, L. M., Thomas, C. G., Jr., Holt, W. A., and Rankin, P.: Hyperthyroidism during pregnancy. *Obst. Gynec.* 36:779, 1970.

109. Emslander, R. F., Weeks, R. E., and Malkasian, G. D., Jr.: Hyperthyroidism and pregnancy. *Med. Clinics N.A.* 58:835, 1974.

110. Ramsay, I. D.: Thyroid therapy in pregnancy, in *Therapeutic Problems in Pregnancy,* ed. P. J. Lewis. University Park Press, Baltimore, 1977, p. 93.

111. Burrow, G. N.: Thyroid diseases, in *Medical Complications During Pregnancy,* ed. Burrow and Ferris. W. B. Saunders Company, 1977, p. 196.

112. Greer, M. A., Kammer, H., and Bouma, D. J.: Short-term antithyroid drug therapy for the thyrotoxicosis of Graves' disease. *N.E.J.M.* 297:173, 1977.

113. Fraser, R., and Wilkinson, M.: Simplified method of drug treatment for thyrotoxicosis. *Brit. Med. J.* 1:481, 1953.

114. Asper, S., and London, F.: Thyrotoxicosis and pregnancy. *J. Amer. Climat. Clin. Assoc.* 72:110, 1960.

115. Herbst, A. L., and Selenkow, H. A.: Combined antithyroid-thyroid therapy of hyperthyroidism in pregnancy. *Obstet. Gynec.* 21:543, 1963.

116. Reinfrank, R. F.: Hyperthyroidism in pregnancy. *Southern Med. J.* 64:299, 1971.

117. Horger, E. O., III, Kenimer, J. G., Azukizawa, M., et al.: Failure of triiodothyronine to prevent propylthiouracil-induced hypothyroidism and goiter in fetal sheep *Obst. Gynec.* 47:46, 1976.

118. Keynes, G.: Obstetrics and gynecology in relation to thyrotoxicosis and myasthenia gravis. *J. Obstet. Gynaec. Brit. Emp.* 59:173, 1952.

119. Ibberstsow, H. K., Seddon, R. J., and Croxson, M. S.: Fetal hypothyroidism complicating medical therapy of thyrotoxicosis in pregnancy. *Clin. Endocrin.* 4:521, 1975.

120. Hamburger, J.: Management of the pregnant hyperthyroid. *Obst. Gynec.* 40:114, 1972.

121. Burrow, G. N., Bartsocas, C., Klatskin, E. H., et al.: Children exposed in utero to propylthiouracil: Subsequent intellectual and physical development. *Am. J. Dis. Child.* 116:161–165, 1968.

122. Milham, S., Jr., and Elledge, W.: Maternal methimazole and congenital defects in children. *Teratology* 5:125, 1972.

123. Levy, C. A., Waite, J. H., and Dickey, R.: Thyrotoxicosis and pregnancy: Use of preoperative propanolol for thyroidectomy. *Am. J. Surg.* 133:319, 1977.

124. Langer, A., Hung, C., Mc A'Nulty, J., et al.: Adrenergic blockade: A new approach to hyperthyroidism during pregnancy. *Obst. Gynec.* 44:181, 1974.

125. Joelsson, I., Barton, M. D., Daniel, S., James, S., and Adamson, K.: The response of the unanesthetized sheep fetus to sympathomimetic aminos and adrenergic blocking agents. *Am. J. Obst. Gynec.* 114:43, 1972.

126. Fiddler, G. I.: Propanolol in pregnancy. *Lancet* 2:722, 1974.

127. Gladstone, G. R., Hordof, A., and Gersony, W.: Propanolol administration during pregnancy: Effects on the fetus. *J. Pediatrics* 86:962, 1975.

128. Man, E. P., Shaver, B. A., and Cooke, R. E.: Studies of children born to women with thyroid disease. *Am. J. Obst. Gynec.* 75:728, 1958.

129. Ginsberg, J., and Walfish, P. G.: Post-partum transient thyrotoxicosis with painless thyroiditis. *Lancet* 1:1125–1128, 1977.

130. Amino, N., Miyai, K., Yamamoto, T., et al.: Transient recurrence of hyperthyroidism after delivery in Graves' disease. *J. Clin. Endoc. Metab.* 44:130, 1977.

131. Tisne, L., Barzelatto, J., and Stevenson, C.: Estudio de la funcion tiroidea durante el estado gravida–puerperal con el yodo radioactivo. *Bol. Soc. Chil. Obstet. Ginecol.* 20:246–251, 1955.

132. Dowling, J. T., Ingbar, S. H., and Freinkel, N.: Iodine metabolism in hydatidiform mole and choriocarcinoma. *J. Clin. Endoc. Metab.* 20:1–12, 1960.

133. Kock, H., van Kessel, H., Stolte, L., and van Leusden, H.: Thyroid function in molar pregnancy. *J. Clin. Endoc. Metab.* 26:1128, 1966.

134. Galton, V. A., Ingbar, S. H., Jimenez-Fonseca, J., and Hershman, J. M.: Alterations in thyroid hormone economy in patients with hydatidiform mole. *J. Clin. Invest.* 50:1345, 1971.

135. Hershman, J. M., and Higgins, H. P.: Hydatidiform mole: A cause of clinical hyperthyroidism: Report of two cases with evidence that the molar tissue secreted a thyroid stimulator. *N.E.J.M.* 284:573, 1971.

136. Higgins, H. P., Hershman, J. M., Kenimer, J. G., Patillo, R. A., Bayley, T. A., and Walfish, P.: The thyrotoxicosis of hydatidiform mole. *Ann. Int. Med.* 83:307, 1975.

137. Nagataki, S., Mizuno, M., Sakamoto, S., et al.: Thyroid function in molar pregnancy. *J. Clin. Endoc. Metab.* 44:254, 1977.

138. Hershman, J. M.: Hyperthyroidism induced by trophoblastic thyrotropin. *Mayo Clin. Proc.* 47:913, 1972.

139. Kenimer, J. G., Hershman, J. M., and Higgins, H. P.: The thyrotropin in hydatidiform moles is human chorionic gonadotropin. *J. Clin. Endoc. Metab.* 40:482, 1975.

140. Nisula, B. C., and Ketelslegers, J.: Thyroid-stimulating activity and chorionic gonadotropin. *J. Clin. Invest.* 54:494, 1974.

141. Miyai, K., Tanizawa, O., Yamamoto, T., et al.: Pituitary-thyroid function in trophoblastic disease. *J. Clin. Endoc. Metab.* 42:254, 1976.

142. Parmelle, A. H., Allen, E., Stein, I. F., and Buxbaum, H.: Three cases of newborn infants with congenital goiter due to ingestion of iodide. *Am. J. Obst. Gynec.* 40:145–147, 1940.

143. Davies, J. R. S.: Sporadic congenital obstructive goiter with recovery following operation in a 13 day old infant. *J. Pediatrics* 22:570–580, 1943.

144. Galina, M. P., Aunet, N. L., and Einborn, A.: Iodides during pregnancy: An apparent cause of neonatal death. *N.E.J.M.* 267:1124–1127, 1962.

145. Carswell, F., Kerr, M. M., and Hutchinson, J. H.: Congenital goitre and hypothyroidism produced by maternal ingestion of iodides. *Lancet* 1:1241–1243, 1970.

146. Begg, T. G., and Hall, R. Q.: Iodine goiter and hypothyroidism. *Quart. J. Med.* 32:351–362, 1963.

147. Packard, G. B., Williams, E. T., and Wheelock, S. E.: Congenital obstructing goiter. *Surgery* 48:422–431, 1960.

148. Shenkman, L., Mitsuma, T., Penna, M., Medeiros-Neto, G. A., Monteiro, K., Pupo, A. A., and Hollander, C. S.: Evidence of hypothyroidism in endemic cretinism in Brazil. *Lancet* 2:67–69, 1973.

149. Buttfield, I. H., Black, M. L., Hoffman, M. J., Mason, E. K., and Ketzel, B. S.: Correction of iodine deficiency in New Guinea natives by iodised oil injections. *Lancet* 2:767, 1965.

150. Pharoah, P. O. D., and Hornabrook, R. W.: Endemic cretinism of recent onset in New Guinea. *Lancet* 2:1038, 1974.

151. Fierro-Benitez, R., Penafield, W., DeGroodt, L. S., and Ramirez, J.: Endemic goiter and endemic cretinism in the Andean region. *N.E.J.M.* 280:296–301, 1969.

152. Pharoah, P. O. D., Ellis, S. M., Ekins, R., and Williams, E. S.: Maternal thyroid function, iodine deficiency and fetal development. *Clinical Endocrinology* 5:159–166, 1976.

153. Halnan, K. E.: Radioiodine uptake of human thyroid in pregnancy. *Clin. Sci.* 17:201, 1958.

154. Weier, D. L., Duggan, H. E., and Scott, D. B.: Total body radiation and dose to the gonads from the therapeutic use of iodine 131. *J. Canada Assoc. Radiologists* 11:50, 1960.

155. Cantalino, S J., Schmickel, R. D., Ball, M., and Cisa, C. F.: Persistent chromosomal aberrations following radioiodine therapy for thyrotoxicosis. *N.E.J.M.* 275:739, 1966.

156. Murray, I. P.: The current status of radioactive iodine. *Practitioner* 199:696, 1967.

157. Ray, E. W., Sterling, K., and Garoner, L. I.: Congenital cretinism associated ith I-131 therapy of the mother. *A.M.A. J. Dis. Child.* 98:506, 1959.

158. Russell, K. P., Rose, H., and Star, P.: The effects of radioactive iodine on maternal and fetal thyroid functions during pregnancy. *Surgery Gynec. Obstet.* 104:560, 1957.

159. Hamill, G. C., Jarman, J. A., and Wynne, M. D.: Fetal effects of radioactive iodine therapy in a pregnant women with thyroid cancer. *Am. J. Obst. Gynec.* 81:1018, 1961.

160. Fisher, W. D., Voorhess, M. L., and Gardner, L. I.: Congenital hypothyroidism in infant following maternal I-131 therapy. *Journal Pediatrics* 62:132–146, 1963.

161. Green, H. G., Gareis, F. V., Shepard, T. H., et al.: Cretinism associated with maternal sodium iodide 131 I therapy during pregnancy. *Am. J. Dis. Child.* 122:247, 1971.

162. Stoffer, S. S., and Hamburger, J. I.: Inadvertent 131-I therapy for hyperthyroidism in the first trimester of pregnancy. *J. Nuclear Med.* 17:146–149, 1976.

163. Van Herle, A. J., Young, R. T., Fisher, D. A., et al.: Intra-uterine treatment of a hypothyroid fetus. *J. Clin. Endoc. Metab.* 40:474, 1975.

164. Lightner, E. S., Fisher, D. A., Giles, H., and Woolfenden, J.: Intraamniotic injection of thyroxine (T4) to a human fetus: Evidence for conversion of T4 to reverse T3. *Am. J. Obst. Gynec.* 127:487–490, 1977.

165. Schou, M., Amdisen, A., Jensen, S., and Olsen, T.: Occurrence of goitre during lithium treatment. *Brit. Med. J.* 3:710, 1968.

166. Emerson, C. H., Dyson, W. L., and Utiger, R. D.: Serum thyrotropin and thyroxine concentrations in patients receiving lithium carbonate. *J. Clin. Endoc. Metab.* 36:338, 1973.

167. McLarty, D. G., O'Boyle, J. H., Spencer, C. A., and Ratcliffe, J. G.: Effect of lithium on hypothalamic-pituitary-thyroid function in patients with affective disorders. *Brit. Med. J.* 3:623–626, 1975.

168. Karlsson, K., Linstedt, G., Lundberg, P. A., and Selstan, U.: Transplacental lithium poisoning: Reversible inhibition of fetal thyroid. *Lancet* p. 1295, June 7, 1975.

169. Krugman, L. G., Hershman, J. M., Chopra, I. J., et al.: Patterns of recovery of the hypothalamic-pituitary-thyroid axis in patients taken off chronic thyroid therapy. *J. Clin. Endoc. Metab.* 41:70, 1975.

170. Cotton, G. E., Gorman, C. A., and Mayberry, W. E.: Suppression of thyrotropin (h-TSH) in serums of patients with myxedema of varying etiology treated with thyroid hormones. *N.E.J.M.* 285:529, 1971.

171. Rasmussen, H.: Parathyroid hormone, calcitonin and the calciferols, in *Textbook of Endocrinology,* Ed. by Williams, R. Philadelphia, W. B. Saunders Co., 1974, pp. 600–773.

172. Hytten, F. E., and Leitch, I.: *The Physiology of Human Pregnancy,* ed. 2. Oxford, Blackwell Scientific Publications, 1971, p. 383.

173. Pitkin, R. M.: Calcium metabolism in pregnancy: A review. *Am. J. Obst. Gynec.* 121:724–737, 1975.

174. Heaney, R. P., and Skillman, T. G.: Calcium metabolism in normal human pregnancy. *J. Clin. Endoc.* 33:661–670, 1971.

175. Cushard, W. G., Jr., Creditor, M. A., Canterbury, J. M., and Reiss, E.: Physiologic hyperparathyroidism in pregnancy. *J. Clin. End.* 34:767–771, 1972.

176. Mull, J. W., and Bill, A. H.: Variations in serum calcium and phosphorus during pregnancy: I. Normal variations. *Am. J. Obst. Gynec.* 27:510, 1934.

177. Newman, R. L.: Blood calcium: A normal curve for pregnancy. *Am. J. Obst. Gynec.* 53:817, 1947.

178. Tan, C. M., Raman, A., and Synnathyray, T. A.: Serum ionic calcium levels during pregnancy. *Obst. Gynec.* 79:694, 1972.

179. Pitkin, R. M., and Gebhardt, M. P.: Serum calcium concentrations in human pregnancy. *Am. J. Obst. Gynec.* 127:775, 1977.

180. Ramberg, C. F., Jr., Delivoria-Papadopoulos, M., Crandall, E. D., and Kronfield, D. S.: Kinetic analysis of calcium transport across the placenta. *J. Applied Physiology* 35:682–688, 1973.

181. Martin, T. J.: Biosynthesis of parathyroid hormone. *Clincs. Endo. Metab.* 3:199–214, 1974.

182. Reiss, E., and Canterbury, J. M.: Emerging concepts of the nature of circulating parathyroid hormone: Implications for clinical research. *Recent Progress Hormone Research* 30:391–429, 1974.

183. Samaan, N. A., Wigoda, C., and Castillo, S. G.: Human serum calcitonin and parathyroid hormone levels in the maternal umbilical cord blood and post-partum, *Endocrinology 1973 (Proceedings of the 4th International Symposium, London, England).* William Heinemann Medical Books Ltd., pp. 364–372.

184. Anast, C. S.: Parathyroid hormone during pregnancy and effect on offspring, in *Diabetes and Other Endocrine Disorders During Pregnancy and in the Newborn,* ed. by M. I. New and R. H. Eiser, Jr., Alan R. Liss, Inc., 1976, pp. 235–248.

185. DeLuca, H. F.: Vitamin D endocrinology. *Ann. Int. Med.* 85:367–377, 1976.

186. Garabedian, M., Holick, M. F., DeLuca, H. F., et al.: Control of 25-hydroxycholcalciferol metabolism by the parathyroid glands. *Proc. Natl. Acad. Sci. U.S.A.* 69:1673–1676, 1972.

187. Fraser, D. R., and Kodicek, E.: Regulation of 25-hydroxycholicalciferol-1-hydroxylase activity in kidney by parathyroid hormone. *Nature* 141:163–166, 1973.

188. Hillman, L. S., and Haddad, J. G.: Perinatal vitamin D metabolism: III. Factors influencing late gestational human serum 25-hydroxyvitamin D. *Am. J. Obst. Gynec.* 125:196–200, 1976.

189. Turton, C. W. G., Stamp, T. C. B., Stanely, P., and Maxwell, J. D.: Altered vitamin D metabolism in pregnancy. *Lancet* 1:222, 1977.

190. Watney, P., Chanee, G., Scott, P., and Thompson, J.: Maternal factors in neonatal hypocalcemia: A study of three ethnic groups. *Brit. Med. J.* 2:432–435, 1971.

191. Ford, J. A., Davidson, D. C., McIntosh, W. B., Fyge, W. M., and Donnigan, M. G.: Neonatal rickets in Asian immigrant population. *Brit. Med. J.* 3:211–212, 1973.

192. Moncrieff, M., and Fadahunsi, J.: Congenital rickets due to maternal vitamin D deficiency. *Arch. Dis. Child.* 49:810–811, 1974.

193. Rosen, J., Roginsky, M., Nathenson, G., and Finberg, L.: The 25-hydroxyvitamin D (Plasma levels in mothers and their premature infants with neonatal hypocalcemia). *Am. J. Dis. Child.* 127:220, 1974.

194. Hillman, L. S., and Haddad, J. G.: Human perinatal vitamin D metabolism: I. 25-hydroxyvitamin D in maternal and cord blood. *J. Pediatrics* 84:742, 1974.

195. Haddad, J. G., and Walgate, J.: 25-Hydroxyvitamin D transport in human plasma: Isolation and partial characterization of calciferol-binding protein. *J. Biol. Chem.* 251:4083, 1976.

196. Imawari, M., Kida, K., and Goodman, DeW. S.: The transport of vitamin D and its 25-hydroxy metabolite in human plasma: Isolation and partial characteristics of vitamin D and 25-hydroxyvitamin D-binding protein. *J. Clin. Invest.* 58:514, 1976.

197. Bouillon, R., Van Baelen, H., and De Moor, P.: 25-Hydroxyvitamin D and its binding protein in maternal and cord serum. *J. Clin. Endoc. Metab.* 45:679, 1977.

198. Committee on Nutrition: The relation between infantile hypercalcemia and vitamin D: Public health implications in North America. *Pediatrics* 40:1050, 1967.

199. Friedman, W. F., and Roberts, W. C.: Vitamin D and the supravalvar aortic stenosis syndrome. *Circulation* 34:77, 1966.

200. Fairney, A., Naughten, E., and Oppe, T. E.: Vitamin D and human lactation. *Lancet* p. 739, Oct. 8, 1977.

201. Queener, S. F., and Bell, N. H.: Calcitonin: A general survey. *Metabolism* 24:555–567, 1975.

202. Stratton Hill, Jr., C., Ibanez, M., Samaan, N., et al.: Medullary (solid) carcinoma of the thyroid gland: An analysis of the M. D. Anderson Hospital experience with patients with the tumor, its special features and its histogenesis. *Medicine* 52:141, 1973.

203. Samaan, N. A., Anderson, G. D., and Adam-Mayne, M. E.: Immunoreactive calcitonin in the mother, neonate, child, and adult. *Am. J. Obst. Gynec.* 121:622–625, 1975.

204. Boonstra, C. E., and Jackson, C. E.: Serum calcium survey for hyperparathyroidism. *Am. J. Clin. Pathology* 55:523–526, 1971.

205. Watson, L.: Primary hyperparathyroidism. *Clin. End. Metab.* 3:215–235, 1974.

206. Purnel, D. C., Smith, L. H., Scholz, D. A., Elveback, L. R., and Arnaud, C. D.: Primary hyperparathyroidism: A prospective study. *Am. J. Med.* 50:670–678. 1971.

207. Pyran, L. N., Hodgkinson, A., and Anderson, C. K.: Primary hyperparathyroidism. *Brit. J. Surg.* 53:245–316, 1966.

208. Johnstone, L. E., II, Kreindler, T., and Johnstone, R. E.: Hyperparathyroidism during pregnancy. *Obst. Gynec.* 50:580–585, 1972.

209. Mallette, I., Bilezikian, J. P., Heath, D. A., and Aurbach, G. D.: Primary hyperparathyroidism: Clinical and biochemical features. *Medicine* 53:127, 1974.

210. Reiss, E., and Canterbury, J. M.: Spectrum of hyperparathyroidism. *Am. J. Med.* 56:794–799, 1974.

211. Watson, L.: Primary hyperparathyroidism. *Clin. End. Metab.,* 3:215–235, 1974.

212. Ludwig, G. D.: Hyperparathyroidism in relation to pregnancy. *N.E.J.M.* 267:637–642, 1962.

213. Petit, D. W., and Clark, R. L.: Hyperparathyroidism in pregnancy. *Am. J. Surgery* 74:860, 1974.

214. Whalley, P.: Hyperparathyroidism and pregnancy. *Am. J. Obst. Gynec.* 86:517, 1963.

215. Norris, E. H.: The parathyroid adenoma: A study of 322 cases. *Arch. Pathol.* 42:261–273, 1946.

216. Friderichsen, D.: Tetany in a suckling with latent osteitis fibrosa in the mother. *Lancet* 1:85, 1939.

217. Delmonico, F. L., Neer, R. M., Cosimi, A., et al.: Hyperparathyroidism during pregnancy. *Am. J. Surgery* 131:328–337, 1976.

218. Bruce, J., and Strong, J. A.: Maternal hyperparathyroidism and parathyroid deficiency in child. *Q. J. Med.* 24:307, 1955.

219. Better, O. S., Levi, J., Greif, E., et al.: Prolonged neonatal parathyroid suppression. *Arch. Surg.* 106:722, 1973.

220. Pedersen, N. T., and Permin, H.: Hyperparathyroidism and pregnancy. *Acta Obstet. Gynec. Scand.* 54:281–283, 1975.

221. Merkatz, I. R., Schwartz, G. H., David, D. S., et al.: Resumption of female reproductive function following renal transplantation. *J.A.M.A.* 216:1749–1754, 1971.

222. Editorial: Pregnancy after renal transplant. *Brit. Med. J.* 1:733–734, 1976.

223. Soyanno, M. A. O., Bell, M., McGeown, M. G., et al.: A case of acute hyperparathyroidism with thyrotoxicosis and pancreatitis presenting as hyperemesis gravidarum. *Postgrad. Med. J.* 44:861–878, 1968.

224. Schenker, J. G., and Kallner, B.: Fatal postpartum hyperparathyroid crisis due to primary chief cell hyperplasia of parathyroidism. *Obst. Gynec.* 25:705–709, 1965.

225. Suki, W. N., Yium, J. J., Von Minden, M., et al.: Acute treatment of hypercalcemia with furosemide. *N.E.J.M.* 283:836–840, 1970.

226. Strott, C. A., and Nugent, C.: Laboratory tests in the diagnosis of hyperparathyroidism in hypercalcemic patients. *Ann. Int. Med.* 68:188, 1968.

227. Gaeke, R. F., Kaplan, E. L., Lindheimer, M. D., et al.: Maternal primary hyperparathyroidism of pregnancy. *J.A.M.A.* 238:508, 1977.

228. Dorey, L. G., and Gell, J. W.: Primary hyperparathyroidism during the third trimester of pregnancy. *Obst. Gynec.* 45:469–472, 1975.

229. Davies, D. R.: The surgery of primary hyperparathyroidsim. *Clinic Endo. Metab.* 3:253–265, 1974.

229a. Montoro, M., Collea, J., and Mestman, J. H.: Oral phosphate in the treatment of hyperparathroidism in pregnancy (submitted for publication).

230. Harrison, H. E.: Hypoparathyroidism. *Modern Treatment* 7:636–648, 1970.

231. Nusynowitz, M. D., Frame, B., and Kolb, F. D.: The spectrum of the hypoparathyroid states. *Medicine* 55:105–119, 1976.

232. Blizzard, R. M., Chee, D., and Davis, W.: The incidence of parathyroid and other antibodies in the sera of patients with idiopathic hypoparathyroidism. *Clin. Exp. Immunol.* 1:119, 1966.

233. Benson, P. F., and Parsons, V.: Hereditary hypoparathyroidism presenting with edema in the neonatal period. *Quart. J. Med.* 33:197, 1964.

234. Gorodischer, R., Aceto, T. J., and Terplan, K.: Congenital familial hypoparathyroidism. *Amer. J. Dis. Child.* 119:74, 1970.

235. Anderson G. W., and Musselman, L.: The treatment of tetany in pregnancy. *Am. J. Obst. Gynec.* 43:547–567, 1942.

236. Graham, W. P., Gordon, G. S., Loken, H. F., et al.: Effect of pregnancy and of the menstrual cycle on hypoparathyroidism. *J. Clin. Endoc. Metab.* 24:512, 1964.

237. Aceto, T., Jr., Batt, R. E., Bruck, E., et al.: Intrauterine hyperparathyroidism: A complication of untreated maternal hypoparathyroidism. *J. Clin. End. Metab.* 26:487–492, 1966.

238. Landing, B. H., and Kamoshita, S.: Congenital hyperparathyroidism secondary to maternal hypoparathyroidism. *J. Pediatrics* 77:842–847, 1970.

239. Bronsky, D., Kiamko, R. T., Moncada, R., et al.: Intrauterine hyperparathyroidism secondary to maternal hypoparathyroidism. *Pediatrics* 42:606–613, 1968.

240. Monif, G. R. G., and Savory, J.: Iatrogenic maternal hypocalcemia following magnesium sulfate therapy. *J.A.M.A.* 219:1469–1470, 1972.

241. O'Leary, J. A., Klaiwer, L. M., and Neuwirth, R. J.: The management of hypoparathyroidism in pregnancy. *Am. J. Obst. Gynec.* 94:1103–1107, 1966.

242. Parfitt, A. M.: Vitamin D treatment in hypoparathyroidism. *Lancet* 2:614–615, 1970.

243. Goodman, L. S., and Gilman, A.: *The Pharmacological Basis of Therapeutics,* 3rd ed. Macmillan, New York, 1966, p. 1692.

244. Woodhouse, N. J. Y.: Hypocalcemia and hypoparathyroidism. *Clin. End. Metab.* 3:323–343, 1974.

245. Wright, A. D., Joplin, G. F., and Dixon, H. G.: Post-partum hypercalcaemia in treated hypoparathyroidism. *Brit. Med. J.* 1:23, 1969.

246. Mestman, J. H., and Cetrulo, C.: Unexplained hypercalcemia in a hypoparathyroid patient immediately postpartum (in preparation).

247. Kooh, S. W., Fraser, D., DeLuca, H. F., et al.: Treatment of hypoparathyroidism and pseudohypo-parathyroidism with metabolites of vitamin D: Evidence for impaired conversion of 25-hydroxyvitamin D to 1,25-dihydroxyvitamin D. *N.E.J.M.* 293:840–844, 1975.

248. Russell, R. G. G., Smith, R., Walton, R. J., et al.: 1,25 Dihydroxycholecalciferol and α-hydroxychole-calciferol in hypoparathyroidism. *Lancet* 2:14, 1974.

249. Goldberg, L. D.: Transmission of a vitamin D metabolite in breast milk. *Lancet* 2:1258–1259, 1972.

250. Heany, R. P.: The osteomalacias, in *Textbook of Medicine.* Beeson, P. B., and McDermott, W. (eds.): W. B. Saunders Co., Philadelphia, 1975, p. 1830.

251. Dent, C. E., Richens, A., Rowe, D. J. F., et al.: Osteomalacia with long term anticonvulsant therapy in epilepsy. *Brit. Med. J.* 4:69–72, 1970.

252. Richens, A., and Rowe, D. J. F.: Disturbing of calcium metabolism by anticonvulsant drugs. *Brit. Med. J.* 4:73–76, 1970.

253. Bouillon, R., Reynaert, J., Claes, J. H., et al.: The effect of anticonvulsant therapy on serum levels of 25-hydroxyvitamin D, calcium, and parathyroid hormone. *J. Clin. End.* 41:1130, 1975.

254. Holmes, A. M., Enouch, B. A., Taylor, J. L., et al.: Occult rickets and osteomalacia among the Asian immigrant population. *Quart. J. Med. New Series XLIII* 165:125–149, 1973.

21
Thyroid and Parathyroid Function and Disorders in the Fetus and Newborn

Delbert A. Fisher, M.D.

During the past three decades our understanding of fetal endocrine physiology has expanded rapidly, more recently because of the availability of radiolabeled hormones and sensitive procedures for radioimmunoassay of hormones. Extensive data in several mammalian species support the concept of fetal endocrine autonomy proposed initially by Jost (1,2). Although steroid hormones can traverse the placental "barrier," it is now clear from studies in several species that this barrier is essentially complete for polypeptide and thyroid hormones (1–8). Moreover, considerable data are available characterizing the patterns of autonomous development of fetal endocrine systems, including the hypothalamic-pituitary-thyroid system and the parathyroid-calcitonin system (8–10). Both are functional during the last trimester of gestation and both are importantly involved in the metabolic adaptations of the newborn to the extrauterine environment.

EMBRYOGENESIS

The thyroid and parathyroid systems of the human fetus develop from the primitive pharyngeal gut (8). The thyroid gland forms from a midline outpouching of the entoderm of the floor of the buccal cavity at 16 to 17 days' gestation. By 24 days the thyroid anlage resembles a deep cup that develops into a flasklike, hollow vesicle as it grows caudally along the ventral neck. By 4 to 5 weeks the pharyngeal pouches are visible on the lateral walls of the pharyngeal gut. The third pouches form the thymus and inferior parathyroid glands, and the fourth pouches the superior parathyroid glands. The fifth pouches contribute paired ultimobranchial bodies that become incorporated into the developing thyroid gland as the parafollicular C cells, the calcitonin-secreting cells.

Between 4 and 7 weeks' gestation the thyroid anlage incorporates the ultimobranchial bodies, and the bilobed mass loses its lumen to become a solid mass of laterally expand-

533

ing tissue (8,10). At 7 weeks the gland has assumed its definitive shape and position in the ventral, lower neck and weighs 1 to 2 mg. There is a progressive increase in thyroid mass thereafter, in rough proportion to the increase in body weight.

The parathyroid glands develop between 5 and 12 weeks (10). The third pouches encounter the migrating thyroid anlage, and the parathyroid anlagen are carried caudally with the thyroid gland. They finally come to lie at the lower poles of the thyroid lobes as the inferior parathyroid glands. The fourth pouches encounter the thyroid anlage later and come to rest at the upper poles of the thyroid gland as the superior parathyroid glands. The parathyroid glands increase in size from less than 0.1 mm in diameter at 14 weeks to some 1 to 2 mm at birth.

The anterior pituitary gland also is a derivative of the primitive buccal cavity (Rathke pouch), and its embryological development parallels that of the thyroid (8). By the fifth week the Rathke pouch makes contact with the infundibular process of the third cerebral ventricle, which has grown ventrally. By 12 weeks the buccal connection is obliterated by the developing sphenoid bone as the pituitary is partially encapsulated in a bony cavity, the sella turcica.

MATURATION OF THYROID FUNCTION

Thyroid gland function is regulated by the hypothalamic-anterior pituitary neuroendocrine transducer. Ontogenesis of thyroid control thus involves maturation of the hypothalamus and the pituitary portal blood vascular system (8). The hypothalamic nuclei become visible histologically between 8 and 16 weeks' gestation and thyrotropin releasing hormone (TRH) is detectable by radioimmunoassay during this time. The primary (hypothalamic) plexus of the pituitary portal vascular system can be identified by 13 to 14 weeks, and continuity of the primary and secondary (pituitary) plexus occurs by 18 to 20 weeks (8). Coincident with the continuity of the pituitary portal plexuses, an increase in fetal serum TSH (thyroid-stimulating hormone) concentration and fetal thyroidal radioiodine uptake are observed, and followed by a progressive increase in fetal serum thyroxine (T4) concentration (8). Fetal serum T4 levels increase from a mean of about 4 μg/dl at 20 weeks to about 9 μg/dl at 30 weeks and 11 μg/dl at term (8,11). Serum thyroxine-binding globulin (TBG) concentrations increase progressively between 10 and 30 weeks and contribute in part to the increase in fetal serum T4, but free T4 concentrations also increase progressively between 20 and 40 weeks, indicating progressive saturation of TBG binding sites for T4 and suggesting a progressive increase in T4 production (8).

Maturation of negative feedback control of TSH secretion also occurs during the last half of gestation. There is a progressive decrease in fetal serum TSH concentration associated with the increase in serum free T4 between 30 and 40 weeks' gestation, and there is a further increase in free T4/TSH serum ratio until 1 month of postnatal life (8,11). Moreover, serum TSH concentrations increase in response to hypothyroxinemia and can be suppressed with exogenous T4 at term (37 to 42 weeks) (8,12).

The final phase of thyroid system ontogenesis in the fetus is maturation of the peripheral, presumably enzymatic, systems for deiodination of thyroxine. The first step in T4 metabolism is monodeiodination to a triiodothyronine. If the beta (hydroxyl) iodothyronine ring is monodeiodinated, 3,5,3'-triiodothyronine (T3) is produced. Monodeiodination of the alpha (alanine) ring produces 3,3',5'-triiodothyronine or

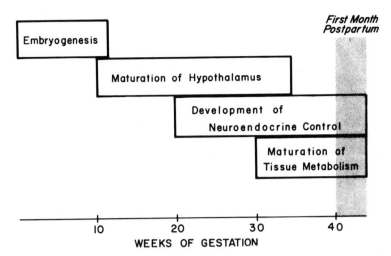

Figure 1. Ontogenesis of hypothalamic-pituitary-thyroid function in the human fetus. Embryogenesis of the thyroid and pituitary glands is complete by 10 to 12 weeks. Histological and functional maturation of the hypothalamus and pituitary portal system occur between 10 and 35 weeks. Neuroendocrine feedback control of TSH secretion matures during the latter half of gestation. Finally the iodothyronine deiodination systems in peripheral tissues mature near term and in the neonatal period.

reverse T3 (rT3) (8). T3 has three to four times the metabolic potency of T4, and rT3 appears to be metabolically inactive. It is now clear that fetal tissues deiodinate T4 predominantly to rT3 (8,13). T3 concentrations in fetal serum are undetectable before 30 weeks and increase progressively thereafter to term (8). The mean level in cord serum is quite low, however (about 50 ng/dl), by either child or adult standards, and a further rapid increase in serum T3 occurs in the early neonatal period (8). The most marked increase occurs in the first 4 hr with a subsequent slower rise to 24 hr (14,15). Present evidence suggests that the increase in serum T3 during the last 10 weeks of gestation is due to maturation of the capacity of tissues to monodeiodinate T4 to T3 (beta ring monodeiodinase activity). The early neonatal increase also is largely due to increased T4 to T3 conversion, although increased secretion also occurs (8).

Figure 1 summarizes the several events of thyroid system ontogenesis in the human fetus relative to gestational and postnatal age.

PARATHYROID-CALCITONIN SECRETION IN THE FETUS

Parathyroid-calcitonin system ontogenesis has been less well studied. It is clear that the fetal parathyroid glands contain parathyroid hormone (PTH) during the last trimester of gestation. Studies in fetal sheep indicate that the fetus responds to EDTA-induced hypocalcemia with an increase in serum PTH concentration as well as increased renal phosphate excretion (16). Thyroid C cells are prominent in the neonatal thyroid gland, and calcitonin (CT) concentrations are 500 to 2000 mU/g tissue, values as much as 10 times greater than those observed in adult glands (17). In addition, the fetal sheep is clearly capable of increasing serum CT in response to induced hypercalcemia (18).

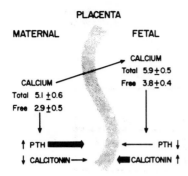

Figure 2. The placenta actively transports calcium in the maternal to fetal direction, maintaining relatively higher total and free plasma calcium concentrations in the fetus. The calcium pump tends to lower maternal plasma calcium levels and stimulates maternal parathyroid hormone (PTH) secretion; maternal calcitonin is inhibited. In the fetus the high plasma calcium tends to inhibit PTH secretion and stimulate calcitonin.

In the term human fetus, mean serum PTH concentrations are low (about 50% of base line adult values) and serum CT concentrations high (about 200% of base line adult values) (9,19,20). Serum total and ionized calcium concentrations are higher than maternal values, and there is evidence that this fetal to maternal gradient of calcium is maintained by an active "pumping" of maternal calcium across the placenta to the fetus (9,10). Since fetal PTH and CT levels are appropriately responsive to changes in serum calcium, the current view of fetal PTH-CT physiology is that the high prevailing fetal ionized calcium concentrations stimulate CT and suppress PTH secretion. This is further supported by the observations of high thyroidal C cell and CT concentrations and the relative preponderance of inactive chief cells in the fetal parathyroid glands (10,17). These concepts are summarized in Figure 2.

ADAPTATION TO EXTRAUTERINE LIFE

Thyroid Function

With the advent of parturition, the newborn infant experiences a transition from a state of T3 deficiency to a state of transient T3 thyrotoxicosis. Cooling in the newborn secondary to extrauterine exposure triggers a marked increase in TSH secretion; serum TSH levels peak at 60 to 120 μU/ml by 30 min of age, and there is a subsequent increase in serum T4 concentration that peaks at 24 to 36 hr (8,14,15). There is a coincident rapid increase in serum T3 levels during the first 4 hr, followed by a more gradual increase to peak concentrations at 24 to 36 hr (8,14,15). The early (4 hr) increase in serum T3 is largely due to further increases in T4 to T3 conversion in peripheral tissues, since it can be dissociated from the TSH surge (8). The subsequent (4 to 24 hr) increase represents both conversion and secretion (8,12).

The mechanism of the increase in T4 to T3 conversion during the perinatal period is not entirely clear. There is evidence to suggest that the prenatal increase is cortisol-induced (8). The early, dramatic postnatal T3 surge appears to correlate with the early increase in catecholamine secretion and may represent conversion linked to the stimulation of catecholamine synthesis (8). Serum rT3 levels are stable during the first few days of life, suggesting that the perinatal changes in T3 metabolism affect only beta ring monodeiodination (8,21).

There is evidence to support the view that the transient hyperthyroid state importantly potentiates catecholamine thermogenesis. The unique brown fat supply of the newborn and the integrated catecholamine–thyroid hormone production systems thus provide for the augmented nonshivering thermogenesis that is critical for survival of the newborn in the extrauterine environment (8,22).

Calcium Homeostasis

With the removal of the placental calcium pump and the chronic source of intravenous calcium at the time of parturition, there is a fall in serum calcium concentration. In the term infant this decrease amounts to about 2 mg/dl (11.5 to 9.5 mg/dl) and reaches its nadir at 24 to 48 hr (9,10). Under similar circumstances in a child or adult a prompt increase in PTH secretion would occur, bone calcium would be mobilized, and serum calcium would return promptly to normal levels. In the newborn, however, serum PTH levels remain low during the first 2 to 3 days, increasing gradually to adult levels by 5 to 7 days (10). The high serum CT concentrations remain high during the first 2 to 3 days, falling gradually to adult levels by 5 to 7 days (10,19,20).

Thus PTH-CT-calcium homeostasis seems impaired in the newborn period, and the low PTH and high CT concentrations predispose to hypocalcemia. Calcium homeostasis in the newborn also is compromised by the low level of renal glomerular filtration, which limits phosphate excretion and predisposes to hyperphosphatemia and hypocalcemia (10).

THYROID DYSFUNCTION

Prematurity

Serum T4 and T3 concentrations decrease progressively with decreasing gestational age in the premature infant, and values are particularly low in infants between 20 and 30 weeks' gestational age (8). Moreover the thyroid responses to extrauterine exposure appear to be relatively reduced, including both the TSH-T4 response to cooling and the T4 to T3 conversion response to extrauterine exposure (23). Normal values for serum T4, T3, and TSH concentrations in premature infants have not been characterized adequately. It is clear that the serum T4 concentration decreases progressively with decreasing gestational age, from about 12 μg/dl at 40 to 45 weeks to about 9 μg/dl at 30 weeks (11). Serum TSH concentrations increase progressively, from about 7 μU/ml at 40 to 45 weeks to about 15 μU/ml at 30 weeks (11). Serum T3 concentrations decrease from about 50 ng/dl at 40 to 45 weeks to less than 15 μU/ml at 30 weeks (8). Precise ranges for these values, however, are not available, and only sketchy information is available below 30 weeks' gestational age.

Neonatal Morbidity

Perinatal stress or acute neonatal disease, like adult morbidity of various kinds, can result in suppression of T4 to T3 conversion and further lowering of serum T3 levels in the newborn period. Only preliminary information is presently available, but low serum T3 concentrations, sometimes with low serum T4 levels, have been reported for premature infants with respiratory distress (23). Two to four weeks may be required before depressed serum T3 levels increase to the normal range (24). Some blunting of the neonatal T4 increment also may occur, suggesting hypothalamic immaturity (23). Such changes are difficult to interpret in the absence of adequate normal standards for test results in small infants. The only indication for thyroid replacement therapy in the newborn with low serum thyroid hormone concentrations at present is an elevation in serum TSH concentration above 20 μU/ml after 3 days of age.

Infant of Thyrotoxic Mother

The maternal thyrotoxic state does not usually harm the fetus, since thyroid hormones do not cross the placenta. However, severe maternal thyrotoxicosis associated with weight loss or failure to gain weight can result in fetal malnutrition. Maternal hypothyroidism also is undesirable, since it compromises placental blood flow and fetal substrate supply. Thus euthyroidism or only mild hyperthyroidism provides the optimal fetal environment in the pregnant woman.

The major risk to the fetus of the woman with Graves disease is the possibility of fetal hypothyroidism produced as a result of maternal treatment: either ablation of the fetal thyroid by inadvertent therapeutic radioiodine or drug-induced fetal hypothyroidism secondary to placental transfer of maternal antithyroid drugs. Several instances of radioiodine-induced fetal hypothyroidism have been reported (25,26). This usually occurs during the second trimester after the fetal thyroid can concentrate radioiodine (10 to 12 weeks) and before pregnancy is obvious. Iodides, propylthiouracil (PTU), and methimazole (MT) cross the placental barrier without difficulty and may produce fetal goiter or hypothyroidism (10,26). The newborn of women with treated Graves disease must be carefully examined for evidence of goiter and hypothyroidism, including measurement of serum T4 and TSH concentrations. The cord serum T4 level should exceed 7 μg/dl, and TSH should be less than 20 μU/ml, although 2 to 3% of normal infants have values as high as 60 μU/ml (27). Neonatal hypothyroidism due to PTU is transient, lasting 1 to 2 weeks, and in the absence of signs or symptoms or a large goiter probably does not require treatment.

Another risk for the infant of the hyperthyroid (Graves disease) mother is neontal Graves disease. In most instances this disorder is transient, lasting 1 to 3 months, and appears, usually, to result from transplacental passage of maternal immunoglobulins capable of stimulating the thyroid gland (28). There is evidence that these IgG antibodies are directed against the TSH receptors on the thyroid follicular cell membranes and, like TSH, stimulate thyroid activity as binding occurs (29,30). The long-acting thyroid stimulator (LATS) was the first of the thyroid-stimulating immunoglobulins (TSI) to be discovered, but other TSI species detected by a variety of in vitro tests have been reported. Since Graves disease usually results from transplacental TSI, the sex ratio for neonatal thyrotoxicosis is 1:1. This is in contrast to a F/M ratio of 8 to 10:1 for the adult disease (28).

In some instances neonatal thyrotoxicosis persists beyond 3 months or recurs in later infancy (31). The etiology of the disease in these cases is not clear. A hereditary predisposition with autonomous production of sensitized lymphocytes and TSI by the newborn is possible (28). Clinical manifestations of neonatal Graves disease may be minimal at birth, probably because of transplacental passage of antithyroid drugs and the fact that T4 is metabolized in the fetus to the inactive metabolite rT3 rather than T3. Also catecholamine secretion in utero probably is minimal (32).

The newborn must be examined carefully for the presence of a goiter, and cord blood should be collected for measurement of T4, T3, and TSH concentrations. The presence of a goiter and suppressed cord serum TSH (less than 3 μU/ml) in the presence of elevated serum T3 levels (more than 80 μU/ml) suggests thyrotoxicosis. Irritability, flushing, supraventricular tachycardia, voracious appetite, poor weight gain or excessive weight loss, and exophthalmos are common signs, and these usually progress in severity with time (28,31). Thrombocytopenia with hepatosplenomegaly, and hepatosplenomegaly with jaundice and hypoprothrombinemia have been observed (10,31). Symptoms of tracheal obstruction may occur if the goiter is large. Mortality, which has been reported as high as 25%, usually relates to cardiac decompensation and arrhythmias (10,31). Careful observation of the newborn of the thyrotoxic mother is indicated for 5 to 7 days, and repeat serum T4, T3, and TSH measurements are helpful (at 4 to 5 days) for assessing the possibility of delayed-onset disease.

The treatment of hyperthyroidism in the newborn includes sedation and digitalization as necessary, an antithyroid drug—PTU 5 to 10 mg/(kg)(day) or MT 0.5 to 1.0 mg/(kg)(day)—usually in combination with iodide—Lugol solution, one drop, 8 mg, three times daily—is prescribed. Propranolol HCl—2 mg/(kg)(day)—is useful in controlling sympathetic overstimulation. If no response is observed within 48 to 72 hr, the PTU or MT dose is increased 50%.

Congenital Hypothyroidism

Hypothyroidism in the newborn can result from many causes (Table I).

Endemic Goiter
In areas of endemic goiter, fetal goiter with or without hypothyroidism is not uncommon (33). The precise incidence is not known, but the incidence of congenital hypothyroidism has been reported to be as high as 6% in areas of severe iodine deficiency. In such areas adult goiter may be present in 70 to 90% of the population (33). Homoki et al. have studied newborn infants with goiter in a mildly endemic goiter area of Germany (34). All the goitrous infants were clinically euthyroid, but about 60% presented with retarded bone maturation, low cord serum T4 levels, and an augmented TSH surge during the first 5 days of life. Thus, subtle hypothyroidism can occur in the newborn infants in areas of endemic goiter. The goiters may be large, and in the series

Table I. Causes of Neonatal Hypothyroidism

Endemic goiter
Thyroid dysgenesis:
   Agenesis
   Hypogenesis
   Ectopia
Secondary hypothyroidism:
   Hypothalamic dysfunction
   Pituitary disease
Drug-induced
Inborn defects in thyroid metabolism

of Homoki et al. 20% of the goitrous infants had goiters large enough to produce stridor (34).

Thyroid Dysgenesis

This is the most common abnormality of newborn thyroid function in nongoitrous regions of the world. The incidence approximates 1 in 5000 births (35,36). About one-quarter of such infants present with thyroid agenesis, and three-quarters with hypogenesis or ectopia (35,36). Ectopic tissue usually is situated in the midline and may exist at the base of the tongue or between the base of the tongue and the usual location of the thyroid at the base of the neck (33). The residual hypoplastic tissue in the usual location or that ectopically placed may vary in volume and may be adequate for significant thyroid hormone production. Present information suggests that most infants with thyroid dysgenesis and residual thyroid tissue are born with detectable hypothyroidism manifest by increased serum TSH concentrations with or without serum T4 levels in the hypothyroid range (33–36). In a few instances the onset of hypothroidism may be delayed until later infancy or early childhood (33).

Most infants with congenital hypothyroidism appear clinically euthyroid at birth. Mean birth length and birthweight are greater than for normal newborns because of a tendency to prolonged gestation; the infants are of average size for gestational age (37). Thus, it seems clear that thyroid hormones are not essential for normal somatic growth in utero. Bone maturation may be somewhat retarded, however. Also, the effect of the congenital hypothyroid state on fetal nervous system development is not yet entirely clear. Some delay in maturation may occur, but present evidence suggests that such delay, if present, is reversible; early postnatal thyroid hormone treatment usually prevents severe mental retardation (28).

The emphasis, therefore, in congenital hypothyroidism is on early diagnosis and therapy. Occasionally the diagnosis can be made on clinical grounds during the first week of life (37). The large birthweight (and prolonged gestation), a large (more than 0.5 cm) posterior fontanelle, hypothermia during the first 24 hr, a tendency to prolonged neonatal jaundice, lethargy, poor feeding, delayed passage of meconium, or a large tongue may be obvious. Each of these signs occurs in about one-third of such infants; so the presence of two or more signs is suggestive.

However, since the clinical diagnosis is usually delayed beyond 6 weeks of age, newborn screening for congenital hypothyroidism has been recently tested. Measurement of cord serum TSH concentrations or T4 or TSH assays in filter paper blood spots collected at 2 to 5 days of age have proved most reliable (27,35,36). Serum TSH concentrations in cord blood in such infants usually exceed 100 μU/ml (the normal value is less than 60); serum T4 concentrations at 2 to 5 days are less than 7 μg/dl and serum TSH levels are greater than 50 μU/ml. Several mass screening programs have been established and have proved to be economically feasible, with the cost approximating $10,000 per diagnosed infant. With such programs, treatment can be instituted before 4 to 8 weeks of age.

Secondary Hypothyroidism

Hypothalamic (TRH) deficiency or pituitary (TSH) deficiency can produce congenital hypothyroidism. These abnormalities may occur in infants with severe forebrain anomalies such as anencephaly, cyclopia, or holoprosencephaly; in such cases secondary hypothyroidism is suspected in association with other pituitary dysfunction (33).

However, secondary hypothyroidism also occurs in phenotypically normal infants; the frequency appears to approximate 1 in 60,000 births (36). The clinical manifestations are similar to those in infants with primary hypothyroidism (thyroid dysgenesis). The diagnosis can be suspected on the basis of low serum or filter paper spot T4 concentrations in screening programs, but since serum TSH levels are not elevated, the diagnosis is more difficult to confirm. Retesting of such infants at 4 to 8 weeks is necessary with demonstration of low serum T4 and free T4 index values and normal or slightly elevated TSH concentrations (36). A hypothalamic or pituitary abnormality is defined with a TRH stimulation test. A normal TRH response implies TRH deficiency; an absent TRH response indicates pituitary TSH deficiency.

Inborn Defects in Thyroid Hormone Metabolism

These defects probably occur with variable frequency, since they are genetically conditioned. In the Quebec screening program, the incidence has been about 1 in 40,000 to 50,000 births (36). Several possible defects have been described (33). These include (1) defective thyroidal TSH responsiveness, (2) inability of the thyroid to concentrate iodide, (3) inability of the thyroid to oxidize iodide or couple iodine to tyrosine (organification defect), (4) inability of the thyroid to deiodinate, and thus recycle, iodotyrosines, (and 5) defects in thyroglobulin structure or metabolism. Of these abnormalities, defective organification and thyroglobulin defects are most frequent. Several recent reviews are available, and review is not attempted here (33,39). Generally, however, these infants present with goiter, low T4 concentrations, and elevated serum TSH levels.

Drug-Induced Goiter

A large number of drugs and chemicals have been shown to be goitrogenic in man, including the thionamides (thiouracil, propylthiouracil, methylthiouracil, carbimazole, and methimazole), iodide, perchlorate, thiocyanate, aminobenzene derivatives, para-aminobenzoic acid, sulfonamides, aminoglutethimide, pyrazine, pyrimazines, cobalt, lithium, and phenylbutazone. Of these, the thionamide drugs, iodides, and perchlorate have been observed to produce fetal goiter or hypothyroidism (33). Careful clinical and laboratory evaluation of the newborn of a mother receiving potentially goitrogenic drugs is mandatory. A small goiter might be missed during a cursory physical examination. Death has been reported in infants with large goiters and associated tracheal obstruction.

Treatment of Congenital Hypothyroidism

Hypothyroidism in the newborn infant with or without goiter usually should be treated promptly with adequate replacement with thyroid hormone. The one exception to this approach is the infant with drug-induced hypothyroidism secondary to treatment of the mother with Graves disease. In these infants therapy should be withheld 7 to 10 days to be sure that neonatal thyrotoxicosis does not occur. The treatment of choice is Na-l-thyroxine; there is no advantage in triiodothyronine (T3) (Cytomel) or combinations of T4 and T3 (33). Intramuscular T4 in three daily doses of 100 μg has been shown to raise serum T4 and lower TSH values within 3 to 4 days; thereafter oral maintenance doses maintain serum T4 concentrations (40). Maintenance doses of 5 to 10 μg/(kg)(day) Na-l-T4 are prescribed.

DISORDERS OF CALCIUM METABOLISM IN THE NEWBORN

Transient Neonatal Hypocalcemia

Perinatal calcium concentration is regulated by a number of endocrine and nonendocrine factors whose complex nature and interactions are poorly understood. Several factors predispose to hypocalcemia (serum Ca less than 7.0 mg/dl) in the neonatal period. In chemical terms these include low serum PTH concentrations, elevated serum calcitonin levels, and elevated serum phosphorus (9,10,20,41). In clinical terms predisposing factors include prematurity, maternal diabetes mellitus, cesarean section delivery, and perinatal asphyxia (10,41). Of the latter factors, asphyxia may be most important and seems to predispose to hypocalcemia in the face of relatively high serum PTH concentrations (41). It may be that asphyxia or other of the clinical factors also is associated with lower circulating levels of active vitamin D analogues such as 1,25-dihydroxycholecalciferol, which might inhibit PTH actions. However, there is little or no information currently available regarding vitamin D metabolism in infants with neonatal hypocalcemia.

Most neonatal hypocalcemia occurs during the first 3 to 4 days of extrauterine life before serum PTH concentrations increase to the normal range. The highest incidence is observed on day 1, in fact during the first 12 hr, and the incidence falls off progressively thereafter (41). Serum calcium concentrations should be serially monitored during the first 3 to 4 days in all predisposed infants. Hypocalcemia is treated with intravenous 10% calcium gluconate 2 to 3 ml/kg (20 to 30 mg elemental calcium/kg). Infants with recurrent or unresponsive hypocalcemia usually can be maintained with oral calcium chloride 0.4 g/(kg)(24 hr) or calcium lactate 0.5 mg/(kg)-(24 hr).

Congenital Hypoparathyroidism

Hypoplasia or aplasia of the parathyroid glands may result in severe and refractory hypocalcemia in the neonatal period. The disorder is sporadic and usually is associated with malformation or aplasia of the thymus gland, the other main structure derived from the third and fourth pharyngeal pouches (10). The III and IV pharyngeal pouch syndrome referred to as the DiGeorge syndrome, involves males and females equally. Anomalies of the aortic arch and heart also occur. In addition to hypocalcemia there may be persistent rhinorrhea, recurrent diarrhea, oral and cutaneous moniliasis, and failure to thrive with absence of delayed hypersensitivity. Mortality may occur in the neonatal period from infection, diarrhea, or the associated severe congenital anomalies. Thymic transplantation may reverse the immunologic deficiencies, at least transiently.

A sex-linked recessive form of congenital hypoparathyroidism may represent an inborn defect in capacity to synthesize or respond to PTH. Hypocalcemia, usually manifest as muscle jerking, twitching, laryngospasm, inspiratory stridor, or convulsions may occur in the neonatal period. Serum calcium levels are low (less than 7 mg/dl) and serum phosphorus concentrations high (greater than 8 mg/dl). The hypocalcemia usually is persistent in both the sporadic and sex-linked disorders. Therapy with vitamin D usually is necessary (10).

Infant of Hyperparathyroid Mother

Friderichsen first described neonatal tetany in the newborn of a mother with undiagnosed hyperparathyroidism in 1938, and many instances have been described subsequently (10,43). In all reported cases the mother has had hypercalcemia and hypophosphatemia, and a parathyroid adenoma was found in each instance where surgery was performed. In some, neonatal tetany was the first clue to the maternal disorder. The risks of perinatal death and neonatal tetany have been considered as high as 25 and 50%, respectively (44). The 50% incidence of marked hypocalcemia in the infant of the hyperparathyroid mother is believed to be due to marked suppression of the fetal parathyroid glands by the prolonged intrauterine hypercalcemia. Marked chronic stimulation of calcitonin may be more important (20). Hypomagnesemia also may occur in these infants and may contribute to the inhibition of PTH secretion as well as its renal effect (10,44). Studies of urinary phosphate excretion have indicated that 3 months may be required for the parathyroid glands of the newborn to regain normal function (44). Most infants have remained asymptomatic without residual sequelae after cessation of therapy.

Infant of the Hypoparathyroid Mother

There have been a few instances of fetal-newborn hyperparathyroidism associated with maternal hypoparathyroidism. In these rare instances the mother had persistent hypocalcemia with a tendency to amelioration during pregnancy (45–47). The infants were small (1000 to 2400 g), with gestational age varying from 28 to 40 weeks. The newborn may manifest hypotonia and hypercalcemia associated with vomiting, pneumonia, respiratory distress, failure to thrive, and death (45–47). Some have had minimal neonatal morbidity. All have had skeletal changes of osteitis fibrosa cystica, in some cases associated with marked bone demineralization. Infants without symptoms tend to have normal serum calcium concentrations, but serum PTH and CT levels have not been measured.

REFERENCES

1. Jost, A.: Anterior pituitary function in foetal life, in Harris, G. W., and Donovan, B. T. (eds.): *The Pituitary Gland.* Butterworths, London, 1966, vol. II, p. 299.

2. Jost, A.: Hormones in development: Past and prospects, in Hamburgh, M., and Barrington, E. J. W. (eds.): *Hormones in Development.* Appleton Century Crofts, New York, 1971, p. 1.

3. Killinger, G. W., Beamer, N. B., Hagemenas, F., Hill, J. D., Baughman, W. L., and Ochsner, A. J.: Evidence for autonomous pituitary adrenal function in the near-term fetal rhesus. *Endocrinology* 91:1037, 1972.

4. Foster, D. L., Karsch, F. J., and Nalbandov, A. V.: Regulation of luteinizing hormone (LH) in the fetal and neonatal lamb: II. Study of placental transfer of LH in the sheep. *Endocrinology* 90:589, 1972.

5. King, K. C., Adam, P. A. J., Schwartz, R., and Teramo, K.: Human placental transfer of human growth hormone. *Pediatrics* 48:534, 1971.

6. Wolf, H., Sabata, V., Frerichs, H., and Stubble, P.: Evidence for impermeability of the human placenta for insulin. *Horm. Meta. Res.* 1:224, 1969.

7. Sperling, M. A., Erenberg, A., Fiser, R. H., Oh, W., and Fisher, D. A.: Placental transfer of glucagon in sheep. *Endocrinology* 93:1435, 1973.

8. Fisher, D. A., Dussault, J. H., Sack, J., and Chopra I. J.: Ontogenesis of hypothalamic-pituitary-thyroid function and metabolism in man, sheep, and rat. *Rec. Prog. Horm. Res.* 33:59, 1977.

9. David, L., and Anast, C. S.: Calcium metabolism in newborn infants. *J. Clin. Invest.* 54:287, 1974.

10. Fisher, D. A.: Endocrine physiology I and II, in Smith, C. A., and Nelson, N. W. (eds.): *The Physiology of the Newborn Infant,* 4th ed. Charles C Thomas, Springfield, 1976, p. 554.

11. Oddie, T. H., Fisher, D. A., Bernard, B., and Lam, R. W.: Thyroid function at birth in infants 30 to 45 weeks gestation. *J. Pediatr.* 90:803, 1977.

12. Hobel, C. J., Sack, J., Cousins, L. M., and Fisher, D. A.: The effect of intraamniotic thyroxine on thyroid function in the human fetus and newborn. *Clin. Res.* 25:189A, 1977.

13. Chopra, I. J., Sack, J., and Fisher, D. A.: 3,3',5' Triiodothyronine (reverse T3) in fetal and adult sheep: Studies of metabolic clearance rate, production rate, serum binding, and thyroidal content relative to thyroxine. *Endocrinology* 97:1080, 1975.

14. Erenberg, A., Phelps, D. L., Oh, W., and Fisher, D. A.: Total and free thyroxine and triiodothyronine concentrations in the newborn period. *Pediatrics* 53:211, 1974.

15. Abuid, J. L., Klein, A. H., Foley, T. P., Jr., and Larsen, P. R.: Total and free triiodothyronine and thyroxine in early infancy. *J. Clin. Endocrinol. Metab.* 39:253, 1974.

16. Smith, F. G., Jr., Alexander, D. P., Button, A. G., Buckle, R. M., and Nixon, D. A.: Parathyroid hormone in fetal and adult sheep: The effect of hypocalcemia. *J. Endocrinol.* 53:339, 1972.

17. Wolfe, H. J., DeLellis, R. A., Voelkel, E. F., and Tashjian, A. H., Jr.: Distribution of calcitonin-containing cells in the normal neonatal human thyroid gland: A correlation of morphology and peptide content. *J. Clin. Endocrinol. Metab.* 41:1076, 1975.

18. Littledike, E. T., Arnaud, C. D., and Whipp, S. C.: Calcitonin secretion in ovine, porcine and bovine fetuses. *Proc. Exp. Biol. Med.* 139:428, 1972.

19. Samaan, N. A., Anderson, G. D., and Adam-Mayne, M. E. Immunoreactive calcitonin in the mother, neonate, child and adult. *Am. J. Obstet. Gynecol.* 121:622, 1975.

20. Dirksen, H. C., and Anast, C. S.: Hypercalcitonemia and neonatal hypocalcemia. *Pediatr. Res.* 11:424, 1977 (Abstr.)

21. Chopra, I. J., Sack, J., and Fisher, D. A.: Circulating 3,3',5' triiodothyronine (reverse T3) in the human newborn. *J. Clin. Invest.* 55:1137, 1975.

22. Fisher, D. A., and Makoski, E.: Temperature adaptation of the newborn to the extrauterine environment. *J. Lancet* 86:85, 1966.

23. Klein, A. H., Foley, B., Ho, R. S., Kenny, F. M., and Fisher, D. A.: Thyroid response to parturition: Relationship to gestational age and the respiratory distress syndrome. *Pediatr. Res.* 11:427, 1977 (Abstr.).

24. Uhrmann, S., Marks, K. H., Marsels, M. J., Friedman, Z., Murray, F., Kulin, H., Kaplan, M., and Utiger R., Thyroid function in infants admitted to a neonatal intensive care unit. *Pediatr. Res.* 11:432, 1977 (Abstr.).

25. VanHerle, A. J., Young, R. T., Fisher, D. A., Uller, R. P., and Brinkman, C. R.: Intrauterine treatment of a hypothyroid fetus. *J. Clin. Endocrinol. Metab.* 40:474, 1975.

26. Selenkow, H. A.: Therapeutic considerations for thyrotoxicosis during pregnancy, in Fisher, D. A., and Burrow, G. N. (eds.): *Perinatal Thyroid Physiology and Disease.* Raven Press, New York, 1975, p. 145.

27. Klein, A. H., Agustin, A. V., and Foley, T. P., Jr.: Successful laboratory screening for congenital hypothyroidism. *Lancet* 2:77, 1974.

28. Fisher, D. A.: Pathogenesis and therapy of neonatal Graves' disease. *Am. J. Dis. Child.* 130:133, 1976.

29. Von Westarp, C., Know, A. J. S., Row, V. V., and Volpe, R.: Comparison of thyroid antigens by the experimental production of precipitating antibodies to human thyroid fractions and by identification of an antibody which competes with long-acting thyroid stimulator (LATS) for thyroid binding. *Acta Endocrinol.* 84:759, 1977.

30. Muphtar, E. D., Smith, B. R., Pyle, G. A., Hall, R., and Vice, P.: Relation of thyroid stimulating immunoglobulins to thyroid function and effects of surgery, radioiodine and antithyroid drugs. *Lancet* 1:713, 1975.

31. Hollingsworth, D. R., and Mabry, C. C.: Congenital Graves' disease, in Fisher, D. A., and Burrow, G. N. (eds.): *Perinatal Thyroid Physiology and Disease.* Raven Press, New York, 1975, p. 163.

32. Jones, C. T., and Robinson, R. O.: Plasma catecholamines in foetal and adult sheep. *J. Physiol.* 248:15, 1975.

33. VanWyk, J. J., and Fisher, D. A.: The thyroid, in Rudolph, A. (ed.): *Pediatrics,* 16th ed. Appleton Century Crofts, New York, 1977, p. 1663.

34. Homoki, J., Birk, J., Loos, V., Rothenbuchner, G., Fazekas, A. T. A., and Teller, W. M.: Thyroid function with congenital goiter. *J. Pediatr.* 86:753, 1975.

35. Klein, A. H., Foley, T. P., Jr., Larsen, P. R., Agustin, A. V., and Hopwood, N. J.: Neonatal thyroid function in congenital hypothyroidism. *J. Pediatr.* 89:545, 1976.

36. Dussault, J. H., Latarte, J., Guyda, H., and Laberge, C.: Thyroid function in neonatal hypothyroidism. *J. Pediatr.* 89:541, 1976.

37. Smith, D. W., Klein, A. H., Henderson, J. R., and Myrianthopoulos, N. C.: Congenital hypothyroidism: Signs and symptoms in the newborn period. *J. Pediatr.* 87:958, 1975.

38. Klein, A., Meltzer, S., and Kenny, M.: Improved prognosis in congenital hypothyroidism treated before age three months. *J. Pediatr.* 81:912, 1972.

39. Stanbury, J. B.: Familial goiter, in Stanbury, J. B., Wyngaarden, J. B., and Fredrickson, D. S. (eds.): *The Metabolic Basis of Inherited Disease,* 3rd ed. McGraw-Hill, 1972, p. 223.

40. Hayek, A., Maloof, F., and Crawford, J.: Thyrotropin behavior in thyroid disorders of childhood. *Pediatr. Res.* 7:28, 1973.

41. Schedewie, H. K., Odell, W. D., Fisher, D. A., Krutzik, S. R., Dodge, M., Cousins, L., and Fiser, W. P.: Parathyroid hormone secretion and perinatal calcium homeostasis. *Pediatr. Res.,* 13:1, 1979.

42. Friderichsen, C.: Hypocalcemie bei einem Brustkind und Hypercalcemie bei der Mutter. *Mschr. Kinderheilk.* 75:146, 1938.

43. Pederson, N. T., and Permin, H.: Hyperparathyroidism and pregnancy. *Acta Obstet. Gynecol. Scand.* 54:281, 1975.

44. Butler, O. S., Levi, J., Greif, E., Tuma, S., Gellei, B., and Erlik, D.: Prolonged neonatal parathyroid suppression. *Arch. Surg.* 106:722, 1973.

45. Aceto, T., Butt, R. E., Bruck, E., Schultz R. B., and Perez, Y. R.: Intrauterine hyperparathyroidism: A complication of untreated maternal hypoparathyroidism. *J. Clin. Endocrinol. Metab.* 26:487, 1966.

46. Bronsky, D., Kiamko, R. T., Moncada, R., and Rosenthal, M.: Intrauterine hyperparathyroidism secondary to maternal hypoparathyroidism. *Pediatrics* 42:606, 1968.

47. Landing, B. H., and Kamoshita, S.: Congenital hyperparathyroidism secondary to maternal hypoparathyroidism. *J. Pediatr.* 77:842, 1970.

22
Hypertension in Pregnancy

Frederick P. Zuspan, M.D.

Hypertension in pregnancy is a broad, encompassing term that includes all forms of hypertension for those patients who are pregnant. It does not define whether or not hypertension antedated pregnancy, began during pregnancy but before 24 weeks of gestation, or was an acute episode after 24 weeks of gestation. A more precise definition is always essential, since it is related to prognosis and therapy. Much has been written about pregnancy-induced hypertension, toxemia of pregnancy, preeclampsia-eclampsia, or acute hypertension of pregnancy, and all these terms are interchangeable. Its onset is characteristically subtle, and the untrained observer will err in making an early diagnosis. It is principally a disease of the primigravida characterized by the sequential development of edema, hypertension, and proteinuria after the twenty-fourth week of pregnancy. The etiology remains obscure in spite of a myriad of investigations and books that have been devoted to this entity. The pathophysiology of pregnancy-induced hypertension is known to affect both the mother and fetus with morbidity and mortality, the most overt problem being death. The therapy of this condition continues to be empiric until the specific etiology is known. The type of therapy has a major impact on the outcome of the fetus (1,2).

Specific categorical diagnoses that have been recommended for hypertension in pregnancy include the following: (1) true preeclampsia (glomeruloendotheliosis), (2) chronic hypertension, (3) renal disease, and (4) transient hypertension—an increase in blood pressure intrapartum and postpartum.

Many scholars of hypertension in pregnancy feel that the diagnosis of true preeclampsia can be made only by using a renal biopsy and the electron microscope to confirm the lesion of glomeruloendotheliosis that was first described by the Chicago Lying-in Hospital, University of Chicago, group (3). The renal lesion in their study was present in at least 75% of primigravida patients with a known clinical diagnosis of preeclampsia and in 25% of multigravida patients with a clinical diagnosis of chronic hypertension and superimposed preeclampsia. It may be difficult to tell clinically at the time of the acute episode whether or not underlying disease is present in the kidney or cardiovascular system, and it is well recognized that combinations of these disease categories can be present, with the final manifestation being hypertension in pregnancy.

547

ACUTE HYPERTENSION IN PREGNANCY

The criteria for classification of acute pregnancy-induced hypertension is hypertension in pregnancy that occurs after the twenty-fourth week of gestation that has one or more of the following present: (1) edema of face or hands, (2) a systolic blood pressure of at least 140 mm Hg or a rise of 30 mm or more above the usual level, (3) a diastolic pressure of 90 mm or more or a rise of 15 mm above the usual level, and (4) proteinuria ($>1+$ on a clean voided specimen). Edema and an increase in blood pressure make the diagnosis more firm.

Acute hypertension can be divided into mild, moderate, and severe. It is the last that is of greatest concern to the fetus and mother. A chronological sequence of events develops in the pathophysiology of pregnancy-induced hypertension. The first sign is edema, usually of hands and face, followed by an increase in blood pressure either an incremental increase in systolic and diastolic or an absolute increase above 140/90. The last finding is the appearance of proteinuria. A characteristic finding in patients who have acute hypertension in pregnancy is the changing characteristic of the blood pressure in that different observers may obtain different blood pressure readings and the same observer may obtain a different blood pressure at different times. The lowest pressure is often taken as the one of most significance when, to the contrary, it should be the highest pressure that is the one of significance. Altered cardiovascular reactivity is a characteristic finding in this disease and may represent the ability of the patient to respond to a form of endogenous pressor substances or exogenous stress (4,5). The characteristic pathophysiologic derangement of acute hypertension or pregnancy-induced hypertension is vasospasm. A number of factors affect the blood pressure, and these are more pronounced with the patient who has pregnancy-induced hypertension. Such things as position of the patient, environment, anxiety, activity, and the time of day all affect the blood pressure, and it is imperative that the clinician understand these manifestations of the cardiovascular reactivity of this pregnant patient. This condition is different from any other condition in human medicine and is cured only by termination of the pregnancy. The Europeans have favored the term "proteinuric hypertension of pregnancy" and do not consider the patient to have preeclampsia unless proteinuria is present in a clean catch specimen. I would like to feel that there is a bell-shaped curve of the disease and that some individuals have edema, whereas others have edema and hypertension, whereas others have edema, hypertension, and proteinuria. I have repeatedly stated that the severe forms of the disease should be preventable, but I have never felt that the mild forms of the disease were preventable (6). If we are astute enough to surmise when patients are going to become ill, interference with appropriate measures could alter the development of more severe disease.

A basic understanding of changes that take place in the cardiovascular system during pregnancy is important. It is known that a decrease in peripheral resistance is present in the midtrimester of pregnancy and that the blood pressure characteristically decreases. Another point of significance is that blood pressure changes during a 24-hr period, being lowest during sleep and highest in the afternoon after activity. These changes coincide with the changes in amine excretion, especially norepinephrine. The increment of 30 mm systolic or 15 mm diastolic is almost a normal increase if you use the lowest second trimester reading; hence, the individual patient must serve as her own control for the development of pregnancy-induced hypertension. The subtle incremental change in blood pressure along with other signs, such as edema of hands and face, are helpful in making a diagnosis of mild preeclampsia. The absolute values of blood pressure are not nearly so important as the change from base line pressures using the midtrimester blood pressure reading for comparison. Unfortunately, we often do not see the patient in the midtrimester of pregnancy and may have only an acute situation to determine a specific diagnosis. The projectoscope is not nearly so accurate as the retrospectroscope in these situations.

A recently described phenomenon known as the roll-over test was described by the Dallas group (Gant et al.). They showed an increase in blood pressure from the side to the back (7). The instructions for doing the roll-over test are to have the patient assume a lateral resting position and after the blood pressure is stabilized, to take the pressure in the upper arm. The patient is then instructed to roll on her back, and another pressure is immediately taken. Then, wait 5 min and check the pressure again with the patient still on her back. If the 5-min reading shows a diastolic increment in blood pressure greater than 20 mm Hg, the patient has a positive roll test. This positive roll test has prognostic significance, since somewhere between 60 and 80% of these patients will subsequently develop overt pregnancy-induced hypertension. More important information is a negative roll test. It is most unusual for anybody with a negative roll test to develop pregnancy-induced hypertension; hence, a negative test may be more clinically important than a positive test. The blood pressure reading that I have always felt is the most important is the one taken immediately after the patient turns to her back. It has been my experience that this is positive before the 5-min roll test is positive and may offer additional prognostic information. The roll test may be positive 3 to 4 weeks before overt clinical symptoms develop, and the test is recommended to be done on all primigravida patients on each visit, preferably no longer than 2 weeks apart, from the twenty-fourth week of gestation to term. It is the only known clinical test at this time that can be easily done and has predictive value of future pregnancy outcome.

SEVERE PREECLAMPSIA

The diagnosis of severe preeclampsia is not difficult to make, but the appreciation of its severity often goes unnoticed. The diagnosis can be made if one of the following signs or symptoms is present: (1) a systolic blood pressure of 160 or a diastolic blood pressure of at least 110 on two occasions, 6 hr apart, with the patient at bed rest; (2) proteinuria of 5 g or more during a 24-hr period (practically speaking this is 3 to 4 plus urinary protein on a quantitative determination); (3) oliguria of less than 400 cc in 24 hr; (4) cerebral or visual disturbances; and (5) pulmonary edema or cyanosis.

When proteinuria of 2 g or more is present, an assumption can be made that a glomerular lesion is present such as glomeruloendotheliosis in pregnancy-induced hypertension (8). Interestingly, the renal lesion continues in spite of all therapy until the pregnancy is terminated. Most patients who have severe preeclampsia are ill enough so that delivery should be accomplished if you can be assured that adequate pulmonary maturity of the fetus is present and a live-born fetus will result. We made a clinical observation in 1961 at the Medical College of Georgia that the offspring of eclamptic patients have less respiratory distress than other patients of comparable gestation. This may be due to intrauterine distress and increased fetal cortisol production to help mature the fetal lung.

The most serious form of acute hypertension in pregnancy is when the patient has severe preeclampsia and then develops seizures. At this point the patient is known to have eclampsia, one of the most dreaded conditions seen in obstetrics. Once the patient develops eclampsia, the prognosis for the fetus and the mother is guarded, since 10 to 15% of maternal deaths occur in patients who have eclampsia and approximately 30% of the fetuses die as a result of this maternal condition. This combined fetal and maternal mortality rate of 40% is one of the highest seen in human medicine for a disease that we earlier said should most likely be completely preventable. The loss of life represents 125 years of productivity to society, since the mother has an additional 50 years and the fetus 75 expected years.

ETIOLOGY

Acute hypertension in pregnancy is known as a disease of theories, since the cause is still unknown.

Dr. Joseph B. DeLee wanted to acknowledge special contributions to reproduction and inscribe the names of great men on shields on a colonnade at Chicago Lying-in Hospital. There is one shield that remains uninscribed to this day. It is reserved for the name of the person who discovers the etiology of eclampsia (Fig. 1).

It would appear that certain apparent factors must be explained in any etiologic theory of preeclampsia or pregnancy-induced hypertension. All too often, individuals get on their own special hobbyhorse to emphasize particular points in the pathogenesis of this disease. The following observations are consistent in patients with acute pregnancy-induced hypertension that develops after the twenty-fourth week of pregnancy: (1) preeclampsia is essentially a disease of the primigravida; (2) the condition occurs more frequently among indigent patients than private patients, but the latter are not immune to the disease; (3) it is more prevalent as term approaches; (4) pregnancy-induced hypertension disappears once the uterus is empty; (5) a renal lesion (glomeruloendotheliosis) is present at least three-fourths of the time and disappears after the pregnancy is completed (reversible); and (6) predisposing factors may trigger the disease in individuals who would not normally have the condition, and these include a multiple pregnancy, hydatidiform mole, hydramnios, and diabetes.

PATHOGENESIS AND EPIDEMIOLOGY

It is indeed fortunate that most pregnant patients do not develop pregnancy-induced hypertension. The incidence of preeclampsia throughout the world is estimated to be 5 to 7% of all pregnancies. The incidence in a given hospital or locale is altered by the number of indigent patients, number of primigravida patients, geographic location, whether the hospital is a level 3 or level 1 or 2 hospital, the method of reporting, and the general level of area economics, i.e., a developed or underdeveloped country.

It has been estimated that in the United States alone at least 100 to 125 deaths per day occur in fetuses whose mothers have developed hypertension during pregnancy. The impact of this loss of life can perhaps be better understood when it is noted that it can be equated to the annual death toll in automobile accidents or from violent means such as murder. This, then, should make hypertension in pregnancy a major concern for all

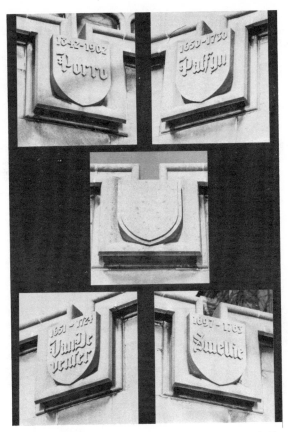

Figure 1. Composite of shields on portico at Chicago lying-on hospital. Empty shield designated for one that discovers etiology of eclampsia.

involved in reproduction, because of this potential loss of life which should be essentially preventable. What is not known is whether or not those newborns who survive from patients who have catastrophic or severe hypertension during pregnancy have as great a potential as is feasible. If we assume that the severe forms of disease are completely preventable, the time has come when a society that is as affluent as ours in this country should not tolerate this disease. One way to help eliminate the disease is patient and doctor education, but once done it is imperative that pregnant patients have better hospital insurance or a mechanism by which hospitalization can be easily accomplished.

Pregnancy is a homeostatic situation that if disrupted may in some way be associated with the onset of pregnancy-induced hypertension (Fig. 2 and 3) (9). The placenta gradually produces increased amounts of progesterone, which in a small way contributes to minor sodium loss. This mild loss of sodium results in contraction of the blood volume in the vascular compartment, which in turn activates the stretch receptor afferent arteriole and juxtaglomerular apparatus to produce more renin. The renin is activated and activates alpha-2 globulin, which is converted to angiotensin I and then by another enzyme to angiotensin II. Angiotensin is one of the most potent of pressor agents known. The angiotensin in turn acts on the adrenal gland in the region of the zona glomerulosa to produce increased amounts of aldosterone as a compensatory

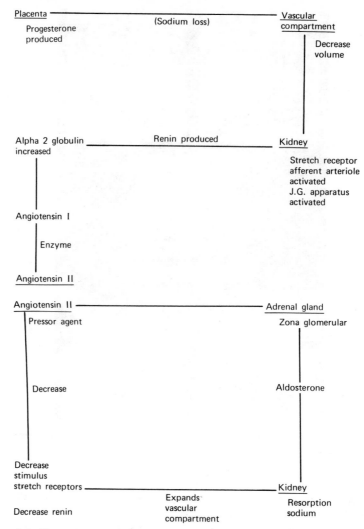

Figure 2 and 3. Homeostatic interaction between placenta, vascular compartment, kidney and adrenal gland.

mechanism to increase the reabsorption of the sodium from the renal tubule. This, then, reexpands the water in the vascular compartment, thus decreasing the stimulus on the stretch receptors, which in turn decreases the renin production. This normal, homeostatic mechanism in pregnancy is in full force, but when acute pregnancy-induced hypertension develops, these feedback mechanisms are altered, and eventually disturbed pathophysiology develops.

The disturbed pathophysiology in pregnancy-induced hypertension includes (1) vasospasm of the arterioles (hypertension, decreased uterine blood flow); (2) altered vascular reactivity (increased sensitivity to pressor agents); (3) compromised metabolic function (retention of sodium); (4) compromised renal function (decreased glomerular filtration rate, oliguria); (5) alterations in the vascular compartment (decrease in blood volume); (6) alterations of the central nervous system (increased irritability, increased reflexes and clonus); and (7) catabolic disease (negative nitrogen balance).

The schematic representation as seen in Figure 4 may well be a partial explanation for the sequence of events that takes place in acute pregnancy-induced hypertension (10). Loop 1 represents normal pregnancy homeostasis that is associated with increased steroid hormones and binding proteins that contribute to the sodium retention and weight gain seen in pregnancy. There is also an increased aldosterone secretion in normal pregnancy that is additionally associated with increased retention of fluid and sodium. We have shown that the mildly affected patient with pregnancy-induced hypertension can easily handle an excess salt load. The beginning pregnancy-induced hypertension may be enhanced by aortic renal compression that is subtle in onset and can be predicted only by using the roll test. Renin activation triggers events that along with sodium retention in vessel walls may contribute to the increased cardiovascular reactivity (Fig. 5). The preeclamptic patient is hyperresponsive to infusions of pressor substances such as epinephrine, norepinephrine, and angiotensin (4,5). Relative uterine ischemia develops and explains to some degree the increased incidence that may occur in primigravida where their uterine vascular tree has never been stretched. The intravascular fibrin deposition is insidious and may contribute to the development of the so-called toxemic lesion known as glomeruloendotheliosis. This renal lesion can explain the decrease in glomerular filtration rate and the increase in proteinuria. The decrease

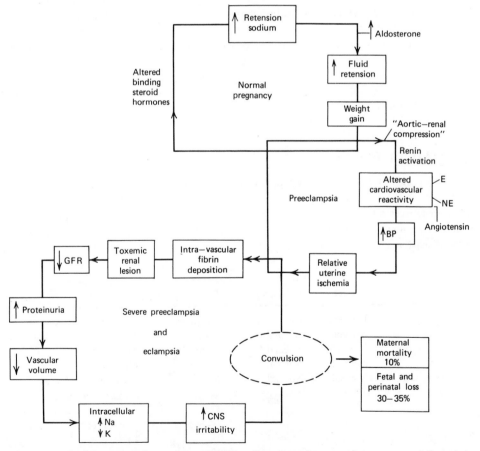

Figure 4. Pathogenesis of preeclampsia. The first loop is normal pregnancy followed by preeclampsia and eclampsia. Organ system changes are identified.

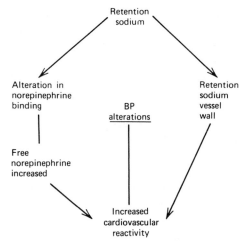

Figure 5. Hypothesis that identifies increased cardiovascular reactivity changes in pregnancy induced hypertension.

in vascular volume can be documented by serial hematocrits in ill patients when hemoconcentration is seen (11). Severe disease is associated with an increased intracellular sodium and decreased intracellular potassium, which is the reverse of normal. The central nervous system becomes more hyperactive and eventually may trigger a convulsion that further worsens the prognosis for both mother and fetus. It is important to underscore the fact that 125 years of productive life exists in the pregnant patient, since the mother will live an additional 50 years and the fetus 75; hence, the fetal and perinatal loss of 30 to 35%, coupled with the maternal mortality of 10% in patients who have eclampsia, makes this one of the most severe of all diseases encountered in medicine.

LABORATORY RESULTS

Laboratory values in cases of pregnancy-induced hypertension in general are within normal limits. The only exception to this is that, in severe cases, alterations in the hematocrit, liver enzymes, serum creatinine, fibrinogen, split products, and proteinuria deviate from normal. The following table indicates the changes that usually take place as the disease worsens:

	Normal	_Mild Preeclampsia_	_Severe Preeclampsia_	_Eclampsia_
Hematocrit	Decreased	Decreased	Increased	Markedly increased
Electrolytes	Normal	Normal	Normal	Normal
Creatinine, serum	Normal	Normal	Normal	Above 0.8
Liver enzymes	Normal	Normal	Normal	Elevated
Fibrinogen, split products	Normal	Normal	Normal	Occasional decrease in fibrinogen and increase in split products
Proteinuria	0	Trace	2+	4+
Estriol	Normal	Normal	Normal	Decreased

CLINICAL COURSE AND COMPLICATIONS

Several premises should be made concerning development of pregnancy-induced hypertension. The most obvious are the following:

1. The onset of the disease is usually insidious, and subtle changes are often disregarded.
2. The most severe forms of the disease, i.e., severe preeclampsia and eclampsia, are completely preventable.

As a generalization an organized sequence of events is seen in development of pregnancy-induced hypertension, with, first, the appearance of edema, second, the appearance of hypertension, and, last, proteinuria. As a generalization, if these signs and symptoms do not appear in this order, other diseases should be entertained.

Once the disease is full-blown, such as a patient who has edema, significant hypertension, and at least 2 plus proteinuria, no form of therapy will reverse her generalized systemic process until the uterus is emptied. The fetus will not prosper in this milieu of disturbed physiology and is often best delivered if mature, as evidenced by an L/S ratio of greater than 3:1 in our laboratories, or if this patient is greater than 34 weeks' gestation.

Once the diagnosis of preeclampsia is made, the only therapy is hospitalization. There is no place for outpatient management of preeclampsia, as procrastination usually leads to the progression of the disease to more severe forms. Patients that have mild preeclampsia often respond to hospital management and may even go home. Caution must be paramount as they return to the environment that created the disease.

MATERNAL COMPLICATIONS

The most overt maternal and fetal complication is death. Severe pregnancy-induced hypertension, i.e., eclampsia, carries with it one of the highest mortality rates in medicine, since the maternal mortality rate varies in the world today from 0 to 13% and the perinatal mortality ranges from 10 to 37%. Perinatal mortality is, however, not the only concern, since it is the morbidity of both mother and fetus that is most significant. The more significant is for the offspring of the patient born of an eclamptic mother, and this is especially tragic when such a disease could have been prevented. The challenge is to deliver a living fetus with its greatest potential in this severe disease and to prevent any residual damage in the mother.

Perinatal mortality depends on the stage of gestation when severe preeclampsia occurs. The eclamptic studies of Pritchard and Stone (2) and Zuspan and Ward (1) show a relatively low perinatal mortality of 10% and no maternal deaths if the fetus is alive when the patient is first seen. Pritchard has recently updated his series of eclamptic patients who now number approximately 350 and these have been treated without a single maternal death (12). The fetal salvage of 90% and a 0% maternal mortality first published by these authors in 1966 and 1964, respectively, are the best salvage rates in the world literature for eclampsia. They continue to be the best results 15 years after publication. Later in this chapter, the specific therapy regimens are outlined. The common denominator in both of these studies was the liberal use of parenteral magnesium sulfate and the relative absence of other medication except for antihypertensive medication to prevent a stroke. Diuretics were not used in either study. It has been suggested that the absence of multiple additional medications may account for the low perinatal mortality, since a better product is presented to the neonatologist for care.

Severe maternal complications are usually not seen in mild preeclampsia. Some of the maternal problems that may present with the more severe forms of the disease are abruptio placenta, hypofibrinogenemia, homolysis, cerebral hemorrhage, ophthalmologic abnormalities, pulmonary edema, and fatty metamorphosis of the liver.

Abruptio placenta is associated in pregnancy with patients who have hypertension and more so with patients who have chronic hypertension rather than acute hypertension. Our studies at the Medical College of Georgia have shown that 23% of the patients with abruptio placenta had preeclampsia-eclampsia (13). The incidence of abruptio placenta tends to be in direct proportion to the incidence of hypertension during pregnancy and more particularly the incidence of preeclampsia-eclampsia. Past studies at Chicago Lying-in Hospital by Dieckmann identified 30% of 186 cases of abruptio placenta to be associated with acute pregnancy-induced hypertension (14).

No serious studies in the human have been done to indicate in a serial manner a decrease in fibrinogen associated with preeclampsia. Usually bleeding does not occur until the fibrinogen level is 100 mg or less. If serial determinations for fibrinogen were done in patients who had severe preeclampsia, it would be my impression that we would more often see changes; but these would be mild changes from the elevated normal levels seen in pregnancy rather than a severe drop. Twenty-three percent of the cases of hypofibrinogenemia at the Medical College of Georgia were associated with preeclampsia; hence, the patient who is identified as having severe toxemia of pregnancy should be critically monitored with fibrinogen and other coagulation determinations (13). A postpartum hemorrhage in a patient with severe pregnancy-induced hypertension may well be due to hypofibrinogenemia.

The patient with severe preeclampsia occasionally exhibits hemolysis that is manifest principally by either jaundice or dark-colored urine. This probably represents hepatocellular damage and red blood cell destruction. The patients are usually so critically ill that detailed studies have not been done to ascertain the specific etiology. It is known that periportal necrosis of the liver is a common autopsy finding in eclampsia and could help explain some of this phenomenon. Hepatocellular changes occur in the liver of patients who have pregnancy-induced hypertension, but often these return to normal within a short time. I have seen at least a half dozen patients with severe preeclampsia with profound hepatocellular damage, clotting defects, and severe hemolysis who eventually recovered and were perfectly normal at follow-up. Oliguria with hemolysis that is manifest by dark-colored urine is a very ominous sign, and aggressive management to interrupt the pregnancy is necessary.

The most dreaded of all problems in acute pregnancy-induced hypertension is cerebral hemorrhage. This usually is preventable, and I would encourage the control of excessive blood pressure in patients who have acute pregnancy-induced hypertension with an antihypertensive agent that you know how to use well. The one that we have used over the years that has proved to be satisfactory has been hydralazine (Apresoline). Apresoline is first given by bolus injection and then by infusion pump from a plastic bag to control the blood pressure. The next alternative if Apresoline does not control the blood pressure is to use intravenous alpha methyl dopa (Aldomet) in conjunction with the Apresoline. I have never seen a patient who could not be controlled with these two modalities of therapy. If the blood pressure is controlled, the diastolic pressure should not be dropped acutely and should ideally hover around 90 to prevent a decrease in uterine blood flow.

A rare complication of acute pregnancy-induced hypertension is the loss of vision. I have seen a number of patients who have manifested this blurring of vision followed by complete loss of vision. Often, this may be associated with hemorrhage in the eye grounds or with acute edema. This acute phenomenon should warn the clinician of an impending cardiovascular accident, and the patient should be vigorously treated with antihypertensive therapy. The loss of vision is usually temporary, and recovery may be expected unless there is retinal detachment.

I have only seen one case of actue pulmonary edema in the 100 eclamptic patients that I have personally observed. This was easily managed by phlebotomy and digitalization.

The lesion known as glomeruloendotheliosis was first described by Spargo et al. at the University of Chicago and was first felt to be a specific lesion for toxemia of pregnancy, since it was seen in 75% of primigravida patients with a clinical diagnosis of preeclampsia (3). It is known now that this is not true and that this is also seen in other conditions associated with D.I.C. The lesion consists of swelling of the endothelial cytoplasm without involvement of other structures and is entirely reversible. Interestingly, in the renal biopsy study done at the University of Chicago it was shown that chronic renal disease (15%) and chronic hypertension may be associated with acute pregnancy-induced hypertension. It is recommended that a renal biopsy not be done during pregnancy, and the time that we recommend is 48 hr or more postpartum.

FETAL COMPLICATIONS

The major problem in acute pregnancy-induced hypertension is the alteration in uterine blood flow that encroaches on the placental reserve and leads toward problems for the fetus. This is related to the profound vasospasm present in patients who have severe pregnancy-induced hypertension. The placenta also shows an increased number of infarcts and premature aging that result in a continued decrease in its functional integrity and additional fetal malnutrition. The degree of intrauterine fetal malnutrition determines the clinical outcome that can be expected, with the most severe being the delivery of a stillborn, or if something less than this is seen, a neonatal death may be present. If the placenta has enough reserve, only intrauterine growth retardation may be the point of concern.

We have shown in a study of 69 eclamptic patients that when a correlation was made between weeks of gestation and the weight of the newborns, fetal malnutrition has taken place in a large number of these newborns. The control curve was from normal gestations of similar socioeconomic backgrounds and illustrates that intrauterine weight retardation can be as much as 400 to 700 g (15). The intrauterine growth retardation or fetal malnutrition results in a weight loss or failure to gain weight and is of major significance in evaluation by the clinician. The obstetrician may be mislead by the small uterus in that he thinks the menstrual period was wrong or the baby is not so mature as it should be; hence he may tend to procrastinate for more time to let the fetus grow, which may be catastrophic for the fetus. We have found that prematurity is a frequent complication of the severe forms of toxemia and the weight of the baby as well as its mature development govern to a great degree the amount of fetal salvage observed. Fetal salvage also is governed by the medication the mother receives to control the preeclampsia during labor as well as the moment of delivery. I have never seen a live-born delivered from an eclamptic patient before 30 weeks of gestation. Ideally, after 32 weeks of gestation the statistical chance of fetal death should be no greater than 10% rather than a figure of increased mortality that is seen in severe pregnancy-induced hypertension.

A serious rethinking is necessary in the mode of delivery of these small babies, especially those who are less than 1500 g. We have found that with appropriate monitoring of the fetus, using supportive care for the mother and specific therapy, namely, magnesium sulfate with control of the blood pressure, good fetal salvage can be expected. If the fetus is less than 1500 g, serious considerations should be given for abdominal delivery so that the neonatologist is presented with the best baby possible. This is in contrast to my earlier thinking, in which I felt all patients should be delivered vaginally by induction, since this is easily achieved. Our salvage rate on our under-1000-g babies at the Ohio State University is now 70%, and this is a figure that is 2½ times greater than expected for the under-1000-g babies (16).

TREATMENT

Prevention

The key to treatment is prevention; however, one of the major problems is to eliminate the ills of society—poor nutrition with low protein intake, overcrowding, limited antenatal care, and poor education on reproduction—to achieve this goal. This approach is impractical; however, we should strive for this, and the health care team's effort should be to identify the patient we know will have a high risk to develop pregnancy-induced hypertension so that a different program for prenatal care can be instituted. Specific characteristics are seen in patients who have an unusual profile and should be considered high risk and are (1) primigravida; (2) low socioeconomic class; (3) low level of education; (4) poor nutrition; (5) often young; (6) associated contributing factors such as diabetes, renal disease, chronic hypertension, twins, and hydramnios. Different degrees of emphasis can be placed on the characteristics above, but the most important is that the primigravida is at serious risk in developing preeclampsia, since approximately 8% of patients in this country now develop pregnancy-induced hypertension.

The major role of the physician should be to develop a profile of suspicion in patients who have the characteristics of predisposition to pregnancy-induced hypertension and realize that hospitalization is mandatory once a clinical diagnosis of preeclampsia can be made. Procrastination has no place in the treatment of this disease, since the patients often develop the disease in a milieu that was not conducive to good prenatal health initially. It has been amply demonstrated that early hospitalization can almost eliminate severe disease. The best example of this statement is the observation in maternal-infant care projects where high-risk patients are identified and early hospitalization encouraged. Vacant beds on obstetrical services in this country could well be used by more liberal admittance policies when patients develop abnormalities of fluid retention and abnormal elevations in their blood pressure. Prevention should be the common goal.

Specific Forms of Therapy

Acute pregnancy-induced hypertension is known as a disease of theories and could also be termed a textbook of different forms of therapy. All therapy for preeclampsia-eclampsia is empiric, since the basic etiologic mechanism is unknown; however, this does not mean that patients should not be treated intelligently, keeping in mind the pathophysiology of (1) vasospasm, (2) retention of sodium, (3) increased central nervous system irritability, (4) altered renal function, (5) decreased vascular volume, and a (6) catabolic disease.

Early hospitalization in patients who have mild preeclampsia certainly will prevent the development of severe manifestations of the disease and will be the major contribution to a decrease in maternal and fetal mortality and morbidity.

There is no specific outlined method of therapy for treating acute pregnancy-induced hypertension, and therapy must be highly individualized. The most important thing is to have guideposts, keeping in mind the disturbed pathophysiology as well as the fact that the condition of the fetus when presented to the neonatologist should be the best possible that can be achieved.

Good prenatal care is without question the single most important issue in the treatment of pregnancy-induced hypertension to prevent severe forms of the disease. I have never been convinced that it is possible to prevent mild preeclampsia, but I am completely convinced that the severe forms can be prevented by astute clinicians and liberal hospitalization policies. There are proponents of the prophylactic and therapeutic use of diuretics during pregnancy, but most reports do not substantiate their beneficial effects on either the fetus, the mother, or the prevention of pregnancy-induced hypertension. Double blind investigations with the prophylactic use of the benzothiadiazine diuretics have shown that all patients on diuretics have less edema but that the onset of preeclampsia is not prevented (17). It is unsound physiologically, and there has been no proof that they are beneficial to either the fetus or the mother.

Identification of the Patient

A major issue is the identification of the patient that you know has a statistically good chance of developing pregnancy-induced hypertension and then outlining a program for her that will alter the occurrence of this disease. The simplest and easiest program is to see the patient more frequently and to encourage two things that I feel are most important in prevention. First, a nutritious diet high in protein and, second, bed rest at midday for at least 1.5 hr on her side regardless of whether the patient works or not.

The working mother or the active mother tends not to rest so much as she could, which in turn is a positive variable in the development of preeclampsia; hence, the patient who has a profile for developing preeclampsia must be encouraged to fulfill the dictum of a nutritious diet and 1.5 hr of bed rest on her side at midday. Patients should be seen frequently, and by this I mean after the twentieth week of pregnancy the primigravida patient should be seen at least every 2 weeks, and the roll test should be done on each visit. A negative roll test is significant in that you can be reasonably assured that the patient will not develop preeclampsia; however, if a patient has a positive roll test, 60 to 80% of these patients later will develop overt pregnancy-induced hypertension. If a patient has a positive roll test, the suggestion should be made that additional bed rest at home is essential, even though there are no overt signs of preeclampsia.

Additionally, I usually suggest that the patient have a diet consisting of high protein intake using fresh and frozen foods and stating that anything out of a bottle or a can should be avoided. This, in essence, gives mild salt sodium restriction and a palatable diet that is nutritious to the patient.

Management Dictums

1. If a patient is hospitalized and under therapy, convulsions should rarely ever occur. Patients who have severe preeclampsia should be treated with therapeutic doses of intravenous magnesium sulfate especially if reflexes are hyperactive. The rule of thumb is to use if in doubt about whether or not magnesium sulfate should be used.

2. Therapy should concern both the fetus and the mother and should assure that neither the fetus nor the mother is harmed by overzealous therapy or poor obstetric judgment. The concern in the preeclamptic patient is primarily for the fetus, since maternal mortality is extremely unusual. The time of the delivery is an issue that can best be determined by the L/S ratio to be certain that the fetus has the greatest chance of salvage once delivery is achieved.

3. Eclampsia is known not to cause residual cardiovascular damage to the mother. A familial history of hypertension makes the patient more prone to develop pregnancy-induced hypertension and to have hypertension later in life. Pure preeclampsia does not seem to predispose subsequent hypertensive vascular disease.

Mild Preeclampsia

A patient with mild preeclampsia when removed from her environmental influence, placed in the hospital at complete bed rest on her side with a nutritious diet, and given a sedative will usually improve in a dramatic fashion in 3 to 5 days. The major aspect of this regimen is to give her only bathroom privileges and to restrict her activity otherwise. Additional measures include an adequate protein intake of 70 g or more per day and a mild sedative such as phenobarbital (30 mg four times a day). Physiologic diuresis is usually achieved within 36 to 48 hr after admittance to the hospital, which can be measured by a decrease in weight of 2 to 4 kg. If there is a mild rise in blood pressure, this usually returns to normal. It is imperative that her blood pressure be taken four times during the day. Any preeclamptic patient does not need diuretics, assuming she has diuresis within 72 hr after admittance to the hospital. The disease usually improves symptomatically within 3 to 5 days, and the patient may then be discharged under careful outpatient observation and should be seen at least twice a week. If her gestation is 38 weeks or more, serious consideration should be given to induction following control of the preeclampsia.

The single most important ingredient in therapy is bed rest, and this is beneficial to both mother and fetus and works with the following hypothesis (Fig. 6). Bed rest increases renal blood flow and thus increases glomerular filtration rate, which presents to the glomerulars an increased sodium load; hence sodium loss and diuresis with decreased weight occurs. An increased sodium loss alters the hyperactive cardiovascular reactivity, and this in turn decreases the blood pressure. At the same time the patient also has a diminution of her own endogenous pressor agent, norepinephrine, which is decreased by bed rest, and this also further decreases her cardiovascular reactivity, with

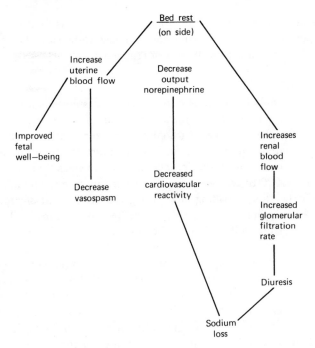

Figure 6. Hypothesis on therapeutic effect of bed rest on pregnancy induced hypertension.

the end result being two measurable components—a decrease in blood pressure and a loss in weight.

Severe Preeclampsia

The individual with severe preeclampsia is seriously ill, and the potential of fetal death and maternal death exists. Many patients with severe preeclampsia are sicker than patients who have eclampsia. Care begins with immediate hospitalization and close supervision. Patients should be placed on their side at bed rest with bathroom privileges only and weighed daily. Base line laboratory studies should be done that include a 24-hr urine specimen for protein and estriol, an amniocentesis for fetal maturity (L/S), a CBC, serum electrolytes, serum creatinine, and blood urea nitrogen. Total protein and serial fibrinogen and liver enzyme determinations are part of the chemical profile.

A decision should be made within a reasonable time concerning delivery in most paitents with severe preeclampsia. The rule of thumb that we have used is if the patient is 34 weeks or more gestation or the fetus has an adequate pulmonary maturity, delivery should be accomplished, since the disease cannot be abated and often worsens under close observation. The fetus usually does not do well in this milieu of severely deranged physiology in the mother and often does better in a neonatal intensive care nursery.

The deep tendon reflexes of the severe preeclamptic patient are usually hyperactive, and this together with symptoms of epigastric pain, headache, and abdominal cramps may herald the onset of a seizure.

The severe preeclamptic patient in all probability will need intravenous magnesium sulfate and may need antihypertensive therapy to prevent a cerebral vascular accident. Intake and output must be meticulous, and a Foley catheter is beneficial in these patients. The following details these treatment regimens:

Magnesium Sulfate

The methods are available for administering magnesium sulfate—either intravenous or intramuscular. We have preferred the intravenous route for the single reason that it is more appropriate for the disturbed pathophysiology that exists in the preeclamptic patient and is less painful for the patient. It is administered by an infusion pump or some form of a controlled administration system. Ten to twenty grams of magnesium sulfate are added to 1000 cc of 5% dextrose in water, and the rate of administration is approximately 1 g/hr after a loading dose of 4 g has been administered. The loading dose of 4 g should be administered slowly over a period of at least 10 min. Practical monitoring of magnesium sulfate level is best achieved by (1) deep tendon reflexes, which should always be present but hypoactive; (2) urinary output, which should exceed 100 cc every 4 hr; and (3) respirations, which should not fall under 10 per min. The therapeutic blood level one attempts to achieve is 6 to 7 mEq/liter. The magnesium sulfate is continued usually until the patient has been delivered and for at least 12 hr following delivery. It is seldom that clinical improvement is so dramatic or gestation so premature that one can discontinue the magnesium sulfate prior to delivery. General information on magnesium sulfate includes: (1) Consider magnesium sulfate a dangerous drug, since it can in toxic doses depress respiration (10 to 12 mEq/liter) as well as cause cardiac arrest (>14 to 15 mEq/liter). It should not be given rapidly. (2) All drugs affect the fetus, but this drug affects the fetus the least; hence, it is the drug of choice in the treatment of severe preeclampsia-eclampsia. (3) Magnesium sulfate is excreted principally by the kidneys; hence, if urinary output is diminished, the dose of magnesium sulfate should be decreased, and conversely if diuresis occurs, additional magnesium sulfate may be needed. (4) Magnesium sulfate overdose can be counteracted by the administration of calcium intravenously (1-g doses intravenously). (5) Magnesium sulfate depresses the activity at the myoneural junction and its major therapeutic modality is to prevent a seizure. (6) The protective effect of magnesium sulfate may be due to an increase in uterine blood flow. This has never been proved in the human; however, this is the case in the monkey. I consider this one of its most effective therapeutic benefits over other drugs in the treatment of this disease. (7) Magnesium sulfate is not a hypotensive agent; however, a transient episode of a decrease in blood pressure may be seen in the first 60 min after the drug is administered. (8) Magnesium sulfate crosses the placenta and is in equilibrium between the mother and the fetus; hence, if a maternal level of magnesium is known, the same exists in the fetus. (9) Magnesium sulfate decreases the variability seen in electronic fetal heart rate monitoring.

Route of Delivery

It can be stated that the fetus has triggered the uterus to respond as increased uterine activity is often seen in the patient with severe pregnancy-induced hypertension. This means that an oxytocin induction given by infusion pump in small doses, i.e., 2 to 4 mU will usually achieve the desired amount of uterine activity. Preeclampsia-eclampsia is one condition in which the condition of the cervix may not predict an easy or a protracted labor. Our studies have shown that an unfavorable cervix in an eclamptic patient is not necessarily associated with a prolonged labor. Most eclamptic patients can be delivered within 18 hr after an induction is started (18,19).

I have recently changed my mind in the approach of the small fetus in the patient with pregnancy-induced hypertension and now recommend that abdominal delivery be reserved for the baby that you estimate to be less than 1500 g. The patient whose fetus is greater than 1500 g can probably be delivered vaginally. We have found now that if we reserve abdominal delivery for the very small baby, especially that which is less than 1000 g, our salvage rate is four times greater than anticipated. The last 12 babies weighing less than 1000 g that we have delivered from hypertensive mothers had a 70% neonatal survival.

Eclampsia

Once a patient develops eclampsia, the survival statistics for both mother and fetus change dramatically. The maternal mortality with eclampsia worldwide is greater than 10% and the fetal mortality greater than 35%. Few conditions in medicine present the major challenge in which the potential loss of life is 45%. This is especially true in conditions that are preventable. As previously stated, this loss of life represents 125 years to society (75 for the fetus and 50 for the mother). The previously outlined therapeutic regimen with intravenous magnesium sulfate has been used for the past 17 years and has resulted in a zero maternal mortality and a 10% fetal mortality if the fetus was alive when the eclamptic patient was first seen. Pritchard recently has presented data in which approximately 350 eclamptic patients have been treated without a maternal death. Our treatment regimens differ only in the fact that he uses intramuscular magnesium sulfate and we have been proponents of intravenous magnesium sulfate. Diuretics are not used, and antihypertensive therapy is used to control any blood pressure in excess of 110 mm Hg diastolic or when it is felt that the patient has the potential for a cerebral vascular accident. These combined results represent the best survival rate in the world literature for both mother and fetus.

Control of Convulsion

Many misconceptions exist in understanding how to control a convulsion in a patient who has eclampsia. The treatment of choice is magnesium sulfate, 4 to 6 g given intravenously, slowly, over a period of 5 to 10 min. Following this the magnesium sulfate is continued at a rate of at least 1 g/hr. Administration should be by infusion pump.

There is no place in the treatment of a convulsing patient for the use of intravenous barbiturates, morphine sulfate, or agents such as paraldehyde, nor for the currently in vogue, intravenous valium. This should not be used, as it has a major adverse effect on the fetus (hypotonia and hypothermia). The usual problem in the patient with eclampsia is that they are undertreated with magnesium sulfate and overtreated with other medications.

The Newborn

The pediatric literature has cast aspersions on the use of magnesium sulfate because of some of the problems that have been encountered in the newborn. If the question is critically examined, there is no good medication; however, magnesium sulfate is the one medication that has the least adverse effect on the fetus. Magnesium sulfate actually provides a protective mechanism for the fetus in this abnormal milieu, since it probably increases uterine blood flow and promotes fetal health. The newborns should receive intensive care observation. Magnesium cord levels are the same as maternal cord levels, and if nothing is done, the magnesium will usually be excreted in the first 4 to 6 hr of newborn life. If the infant is severely hypotonic, calcium supplementation may be necessary, but this is infrequent. It has been our impression over the years that fewer newborns from severe preeclamptic-eclamptic mothers develop RDS than newborns of comparable gestational age and weight than from nontoxemic mothers.

Decision for Delivery

The severe preeclamptic-eclamptic patient needs to be delivered within a reasonable time, as her condition will usually not improve to any great degree with therapy. The major concern for the fetus is death and for the mother a stroke, and both should be prevented. The earlier the gestation, the more dreaded the prognosis; and I have yet to see a fetus live from a mother who was less than 30 weeks, gestation who had eclampsia. If maternal conditions permit in severe preeclampsia-eclampsia, in the patients who are 30 to 32 weeks' gestation, induction of labor may be delayed until pulmonary maturity is reached in a fetus. We have given intravenous hydrocortisone (1 g every 6 hr for four doses) to the mother and waited 48 hr for pulmonary maturity as judged by an L/S ratio increase (19). This has been done in carefully selected preeclamptic-eclamptic patients. Amniocentensis with L/S ratio in our laboratory of greater than 3 : 1 is desirable, since we see no cases of severe RDS with this value. If the gestation is 34 weeks or longer or if the L/S ratio is greater than 3 : 1, the patient should undergo delivery as soon as possible after good therapeutic control is acheived. The decision in these very ill patients should be made soon after the patient is admitted to the hospital, since delay leads only to procrastination and does not favor the fetus. Induction of labor is performed by an infusion pump administering oxytocin and an amniotomy done at the appropriate time. The small fetus, i.e., less than 1500 g, should seriously be considered for abdominal delivery. As previously stated, the condition of the cervix, i.e., ripe or unripe, does not necessarily mean that the patient will or will not achieve a vaginal delivery. We found that in 51 eclamptic patients that were classified according to the condition of their cervices all except 4 patients regardless of the condition of the cervix delivered vaginally after 12 hr of oxytocin induction. Twelve hours can be used as a guidepost for appropriate progress, and if delivery has not been achieved by then, an abdominal delivery should be considered.

Anesthesia for Delivery

Major conduction anesthesia—spinal, caudal, epidural—is contraindicated in pregnancy-induced hypertension, since this may be associated with decreased uterine blood flow and harmful to the fetus. The patient with severe disease also has a diminished blood volume, and this would be even more hazardous when a sympathetic blockade takes place with major conduction anesthesia. Pudenal block with nitrous oxide supplementation is the anesthetic of choice. Pericervical block should seldom be used, and if used, only one-half the usual dose should be given, since it may result in increased decelerations on electronic monitoring.

All our patients in labor, if they can swallow, receive a chilled antacid every 3 hr, and this is especially important in the patient who has preeclampsia, as a convulsion may occur and aspiration then take place. The neutralization of gastric acidity helps prevent fatal aspiration pneumonitis.

If cesarean section is done, balanced general anesthesia, using pentothal, nitrous oxide, and anectine, works very well. Remember to caution the anesthesiologist that magnesium sulfate and long-acting curari-like drugs are synergistic and are contraindicated. It is imperative that patients who have severe preeclampsia-eclampsia be referred to a tertiary care center where a neonatal intensive care center is also available.

Prognosis

The mild forms of preeclampsia are not associated with an increase in fetal or maternal loss; however, the severe forms of preeclampsia-eclampsia are associated with an increased fetal loss and an occasional maternal mortality. Factors that increase maternal and fetal morbidity and mortality include abruptio placenta, hypofibrinogenemia, and prematurity. We know that the long-term prognosis is excellent, since preeclampsia-eclampsia does not cause later hypertension and that recurrent preeclampsia is indeed rare and should not occur more than 10% of the time in subsequent pregnancies (20,21). Recurrence is usually associated with patients who have a genetic component for hypertension. The prognosis for the fetus needs critical evaluation, since morbidity and residues resulting from toxemia itself need to be accurately documented. If a diagnostic problem exists in the hypertensive pregnant patient, a renal biopsy within the first 5 days postpartum is helpful in establishing the diagnosis of preeclampsia-eclampsia, hypertensive cardiovascular disease, or latent renal disease and is useful in counseling the patient for further childbearing. The renal biopsy should not be performed during pregnancy.

CHRONIC HYPERTENSION

Pregnancy tends to be provocative for two conditions. One, the unmasking of chronic hypertensive disease and, the other, an alteration of carbohydrate metabolism, which unmasks diabetes. Thus pregnancy is said to be diabetogenic and hypertensogenic. This phenomenon should not be overlooked and can best be detected by a persistent mildly elevated diastolic blood pressure. Chronic hypertension is seen more commonly in the multigravid patient, but the primigravida should not be excluded. This is frequently the first time hypertension may be seen in this particular group of patients. A very important criterion when trying to establish the diagnosis of chronic hypertensive vascular disease during pregnancy is the knowledge of nonpregnant blood pressure values. It is important that these be established by contacting the referring physician, the pediatrician, etc., if you have not been following this patient in her prepregnancy state. Another important point of substantiating this suspicion is a strong family history of hypertension. This is significant if the history is positive, but often the patient may not know the blood pressure of her parents. The only important way to answer questions concerning patients who manifest hypertension during pregnancy is long-term follow-up. We have shown that eclampsia does not result in an increased incidence of chronic vascular disease later in life; hence, the issue for the patient who has acute pregnancy-induced hypertension is the immediacy of the acute problem for the mother and fetus and not the long-term effect of this disease.

There has been some concern by scholars who study hypertension in pregnancy as to whether or not patients with chronic hypertension, i.e., known hypertension that has occurred before the twenty-fourth week of pregnancy, can actually develop superimposed preeclampsia. It is reasonable to assume that such a condition does exist and should be considered one of the most serious complications in the patient who has chronic hypertension and is pregnant. This is the patient who may have a stroke. We have shown at the Chicago Lying-in Hospital that the following generalizations can be made concerning patients with chronic hypertension. These patients have a worse prognosis for the fetus than those who do not (9). The following table emphasizes this particular point:

	Normal Pregnancy	Mild Chronic Hypertension	Severe Hypertension (Greater than 160/100)
Fetal wastage	10%	16%	40%

The hazards for mother and fetus are greatest in patients who have severe hypertension prior to the twenty-fourth-week of pregnancy, and consideration should be given if the patient is seen early as to whether or not the pregnancy should continue. If the patient has chronic hypertension that is not surgically correctable, serious consideration should be given to a permanent form of contraception following the completion of pregnancy. These patients do not do well on oral contraceptives, and the most sure means of contraception is essential to their continued health.

The patient with chronic hypertension is very difficult to manage; thus it is impossible to outline a single therapy regimen. All the laboratory aids available are necessary to assure adequate antenatal assessment such as VMA, serum creatinine, BUN, electrolytes, EKG, chest x-ray, urinary and serum estriol and protein, HPL, O.C.T., and L/S. Plan on investing much time with each of these patients, since they need to be seen at 1- to 2 week-intervals. A nutritious diet and bed rest, 1 hr in the morning and 2 hr in the afternoon, are essential. Most patients need pharmacotherapy to control their hypertension. The decision for pharmacotherapy in controlling their hypertension can be determined only on an individual basis and related to their progress during pregnancy. Most patients with chronic hypertensive vascular disease need additional bed rest, sedatives (Phenobarbital), and a diuretic (Diazide, hydrochlorithiazed, etc.). Some patients require additional agents, and I have found that alpha methyl dopa is a satisfactory agent causing no major problems in the fetus.

REFERENCES

1. Zuspan, F. P., and Ward, M. C.: Improved fetal salvage in eclampsia. *Obstet. Gynecol.* 26:893, 1965.
2. Pritchard, J. A., and Stone, S. R.: Clinical and laboratory observations in eclampsia. *Am. J. Obstet. Gynec.* 99:754, 1967.

3. Spargo, B., McCartney, C. P., and Winemiller, R.: Glomerular capillary endotheliosis in toxemia of pregnancy. *Arch. Pathol.* 68:593, 1959.

4. Zuspan, F. P., Nelson, G. H., and Ahlquist, R. P.: Epinephrine infusions in normal and toxemic pregnancy: I. Nonesterified fatty acids and cardiovascular alterations. *Am. J. Obstet. Gynec.* 90:88, 1964.

5. Talledo, O. E., Chesley, L. C., and Zuspan, F. P.: Renin-angiotensin system in normal and toxemic pregnancies: III. Differential sensitivity to angiotensin II and norepinephrine in toxemia of pregnancy. *Am. J. Obstet. Gynec.* 100:218, 1968.

6. Zuspan, F. P.: Treatment of severe preeclampsia and eclampsia. *Clin. Obstet. Gynecol.* 9:954, 1966.

7. Gant, N. F., Chand, S., Worley, R. J., Whaley, P. J., Crosby, V. D., and MacDonald, P. C.: A clinical test useful for predicting the development of acute hypertension in pregnancy. *Am. J. Obstet. Gynec.* 120:1, 1974.

8. Sheehan, H., personal communication.

9. Zuspan, F. P.: Toxemia of pregnancy, in *Textbook of Obstetrics,* Sciarra, J., and Gerbie, A. (eds.). F. A. Davis, 1972.

10. Zuspan, F. P.: Pregnancy induced hypertension, in *Perinatology,* Behrman, R., and Seeds, A (eds.). C. V. Mosby Co., St. Louis, 1977.

11. Pritchard, J., personal communication.

12. Pritchard, J. A.: Changes in blood volume during pregnancy and delivery. *Anesthesiology* 26:393, 1965.

13. Madry, J. T.: Blood coagulation defects during pregnancy. *Obstet. Gynecol.* 20:235, 1962.

14. Dieckmann, W. J.: *Toxemias of Pregnancy,* Zuspan, F. P. (ed.). C. V. Mosby Co., St. Louis, 1951.

15. Zuspan, F. P.: Treatment of severe preeclampsia and eclampsia. *Clin. Obstet. Gynecol.* 9:954, 1966.

16. Cordero, L., personal communication.

17. Kraus, G. W., Marchese, J. R., and Yen, S. C.: Prophylactic use of hydrochlorothiazide in pregnancy. *J.A.M.A.* 198:1150, 1966.

18. Zuspan, F. P., and Talledo, O. E.: Factors affecting delivery in eclampsia: Condition of the cervix and uterine activity. *Am. J. Obstet. Gynec.* 100:672, 1968.

19. Talledo, O. E., and Zuspan, F. P.: Spontaneous uterine contractions in eclampsia. *Clin. Obstet. Gynecol.* 9:910, 1966.

20. Zuspan, F. P., Cordero, L., and Semchyshyn, S.: Hydrocortisone therapy and L/S ratio. *Am. J. Obstet. Gynec.,* in press.

21. Bryans, C. I., Jr., Southerland, W. L., and Zuspan, F. P.: Eclampsia: A long-term follow-up study. *Obstet. Gynecol.* 21:701, 1963.

23
The Hemoglobinopathies

Herbert C. Schwartz, M.D.

The hemoglobin molecule because of its essential function in oxygen transport, has been of fundamental interest to scientists for over 100 years. Since there exist disorders of hemoglobin ranging from point mutations, e.g., sickle cell anemia, to a wide variety of abnormalities in protein synthesis, e.g., the thalassemias, an understanding of these diseases offers some preview of the future elucidation of other hereditary diseases. The hemoglobinopathies and the various thalassemia syndromes are of particular significance to perinatal medicine, for they represent worldwide clinical disorders that reflect the effect of genetic abnormalities on biochemical development. The basis for understanding these diseases is knowledge of the structure and synthesis of the hemoglobin molecule.

HEMOGLOBIN BIOCHEMISTRY

Hemoglobin has a molecular weight of 64,400. It has four polypeptide chains, to each of which a heme group is attached. The heme groups are the "functioning" part of the molecule. They consist of the tetrapyrrole, protoporphyrin IX, with an iron atom in coordinate linkage to the central nitrogens of the pyrrole ring. It is the iron atom to which oxygen is reversibly bound. In normal adult human hemoglobin (Hb A), the globin moiety consists of two identical pairs of polypeptide chains, which have been designated alpha and beta chains. Thus, hemoglobin A has two alpha and two beta chains ($\alpha_2\beta_2$). Evidence from x-ray crystallographic studies indicates that the secondary and tertiary structures—the spatial or three-dimensional shape— of the alpha and beta chains are quite similar. However the primary structures—the sequence of amino acid residues—of human alpha and beta chains are different. For example, the alpha chain, which has 141 residues, has valylleucylserine as its amino-terminal sequence and seryllysyltyrosylarginine as its carboxyl-terminal sequence. The beta chain, which has 146 residues, has valylhistidylleucine as its amino-terminal sequence and histidyllysyltyrosylhistidine as its carboxyl-terminal sequence. The amino acids are held together by covalent bonds; however, the chains are held in their molecular relationship by hydrogen, ionic, and other weak bonds.

In addition to adult hemoglobin A, a fetal hemoglobin (Hb F) exists in the fetus and newborn. As early as 1866, Körber had noted the resistance or cord blood (Hb F) to alkali denaturation, when compared with blood from adults (Hb A). Hemoglobin F comprises more than 90% of the hemoglobin in the fetus and more than 50% in the newborn. Although its concentration decreases rapidly in the first 6 months of life, the alkali-resistant hemoglobin fraction may be as high as 2.5% in normal children and adults. The oxygen-dissociation curve for fetal red blood cells is shifted to the left, a position that is advantageous for the transplacental exchange of oxygen. This advantage is due to the decreased reactivity of Hb F to 2,3-diphosphoglycerate (2,3-DPG). Since the oxygen affinity of hemoglobin is inversely related to the amount of 2,3-DPG binding, the hemoglobin F molecule has an increased affinity for oxygen and a left-shifted oxygen-dissociation curve.

Hemoglobin F, like hemoglobin A, has four heme groups and four polypeptide chains. One pair, the alpha chains, are identical with the chains in hemoglobin A; however, the second pair, designated as gamma chains, have an amino acid sequence that is different from the beta chains of hemoglobin A. Thus, hemoglobin F has two alpha and two gamma chains ($\alpha_2\gamma_2$). However, two types of gamma chains exist: one with glycine (G_γ) at amino acid position 136 and the other with alanine (A_γ) at that position. The ratio of G_γ to A_γ is 3 in the newborn, whereas in the Hb F present in the adult it is less than 1. Variations in this ratio have been described in various clinical disorders. In addition, hemoglobin F exists as Hb F_{II} and an acetylated form Hb F_I ($\alpha_2\gamma_2^{\text{N-acetyl}}$).

The structural differences between hemoglobins A and F are reflected not only in their electrophoretic, chromatographic, and immunologic properties but in such chemical characteristics of hemoglobin F as the presence of a tryptophane notch in the ultraviolet absorption spectrum at 289 mμ and the resistance to alkali denaturation. It is the latter property which historically made it possible to determine hemoglobin F concentrations readily. Recently immunochemical techniques have been developed that allow more precise quantitation of Hb F. It is noteworthy that the level of Hb F rises during pregnancy. Although fetal-maternal bleeds may contribute to this rise, most of the hemoglobin F appears to be accounted for by stimulation of a separate clone of "hemoglobin F cells" during the second trimester.

There exist normally several minor hemoglobin components. Except for hemoglobin A_2 and Hb A_{Ic}, the chemical structure and clinical significance of most of these have not been determined. Hemoglobin A_2, which is increased in β thalassemia trait, has a pair of alpha chains that are identical with the alpha chains of hemoglobin A and F; however, the other pair of chains is different from both beta and gamma chains. These chains have been designated as delta chains. Thus, hemoglobin A_2 has two alpha chains and two delta chains ($\alpha_2\delta_2$). Hemoglobin A_2 normally comprises 2.5% of the total hemoglobin.

Hemoglobin A_{Ic} (Hb A_{Ic}) is a normal minor variant of Hb A and amounts to 5% of the total hemoglobin. Its alpha and beta chains are identical with Hb A; however, it differs from Hb A in that a glucose is linked to the N-terminal valine of the beta chain. Hb A_{Ic} has an increased affinity for oxygen, since the glucose interferes with the binding site for 2,3-DPG. An elevation of Hb A_{Ic} to twice normal occurs in diabetes mellitus. Less striking elevations have been observed in pregnant normals and pregnant diabetics. These changes probably reflect maternal blood glucose control and may have a significant effect on maternal-fetal oxygen transport in infants of diabetic mothers.

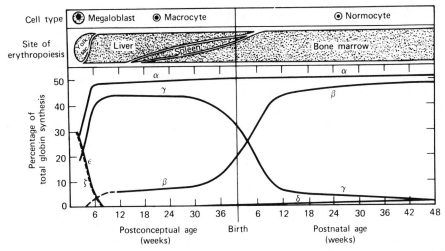

Figure 1. Developmental pattern of the hemoglobin chains. [After Huehns and Shooter (1965) and Kleihauer (1970), with permission from Wood, W.G., *Brit. Med. Bull.* 32:282, 1976.]

Several embryonic hemoglobins have been observed in fetuses with C-R lengths of less than 100 mm. Hemoglobin Gower 1 has two ζ chains and two ϵ chains ($\zeta_2\epsilon_2$). Hemoglobin Gower 2 has two α chains and two ϵ chains ($\alpha_2\epsilon_2$). Hemoglobin Portland has two ζ chains and two γ chains ($\zeta_2\gamma_2$).

These embryonic hemoglobins are probably synthesized in an early primitive red blood cell in the yolk sac and early embryo. As the embryo develops, a definitive red blood cell with distinctly different morphology produces hemoglobin in the fetal liver, spleen, and bone marrow. The switch from Hb F to Hb A appears to occur in the same cell of the definitive line and is independent of cell locus.

The developmental pattern of the hemoglobin chains is shown in Figure 1.

SICKLE CELL TRAIT AND SICKLE CELL DISEASE

For several centuries sickle cell anemia has been recognized in West Africa as a "severe" disease that might affect children of seemingly normal black parents. In America, sickle cell anemia was first observed in 1904 by a Chicago physician, James B. Herrick, who noted a "freakish poikilocytosis" in the blood of an anemic, black West Indian student. In 1917, Emmel found that the number of sickled cells gradually increased when a drop of blood from a patient with sickle cell anemia was placed under a coverslip. However it was not until 1927 that Hahn and Gillespie discovered that the sickling phenomenon was related to the oxygen desaturation of the red blood cell.

In contrast to those blacks with sickle cell anemia, others with a benign form of the disease were also described. They were asymptomatic, did not have any anemia, and sickling of their red blood cells required a greater degree of oxygen desaturation. It became apparent in 1949, from the genetic studies of black populations by Neel, that people who are heterozygous for the sickle gene have the benign form, sickle cell trait, whereas those with sickle cell anemia are homozygous. Thus, both parents of a child with sickle cell anemia have sickle cell trait.

In 1948 Watson observed that the presence of Hb F in newborns with sickle cell anemia delayed the onset of in vitro–induced sickling and suggested that the disease was associated with "the adult type of hemoglobin which possesses the sickling property." In 1949, Pauling and Itano found a difference in the electrophoretic mobility of hemoglobin obtained from normal adults (hemoglobin A) and patients with sickle cell anemia (hemoglobin S). Hemoglobin S had two more net positive charges per molecule than hemoglobin A. When they compared the concentrations of hemoglobins A and S, the homozygotes had 100% S, the heterozygotes approximately 40% S and 60% A, and the normals 100% A. This study provided a major breakthrough in the investigation and understanding of molecular diseases.

The abnormal electrophoretic mobility and decreased solubility of reduced hemoglobin S prompted Ingram to compare the primary structures of hemoglobins S and A. He prepared tryptic digests of these two hemoglobins and compared the peptide patterns ("fingerprints") obtained after analysis on paper by electrophoresis in a horizontal direction followed by chromatography in the vertical direction. Only 1 of the 28 peptides obtained from hemoglobins A and S differed. Subsequent analysis of the amino acid sequence of this peptide revealed that glutamic acid, the sixth residue from the amino-terminal end of the hemoglobin A beta chain, was replaced by a neutral amino acid, valine, in hemoglobin S. This substitution of a single amino acid in each of the beta chains accounts for the net charge difference between hemoglobins S and A. This is the primary genetic alteration in the hemoglobin S molecule and is the result of a missense mutation in the structural gene for beta globin. More than 200 such amino acid substitutions in the alpha or beta chains are known. The codons for these mutants differ from normal by a change in one DNA base, and the clinical alterations may be silent or severe, e.g., hemolytic anemia, cyanosis, or polycythemia.

PATHOPHYSIOLOGY

The biochemical advances and recent studies on the rheology of the sickled cell permit an understanding of all the signs and symptoms of sickle cell anemia. The single amino acid substitution affects the secondary and tertiary structure in such a way that hemoglobin S in the reduced state is less soluble and prone toward molecular aggregation, tactoid formation, and gelling. As the erythrocyte traverses the capillary bed, and the oxygen tension decreases, this molecular aggregation occurs, and the stroma collapses around the tactoids into the characteristic sickle cell. The sickled cells increase blood viscosity and retard capillary flow, permitting hydrogen ion accumulation, deoxygenation, and further sickling. In the areas of venous stasis, where such conditions exist for several minutes, the erythrocytes become irreversibly sickled and may thrombose the vessels. This occurs only in exceptional circumstances, since capillary transit time is usually much more rapid. However, even cells that traverse the circulation may become irreversibly sickled by losing segments of membrane. These permanently deformed cells, irreversibly sickled cells, have a rigidity associated with calcium loading of the erythrocyte membrane. Such cells, even at physiologic oxygen tensions, have increased osmotic and mechanical fragility and cause continuous hemolysis. The erythrocytes from patients with sickle cell trait, because their concentration of hemoglobin S is much lower, undergo such changes only at nonphysiological oxygen tensions.

SIGNS AND SYMPTOMS

Sickle cell trait, the heterozygous state, is present in 8% of American blacks. In general, such patients are asymptomatic and have neither physical nor hematological abnormalities. The trait is identified by a positive in vitro test for sickling and the typical electrophoresis pattern of hemoglobin A and hemoglobin S. Occasional patients have an inability to concentrate their urine, and rarely gross hematuria occurs. Severe hypoxia, such as is associated with high-altitude flying in nonpressurized cabins, may result in splenic infarctions. The main problem is the risk to offspring of having sickle cell anemia when both parents have sickle cell trait.

Sickle cell (anemia) disease, the homozygous state, is present in 0.3% of American blacks. Since this is a severe hemolytic anemia, the signs and symptoms are in part those which accompany any such process. The anemia is generally compensated, and the child so well adapted that weakness and dyspnea are minimal. Prominent physical findings are small stature, thin extremities, pallor of the mucous membrane, scleral icterus, cardiomegaly, and hepatosplenomegaly. The spleen may be very large in infancy, and although it is usually palpable under the age of 10, it is rarely palpable in older children. Laboratory examination reveals a normocytic normochromic anemia, polymorphonuclear leucocytosis, and anisocytosis, poikilocytosis, polychromatophilia, stippling, normoblasts, and sickle cells on the blood smear. There is reticulocytosis and erythroid hyperplasia of the bone marrow. The increased destruction of hemoglobin is evidenced by increased unconjugated bilirubin, increased urine, and stool urobilinogen and a shortened red blood cell survival time. The sickle cell preparation is positive, and electrophoresis reveals a single focus of hemoglobin S.

The most distinctive feature of this disease is the presence of recurrent crises. These are usually thrombotic in etiology and characterized by the sudden onset of severe pain, usually in the abdomen, back, or extremities, with fever and leucocytosis. The signs may well mimic those of an acute surgical abdomen. Crises are usually self-limiting and disappear in 5 to 7 days; however, shock and sudden death may ensue. The clinical manifestations are determined by the sites of thromboses and may vary from those of splenic or pulmonary infarctions to bony infarctions of the head of the femur with subsequent aseptic necrosis. There may be central nervous system involvement with paresis, hemiplegia, or encephalopathy. Chronic skin ulcers may occur over the lower third of the leg in adolescents. In contrast to thrombotic crises, aregenerative or aplastic crises may develop following infections in which reticulocytopenia and erythroid hypoplasia of the bone marrow cause an increase in the severity of the anemia. Rarely a crisis characterized by increased jaundice and accelerated hemolysis may occur. Such crises are more common in children who also have glucose-6-phosphate dehydrogenase (G6PD) deficiency.

Children with sickle cell anemia have an increased susceptibility to infections, and osteomyelitis from a variety of infectious agents, including salmonella, may occur. Cholelithiasis can complicate the continued hemolysis, and congestive failure can result from the profound anemia.

In pregnancy the risk to the fetus and mother with a sickle cell hemoglobinopathy is considerable. The perinatal wastage rate is up to 55% in patients with sickle cell anemia or hemoglobin S-C disease. The pathophysiologic process of hypoxia, which induces sickling, may produce thrombosis in many maternal organs and cause placental infarctions. This may induce severe intrauterine hypoxia in the uterine arcuate and decidual arterioles and result in stillbirth or abortion. When the hypoxia is minimal but frequent, growth retardation may occur.

In early infancy, the manifestations of the disease are minimal, since the high concentration of fetal hemoglobin inhibits sickling. However certain nonspecific symptomatology in the first year of life should suggest the diagnosis in a black infant. These symptoms include irritability with no apparent cause, colic, abdominal distention, failure to thrive, recurrent fever, jaundice, vomiting, and anemia with splenomegaly. A frequent presentation is the occurrence of painful swelling in the hands and feet described as "hand-foot syndrome."

It has been increasingly evident that both high morbidity and high mortality occur among infants with sickle cell anemia in the first year of life. This has prompted diagnosis in the neonatal period so that such infants can be selected for careful follow-up and prompt treatment of infections, dehydration, or other complications. Black pregnant women and their husbands should be screened for sickle cell trait. If both are positive or if the mother is positive and the father was not screened, the infant's hemoglobin should be electrophoresed by a starch or agar gel technique that permits the separation of hemoglobins A and S from F. It is noteworthy that screening tests for hemoglobin S are negative because of the high concentration of hemoglobin F. Many of the routine electrophoretic techniques used in clinical laboratories are also unsatisfactory for diagnosing sickle cell anemia in the newborn period. If one parent screens positive and the other negative, the parent's blood smears should be examined, and electrophoretic studies should be done to rule out other interacting abnormal genes, e.g., Hb C, thalassemia.

Several research centers have been able to diagnose sickle cell anemia prenatally. Fetal erythrocytes synthesize alpha, beta, and gamma chains. The chains can be quantitated by using a radioactive ^{3}H-leucine (tritiated leucine) label of the chains and separation by column chromatography. With this technique, sickle cell trait can be differentiated from both sickle cell anemia and normal hemoglobin in a 16-week fetus; the method has been used successfully in a 19-week fetus. The application of this technique is dependent on the development of safe obstetrical techniques. Satisfactory samples have been obtained by using ultrasound to localize the placenta. Anterior placentas have been aspirated directly for fetal blood in utero. Posterior placental aspiration has been obtained from chorionic vessels after visualization using a Dyonics needlescope. At present, these are research techniques.

TREATMENT

Since the hemolytic anemia is compensated, an equilibrium having been established between the production and destruction of red blood cells, transfusion therapy is rarely of benefit. Transfusions are indicated when signs of anemia develop, especially during an aregenerative crisis. There are several clinical circumstances where transfusions are indicated in order to raise the amount of circulating hemoglobin A to a level where gelling and hyperviscosity are prevented. This is accomplished when the hemoglobin A is 30 to 50% of the total hemoglobin. It is recommended in the third trimester of pregnancy in order to minimize the risk of placental infarctions as well as the complications of anesthesia. This may require a partial exchange transfusion. Transfusion is also the treatment of choice for priapism and a variety of acute neurological episodes that may be associated with reversible abnormalities of the large cerebral arteries.

The treatment of thrombotic crises is supportive. It is important to be constantly aware that a crisis may mimic an acute abdominal condition. However, unnecessary surgical intervention is to be avoided. Occasionally in the first few years of life, children who require frequent transfusions and who have markedly enlarged spleens benefit from splenectomy. However, in most patients, by the age of 10 years there have been recurrent splenic infarcts and autosplenectomy. The use of antisickling agents, e.g., cyanate, is promising but highly experimental. As with all severe hereditary hemolytic anemias, children with sickle cell anemia should receive folic acid.

HEMOGLOBIN C

After the electrophoretic differences between hemoglobins A and S had been demonstrated, similar studies were performed in patients whose manifestations of the sickle cell syndromes were atypical. Many were found to have hemoglobin C. This hemoglobin, on electrophoresis, has a net positive charge that is four units more than hemoglobin A and two units more than hemoglobin S. The same glutamyl residue in hemoglobin A, which is replaced by valine in hemoglobin S, is replaced by the basic amino acid, lysine, in hemoglobin C.

This hemoglobin is present in 2 to 3% of American blacks. In hemoglobin C trait, the heterozygous state, there are an increased number of target cells; however, there is no anemia or splenomegaly, and such patients are asymptomatic. They have from 28 to 44% hemoglobin C, and the remainder hemoglobin A.

Hemoglobin C disease, the homozygous state, is quite rare. There is a moderate, compensated hemolytic anemia, characterized by almost 100% target cells, splenomegaly, and only hemoglobin C on electrophoresis. The prognosis is good.

A more common and disabling syndrome is that associated with double heterozygosity for the hemoglobin S and C genes, sickle cell–hemoglobin C disease. The clinical manifestations vary from a mild, compensated hemolytic anemia in some children to a severe anemia with crises and all the complications of sickle cell disease in others. There are usually splenomegaly and an increased number of target cells. The sickle cell preparation is positive, and the hemoglobin on electrophoresis is 50 to 60% C and the remainder S. Family studies generally reveal that one parent is heterozygous for the hemoglobin C gene, the other for the hemoglobin S gene. The woman with hemoglobin SC disease who is in the third trimester of pregnancy is at a greater risk for the vasoocculsive pulmonary, placental, and anesthetic complications than women with the more severe anemia of hemoglobin S disease. This is probably related to the increased viscosity associated with a higher volume of packed red cells, even though the increased tendency to molecular aggregation and gelling is less than in hemoglobin S disease. Such women should be on folate therapy and in the third trimester may require a partial exchange transfusion. The latter procedure may decrease the high incidence of stillbirths, prematurity, and intrauterine growth retardation that are associated with hemoglobin SS and SC disease.

OTHER ABNORMAL HEMOGLOBINS

More than 200 different abnormal hemoglobins have been described. Many have alpha chain abnormalities; these include the rare hemoglobins G$_{Philadelphia}$, G$_{Bristol}$,

$G_{Honolulu}$, and G_{Ibadan}. Others, like hemoglobins $G_{San Jose}$ and G_{Accra}, have beta chain abnormalities. The G hemoglobins are not associated with any clinical or hematologic manifestations.

Hemoglobin D, which occurs in 0.4% of some black populations in the United States, is also not associated with any clinical abnormalities. It has an electrophoretic mobility like hemoglobin S, but neither tactoid formation nor sickling can be induced. In contrast to hemoglobin S, it has normal solubility in the reduced state. The more common form of this hemoglobin (D_{Punjab}) has a glutaminyl residue substituted for a glutamyl residue in the beta chain.

Although rare in the United States, hemoglobin E is common among certain groups in Southeast Asia. In hemoglobin E trait, 35 to 50% of the hemoglobin is type E; however, there are no other abnormalities. Hemoglobin E disease, the homozygous state, is a mild, compensated hemolytic anemia. The spleen may be slightly enlarged. The erythrocytes are microcytic and normochromic; 10 to 50% are target cells. There is increased resistance to osmotic lysis. More than 90% of the hemoglobin is type E. The structural abnormality is in the alpha chain, where a glutamyl residue is replaced by a lysyl residue.

In contrast to the increased levels of hemoglobin F that occur with abnormalities involving the rate of globin synthesis, i.e., the thalassemias, or with increased production of F cells, i.e., pregnancy and the leukemias, more than 15 structural variants of the gamma chain have been described. When hemolytic anemia occurs in the neonatal period because of a gamma chain mutation, the subsequent developmental switch to beta chain synthesis results in decrease in the hemolytic process. A similar resolution of a marked hemolytic anemia in a premature infant with hemoglobin Hasharon, an alpha chain mutant, has been observed. The Hasharon alpha chain was probably more stable when combined with beta than with gamma chains.

Hemoglobin H disease occurs when there is double heterozygosity for the alpha$_1$ and alpha$_2$ thalassemia genes. Hemoglobin H is unique in that it does not have any alpha chains but is composed of four normal beta chains (β_4). This hemoglobin has a hyperbolic oxygen-dissociation curve, an increased affinity for oxygen, and a tendency to rapid denaturation, which is demonstrable by the formation of intraerythrocytic inclusions after in vitro incubation with cresyl blue. This abnormal hemoglobin results from a decreased synthesis of normal alpha chains and is associated with a moderate hemolytic anemia. The newborn with this disease synthesizes hemoglobin Bart's (γ_4).

Hemoglobin M is clinically mainfest by cyanosis and methemoglobinemia. In the heterozygous state 20 to 30% of the hemoglobin is M, the remainder A. In this syndrome, as distinguished from the methemoglobinemias associated with deficiencies of glutathione or diaphorese I (NADH-dependent methemoglobin reductase), various structural abnormalities of the globin moiety may exist.

For example, hemoglobins $M_{Saskatoon}$ ($\alpha_2\beta_2^{63\ His\rightarrow Tyr}$) and $M_{Milwaukee}$ ($\alpha_2\beta_2^{67\ Glu\rightarrow Val}$) have β chain defects, whereas hemoglobins M_{Boston} ($\alpha_2^{58\ His\rightarrow Tyr}\beta_2$) and M_{Iwate} ($\alpha_2^{87\ His\rightarrow Tyr}\beta_2$) have α chain defects. These defects are so located in contiguity with the heme groups as to affect their reactivity. In each of these hemoglobin M's, tyrosine is substituted for either the proximal or distal histidine. The tyrosine phenolic group probably forms an internal complex that stabilizes the heme iron in the ferric form. The resulting methemoglobin leads to cyanosis.

More than 25 mutants with an increased affinity for oxygen or instability have been described. These are particularly interesting in perinatology, since a pregnant mother with a high-affinity mutant might be expected to have altered transport of oxygen to the fetus. This apparently does not occur, for the secondary polycythemia in the mother compensates sufficiently to deliver a normal oxygen supply to the fetus. However, it is noteworthy that in certain high-risk pregnancies in which the infant suffers from hypoxia, an increase in the oxygen affinity of maternal hemoglobin may put the fetus in jeopardy. Such may be the case in infants of diabetic mothers who have elevated levels of hemoglobin A_{Ic}. This glycosylated hemoglobin, which has an increased affinity for oxygen, may in addition to vascular placental changes contribute to the hypoxia of the infant by decreasing the maternal-fetal gradient for oxygen. This would have special significance in ketoacidosis, where the hypophosphatemia, decrease in 2,3-DPG, and shift of the oxygen-dissociation curve to the left probably cause intrauterine hypoxia.

WORLD DISTRIBUTION

These hereditary abnormalities have been of broad genetic and anthropologic interest. Although many of the rare abnormal hemoglobins represent isolated occurrences, the genes for hemoglobins S, C, D, and E exist in high frequency in circumscribed population groups.

The hemoglobin S gene occurs in 8% of blacks in North America, but its incidence varies widely in different areas. In these areas the gene is probably of West African origin. A frequency of 20% for the gene is present in a broad belt extending across central Africa. The gene frequency varies among different tribes, being as high as 40% in some areas of East Africa. Although there appears to have been a spread westward from the original mutation in East Africa, the presence of the hemoglobin S gene in certain primitive tribes of India has suggested a common Middle East origin of the S mutation.

Despite the high incidence of the sickling trait in Africa, the incidence of sickle cell anemia in older children and young adults is very low. There must be, therefore, a continuous loss of the hemoglobin S gene through the high infant mortality of the homozygote. Since the mutation rate appears to be inadequate for the maintenance of so high a gene frequency, attention has focused on certain factors that might selectively favor the heterozygote and lead to a balanced polymorphism. Such a factor is the increased resistance of individuals with hemoglobin S trait to falciparum malaria. The more favorable conditions for the anopheles mosquito, which have resulted in Africa from the gradual destruction of forests and creation of agricultural lands, may well have influenced the spread of the selectively advantageous hemoglobin S gene. It is not known why erythrocytes with hemoglobin S are less effectively parasitized or why falciparum malaria is less severe and causes fewer fatalities, especially deaths from cerebral involvement, in individuals with hemoglobin S trait.

Similar advantages for the other abnormal hemoglobins have not been recognized. In contrast to hemoglobin S, hemoglobin C occurs in 10% of West African blacks but is not seen in East Africa or Zaire. Hemoglobin D is present in 2% of the Sikhs in north-central India. Hemoglobin E exists commonly in Southeast Asia, where frequencies as high as 35% are encountered.

THE THALASSEMIAS

In contrast to the abnormal hemoglobins, where a mutation in a DNA base results in a single amino acid substitution and the consequent clinical manifestations, the thalassemia syndromes are a heterogeneous group of genetically determined disorders in which there is an unbalanced synthesis of globin chains. In the α-thalassemias, which occur in highest incidence among Southeast Asians, there is a decreased synthesis of α chains; β chains are produced in excess. In the β-thalassemias, which occur predominantly in Italians and Greeks, there is a decreased synthesis of β chains; α chains are produced in excess. The clinical manifestations extend from "silent" mutations to severe hemolytic anemias. This group of disorders is particularly important to perinatal medicine because of the high frequency and worldwide distribution of the thalassemia genes.

MOLECULAR PATHOLOGY

The anemia results from both ineffective erythropoiesis and hemolysis. The unbalanced chain synthesis leads to precipitation of excess chains. These form inclusion bodies that prevent the normal maturation and release of erythrocyte precursors from the bone marrow with resulting ineffective erythropoiesis. Those red cells with inclusion bodies that do enter the circulation are sequestered in the spleen or other parts of the reticuloendothelial system, resulting in a shortened red cell survival and hemolytic anemia.

Virtually every possible defect in the molecular control of protein synthesis has been observed in some variant of thalassemia.

α^0-Thalassemia: Deletion of the α-Globin Gene

Homozygotes with α^0-thalassemia have a syndrome known as hydrops fetalis, make no α-globin chains, and usually die before birth or soon thereafter. All α globin genes are deleted, and no α-globin mRNA is detectable in the RNA extracted from the hepatic or splenic erythroblasts of these babies.

The heterozygote with 1 of 4 α globin genes deleted (α-thal$_2$) appears normal but is a "silent" carrier. When 2 of 4 α globin genes are deleted (α-thal$_1$), microcytic, hypochromic erythrocytes result. When 3 of 4 α globin genes are deleted, a moderate hemolytic anemia with hemoglobin H occurs:

Genetic Condition			*Result*
Normal	α	α	Normal hemoglobin synthesis
Normal	α	α	
α-thal$_1$	–	–	α-thal$_1$ trait
Normal	α	α	
α-thal$_2$	–	α	α-thal$_2$ trait
Normal	α	α	
α-thal$_2$	–	α	Hemoglobin H disease, variable
α-thal$_1$	–	–	anemia, 5 to 30% Hbβ_4, remainder Hb A
α-thal$_1$	–	–	Hydrops fetalis, lethal,
α-thal$_1$	–	–	no α-globin

β^0-Thalassemia: A Defect in Messenger Synthesis or Function

In homozygotes for β^0-thalassemia, there is no β globin. However, in contrast to α-thalassemia, the β gene is present. In the form of thalassemia that is seen most commonly in Greeks and Italians, no mRNA is made. However in two variant forms of thalassemia major reported in certain Italians (Ferrara) and Chinese populations, there is 15 to 20% of normal mRNA present. The heterozygotes may be normal or have mild hemolytic anemia; however, the red cells are microcytic and hypochromic with prominent basophilic stippling and target cells. The hemoglobin A_2 ($\alpha_2\delta_2$) is increased to 5% of the total hemoglobin in contrast to normal values of 2.5%.

Elongated Hemoglobins and Chain Termination

Thalassemia variants that contain α or β subunits elongated at their C-terminal ends result from a failure of polypeptide chain termination. Hemoglobin Constant Spring, which occurs with a high frequency in Thailand, has 31 residues beyond the C-terminal arginine of the normal α chain. A number of other abnormal hemoglobins—Icaria, Koya Dora, and Wayne—have elongated β chains. Two elongated β-chain variants, hemoglobins Cranston and Tak, have 10 additional residues at the C-terminal end of the β chain, which is normally 146 residues long. These inherited C-terminal elongations of α and β globins result from a failure of normal chain termination due to either a base substitution in the normal UAA termination codon or deletions or insertions before the termination codon that shift the reading frame. Translation continues until the next termination codon is reached.

Fusion Hemoglobins

The chains β, δ, and γ have closely related amino acid sequences. Of their 146 amino acids, δ chains differ from β at 10 positions and γ chains differ from β at 37 positions. Thus the nucleotide sequences in the three corresponding genes are likely to be similar over most of their lengths. Family pedigrees show that the β, γ, and δ genes are closely linked to one another. No definite example of a crossing over between the γ and δ genes has been observed. However, unequal crossing over between the δ and β genes gives rise to a fusion of these genes, which, in turn, codes for a "fusion protein." Hemoglobins Lepore, Hollandia, Baltimore, Washington, Nilotic, and Miyada are the products of δ-β gene fusions.

Hemoglobin Kenya, which arose by unequal crossing over between the γ and β genes, has an N-terminal sequence like the first part of a normal γ chain and a C-terminal sequence like a normal β chain.

Hereditary Persistence of Fetal Hemoglobin (HPFH)

A person who inherits the HPFH mutation continues to produce hemoglobin F into adult life. Since Hb F can transport oxygen, such individuals are normal. The hemoglobin F is distributed homogeneously in the red blood cells. This disorder results from a β globin gene deletion.

SIGNS AND SYMPTOMS

The clinical aspects of the α- and β-thalassemias are summarized in Tables I and II. The manifestation of the homozygous state, thalassemia major, were described in 1925 by Thomas Cooley, a pediatrician in Detroit. The disorder is also known as Cooley or Mediterranean anemia.

The diagnosis is usually made during infancy when pallor, poor feeding, and splenomegaly become evident. Older children have symptoms of anemia, marked pallor and a yellowish tinge to the skin, short stature, and a characteristic "mongoloid facies" with slight slanting of the eyes, epicanthal folds, and prominent malar eminences. The head is enlarged with frontal and parietal bossing. The heart is enlarged, and hemic murmurs are present. Hepatomegaly and splenomegaly are prominent features, with the spleen sometimes enlarging to a disabling proportion. The severe anemia is characterized by microcytic, hypochromic erythrocytes with marked anisocytosis, poikilocytosis, and the presence of target cells. There is increased resistance to osmotic lysis with hypotonic saline. All the signs of active regeneration that are associated with a severe hemolytic process are evident; these include basophilic stippling, polychromatophilia, normoblastosis, reticulocytosis, leukocytosis, and erythroid hyperplasia of the bone marrow. Red blood cell survival time is shortened, and accelerated breakdown of hemoglobin is evident in the increased unconjugated bilirubin and in fecal and urinary urobilinogen. Roentgenographic examinations of the skull reveal thickened diploë with a "hair on end" appearance. The long bones have a widened medullary cavity due to overgrowth of the hyperactive marrow. X-Ray examination reveals marked rarefaction and thinning of the cortex.

TREATMENT

The clinical course varies from children with a compensated hemolytic process who have a fairly good prognosis to those who require transfusion support regularly and whose life expectancy rarely exceeds the third decade. In such patients, maintaining the hemoglobin between 9 and 13 g % minimizes the growth problems during the first decade. If the size of the spleen causes pressure symptoms or if transfusion requirements become increased because of an extra corpuscular defect, splenectomy is indicated. Such children should be maintained on penicillin prophylaxis.

In the second decade, the complications of transfusion hemosiderosis develop. Recent studies on the efficacy of desferrioxamine in chelating iron when infused continuously with a portable pumping system and the development of new chelating agents are promising approaches. Certain research centers have been able to diagnose homozygous α- and β-thalassemia prenatally in fetuses of less than 20 weeks' gestation. This technique is highly experimental.

As with sickle cell anemia, detection of the heterozygote, an intensive program of education, and genetic counseling are important to the prevention of the disease.

MIXED THALASSEMIA SYNDROMES

Various double heterozygous conditions exist in which the affected child inherits the thalassemia gene from one parent and an abnormal hemoglobin gene from the other.

Table I. Clinical Aspects of α-Thalassemias

Condition	Parental Genotype	Risk	Hemoglobin Pattern	Severity	α mRNA	Genes
Homozygous: α-Thalassemia (hydrops fetalis with Hb Bart's)	Both α-thalassemia trait	1/4	80% Hb Bart's; remainder, Hb H and Portland	Lethal	Absent	All α genes deleted
Hb H disease	(i) α-Thalassemia trait, silent carrier	1/4	4–30% Hb H in adults: approximately 25% Hb Bart's in cord blood; when Hb CS gene present, 2–3% Hb CS	Variable, usually thalassemia intermedia	Marked deficiency	(i) 3 of 4 α genes deleted
	(ii) α-Thalassemia trait, Hb CS heterozygote	1/4				(ii) 2 of 4 deleted; 1 normal; 1 Hb CS gene
Heterozygous: α-Thalassemia (α-thal trait)	α-thalassemia trait, normal	1/2	Approximately 5% Hb Bart's in cord blood	Mild; very mild in blacks	Presumed deficiency	2 of 4 α genes deleted; (?) 1 of 3 deleted in blacks
Silent carrier	Silent carrier, normal	1/2	Approximately 1–2% Hb Bart's in cord blood	0	Presumed slight deficiency	1 of 4 α genes deleted
Heterozygous: Hb Constant Spring (CS)	Hb CS heterozygote, normal	1/2	Approximately 1% Hb CS	0	Presumed deficiency	3 of 4 α genes present; 1 Hb CS gene

SOURCE: With permission from Orkin, S. H., and Nathan, D. G. *N. Eng. J. Med.* 295:710, 1976.

Table II. Clinical Aspects of β-Thalassemias

Condition	Parental Genotypes	Risk	Hemoglobin Pattern	Severity	β mRNA	Genes
Homozygous:						
β⁺-Thalassemia	Both β^+/β	1/4	↓Hb A, ↑Hb F, variable Hb A₂	Variable, usually Cooley anemia	Marked deficiency of β mRNA	β genes present
β⁰-Thalassemia	both β^0/β	1/4	0 Hb A, variable; Hb A₂, residual; Hb F	Cooley anemia	(i) Absent β mRNA (ii) Mutant, nonfunctional β mRNA present in rare Oriental cases	β genes present
δβ⁰-Thalassemia	Both $\delta\beta^0/\delta\beta$	1/4	0 Hb A, Hb A₂; 100% Hb F	Thalassemia intermedia	δ and β mRNA's absent	β genes deleted; probable δ-gene deletion
Hb Lepore	Both Hb Lepore/β	1/4	0 Hb A, Hb A₂; 75% Hb F, 25% Hb Lepore	Cooley anemia	β-like mRNA present in reduced amount	β-δ fusion genes present; no normal β or δ genes

Heterozygous:

β^+-Thalassemia	β^+/β, normal	1/2	↑Hb A_2, slight ↑Hb F	Thalassemia minor	Deficient β mRNA	β genes present
β^0-Thalassemia	β^0/β, normal	1/2	↑Hb A_2, slight ↑Hb F	Thalassemia minor	Deficient β mRNA or rarely non-functional β mRNA present	β genes present
$\delta\beta^0$-Thalassemia	$\delta\beta^0/\delta\beta$, normal	1/2	5–20% Hb F	Thalassemia minor	Presumed deficiency of β and δ mRNA's	β and probable δ gene deletion on 1 homologous chromosome
Hb Lepore	Hb Lepore/β, normal	1/2	↑Hb F, Hb A_2, 5–15% Hb Lepore	Thalassemia minor	β-like mRNA present	Hb Leopre gene replaces normal β and δ genes on 1 chromosome

SOURCE: With permission from Orkin, S. H., and Nathan, D. G. *N. Eng. J. Med.* 295:710, 1976.

The most common and most severe of these is hemoglobin S–β-thalassemia disease. This condition is characterized by a moderate hemolytic anemia, splenomegaly, and crises similar to those seen in sickle cell anemia. The erythrocyte morphology is that associated with thalassemia; however, the sickling preparation is positive. On electrophoresis, hemoglobin S predominates, hemoglobin F is increased, and small amounts of hemoglobin A are present. The manifestations of the disease are usually less severe than either sickle cell anemia or thalassemia major. Hemoglobin C–β-thalassemia disease is a mild, hemolytic anemia with splenomegaly. The erythrocytes are microcytic and hypochromic, and an increased number of target cells are present. Most of the hemoglobin is C, with increased amounts of F. Hemoglobin E–β-thalassemia disease is common in Thailand. The clinical and hematologic manifestations may be indistinguishable from thalassemia major.

REFERENCES

1. Alperin, J. B.: Folic acid deficiency complicating sickle cell anemia. *Arch. Intern. Med.* 120:298, 1967.
2. Alter, B. P., Rappeport, J. M., Huisman, T. H. J., Schroeder, W. A., and Nathan, D. G.: Fetal erythropoiesis following bone marrow transplantation. *Blood* 48:843, 1976.
3. Bellingham, A. J.: Hemoglobins with altered oxygen affinity. *Brit. Med. Bulletin* 32:193, 1976.
4. Benz, E. J., and Forget, B. G.: The biosynthesis of hemoglobin. *Seminars Hematology* 11:463, 1974.
5. Boyer, S. H., Belding, T. K., Margolet, L., Noyes, A. N., Burke, P. J., and Bell, W. R.: Variations in the frequency of fetal hemoglobin-bearing erythrocytes (F-cells) in well adults, pregnant women, and adult leukemics. *The Johns Hopkins Medical Journal* 137:105, 1975.
6. Castle, W. B.: From man to molecule and back to mankind. *Seminars Hematology* 13:159, 1976.
7. Clark, M. R., Greenquist, A. C., and Shohet, S. B.: Stabilization of the shape of sickled cells by calcium and A23187. *Blood* 48:899, 1976.
8. Conley, C. L., Weatherall, D. J., Richardson, S. N., Shepard, M. K., and Charache, S.: Hereditary persistence of fetal hemoglobin: A study of 79 affected persons in 15 Negro families in Baltimore. *Blood* 21:261, 1963.
9. Defuria, F. G., Miller, D. R., Cerami, A., and Manning, J. M.: The effects of cyanate *in vitro* on red blood cell metabolism and function in sickle cell anemia. *J. Clin. Invest.* 51:566, 1972.
10. Forget, B. G.: The molecular basis of thalassemia. *CRC Crit. Rev. Biochem.* 2:311, 1974.
11. Forget, B. G., Hillman, D. G., Lazarus, H., et al.: Absence of messenger RNA and gene DNA for beta globin chains in hereditary persistence of fetal hemoglobin. *Cell* 7:323, 1976.
12. Frick, P. G., Hitzig, W. H., and Betke, K.: Hemoglobin Zürich: I. A new hemoglobin anomaly associated with acute hemolytic episodes with inclusion bodies after sulfonamide therapy. *Blood* 20:261, 1962.
13. Gerald, P. S., and Diamond, L. K.: A new hereditary hemoglobinopathy (the Lepore trait) and its interaction with thalassemia trait. *Blood* 13:835, 1958.
14. Gerald, P. S., and Diamond, L. K.: The diagnosis of thalassemia trait by starch block electrophoresis of hemoglobin. *Blood* 13:61, 1958.
15. Gerald, P. S., and Efron, M. L.: Chemical studies of several varieties of Hb M. *Proc. Natl. Acad. Sci. U.S.* 47:1758, 1961.
16. Graziano, J. H., and Cerami, A.: Chelation therapy for the treatment of thalassemia. *Seminars Hematology* 14:127, 1977.
17. Hahn, E. V., and Gillespie, E. B.: Sickle cell anemia: Experimental study of sickle cell formation. *Arch, Sub. Med.* 39:233, 1927.
18. Ham, T. H., and Castle, W. B.: Relation of increased hypotonic fragility and of erythrostasis to mechanism of hemolysis in certain anemias. *Trans. Assoc. Am. Physicians* 55:127, 1940.

19. Harris, J. W.: Studies on the destruction of red blood cells: VIII. Molecular orientation in sickle cell hemoglobin solutions. *Proc. Soc. Exp. Biol. Med.* 75:197, 1950.

20. Hercules, J. I., et al. (eds.): *Proceedings of the First National Symposium on Sickle Cell Disease.* DHEW Publication No. (NIH) 75-723.

21. Herrick, J. B.: Peculiar elongated and sickle-shaped red blood corpuscles in a case of severe anemia. *Arch. Sub. Med.* 6:517, 1910.

22. Hill, R. L., Swenson, R. T., and Schwartz, H. C.: The chemical and genetic relationships between hemoglobins S and G$_{San Jose}$. *Blood* 19:573, 1962.

23. Hollenberg, M. D., Kaback, M. M., and Kazazian, H. H.: Adult hemoglobin synthesis by reticulocytes from the human fetus at midtrimester. *Science* 174:698, 1971.

24. Huehns, E. R., Flynn, F. V., Butler, E. A., and Shooter, E. M.: The occurence of haemoglobin "Bart's" in conjunction with haemoglobin H. *Brit. J. Haematol.* 6:388, 1960.

25. Huehns, E. R., and Shooter, E. M.: Human Haemoglobins. *J. Med. Genet.* 2:48, 1965.

26. Huisman, T. H. J., and Schroeder, W. A.: New aspects of the structure, function, and synthesis of hemoglobins. *CRC Crit. Rev. Clin. Lab. Sci.,* 1971.

27. Ingram, V. M.: A specific chemical difference between the globins of normal human and sickle-cell anemia haemoglobin. *Nature* 178:792, 1956.

28. Jensen, W. N.: Fragmentation and the "freakish poikilocyte." *Am. J. Med. Sci.* 257:355, 1969.

29. Kan, Y. W., Dozy, A. M., Alter, B. P., et al.: Detection of the sickle gene in the human fetus: Potential for intrauterine diagnosis of sickle cell anemia. *N. Engl. J. Med.* 287:1, 1972.

30. Kan, Y. W., Golbus, M. S., Klein, P., et al.: Successful application of prenatal diagnosis in a pregnancy at risk for homozygous β-thalassemia. *N. Engl. J. Med.* 292:1096, 1975.

31. Kan, Y. W., Golbus, M. S., and Trecartin, R.: Prenatal diagnosis of sickle cell anemia. *N. Engl. J. Med.* 294:1039, 1976.

32. Kan, Y. W., Holland, J. P., Dozy, A. M., et al.: Deletion of the β-globin structural gene in hereditary persistence of foetal haemoglobin. *Nature* 258:162, 1975.

33. Kleihauer, E.: *The Hemoglobins in Physiology of the Perinatal Period,* edited by U. Stave. 1970, chap. 9, p. 255.

34. Kleihauer, E., Braun, H., and Betke, K.: Demonstration von fetalem hamoglobin in den erythrocyten eines blutasstrichs. *Klin. Wschr.* 35:637, 1957.

35. Konotey-Ahulu, F. I. D.: The sickle cell diseases: Clinical manifestations including the "sickle crises." *Arch. Intern. Med.* 133:611, 1974.

36. Levine, R. L., Lincoln, D. R., Buchholz, W. M., Gribble, T. J., and Schwartz, H. C.: Hemoglobin Hasharon in a premature infant with hemolytic anemia. *Ped. Res.* 9:7, 1975.

37. Morrison, J. C., and Wiser, W. L.: The effect of maternal partial exchange transfusion on the infants of patients with sickle cell anemia. *J. Pediat.* 89:286, 1976.

38. Nalbandian, R. M., Henry, R. L., Barnhart, M. I., Nichols, B. M., Carip, F. R., and Wolf, P. L.: Sickling reversed and blocked by urea in invert sugar. *Amer. J. Path.* 64:405, 1971.

39. Neel, J. V.: The inheritance of sickle cell anemia. *Science* 110:64, 1949.

40. Orkin, S. H., and Nathan, D. G.: The thalassemias. *N. Engl. J. Med.* 295:710, 1976.

41. Ottolenghi, S., Lanyon, W. G., Paul, J., et al.: The severe form of α-thalassaemia is caused by a haemoglobin gene deletion. *Nature* 251:389, 1974.

42. Pauling, L., Itano, H. A., Singer, S. J., and Wells, I. C.: Sickle-cell anemia: A molecular disease. *Science* 110:543, 1949.

43. Pearson, H. A., and O'Brien, R. T.: The management of thalassemia major. *Seminars Hematology* 12:255, 1975.

44. Perutz, M. F.: Structure and mechanism of hemoglobin. *Brit. Med. Bulletin* 32:195, 1976.

45. Propper, R. D., Shurin, S. B., and Nathan, D. G.: Reassessment of the use of desferrioxamine B in iron overload. *N. Engl. J. Med.* 294:1421, 1976.

46. Schroeder, W. A., Huisman, T. H. J., Shelton, J. R., Shelton, J. B., Kleihauer, E. F., Dozy, A. M., and Robberson, B.: Evidence for multiple structural genes for the γ chain of human fetal hemoglobin. *Proc. Natl. Acad. Sci. U.S.* 60:537, 1968.

47. Schwartz, H. C., King, K. C., Schwartz, A. L., Edmunds, D., and Schwartz, R.: Effect of pregnancy on hemoglobin A_{Ic} in normal, gestational diabetic and diabetic women. *Diabetes* 25:1118, 1976.

48. Widness, J. A., Schwartz, H. C., Thompson, D., Kahn, C. B., Oh, W., and Schwartz, R.: Haemoglobin A_{Ic} (glycohaemoglobin) in diabetic pregnancy: an indicator of glucose control and fetal size. *Brit. J. Obs. & Gyn.* 85:812, 1978.

49. Sherman, L. J.: The sickling phenomenon, with special reference to the differentiation of sickle cell anemia from the sickle cell trait. *Bull. J. Hopkins Hosp.* 67:309, 1940.

50. Sydenstricker, V. P.: Further observations on sickle cell anemia. *J.A.M.A.* 83:12, 1924.

51. Taylor, J. M., Dozy, A., Kan, Y. W., et al.: Genetic lesion in homozygous α-thalassaemia (hydrops fetalis). *Nature* 251:392, 1974.

52. Tolstoshev, P., Mitchell, J., Lanyon, G., et al.: Presence of gene for β globin in homozygous β^0-thalassaemia. *Nature* 259:95, 1976.

53. Trivelli, L. A., Ranney, H. M., and Lai, H.: Hemoglobin components in patients with diabetes mellitus. *N. Engl. J. Med.* 284:353, 1971.

54. Watson, J.: The significance of the paucity of sickle cells in newborn Negro infants. *Am. J. Med. Sci.* 215:419, 1948.

55. Watson, R. T., Burko, H., Hercules, M., and Robinson, M.: The hand-foot syndrome in sickle-cell disease in young children. *Pediatrics* 31:975, 1963.

56. Weatherall, D. J. (ed.): Hemoglobin: Structure, function and synthesis. *Brit. Med. Bulletin,* vol. 32, 1976.

57. Weatherall, D. J., and Clegg, J. B.: *The Thalassaemia Syndromes,* 2nd ed. Oxford, Blackwell Scientific Publications, 1972.

58. White, J. M.: The unstable hemoglobins. *Brit. Med. Bulletin* 32:219, 1976.

59. Wood, W. G.: Hemoglobin synthesis during human fetal development. *Brit. Med. Bulletin* 32:282, 1976.

24
Diabetes Mellitus in Pregnancy

Steven G. Gabbe, M.D.

In 1949, Dr. Priscilla White commented: "Much that is controversial still exists in this problem of pregnancy complicating diabetes" (1).

Many unanswered questions remain with us today. What factors contribute to the intrauterine deaths and congenital malformations responsible for much of the perinatal mortality? Which methods most accurately assess fetal well-being in the antepartum period? How should one treat the pregnant patient with gestational diabetes?

Despite these uncertainties, remarkable improvement has been made in reducing morbidity and mortality for the pregnant diabetic woman and her infant. Prior to the discovery of insulin in 1921, few diabetic women survived long enough to become pregnant. Maternal mortality due to ketoacidosis or the delivery of a macrosomic still-born was common in those who did conceive. Careful control of the diabetic state, thereby safeguarding the life of the pregnant patient, was an important achievement. Thereafter, a reduction in perinatal deaths became the foremost concern.

Dr. Priscilla White and her mentor, Dr. Elliott Joslin, pioneered the development of successful treatment programs for the pregnant diabetic woman in the United States. Throughout this chapter, many of their early observations are cited. It is hoped that these quotations will illustrate important principles established in the past as well as indicate areas to be explored in the future.

CARBOHYDRATE METABOLISM IN PREGNANCY

[O]ne must never forget the lesson of Carlson's pregnant dog, who survived complete pancreatectomy until the protecting pancreases of her fetuses were lost to her at their birth (2).

Dr. Elliott Joslin, 1923

The fetal pancreas does not ameliorate maternal diabetes. Exogenous insulin therapy must be carefully combined with dietary supervision to manage the mother's insulin-deficient state. An understanding of carbohydrate metabolism is essential in developing such a plan.

During pregnancy, maternal metabolism is restructured to provide adequate nutrition for the mother and the growing fetoplacental unit. At term, the human fetus requires approximately 30 g of glucose daily (3). It not only depletes the maternal compartment of this nutrient but also removes alanine, the key precursor in gluconeogenesis. When fasted, the pregnant woman rapidly develops hypoglycemia, hypoinsulinemia, and ketosis (4). Maternal mechanisms to offset this state of "accelerated starvation" include increased protein catabolism and accelerated renal gluconeogenesis (5).

Fats become an important maternal fuel (6). Human placental lactogen (HPL), a polypeptide hormone produced by the syncytiotrophoblast, stimulates lipolysis in adipose tissue (7,8). The subsequent release of glycerol and fatty acids leads to a reduction in glucose utilization by maternal tissues and spares glucose for the fetus. HPL levels change with alterations in maternal food intake, rising when the mother is fasted but falling when she is fed and adequate glucose is available (9).

The actions of HPL are responsible, in part, for the "diabetogenic state" of pregnancy (10–12). The latter is characterized by an exaggerated rate and amount of insulin release associated with an apparent decrease in sensitivity to insulin at the cellular level. Other hormones that modify maternal pancreatic function include elevated levels of free cortisol, estrogen, and progesterone (13–15). In addition, the placenta produces enzymes capable of destroying insulin (16,17). As placental size increases, larger amounts of these contrainsulin factors are synthesized. In most pregnancies, the maternal β-cell hyperplasia is induced, insulin production increases, and normal insulin-glucose homeostasis is maintained (18). A woman with overt diabetes cannot respond to the stress and needs additional insulin replacement as pregnancy progresses. If a pregnant patient has a borderline pancreatic reserve, it is possible that her endogenous insulin production will fail to meet this diabetogenic challenge. Diabetes mellitus may be revealed for the first time.

Despite its glycogenolytic and gluconeogenic actions, glucagon does not contribute to the diabetogenic stress of pregnancy. Glucagon levels change little throughout gestation (11). Daniel and his coworkers have demonstrated heightened suppressibility of circulating glucagon following glucose administration to normal pregnant women (19). This phenomenon would result in more prolonged hyperglycemia and hyperinsulinemia after feeding and would permit periods of "facilitated anabolism" to counterbalance the "accelerated starvation" observed during fasting (20).

The placenta not only produces hormones that markedly alter maternal metabolism but also controls the transport of nutrients and protein hormones to the fetal compartment. The placenta is essentially impermeable to protein hormones such as insulin, glucagon, growth hormone, and HPL (21,22). Maternal glucose probably reaches the fetus by the process of facilitated diffusion, crossing the placenta at a faster rate than would be expected on physicochemical grounds alone (23). Fetal blood glucose levels usually remain 20 to 30 mg% lower than those in the maternal compartment (24). A close correlation has been documented among fetal glucose uptake, maternal blood glucose concentration, and the maternal-fetal concentration gradient (25–27). Ketone bodies diffuse freely across the placenta and may be an important fetal fuel during maternal fasting (4).

The fetus is a passive recipient of maternal glucose but not maternal insulin. Fetal glucose levels are normally maintained within narrow limits because the maternal pancreas so meticulously regulates maternal glucose levels. The fetal pancreas itself plays a limited role in controlling fetal glucose concentrations (18,28). Although insulin is present in the fetal pancreas by 8 to 9 weeks' gestation, its release is not triggered by changing glucose levels until late in pregnancy (29,30). The fetal pancreas does respond to the amino acids leucine and arginine, stimuli that activate the formation of cyclic AMP (31,32).

Fetal anabolism is regulated by insulin. Insulin can increase fetal glycogen and protein synthesis and stimulate glucose uptake (33–35). Insulin receptors have also been found in the human placenta (36). In vitro experiments have revealed stimulation of placental glycogen and protein synthesis in response to insulin administration (37,38).

PATHOPHYSIOLOGY OF DIABETES MELLITUS IN PREGNANCY

The size of the baby is one of the greatest dangers. The high glucose content of placental blood in diabetes . . . is probably an etiological factor (39).

Dr. Priscilla White, 1928

Maternal hypoinsulinemia initiates a series of events that lead to marked derangements in fetal homeostasis. Sustained maternal hyperglycemia and rapid fluctuations in maternal glucose levels are accompanied by similar changes in the fetal compartment. Even with optimal therapy, the diurnal glucose variation in insulin-dependent pregnant diabetics is much greater than that seen in normal woman (40). Over 20 years ago, Pedersen proposed that maternal hyperglycemia led to fetal hyperglycemia and finally to fetal hyperinsulinemia (41). The fetal pancreas usually demonstrates the consequences of this excessive stimulation. Hyperplasia of fetal islets with increased numbers of β cells and elevated insulin levels have been found in 80% of infants of diabetic women (42,43). Fibrosis within the islets of Langerhans has also been reported (44).

Fetal macrosomia is a result of this hyperglycemic-hyperinsulinemic state. Increased deposition of fat, protein, and glycogen leads to birthweights over 4000 g in one-fourth of pregnancies complicated by diabetes (45). Although maternal hyperglycemia may be correlated with birthweight, other causes for this gigantism have been proposed. Szabo has demonstrated a relationship between the elevated free fatty acid levels found in diabetic women and subsequent macrosomia (46). He hypothesizes that glucose serves primarily as a precursor for the α-glycerophosphate used in triglyceride synthesis. Persson has also questioned the correlation between control of maternal glycemia and macrosomia, proposing that increased amino acid utilization may be important (47).

The placenta and umbilical cord share in the gigantism characteristic of the infant of the diabetic (48). The increase in placental size is due to cellular hyperplasia (49). Glycogen concentrations are significantly elevated in placentas of diabetic women (50). Microscopic examination of the placental villi reveals they are large and edematous with a thickened basement membrane (51,52). Fetal stem arteries often demonstrate an obliterative endarteritis. In diabetic women with vascular disease, the placenta may be small and decidual vessels narrowed by hyalinization and fibrinoid necrosis (48).

Macrosomia is only one of many manifestations of fetal hyperglycemia and hyperinsulinemia. The perinatal mortality arising from intrauterine deaths, congenital malformations, and functional immaturity may be directly or indirectly related to derangements in fetal carbohydrate metabolism.

MATERNAL MORBIDITY AND MORTALITY

Before insulin, coma was the end result of the pregnant diabetic (39).

Dr. Priscilla White, 1928

Insulin is your life insurance policy (53).

Dr. Elliott Joslin, 1929

The changing metabolic demands of pregnancy remain the greatest threat for the pregnant woman with diabetes. Before the availability of insulin, maternal mortality ranged from 6 to 45% (54,55). During the past 50 years, this figure has been reduced to approximately 0.5%, a rate which is still 20 times higher than that of the general obstetrical population.

Ketoacidosis and hypoglycemia are important and often avoidable causes of maternal death in diabetes mellitus. During the period 1957–1974, 24 pregnant diabetic women died in Los Angeles County (56). Fatal ketoacidosis occurred in four women, and hypoglycemia was responsible for three mortalities. The pregnant woman with diabetes mellitus is at greatest risk for developing ketoacidosis in the second and third trimesters. Insulin requirements may rise 60 to 70% at this time in response to increased placental production of HPL, progesterone, estrogen, and insulinase. White observed that ketoacidosis in pregnancy has a rapid onset, occurs at a relatively low blood sugar, and may be refractory to insulin treatment (57). A perinatal mortality rate of 30 to 70% has been reported after ketoacidosis (13). Fetal oxygenation may be decreased during acidosis by a reduction in maternal erythrocyte 2,3-diphosphoglycerate (58).

Hypoglycemic complications occur in the first trimester or postpartum period. Nausea and vomiting early in pregnancy lead to a decrease in caloric intake and necessitate reduction of insulin doses. The diabetic woman may be unaware that glycosuria occurs commonly in pregnancy. She administers additional insulin to treat her "bad tests" and produces a hypoglycemic reaction. In the postpartum period, absence of placental hormones, changes in insulin antibody action (59), and possibly a blunted growth hormone response (60) create a relatively diabetes-free state. Thus, insulin doses must be reduced.

Deaths due to vascular disease occur more frequently in the pregnant diabetic. Fatal myocardial infarctions have been reported in patients over the age of 30 (61). The incidence of deaths attributable to preeclampsia may also be increased (13). In addition, the diabetic woman is often obese and at greater risk for a fatal pulmonary embolism (62).

Fetal macrosomia and fetal distress increase the incidence of cesarean section and traumatic vaginal delivery (56). Both procedures may lead to mortality from hemorrhage, sepsis, and complications of anesthesia.

PERINATAL MORBIDITY AND MORTALITY

It is evident that our problem must concern the investigation of the causes and the means to prevent premature delivery of the infant of the diabetic mother . . . and, secondly, the termination of the pregnancy at the point of viability and before the dreaded late intrauterine accident can occur (1).

Dr. Priscilla White, 1949

The most tragic of the harmful influences—tragic because it is unpredictable—is the occurrence of the congenital fatal defect (1).

Dr. Priscilla White, 1949

The fetus of a diabetic patient, for reasons that remain unclear, can die suddenly and unexplainedly in the final trimester of pregnancy. Stillbirths may occur 10 to 20 times more frequently than in the normal population (63). These deaths appear to be most common in the poorly controlled patient, in association with fetal macrosomia, in pregnancies complicated by preeclampsia, and in those women who have had a previous stillbirth. Autopsy data provide little help in solving this mystery. Several investigators have suggested that fetal hyperinsulinemia may produce fatal hypoglycemia (64). This theory is supported by the clinical observation that deaths often occur during the night, when both mother and fetus are apt to be hypoglycemic. Cardiac failure due to excessive glycogen deposition in the fetal myocardium (65) or cardiac arrhythmias resulting from hypokalemia have been implicated as causes of death (66). Acute villous edema might decrease the volume of the intervillous space, increase the diffusion distance for oxygen, and lead to fetal asphyxia (67).

Recent data from Shelley and her coworkers indicate that these unexplained intrauterine deaths may be caused by lactic acidosis (68). Hyperglycemia in normally oxygenated lambs produces a small increase in plasma lactate and little change in pH. Hyperglycemia in slightly hypoxic lambs, however, results in a marked rise in plasma lactate with a rapid fall in pH. The lambs fail to recover if their arterial pH drops below 7.1. Hyperglycemia certainly occurs in the fetus of the diabetic woman, and the findings of extramedullary hematopoiesis and cardiac hypertrophy suggest chronic intrauterine hypoxia (48). Could lactic acidosis account for the "dreaded late intrauterine accident"?

In an attempt to reduce the incidence of stillbirths, early delivery was usually planned for diabetic women. Fetal macrosomia, hydramnios, and maternal obesity thwarted the obstetrician's efforts to estimate fetal size and assess gestational age. Often he would deliver a large but premature infant who developed respiratory distress syndrome and died (69). Even infants thought to be near term by well-established menstrual histories and clinical milestones appeared functionally immature. Hyperinsulinemia may be responsible for this delay in cellular maturation. Smith and his coworkers have found that insulin abolishes the stimulatory effect of cortisol on lecithin synthesis in cultures of rabbit fetal lung (70). Histologic measures of lung maturation are also retarded in some infants of diabetics (71). These findings could explain the five to sixfold increase in the incidence of the respiratory distress syndrome (RDS) reported in a retrospective study of pregnancies complicated by diabetes (72).

Birth trauma has accounted for almost 10% of perinatal mortality in infants of diabetic women (73). The traumatic morbidity associated with a birthweight over 4000 g may be as high as 15% (74).

During the past 5 years, improvements in the assessment of fetal maturity and well-being, more liberal use of cesarean section, and advances in neonatal care have significantly decreased perinatal mortality due to intrauterine death, prematurity, and birth injury. In many centers, congenital malformations have emerged as the most important cause of perinatal death, accounting for 40 to 50% of all losses (75). Anomalies occur two to three times more frequently in children of overt diabetic women (76). Pedersen's group demonstrated a significant increase in the number of total, major, fatal, and multiple malformations (77). Several studies report a 2 to 3% incidence of fatal anomalies (54,78). Women whose diabetes begins early in life, who have had the disease for at least 5 years, or who have renal disease have a higher incidence of malformed offspring (76,77,79). Infants of gestational diabetics and infants of diabetic fathers do not have an increased frequency of anomalies (76). Apparently, the more severe the derangement in maternal metabolism, the greater the teratogenic effect. Malformations of the cardiovascular, skeletal, central nervous, and genitourinary systems are especially common. The syndrome of phocomelic diabetic embryopathy or caudal dysplasia may be the anomaly most specific for diabetes mellitus (80). Our ability to prevent or predict "the most tragic of the harmful influences" has improved little in the past 30 years.

The stigmata of development in an abnormal intrauterine environment characterized by hyperglycemia and hyperinsulinemia are seen during the nursery course of the infant of the diabetic woman. This morbidity includes hypoglycemia, hypocalcemia, hyperbilirubinemia, RDS, polycythemia, renal vein thrombosis, and necrotizing enterocolitis (81). Infants may be growth-retarded in pregnancies complicated by vascular disease.

CLASSIFICATION AND RISK ASSESSMENT

> If a pregnant woman acquires diabetes, my advice would be to allow the pregnancy to continue. . . . If a diabetic becomes pregnant, it is more serious (2).
>
> *Dr. Elliott Joslin, 1923*

> [I]t is evident that age at onset of diabetes, duration, severity and degree of maternal vascular disease all influence the fetal survival unfavorably (1).
>
> *Dr. Priscilla White, 1949*

Counseling a pregnant patient and formulating a plan of management require careful assessment of maternal and fetal risk. For the pregnant woman with diabetes mellitus, the factors in the quote above by Dr. White appear most important. Initially the Joslin group was most concerned with a classification based on levels of estrogen, progesterone, and human chorionic gonadotropin. Imbalance in these hormones was thought to predict a poor outcome. In 1948, a clinical grading was added to the chemical assessment, and the former has had wide application (Table I).

Class A "includes patients in whom the diagnosis of diabetes was made upon a glucose tolerance test which deviates but slightly from the normal. Such patients require no insulin and little dietary regulation" (1). White added in a subsequent paper that "fasting values are normal or near normal" (82). The use of terms such as prediabetes, potential diabetes, chemical diabetes, latent diabetes, and gestational diabetes has created considerable confusion in risk assessment and patient management. Latent diabetes describes a state in which glucose tolerance is normal except under stress, such as the stress of infection, surgery, or pregnancy (83). Gestational diabetes is a form of latent diabetes. The pregnant patient demonstrates a disorder of carbohydrate metabolism but returns to normal after delivery. The term gestational diabetes fails to specify whether the patient requires diet alone, has abnormal fasting blood sugars, or must be given insulin. This distinction is critical. Those patients who remain normoglycemic in the fasting state or who maintain a normal 2-hr postprandial glucose

Table I. White Classification of Pregnant Diabetic Women

| | Diabetes | | | | |
Class	Onset Age (Years)		Duration (Years)	Vascular Disease	Insulin Needs
A	Any		Any	0	0
B	>20		<10	0	+
C	10–19	or	10–19	0	+
D	<10	or	>20	+	+
F	Any		Any	+	+
R	Any		Any	+	+

have a low perinatal mortality rate (45,84,85). They may be safely delivered at term without an increased incidence of intrauterine deaths (86–88). Gestational diabetics with abnormal fasting glucoses or women receiving insulin are at much greater risk for a poor outcome (89,90). At Los Angeles County (LAC) Women's Hospital the term class A diabetes is used for those pregnant women who have a normal fasting serum glucose, an abnormal glucose tolerance test (GTT), and who require little dietary regulation.

Patients requiring insulin are designated by the letters B, C, D, R, and F.

Class B patients are those whose disease had its onset after age 20. They have been diabetic less than 10 years and have no vascular disease. At LAC Women's Hospital, approximately 10% of pregnant patients who develop abnormal fasting glucoses may be managed by strict dietary therapy if they remain hospitalized. The risk of intrauterine death in these women exceeds that for class A patients, and careful antepartum surveillance is, therefore, required. Although not on insulin, this small group is considered to be in class B.

Class C patients have the onset of their disease between the ages of 10 and 19 or have had diabetes for 10 to 19 years. They have no demonstrable vascular disease.

Class D includes women whose diabetes is of 20 or more years' duration, or whose onset occurred before the age of 10, or who have benign retinopathy. The last includes retinal vein dilatation, exudates, and microaneurysms.

Class F applies to those women who have developed nephropathy with proteinuria and a reduction in creatinine clearance.

Class R designates patients with proliferative retinopathy. Both nephropathy and retinopathy may intensify in pregnancy, and one must seriously consider maternal risk in these classes.

Although other classes have been suggested, the six described above have had the widest use. One may actually divide pregnant diabetics into three functional groups. As White has emphasized, the course of pregnancy for an obese, elderly, multiparous patient with diabetes of recent onset is different from that of a young primipara who has developed hypertension after 15 years of diabetes. Class A patients represent a population with a relatively low risk for poor fetal outcome. They do require dietary management. Classes B and C have diabetes of relatively recent onset and so require intensive education and supervision. If neglected, they may have an extremely high perinatal mortality. Classes D, F, and R require, and usually receive, intensive therapy for their diabetes and careful antepartum surveillance of fetal well-being. Preeclampsia may occur frequently in these patients.

One can improve risk assessment using the Prognostically Bad Signs in Pregnancy (75). Pedersen has found that perinatal mortality increases if a pregnant diabetic woman develops clinically apparent pyelonephritis, severe acidosis, or preeclampsia. Furthermore, if she does not come for regular care, a group that Pedersen has termed neglectors, the risk is also heightened. Pedersen has not observed an increase in perinatal mortality if hydramnios is present (91).

DETECTION OF DIABETES IN PREGNANCY

That the warning of glycosuria in pregnancy must not be ignored as a starting point of diabetes is evidenced by the fact that 33 of our 58 pregnant diabetic women developed diabetes during pregnancy (39).

Dr. Priscilla White, 1928

Diabetes mellitus complicates 1 to 2% of all pregnancies (64). Although those women who have a past history of diabetes or who present with symptomatic overt disease present little diagnostic difficulty, they represent only one-tenth of all cases. The recognition of patients with class A diabetes remains an important diagnostic challenge. Their detection will select a population at significant risk for developing diabetes later in life (92–94). O'Sullivan has reported that over 30% of these women will become diabetic in the 12 years following their pregnancy.

Because class A patients exhibit an abnormal insulin response to a glucose load but remain normoglycemic in the fasting state, some evaluation of glucose tolerance is required. Initially, however, the physician should seek out those patients with certain historical and clinical clues (95). These include a family history of diabetes, a history of an unexplained stillbirth, malformed infant, or neonatal death due to trauma, and the delivery of a baby weighing 4000 g or more (74). Clinical "red flags" might be obesity, hypertension, or glycosuria. The last is common in pregnancy due to an increase in the glomerular filtration rate (96). Glycosuria must not be overlooked as a sign of diabetes and is most significant when found in the second-voided morning urine of the fasting patient (97). O'Sullivan has reported that over 50% of patients who subsequently have an abnormal GTT are not detected by historical and clinical screening (98). He advocates evaluating all patients with a 1 hr blood sugar after ingestion of 50 g of glucose. Levels greater than 130 mg% for whole blood or 150 mg% for plasma or serum are abnormal. It should be noted that plasma or serum values are 15% higher than those for whole blood. Several investigators have emphasized the evaluation of women over 25 to 30 years of age (99,100). O'Sullivan believes this older age group is at greatest risk for perinatal mortality.

Women with positive historical or clinical screening criteria are best evaluated by a glucose determination performed 2 hr after ingestion of a 100-g carbohydrate load (100). If patients are not eating an adequate carbohydrate diet prior to this test, they should prepare by consuming 300 g of carbohydrate daily for 3 days. Although by no means specific for diabetes, this evaluation is very sensitive and misses few patients who subsequently have an abnormal GTT. Glucose values at 2 hr should not exceed 120 mg% for whole blood or 140 mg% for plasma. If the initial test is normal, a repeat test

Table II.   Normal Oral GTT Values

Hour	O'Sullivan (Whole Blood) (mg %)	Mestman (Plasma) (mg %)
Fasting	90	110
1	165	200
2	145	150
3	125	130

is scheduled by 34 weeks' gestation. As placental hormone production increases, the patient's pancreatic reserve is further stressed. Therefore, the closer the patient gets to term, the more easily will her abnormality be detected (65).

An abnormal glucose value on screening should be followed by a GTT (102). Some investigators favor the oral GTT (85,103). They believe it is more physiologic and assesses the gastrointestinal factors involved in insulin secretion. Furthermore, the oral GTT appears to be more sensitive, has been well standardized, and demonstrates better correlation with other parameters of carbohydrate metabolism than the intravenous technique. Critics of the oral method cite the pregnancy-related changes in gastrointestinal function that can modify the study and feel that this technique yields many false positive results. O'Sullivan and Mestman have had extensive experience evaluating the 3 hr oral GTT after a 100-g glucose load (104,105). The normal values in their clinics are listed in Table II. The patient must have a normal fasting glucose and two abnormal values to be designated a class A diabetic. Should the initial oral GTT be normal, a repeat test is scheduled by 34 weeks' gestation.

Is an abnormal oral GTT associated with significant fetal risk? Although perinatal mortality is not increased in class A pregnancies, neonatal morbidity may arise from hyperbilirubinemia, hypoglycemia, or trauma (45). Gillmer and his coworkers have shown a significant correlation between the total area under the oral GTT curve or the plasma glucose level at 2 hr and subsequent neonatal hypoglycemia (106,107). The total area also correlates well with mean diurnal plasma glucose concentrations, thus reflecting glucose levels throughout the day. Hyperglycemia during the oral GTT has been associated with increased placental growth and hypoglycemia may be related to placental and fetal growth retardation (108,109). Further correlations between glucose tolerance testing and fetal outcome must be sought.

Very often, the patient who has delivered a macrosomic infant or stillborn will have had no evaluation for diabetes during pregnancy. An oral GTT performed in the immediate postpartum period can be unreliable (87,110). The physician may rule out overt diabetes by determining a fasting glucose. An oral GTT should be performed at a later date, before allowing the diabetes suspect to begin oral contraceptives.

PRINCIPLES OF TREATMENT

In general, close and persistent supervision of the patient by both internist and obstetrician is the most important part of the treatment (39).

Dr. Priscilla White, 1928

The diabetic woman will most often have a successful pregnancy if her care is directed by an experienced team. Each member—the obstetrician, internist, pediatrician, nurse, and dietitian—must pay careful attention to detail. In several large centers throughout Europe and the United States, this approach has yielded a perinatal mortality rate of 5% or less for pregnancies complicated by overt diabetes mellitus (73,111–115). The important goals for the treatment team include control of maternal glycemia, elimination of complications due to trauma, prevention of iatrogenic prematurity, and detection of intrauterine distress before fetal damage or death occur.

CONTROL OF MATERNAL GLYCEMIA

Controlled diabetes is essential to fetal welfare (39).

Dr. Priscilla White, 1928

Normalization of the intrauterine environment may be achieved by precise regulation of maternal diabetes. Such control may be the most important objective in the treatment program (111,112,115). Maintenance of maternal normoglycemia has been correlated with improved perinatal mortality rates. Karlsson and Kjellmer demonstrated a significant decrease in fetal loss if mean maternal blood sugars were maintained below 100 mg% during the last 10 to 12 weeks of pregnancy (116). A reduction in fetal macrosomia as well as perinatal mortality has also been reported by Roversi and his coworkers. They use a "maximal tolerated dose" of insulin, progressively increasing the dose until minor symptoms of hypoglycemia appear (111). Although occasional hypoglycemic episodes have not been associated with fetal compromise (117), this aggressive approach may interfere with the patient's daily activities.

The danger of reduction of diet and increase of insulin dosage on urine tests alone cannot . . . be over-emphasized (39).

Dr. Priscilla White, 1928

Postprandial glycosuria is common. A profile of blood glucose values obtained throughout the day must be used to determine the adequacy of therapy and the need for changing insulin dose or diet (118). Treatment must be individualized. Patients can often be managed with a single prebreakfast injection of NPH insulin. Some will require twice daily combinations of NPH and regular insulin for good control. What is good control? In general, fasting plasma glucose should be maintained near 100 to 110 mg% and postprandial values at 140 to 150 mg%.

A glycosylated hemoglobin, hemoglobin A_{Ic}, may be useful in assessing diabetic control over previous weeks and months (119). Hemoglobin A_{Ic} levels are normally elevated during the third trimester of pregnancy. They are significantly higher in pregnancies complicated by overt and gestational diabetes. Schwartz and his associates have found a striking decrease in the hemoglobin A_{Ic} levels of pregnant diabetics as compared with nonpregnant diabetic women (120). These lower levels could reflect better control during pregnancy.

A diet containing 30 cal/kg actual body weight should be used (83). Approximately 25% of the calories are consumed at breakfast, 30% at lunch, 30% at supper, and 15% as a prebedtime snack. Carbohydrates may comprise 40 to 50% of the total calories, fat 25 to 30%, and protein 25 to 30%. Weight reduction should be discouraged and ketonuria avoided. Studies by Churchill and Berendes have linked ketonuria, whether due to inadequate caloric intake or poor diabetic control, to significantly lower IQ scores in offspring (121). Such ketonuria might reflect a suboptimal environment for fetal nutrition and brain development.

Xanthurenic acid forms a stable complex with insulin and acts as an insulin antagonist (11). Its synthesis is increased in pyridoxine-deficient states such as pregnancy. Treatment with pyridoxine has been reported to improve oral glucose tolerance in a small group of gestational diabetics and could prove to be valuable in dietary management (122).

Oral hypoglycemics should be avoided. Not only may these drugs be teratogenic, but they can produce profound neonatal hypoglycemia (123).

Hospitalization during the 4 to 6 weeks prior to delivery has been considered an important part of the management program in many centers. Is it essential? Hospitalization is not only expensive but disruptive to the patient's family life. Nevertheless, it permits optimal stabilization with insulin and diet, enables the patient to remain at bed rest, and allows more intensive antepartum surveillance. In selected, well-motivated patients, an outpatient approach may be successfully used (118). For the majority of women with overt diabetes, several weeks of hospital care are necessary.

ELIMINATION OF TRAUMA

Unless the patient is multiparous, has had diabetes for a short time and has had a pregnancy which is normal clinically and chemically, we believe she is best delivered by cesarean section (124).

Dr. Priscilla White, 1946

Determining when a diabetic patient will deliver is more important than the method of delivery used. Some have recommended cesarean section for all patients (112) and appear willing to accept the increased maternal morbidity. Many patients, however, can be delivered vaginally (125). A serial induction should be avoided, as it permits deterioration of diabetic control and often interrupts antepartum surveillance. Labor must progress normally and shoulder dystocia must be anticipated. During labor, continuous electronic monitoring of fetal heart rate and uterine activity must be used. Early detection and treatment of intrapartum distress can decrease neonatal morbidity and mortality (126). If the fetus is thought to weigh over 4000 g, a cesarean section should be considered. Determinations of fetal weight by ultrasound should prove more useful than clinical estimates (127).

General anesthesia is preferred for cesarean section. Infants of diabetics delivered after general anesthesia demonstrate a normal acid-base state. Spinal anesthesia may produce a significantly lower pH and greater base deficit (128).

ELIMINATION OF IATROGENIC PREMATURITY; DETECTION OF INTRAUTERINE DISTRESS

The indication for early delivery is prevention of late intrauterine death characteristic of diabetic pregnancies (124).

Dr. Priscilla White, 1946

[F]atalities have resulted . . . from neonatal deaths in large infants who were premature by date, structure, and behavior (129).

Dr. Priscilla White, 1952

Careful control of diabetes and a team approach decreased perinatal mortality rates to 10% for classes B, C, and D and 20 to 30% for classes F and R (82). Many of these deaths were attributable to iatrogenic prematurity. Obstetricians could not determine when the fetus was functionally mature or distinguish the healthy fetus from one that was deteriorating. Early termination of all diabetic pregnancies saved some infants from intrauterine death but led to neonatal mortality from hyaline membrane disease (HMD) in others.

The lecithin/sphingomyelin (L/S) ratio fulfilled the need for a reliable indicator of fetal pulmonary maturity. Although its prognostic value has been questioned in pregnancies complicated by diabetes mellitus (130), several investigators have reported a low incidence of RDS with an L/S ratio of 2.0 or greater (131,132). In a recent study at LAC Women's Hospital, the L/S ratio was determined in 210 pregnancies complicated by overt diabetes. These data were retrospectively correlated with the occurrence of RDS or HMD. Only 4 cases of RDS and 2 cases of HMD were observed in 200 patients with an L/S ratio of 2.0 or greater prior to delivery. This 3% incidence of complications was no higher than that of the nondiabetic population (133). Only 1 infant of 43 delivered within 24 hr after determination of a mature L/S ratio developed RDS. However, 7 of 10 neonates with an antenatal L/S ratio of 1.5 to 1.9 did develop mild RDS. In a prospective study, no cases of RDS have been observed in over 100 infants of overt diabetic women delivered with an L/S ratio of 2.0 or greater.

Gluck reported accelerated pulmonary maturation in diabetic pregnancies complicated by vascular disease or preeclampsia. He believes this process is retarded in class A, B, or C pregnancies (134). The study at LAC Women's Hospital has not supported these observations.

Other markers of fetal pulmonary maturity, phosphatidylinositol and phosphatidylglycerol, may prove to be valuable in pregnancies complicated by diabetes (135).

Do infants of diabetics develop RDS if the L/S ratio is mature? RDS can occur despite adequate pulmonary surfactant if the neonate is asphyxiated (133). Epstein and his coworkers have found higher L/S ratios and increased rates of lecithin synthesis in pregnant rhesus monkeys with glucose intolerance (136). However, fetal lung lecithin concentrations were decreased. The fetus would then have a mature L/S ratio but an inadequate lung lecithin reservoir and could be at greater risk for RDS. Whether these derangements occur in infants of diabetics remains unknown.

To prevent unnecessary intervention and detect antepartum distress, the clinician must have reliable indices of fetal well-being. Biochemical tests of placental function such as HPL, diamine oxidase, heat-stable alkaline phosphatase, human chorionic gonadotropin, urinary pregnanediol, and oxytocinase are of little value (125,137). At the present time, many centers use both a biophysical evaluation, the contraction stress test (CST), and a biochemical test, 24-hr urinary estriol excretion, for antepartum surveillance (113,114,138). A negative CST, one without evidence of fetal distress, has been associated with few unexplained intrauterine deaths. Delivery can be safely delayed while awaiting fetal maturation. A positive CST is often associated with fetal compromise, although false positive tests do occur. The CST is usually performed at weekly intervals, but decreased fetal activity or unstable diabetic control may necessitate more frequent examinations. A rising curve of 24 hr urinary estriol excretion, like a negative CST, usually reflects fetal well-being (141,142). Unless these assays are done meticulously and are available daily, fetal distress will be missed (143). Each laboratory must determine what constitutes a significant fall in estriol excretion. At LAC Women's Hospital, Goebelsmann has found that a 35% fall in estriol excretion from the mean of the 3 previous days in association with a concomitant decrease in estriol/creatinine ratio can reflect fetal jeopardy (142). Unconjugated plasma estriol determinations may eventually eliminate many of the problems associated with 24 hr urinary estriols (144). A prospective, blinded study of 62 diabetic pregnancies revealed that the unconjugated plasma estriol more accurately predicted fetal status than total plasma estriol or 24 hr urinary estriol excretion (145).

Fetal growth may be assessed by serial measurements of the biparietal diameter of the fetal head. There are no differences in biparietal diameter between the fetuses of diabetic women and normal fetuses from the thirtieth to the thirty-seventh week (146). After this time, biparietal diameters in the diabetic pregnancies are significantly larger.

If performed properly and interpreted accurately, the CST, L/S ratio, estriol assays, and biparietal diameter measurements are valuable aids in monitoring the diabetic pregnancy. Done carelessly and used without full knowledge of the clinical situation, they lead to unexplained intrauterine deaths, unnecessary intervention, and iatrogenic prematurity.

MANAGEMENT AND OUTCOME OF DIABETES MELLITUS AT LAC WOMEN'S HOSPITAL

Class A

In 1970, the following plan of management was adopted for the class A diabetic patient at LAC Women's Hospital: Once identified, she would be followed in diabetes clinic every 2 weeks. Fasting serum glucose would be measured at each visit to the clinic. The patient was also asked to test a second-voided morning urine for sugar daily. In this way, those women who developed overt diabetes during pregnancy could be detected. Approximately 10 to 15% of class A diabetics may demonstrate such a change. Early delivery was to be avoided, and patients would be allowed to go to 40 weeks' gestation. If the patient had poor dates or an unripe cervix and was undelivered at 40 weeks, twice weekly 24 hr urinary estriols would be started. This surveillance would continue until the pregnancy ended. Primary cesarean section would be performed if the estimated fetal weight was more than 4000 g.

Two groups of class A patients were thought to be at greater risk for perinatal mortality: women who had had a previous stillbirth and those who developed preeclampsia. Such patients were managed as if they had overt diabetes—with weekly clinic visits, hospitalization at 34 weeks' gestation, daily urinary estriols, and weekly contraction stress tests.

During the 3-year period 1970–1972, 27,261 deliveries were recorded at LAC Women's Hospital. One percent or 261 occurred in diagnosed class A diabetics. Of these, 196, or 75%, had uncomplicated class A diabetes. Thirty-four, or 13%, had had a previous stillbirth; and 31, or 12%, developed preeclampsia during their pregnancy.

Thus, 25% of the patients were thought to be at greater risk for fetal loss and were managed as if they were overt diabetics.

Between 1970 and 1972, the perinatal mortality rate at LAC Women's Hospital was 32/1000. In class A diabetics, it was not significantly different, 19/1000 (45).

Five perinatal deaths occurred in this study—one stillbirth and four neonatal deaths. The uncomplicated class A patients accounted for two of these deaths. Three losses occurred in those class A women with a history of a previous stillbirth for a significantly higher perinatal mortality rate of 88/1000 ($p < .005$). No deaths were observed in the preeclamptic group.

Of the four neonatal mortalities, two were related to congenital malformations, and only one occurred in an infant over 2500 g. There was not a single perinatal mortality related to iatrogenic prematurity or trauma. The only stillbirth was preceded by an unrecognized 50% fall in urinary estriol. The infant weighed 3200 g and had multiple anomalies, including a cleft lip and palate.

Ninety-seven percent of the class A patients delivered at or beyond 36 weeks' gestation, 76% after 38 weeks, and 26% at or beyond 40 weeks.

Approximately two-thirds of the class A diabetics went into labor spontaneously, and one-third required some intervention. Almost 90% of the total interventions were performed for general clinical indications, including elective inductions (12 cases), inductions for post-dates (15 cases), premature ruptured membranes (20 cases) or preeclampsia (5 cases), elective repeat cesarean sections (23 cases), or elective primary sections (8 cases). Only 9% of the total interventions in the class A population were for specific fetal indications, including falling or low urinary estriols (5 cases) or a positive contraction stress test (3 cases). Of these 8 cases, 6 had a good outcome, and 2 infants, both in the preeclampsia group, were growth-retarded.

Approximately one-fourth of infants of class A mothers did experience some morbidity, primarily hyperbilirubinemia and hypoglycemia. Although the overall incidence of traumatic morbidity was only 3%, it rose to 10% in infants weighing over 4000 g who were delivered vaginally.

These data indicate a relatively low risk of perinatal mortality if one is dealing with a population of women who are normoglycemic in the fasting state. As long as the fasting serum glucose remains normal, an unexplained intrauterine death is a rare event, and there is no need for premature intervention. A high-risk group of patients who have had a previous stillbirth or who develop preeclampsia deserve closer scrutiny for fetal well-being.

Classes B to F

At LAC Women's Hospital, all insulin-dependent diabetics are hospitalized when they are first seen in clinic. This hospitalization permits establishment of optimal control. In addition, we obtain a urine culture, determine the patient's renal threshhold, order retinal photographs if indicated, calculate a base line creatinine clearance, and educate the patient about her diet, her insulin requirements, and what the remainder of her pregnancy will bring. Base line ultrasound studies may also be performed. This hospitalization lasts 3 to 5 days.

Patients are then discharged and followed weekly in the clinic. They are asked to check their double-voided urines four times daily and have a fasting serum glucose determined at each visit. Urine cultures are repeated every 4 to 6 weeks. During the second trimester, 10 to 15% of the patients may require an additional hospitalization for correction of poor control, evaluation of hypertension, or treatment of pyelonephritis.

Weekly 24-hr urinary estriol determinations are begun at 30 weeks to establish base line excretion.

Women in classes B to F are hospitalized again at 34 weeks. They are placed at bed rest, and their diabetes is carefully regulated. Intensive antepartum surveillance of fetal well-being is begun, using daily 24-hr urinary estriol assays and weekly contraction stress tests. An L/S ratio is determined before the elective delivery of any patient. Termination of pregnancy is considered (1) if a patient reaches 38 weeks' gestation and has an L/S ratio of 2.0 or greater, (2) if estriol excretion falls significantly or the CST is positive and an L/S ratio is mature or, (3) if estriol values drop and the CST is positive even with an immature L/S ratio.

Patients receive approximately one-third of their prepregnancy insulin dose on the morning of elective induction or cesarean section. A controlled infusion of 5% glucose at a rate no greater than 150 cc/hr is maintained (147). Blood sugars are monitored every 4 to 6 hours as well as at delivery, and regular insulin is administered if necessary.

During the period 1971–1976, 323 women with overt diabetes mellitus were treated with the protocol above. Their classification by White's criteria was class B, 239; class C, 46; class D, 29; class F, 6; and class R, 3. Fourteen percent of these patients had had a previous intrauterine death.

Perinatal mortality for classes B to F was not significantly higher than that of the general population during this 6-year period, 38/1000 as compared with 23/1000. Three stillbirths and nine neonatal deaths occurred in the diabetic patients. The fetal death rate was no greater than that of the general population. There were no intrapartum deaths, and no infants were lost because of trauma or iatrogenic prematurity. Congenital malformations were responsible for four neonatal deaths, necrotizing enterocolitis for two, and hyaline membrane disease for only one.

Our approach of expectant management yielded a mean gestational age of 38 weeks with only 35 births before 36 weeks. Forty-six percent of all patients were vaginally delivered. Almost 90% of the cesarean sections performed were primary procedures, and more than half were undertaken for suspected fetal jeopardy. One-third of the patients went into spontaneous labor, and 47% were delivered for general clinical indications, including elective inductions (106 cases) and inductions for ruptured membranes (39 cases) or preeclampsia (8 cases).

Sixty-five pregnancies were terminated for fetal indications. Thirty-one women were delivered for low or falling estriols, 18 for a positive CST, and 16 for both a positive CST and abnormal estriols. None of the 268 patients who had a negative CST had an intrauterine death within 1 week of that test. Only 1 of 239 women with normal urinary estriol excretion suffered an intrauterine death. Although urinary estriols were normal in this patient, unconjugated plasma estriol levels had fallen 40%. Two patients who had not been evaluated by the CST had intrauterine deaths heralded by significant falls in estriol excretion that were unrecognized. The incidence of perinatal mortality, low birthweight, and previous stillbirths was significantly increased in patients with abnormal antepartum tests. Low Apgar scores, late decelerations in labor, and subsequent RDS were higher in this group but did not attain statistical significance.

Neonatal morbidity correlated significantly with gestational age, occurring in 80% of the preterm and 40% of the term infants. The overall incidence of complications was hyperbilirubinemia, 37%; hypoglycemia, 34%; and hypocalcemia, 13%. RDS occurred in only 5% and traumatic morbidity in 2%.

This plan of expectant management has not only eliminated deaths due to iatrogenic prematurity but reduced the fetal death rate to less than 1%. Congenital malformations are now the leading cause of mortality.

COUNSELING THE DIABETIC WOMAN

Should a diabetic marry? No diabetic girl or boy should get married unless sufficient capital is available to provide for a "sick fund" in case of an emergency or pregnancy (53).

Dr. Elliott Joslin, 1929

The foundation for a successful pregnancy must be built before the diabetic woman conceives. Each pregnancy must be carefully planned. A program of birth control is essential, using either oral contraceptives or, in patients with vascular disease or class A diabetes, an intrauterine device (148). Diabetic women should be encouraged to complete their childbearing early in life, and sterilization should be considered after two or three pregnancies. Those patients with active proliferative retinopathy, advanced nephropathy, or a history of myocardial infarction are candidates for therapeutic abortion.

As noted by Joslin almost 50 years ago, pregnancy is a great financial burden for the diabetic woman. She must consider this problem with her family and plan for her often lengthy hospitalization.

Patients frequently ask if their children will be diabetics. Zonana and Rimoin have emphasized that, at the present time, accurate genetic counseling in diabetes is impossible (149). The pattern of inheritance is not simply autosomal recessive.

If the tragedy of intrauterine death or fatal congenital malformation occurs, the health care team must be supportive (150,151). The parents should be encouraged to discuss their loss, to see the baby if they wish, and to mourn for their child.

THE FUTURE

[O]nly when the entire genetic and vascular problem of diabetes is solved will our total experience be equal to the best in non-diabetic pediatric and obstetrical experience (129).

Dr. Priscilla White, 1952

The discovery of insulin permitted the diabetic woman to survive pregnancy and frequently bear a healthy infant. Perinatologists and neonatologists next developed methods to monitor fetal well-being and care for the sick neonate. Today, our treatment must go beyond assuring maternal and fetal survival. We must examine the residual morbidity diabetes mellitus imposes on the reproductive process and determine the quality of life that may be predicted for the pregnant diabetic and her infant. Certainly, the etiologies of intrauterine death and fatal congenital malformation are challenging enigmas. Complications such as hypoglycemia, hyperbilirubinemia, and hypocalcemia must also be considered and their long-term effects discovered. It appears that better methods of diabetic control will prove important in reducing this morbidity. Insulin treatment of class A patients and constant insulin infusions during labor are two approaches that may be helpful. The ultimate treatment for the pregnant diabetic and her fetus could be an artificial pancreas or β-cell transplant.

REFERENCES

1. White, P.: Pregnancy complicating diabetes. *Am. J. Med.* 7:609, 1949.

2. Joslin, E. P.: Pregnancy and diabetes, in *The Treatment of Diabetes Mellitus,* Joslin, E. P. Philadelphia, Lea and Febiger, 1923, p. 649.

3. Crenshaw, C., Jr.: Fetal glucose metabolism. *Clin. Obstet. Gynecol.* 13:579, 1970.

4. Felig, P.: Maternal and fetal fuel homeostasis in human pregnancy. *Am. J. Clin. Nutr.* 26:998, 1973.

5. Freinkel, N., Metzger, B. E., Nitzan, M., Hare, J. W., Shambaugh, G. E., III, Marshall, R. T., Surmaczynska, B. Z., and Nagel, T. C.: "Accelerated starvation" and mechanisms for the conservation of maternal nitrogen during pregnancy. *Isr. J. Med. Sci.* 8:426, 1972.

6. Girard, J. R.: Metabolic fuels of the fetus. *Isr. J. Med. Sci.* 11:591, 1975.

7. Spellacy, W. N: Human placental lactogen (HPL): The review of a protein hormone important to obstetrics and gynecology. *South Med. J.* 62:1054, 1969.

8. Kaplan, S. L.: Human chorionic somatomammotropin: Secretion, biologic effects, and physiologic significance, in *The Endocrine Milieu of Pregnancy, Puerperium and Childhood,* ed. Jaffe, R. B. Columbus, Ohio, Ross Laboratories, 1974, p. 75.

9. Gaspard, U., Sandront, H., and Luyckx, A.: Glucose-insulin interaction and the modulation of human placental lactogen (HPL) secretion during pregnancy. *J. Obstet. Gynaecol. Br. Commonw.* 81:201, 1974.

10. Yen, S. S. C.: Endocrine regulation of metabolic homeostasis during pregnancy. *Clin. Obstet. Gynecol.* 16:130, 1973.

11. Spellacy, W. N.: Maternal and fetal metabolic interrelationships, in Carbohydrate Metabolism in Pregnancy and the Newborn, ed. Sutherland, H. W., and Stowers, J. M. Edinburgh, Churchill Livingstone, 1975, p. 42.

12. Burt, R. L., and Davidson, I. W. F.: Insulin half-life and utilization in normal pregnancy. *Obstet. Gynecol.* 43:161, 1974.

13. Kyle, G. C.: Diabetes and pregnancy. *Ann. Intern. Med.* 59 (Suppl. 3):1, 1963.

14. Ajabor, L. N., Tsai, C. C., Vela, P., and Yen, S. S. C.: Effect of exogenous estrogen on carbohydrate metabolism in postmenopausal women. *Am. J. Obstet. Gynecol.* 113:383, 1972.

15. Costrini, N. V., and Kalkhoff, R. K.: Relative effects of pregnancy, estradiol and progesterone on plasma insulin and pancreatic islet secretion. *J. Clin. Invest.* 50:992, 1971.

16. Freinkel, N., and Goodner, C. J.: Carbohydrate metabolism in pregnancy: I. The metabolism of insulin by human placental tissue. *J. Clin. Invest.* 39:116, 1960.

17. Posner, B. I.: Insulin metabolizing enzyme activities in human placental tissue. *Diabetes* 22:552, 1973.

18. VanAssche, F. A., Hoet, J. J., and Jack, P. M. B.: The endocrine pancreas of the pregnant mother, fetus, and newborn, in *Fetal Physiology and Medicine,* ed. Beard, R. W., and Nathanielsz, P. W. London, W. B. Saunders, 1976, p. 121.

19. Daniel, R. R., Metzger, B. E., Freinkel, N., Faloona, G. R., Unger, R. H., and Nitzan, M.: Carbohydrate metabolism in pregnancy: XI. Response of plasma glucagon to overnight fast and oral glucose during normal pregnancy and in gestational diabetes. *Diabetes* 23:771, 1974.

20. Freinkel, N., and Metzger, B. E.: Some considerations of fuel economy in the fed state during late human pregnancy, in *Early Diabetes in Early Life,* ed. Camerini-Davalos, R. A., and Cole, H. S. New York, Academic Press Inc., 1975, p. 289.

21. Adam, P. A. J., King, K. C., Schwartz, R., and Teramo, K.: Human placental barrier to ^{125}I-glucagon early in gestation. *J. Clin. Endocrinol. Metab.* 34:772, 1972.

22. Kalhan, S. C., Schwartz, R., and Adam, P. A. J.: Placental barrier to human insulin-I[125] in insulin-dependent diabetic mothers. *J. Clin. Endocrinol. Metab.* 40:139, 1975.

23. Widdas, W. F.: The inability of diffusion to account for placental glucose transfer in the sheep and consideration of the kinetics of a possible carrier. *J. Physiol. (Lond.)* 118:23, 1952.

24. Shelley, H. J.: Glucose metabolism in the foetus in physiological and pathological circumstances, in *Physiology and Pathology in the Perinatal Period,* ed. Gevers, R. H., and Ruys, J. H. Netherlands, 1971, Springer Verlag, Leiden University Press, p. 13.

25. Beard, R. W., Turner, R. C., and Oakley, N. W.: Fetal response to glucose loading. *Postgrad. Med. J.* 47:68, 1971.

26. James, E. J., Raye, J. R., Gresham, E. L., Makowski, E. L., Meschia, G., and Battaglia, F. C.: Fetal oxygen consumption, carbon dioxide production, and glucose uptake in a chronic sheep preparation. *Pediatrics* 50:361, 1972.

27. Boyd, R. D., Morris, F. H., Jr., Meschia, G., Makowski, E. L., and Battaglia, F. C.: Growth of glucose and oxygen uptake by fetuses of fed and starved ewes. *Am. J. Physiol.* 225:897, 1973.

28. Adam, P. A. J., Teramo, K., Raiha, N., Gitlin, D., and Schwartz, R.: Human fetal insulin metabolism early in gestation: Response to acute elevation of the fetal glucose concentration and placental transfer of human insulin-I-[131]. *Diabetes* 18:409, 1969.

29. Reynolds, W. A., and Pitkin, R. M.: Fetal insulin response to glucose: A re-examination. *Gynecol. Invest.* 7:48, 1976.

30. Bassett, J. M., and Madill, D.: The influence of maternal nutrition on plasma hormone and metabolite concentrations of foetal lambs. *J. Endocrinol.* 61:465, 1974.

31. Milner, R. D. G.: The development of insulin secretion in man, in *Metabolic Processes in the Foetus and Newborn Infant,* ed. Jonxis, J. H. P., Vissei, H. K. A., and Troelstra, J. A. Leiden, Holland, H. E. Stenfert Kroese, Williams and Wilkins, 1971, p. 193.

32. Chez, R. A., Mintz, D. H., and Hutchinson, D. L.: Effect of theophylline on glucagon and glucose-mediated plasma insulin responses in subhuman primate fetus and neonate. *Metabolism* 20:805, 1971.

33. Bocek, R. M., and Beatty, C. H.: Effect of insulin on carbohydrate metabolism of fetal rhesus monkey muscle. *Endocrinology* 85:615, 1969.

34. Clark, C. M., Jr.: The stimulation by insulin of amino acid uptake and protein synthesis in the isolated fetal rat heart. *Biol. Neonate* 19:379, 1971.

35. Eisen, H. J., Glinsmann, W. H., and Sherline, P.: Effect of insulin on glycogen synthesis in fetal rat liver in organ culture. *Endocrinology* 92:584, 1973.

36. Posner, B. I.: Insulin receptors in human and animal placental tissue. *Diabetes* 23:209, 1974.

37. Demers, L. M., Gabbe, S. G., Villee, C. A., and Greep, R.: The effects of insulin on placental glycogenesis. *Endocrinology* 91:270, 1972.

38. Villee, D. B.: Discussion, in *Early Diabetes in Early Life,* ed. Camerini-Davalos, R. A., and Cole, H. S. New York, Academic Press, Inc., 1975, p. 78.

39. White, P.: Diabetes in pregnancy, in *The Treatment of Diabetes Mellitus,* Joslin, E. P. Philadelphia, Lea and Febiger, 1928, p. 861.

40. Gillmer, M. D. G., Oakley, N. W., Brooke, F. M., and Beard, R. W.: Metabolic profiles in pregnancy. *Isr. J. Med. Sci.* 11:601, 1975.

41. Pedersen, J., Bojsen-Møller, B., and Poulsen, H.: Blood sugar in newborn infants of diabetic mothers. *Acta Endocrinol.* (kbh) 15:33, 1954.

42. Steinke, J., and Driscoll, S. G.: The extractable insulin content of pancreas from fetuses and infants of diabetic and control mothers. *Diabetes* 14:573, 1963.

43. VanAssche, F. A.: The fetal endocrine pancreas, in *Carbohydrate Metabolism in Pregnancy and the Newborn,* ed. Sutherland, H. W., and Stowers, J. M. Edinburgh, Churchill Livingstone, 1975, p. 68.

44. Hultquist, G. T., and Olding, L. B.: Pancreatic-islet fibrosis in young infants of diabetic mothers. *Lancet* 2:1015, 1975.

45. Gabbe, S. G., Mestman, J. H., Freeman, R. K., Anderson, G. V., and Lowensohn R. I.: Management and outcome of Class A diabetes mellitus. *Am. J. Obstet Gynecol.* 127:465, 1976.

46. Szabo, A. J., Oppermann, W., Hanover, B., Gugliucci, D., and Szabo, O.: Fetal adipose tissue development: Relationship to maternal free fatty acid levels, in *Early Diabetes in Early Life,* ed. Camerini-Davalos, R. A., and Cole, H. S. New York, Academic Press Inc. 1975, p. 167.

47. Persson, B.: Assessment of metabolic control in diabetic pregnancy, in *Size at Birth,* ed. Elliott, K., and Knight, J. Ciba Foundation Symposium N.S. No. 27. Amsterdam, Associated Scientific Publishers, 1974, p. 247.

48. Driscoll, S. G.: The pathology of pregnancy complicated by diabetes mellitus. *Med. Clin. North Am.* 49:1053, 1965.

49. Winick, M., and Noble, A.: Cellular growth in human placenta: II. Diabetes mellitus. *J. Pediatr.* 71:216, 1967.

50. Gabbe, S. G., Demers, L. M., Greep, R. O., and Villee, C. A.: Placental glycogen metabolism in diabetes mellitus. *Diabetes* 21:1185, 1972.

51. Jones, C. J. P., and Fox, H.: An ultrastructural and ultrahistochemical study of the placenta of the diabetic woman. *J. Path.* 119:91, 1976.

52. Fox, H.: Pathology of the placenta in maternal diabetes mellitus. *Obstet. Gynecol.* 34:792, 1969.

53. Joslin, E. P.: *A Diabetic Manual.* Philadelphia, Lea and Febiger, 1929, pp. 25, 140.

54. Gellis, S. S., and Hsia, D. Y.: The infant of the diabetic. *Am. J. Dis. Child.* 97:1, 1959.

55. Williams, J. W.: *Obstetrics,* 4th ed. New York, Appleton, 1920, p. 533.

56. Gabbe, S. G., Mestman, J. H., and Hibbard, L. T.: Maternal mortality in diabetes mellitus. *Obstet. Gynecol.* 48:549, 1976.

57. White, P.: Pregnancy and diabetes: medical aspects. *Med. Clin. North Am.* 49:1015, 1965.

58. Bleicher, S. J., and Pang, S.-J.: Oxygen transport and the role of erythrocyte 2,3-diphosphoglycerate, in *Early Diabetes in Early Life,* ed. Camerini-Davalos, R. A., and Cole, H. S. New York, Academic Press Inc., 1975, p. 243.

59. Lev-Ran, A.: Sharp temporary drop in insulin requirement after cesarean section in diabetic patients. *Am. J. Obstet. Gynecol.* 120:905, 1974.

60. Mintz, H. D., Stock, R., Finster, J. L., and Taylor, A.: The effects of normal and diabetic pregnancies on growth hormone responses to hypoglycemia. *Metabolism* 17:54, 1968.

61. White, P.: Life cycle of diabetes in youth. *J. Am. Med. Women's Assoc.* 27:293, 1972.

62. Maeder, E. C., Barno, A., and Mecklenburg, F.: Obesity: A maternal risk factor. *Obstet. Gynecol.* 45:669, 1975.

63. Hagbard, L.: Pregnancy and diabetes mellitus. *Acta Obstet. Gynec. Scand.* 35(suppl. 1), chap. 4, 1956.

64. Beard, R. W., and Oakley, N. W.: The fetus of the diabetic, in *Fetal Physiology and Medicine,* ed. Beard, R. W., and Nathanielsz, P. W. London, W. B. Saunders, 1976, p. 137.

65. Spellacy, W. N.: Diabetes mellitus complicating pregnancy, chap. 72, *Davis' Gynecology and Obstetrics.* Hagerstown, Maryland, Harper and Row Publishers Inc., 1972, p. 1.

66. Farquhar, J. W.: The infant of the diabetic mother. *Clinics Endocrinology Metabolism* 5:237, 1976.

67. Adamsons, K., and Myers, R. E.: Circulation in the intervillous space: Obstetrical considerations in fetal deprivation, in *The Placenta and Its Maternal Supply Line,* ed. Gruenwald, P. Baltimore, University Park Press, 1975, p. 158.

68. Shelley, H. J., Bassett, J. M., and Milner, R. D. G.: Control of carbohydrate metabolism in the fetus and newborn. *Br. Med. Bull.* 31:37, 1975.

69. Driscoll, S. G., Benirschke, K., and Curtis, G. W.: Neonatal deaths among infants of diabetic mothers. *Am. J. Dis. Child.* 100:818, 1961.

70. Smith, B. T., Giroud, C. J. P., Robert, M., and Avery, M. E.: Insulin antagonism of cortisol action on lecithin synthesis by cultured fetal lung cells. *J. Pediatr.* 87:953, 1975.

71. Naeye, R. L.: Fetal lung and kidney maturation in abnormal pregnancies. *Arch. Pathol.* 99:533, 1975.

72. Robert, M. F., Neff, R. K., Hubbell, J. P., Taeusch, H. W., and Avery, M. E.: Maternal diabetes and the respiratory-distress syndrome. *N. Engl. J. Med.* 294:357, 1976.

73. Brudenell, M.: Care of the clinical diabetic woman in pregnancy and labour, in *Carbohydrate Metabolism in Pregnancy and the Newborn,* ed. Sutherland, H. W., and Stowers, J. M. Edinburgh, Churchill Livingstone, 1975, p. 221.

74. Horger, E. O., III, Miller, M. C., III, and Conner, E. D.: Relation of large birthweight to maternal diabetes mellitus. *Obstet. Gynecol.* 45:150, 1975.

75. Pedersen, J., Pedersen, L. M., Andersen, B.: Assessors of fetal perinatal mortality in diabetic pregnancy. *Diabetes* 23:302, 1974.

76. Chung, C. S., and Myrianthopoulos, N. C.: Factors affecting risks of congenital malformations: II. Effect of maternal diabetes in birth defects, in *Original Article Series: The National Foundation March of Dimes,* ed. Bergsma, D. Miami, Symposia Specialists, 1975, p. 23.

77. Pedersen, L. M., Tygstrup, I., and Pedersen, J.: Congenital malformations in newborn infants of diabetic women. *Lancet* I:1124, 1964.

78. Farquhar, J. W.: Prognosis for babies born to diabetic mothers in Edinburgh. *Arch. Dis. Child.* 44:36, 1969.

79. Soler, N. G., Walsh, C. H., and Malins, J. M.: Congenital malformations in infants of diabetic mothers. *Quart. J. Med.* XLV(178):303, 1976.

80. Passarge, E., and Lenz, W.: Syndrome of caudal regression in infants of diabetic mothers: Observations of further cases. *Pediatrics* 37:672, 1966.

81. Cornblath, M., and Schwartz, R.: Infant of the diabetic mother, in *Disorders of Carbohydrate Metabolism in Infancy,* ed. Cornblath, M., and Schwartz, R. Philadelphia, W. B. Saunders, 1976, p. 115.

82. White, P.: Pregnancy and diabetes, in *Joslin's Diabetes Mellitus,* ed. Marble, A., White, P., Bradley, R. F., and Krall, L. P. Philadelphia, Lea and Febiger, 1971, p. 581.

83. Felig, P.: Diabetes mellitus, in *Medical Complications During Pregnancy,* ed. Burrow, G. N., and Ferris, T. F. Philadelphia, W. B. Saunders, 1975, p. 176.

84. Zarowitz, H. and Moltz, A.: Management of diabetes in pregnancy. *Obstet. Gynecol.* 27:820, 1966.

85. Carrington, E. R., Reardon, H. S., and Schuman, C. R.: Recognition and management of problems associated with prediabetes during pregnancy. *J.A.M.A.* 166:245, 1958.

86. Shea, M. A., Garrison, D. L., and Tom, S. K. H.: Diabetes in pregnancy. *Am. J. Obstet. Gynecol.* 111:801, 1971.

87. Khojandi, M., Tsai, M., and Tyson, J. E.: Gestational diabetes: The dilemma of delivery. *Obstet. Gynecol.* 43:1, 1974.

88. Stallone, L. A., and Ziel, H. K.: Management of gestational diabetes. *Am. J. Obstet. Gynecol.* 119:1091, 1974.

89. Cassady, G., Hinkley, C., Barley, P., Blake, M., and Younger, B.: Amniotic fluid creatinine in pregnancies complicated by diabetes. *Am. J. Obstet. Gynecol.* 122:13, 1975.

90. Miller, H. C., Hurwitz, D., and Kuder, K.: Fetal and neonatal mortality in pregnancies complicated by diabetes mellitus. *J.A.M.A.* 124:271, 1944.

91. Pedersen, J., and Jorgensen, G.: Hydramnios in diabetes. *Acta Endocrinol.* 15:333, 1954.

92. O'Sullivan, J. B.: Gestational diabetes. *N. Engl. J. Med.* 264:1082, 1961.

93. Dandrow, R. V., and O'Sullivan, J. B.: Obstetric hazards of gestational diabetes. *Am. J. Obstet. Gynecol.* 96:1144, 1966.

94. Mestman, J. H., Anderson, G. V., and Guadalupe, V.: Follow-up study of 360 subjects with abnormal carbohydrate metabolism during pregnancy. *Obstet. Gynecol.* 39:421, 1972.

95. Chen, W., Palar, A., and Tricomi, V.: Screening for diabetes in a prenatal clinic. *Obstet. Gynecol.* 40:567, 1972.

96. Zarowitz, H. and Newhouse, S.: Renal glycosuria in normoglycemic glycosuric pregnancy: A quantitative study. *Metabolism* 22:755, 1973.

97. Sutherland, H. W., Stowers, J. M., and McKenzie, C.: Simplifying the clinical problem of glycosuria in pregnancy. *Lancet* 1:1069, 1970.

98. O'Sullivan, J. B., Mahan, C. M., Charles, D., and Dandrow, R. V.: Screening criteria for high-risk gestational diabetic patients. *Am. J. Obstet. Gynecol.* 116:895, 1973.

99. O'Sullivan, J. B., Charles, D., Mahan, C. M., and Dandrow, R. V.: Gestational diabetes and perinatal mortality. *Am. J. Obstet. Gynecol.* 116:901, 1973.

100. Macafee, C. A. J., and Beischer, N. A.: The relative value of the standard indications for performing a glucose tolerance test in pregnancy. *Med. J. Aust.* 1:911, 1974.

101. Hohe, P. T.: Glucose tolerance testing during pregnancy. *Obstet. Gynecol.* 38:693, 1971.

102. Hadden, D. R.: Glucose tolerance tests in pregnancy, in *Carbohydrate Metabolism in Pregnancy and the Newborn,* ed. Sutherland, H. W., and Stowers, J. M. Edinburgh, Churchill Lingingstone, 1975, p. 19.

103. Benjamin, F., and Casper, D. J.: Comparative validity of oral and intravenous glucose tolerance tests in pregnancy. *Am. J. Obstet. Gynecol.* 97:488, 1967.

104. O'Sullivan, J. B.: Prospective study of gestational diabetes and its treatment, in *Carbohydrate*

Metabolism in Pregnancy and the Newborn, ed. Sutherland, H. W., and Stowers, J. M. Edinburgh, Churchill Livingstone, 1975, p. 195.

105. Mestman, J.: Medical management of the pregnant diabetic. *Contemp. OB/Gyn* 1:61, 1973.

106. Gillmer, M. D. G., Beard, R. W., Brooke, F. M., and Oakley, N. W.: Carbohydrate metabolism in pregnancy: Part I. Diurnal plasma glucose profile in normal and diabetic women. *Br. Med. J.* 3:399, 1975.

107. Gillmer, M. D. G., Beard, R. W., Brooke, F. M., and Oakley, N. W.: Carbohydrate metabolism in pregnancy: Part II. Relation between maternal glucose tolerance and glucose metabolism in the newborn. *Br. Med. J.* 3:402, 1975.

108. Abell, D. A., and Beischer, N. A.: Evaluation of the three-hour oral glucose tolerance test in detection of significant hyperglycemia and hypoglycemia in pregnancy. *Diabetes* 24:874, 1975.

109. Editorial, Hyperglycaemia and hypoglycaemia in pregnancy. *Lancet* II:889, 1976.

110. Love, E. J., Stevenson, J. A. F., and Kinch, R. A. H.: Evaluation of oral and intravenous glucose tolerance tests for the diagnosis of "prediabetes" in the puerperium. *Am. J. Obstet. Gynecol.* 88:283, 1964.

111. Roversi, G. D., Canussio, V., Garguilo, M., and Candiani, G. B.: The intensive care of perinatal risk in pregnant diabetics (136 cases): A new therapeutic scheme for the best control of maternal disease. *J. Perinat. Med.* 1:114, 1973.

112. Tyson, J. E., and Hock, R. A.: Gestational and pregestational diabetes: An approach to therapy. *Am. J. Obstet. Gynecol.* 125:1009, 1976.

113. Gugliucci, C. L., O'Sullivan, M. J., Opperman, W., Gordon, M., and Stone, M. L.: Intensive care of the pregnant diabetic. *Am. J. Obstet. Gynecol.* 125:435, 1976.

114. Francois, R., Picaud, J. J., Ruitton-Uglieno, A., David, L., Cartal, M. J., and Bauer, D.: The newborn of diabetic mothers. *Biol. Neonate* 24:1, 1974.

115. Persson, B., Feychting, H., and Gentz, J.: Management of the infant of the diabetic mother, in *Carbohydrate Metabolism in Pregnancy and the Newborn,* Sutherland, H. W., and Stowers, J. M., (eds.). Edinburgh, Churchill Livingstone, 1975, p. 232.

116. Karlsson, K., and Kjellmer, I.: The outcome of diabetic pregnancies in relation to the mother's blood sugar level. *Am. J. Obstet. Gynecol.* 112:213, 1972.

117. Churchill, J. A., Berendes, H. W., and Newmore, J.: Neuropsychological deficits in children of diabetic mothers. *Am. J. Obstet. Gynecol.* 105:257, 1969.

118. Lewis, S. B., Murray, W. K., Wallin, J. D., Coustan, D. R., Daane, T. A., Tredway, D. R., and Navins, J. P.: Improved glucose control in nonhospitalized pregnant diabetic patients. *Obstet. Gynecol.* 48:260, 1976.

119. Koenig, R. J., Peterson, C. M., Jones, R. L., Saudek, C., Lehrman, M., and Cerami, A.: Correlation of glucose regulation and hemoglobin A_{1c} in diabetes mellitus. *N. Engl. J. Med.* 295:417, 1976.

120. Schwartz, H. C., King, K. C., Schwartz, A. L. Edmunds, D., and Schwartz, R.: Effects of pregnancy on hemoglobin A_{1c} in normal, gestational diabetic and diabetic women. *Diabetes* 25:1118, 1976.

121. Churchill, J. A., and Berendes, H. W.: Intelligence of children whose mothers had acetonuria during pregnancy, in *Perinatal Factors Affecting Human Development.* Scientific Publication No. 185, Pan American Health Organization, 1969, p. 30.

122. Coellingh Bennink, H. J. T., and Schreurs, W. H. P.: Improvement of oral glucose tolerance in gestational diabetes by pyridoxine. *Br. Med. J.* 3:13, 1975.

123. Adam, P. A. J., and Schwartz, R.: Diagnosis and treatment: Should oral hypoglycemic agents be used in pediatric and pregnant patients? *Pediatrics* 42:819, 1968.

124. White, P.: Pregnancy complicating diabetes, in *The Treatment of Diabetes Mellitus,* ed. Joslin, E. P., Root, H. F., White, P., Marble, A., and Barley, C. C. Philadelphia, Lea and Febiger, 1946, p. 769.

125. Beard, R. W., and Brudenell, J. M.: Fetal monitoring in diabetic pregnancy, in *Early Diabetes in Early Life,* Camerini-Davalos, R. A., and Cole, H. S. New York, Academic Press, Inc., 1975, p. 523.

126. Hon, E. H., Zanini, B., and Quilligan, E. J.: The neonatal value of fetal monitoring. *Am. J. Obstet. Gynecol.* 122:508, 1975.

127. Kurjak, A., and Breyer, B.: Estimation of fetal weight by ultrasonic abdominometry. *Am. J. Obstet. Gynecol.* 125:962, 1976.

128. Datta, S., Brown, W. U., Jr., and Alper, M. H.: Acid-base balance in diabetics after general or spinal anesthesia for cesarean section, American Society of Anesthesiologists, 1976 Meeting, San Francisco, California, p. 251.

129. White, P.: Pregnancy complicating diabetes, in *The Treatment of Diabetes Mellitus*, ed. Joslin, E. P., Root, H. F., White, P., and Marble, A. Philadelphia, Lea and Febiger, 1952, p. 676.

130. Farrell, P. M. Indices of maturation in diabetic pregnancy. *Lancet* 1:596, 1976.

131. Aubry, R. H., Rourke, J. E., Almanza, R., Cantor, R. M., and Van Doren, J. E.: The lecithin/sphingomyelin ratio in a high-risk obstetric population. *Obstet. Gynecol.* 47:21, 1976.

132. Tchobroutsky, C., Cédard, L., Rouvillois, J. L., and Amiel-Tison, C.: The lecithin/sphingomyelin ratio in amniotic fluid in diabetic pregnancies treated with insulin. *J. Gyn. Obst. Biol. Repr.* 4:93, 1975.

133. Donald, J. R., Freeman, R. K., Goebelsmann, U., Chan, W. H., and Nakamura, R. M.: Clinical experience with the amniotic fluid lecithin/sphingomyelin ratio: I. Antenatal prediction of pulmonary maturity. *Am. J. Obstet. Gynecol.* 115:547, 1973.

134. Gluck, L., and Kulovich, M. V.: Lecithin/sphingomyelin ratios in amniotic fluid in normal and abnormal pregnancy. *Am. J. Obstet. Gynecol.* 115:539, 1973.

135. Hallman, M., Kulovich, M., Kirkpatrick, E., Sugarman, R. G., and Gluck, L.: Phosphatidylinositol and phosphatidylglycerol in amniotic fluid: Indices of lung maturity. *Am. J. Obstet. Gynecol.* 125:617, 1976.

136. Epstein, M. F., Farrell, P. M., and Chez, R. A.: Fetal lung lecithin metabolism in the glucose-intolerant rhesus monkey pregnancy. *Pediatrics* 57:722, 1976.

137. Soler, N. G., Nicholson, H. O., and Malins, J. M.: Serial determinations of human placental lactogen in the management of diabetic pregnancy. *Lancet* II:54, 1975.

138. Greene, J. W., Jr.: Diabetes mellitus in pregnancy. *Obstet. Gynecol.* 46:724, 1975.

139. Freeman, R. K.: The use of the oxytocin challenge test for antepartum evaluation of uteroplacental respiratory function. *Am. J. Obstet. Gynecol.* 121:481, 1975.

140. Freeman, R. K., Goebelsmann, U., Nochimson, D., and Cetrulo, C.: An evaluation of the significance of a positive oxytocin challenge test. *Obstet. Gynecol.* 47:8, 1976.

141. Rivlin, M. E., Mestman, J. H., Hall, T. D., Weaver, C. P., and Anderson, G. V.: Value of estriol estimations in the management of diabetic pregnancy. *Am. J. Obstet. Gynecol.* 106:875, 1970.

142. Goebelsmann, U., Freeman, R. K., Mestman, J. H., Nakamura, R. M., and Woodling, B. A.: Estriol in pregnancy: II. Daily urinary estriol in the management of the pregnant diabetic woman. *Am. J. Obstet. Gynecol.* 115:795, 1973.

143. Dumont, M., Cohen, M., Cohen, H., and Bertrand, J.: Diagnosis of fetal distress in utero by determination of plasma levels of nonconjugated estrogens: Advantages and limits. *Rev. Franc. Gynec.* 70:171, 1975.

144. Katagiri, H., Distler, W., Freeman, R. K., and Goebelsmann, U.: Estriol in pregnancy: IV. Normal concentrations, diurnal and/or episodic variations, and day-to-day changes of unconjugated and total estriol in late pregnancy plasma. *Am. J. Obstet. Gynecol.* 124:272, 1976.

145. Gabbe, S. G., Distler, W., Freeman, R. K., Mestman, J. H., and Goebelsmann, U.: Comparison of unconjugated and total plasma with 24-hr. urinary estriols in management of the pregnant diabetic. Society for Gynecologic Investigation, 1977, Tuscon, Arizona.

146. Murata, Y., and Martin, C. B., Jr.: Growth of the biparietal diameter of the fetal head in diabetic pregnancy. *Am. J. Obstet. Gynecol.* 115:252, 1973.

147. Light, I. J., Keenan, W. J., and Sutherland, J. M.: Maternal intravenous glucose administration as a cause of hypoglycemia in the infant of the diabetic mother. *Am. J. Obstet. Gynecol.* 113:345, 1972.

148. Oakley, N. W., and Beard, R. W.: Conception control in diabetes mellitus, in *Early Diabetes in Early Life,* Camerini-Davalos, R. A., and Cole, H. S. New York, Academic Press, Inc., 1975, p. 345.

149. Zonana, J., and Rimoin, D. L.: Current concepts: Inheritance of diabetes mellitus. *N. Engl. J. Med.* 295:603, 1976.

150. Lewis, E.: The management of stillbirth: Coping with an unreality. *Lancet* II:619, 1976.

151. Kowalski, K., and Bowes, W. A., Jr.: Parents' response to a stillborn baby. *Contemp. OB/Gyn* 8:53, 1976.

25

Infant of the Diabetic Mother*

Marvin Cornblath, M.D.
Robert Schwartz, M.D.

These infants are remarkable not only because like foetal
versions of Shadrach, Meshach and Abednego, they
emerge at least alive from within the fiery metabolic
furnace of diabetes mellitus, but because they resemble
one another so closely that they might well be related.
They are plump, sleek, liberally coated with vernix caseosa,
full-faced and plethoric. The umbilical cord and the
placenta share in the gigantism. During their first 24 or
more extrauterine hours they lie on their backs, bloated
and flushed, their legs flexed and abducted, their lightly
closed hands on each side of the head, the abdomen
prominent and their respiration sighing. They convey a
distinct impression of having had such a surfeit of both
food and fluid pressed upon them by an insistent hostess
that they desire only peace so that they may recover from
their excesses. And on the second day their resentment of
the slightest noise improves the analogy while their
trembling anxiety seems to speak of intrauterine
indiscretions of which we know nothing (1) (Fig. 1).

The infant of the diabetic mother, so exquisitely described by Farquhar (1), has
survived an unusual genetic and environmental ordeal. This description now applies to
fewer newborn infants of both insulin-dependent and gestational diabetic mothers.
Advances in understanding the intrauterine environment, the precise definition of metabolic control, awareness of the advantages of prolonged controlled hospitalization, and
the recognition and treatment of gestational diabetics have reduced the number of
oversized infants, as well as their perinatal and neonatal mortality and morbidity. The
ability to conceive does not apparently differ between diabetic and nondiabetic women.

* Modified from Cornblath, M., and Schwartz, R. *Disorders of Carbohydrate Metabolism in Infancy*, 2nd
ed. W. B. Saunders Co., Philadelphia, 1976.

609

Fetal wastage, neonatal mortality, and morbidity in these babies, although of a higher incidence than those in nondiabetics, have steadily declined over the past three decades (2–8). In a prospective study, O'Sullivan and associates (3) found a perinatal mortality of 6.4% in gestational diabetes compared with 1.5% in controls. Women over 25 years of age were found to be at highest risk. In this high-risk group, treatment with diet and insulin initiated before 32 weeks of gestation significantly reduced the frequency of large babies and viable losses (9).

Pedersen et al. (2,10) reviewed the perinatal fetal mortality in 1332 diabetic pregnancies from 1946 to 1972. He observed a declining rate, from 22.1% in the period 1946–1955 to 7.4% in 1970–1972. He classified patients according to factors evident only during pregnancy that carried a poor prognosis, i.e., prognostic bad signs in pregnancy (PBSP). Of these PBSP, four were of major importance: (1) clinical pyelonephritis, (2) precoma or severe acidosis, (3) toxemia, and (4) "neglectors" (women who have not followed the recommended regimen). He observed that the presence of PBSP was associated with a greater mortality and was of better predictive value if combined with the classification of White (Table I). White's classification emphasizes duration of diabetes and vascular complications prior to pregnancy. In particular, the presence of advanced vascular disease, especially nephropathy, is associated with low birthweight infants and poor perinatal outcome. The improvement in overall survival rates in recent years appears to be the result of combined careful medical, obstetric, and pediatric management.

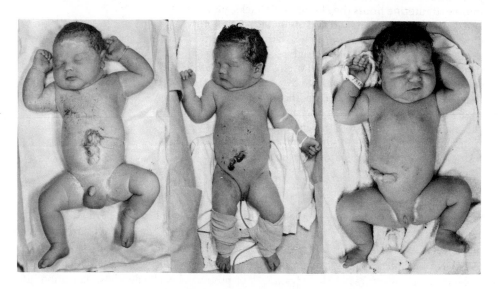

. . . for some of us are out of breath
And all of us are fat. (Lewis Carroll)

Figure 1. Unrelated infants of diabetic mothers observed by J. W. Farquhar. [From *Arch. Dis. Childhood* 34:76, 1959, with the kind permission and cooperation of Dr. Farquhar.]

Table I.   PBSP and White's Classifications Combined for 920 Infants (1959–1972)

White's Class	PBSP Present			PBSP Absent		
	No. of Cases	Perinatal Mortality No.	Perinatal Mortality Percentage	No. of Cases	Perinatal Mortality No.	Perinatal Mortality Percentage
A	35	5	14.3 ⎱ 17.1	132	4	3.0 ⎱ 3.4
B	47	9	19.1 ⎰	132	5	3.8 ⎰
C	68	20	29.4 ⎱ 26.7	155	14	9.0 ⎱ 9.8
D	119	30	25.2 ⎰	171	18	10.5 ⎰
F	48	18	37.5	13	4	30.8
Total	317	82	25.9	603	45	7.5

SOURCE: Pedersen, J., Mølsted-Pedersen, L., and Andersen, B. Assessors of fetal perinatal mortality in diabetic pregnancy. *Diabetes* 23:302, 1974.

PROBLEMS OF THE NEWBORN INFANT: IDM, INFANT OF INSULIN-DEPENDENT MOTHER, AND IGDM, INFANT OF GESTATIONAL DIABETIC MOTHER

The infant of the diabetic mother has survived diverse metabolic alterations that have profoundly affected his intrauterine growth and development. These infants may have obvious physical stigmata and multiple metabolic alterations. Although some have a prolonged stormy course, a significant number—40 to 60% of IDMs and 80% of IGDMs—have an uneventful neonatal period. The overall survival rate is 85 to 95%. Although survival is essential, the ultimate goal is a normal child. Therefore, morbidity cannot be disregarded. The consequences of congenital anomalies, respiratory distress syndrome, hypoglycemia, hypocalcemia, electrolyte abnormalities, hyperbilirubinemia, heart failure, renal vein thrombosis, and hypoparathyroidism must be considered in the management and ultimate evaluation of success of a therapeutic regimen. The frequency of complications varies between infants of gestational diabetic mothers and those of insulin-dependent diabetics (Table II).

SIZE, WEIGHT, AND WATER

In addition to their obese, plethoric, and cushingoid appearance, infants from poorly controlled mothers often have visceromegaly involving the heart, liver, and spleen and hypertrophy of the umbilical cord. Not only are they overweight for gestational age, they have increased length as well. At 260 days of gestation, the infant of the diabetic mother may be comparable with a normal infant at term with respect to weight and length. Careful obstetric-medical management tends to minimize the excess weight gain. It must be noted, however, that the small-for-gestational-age infant is at a greater risk than the larger obese infant.

Table II.   Clinical Course and Frequency of Complications (In Percent)

Complications	IDM*	IGDM†	IDM and IGDM
Uneventful course	50	80	—
Respiratory distress	30	10	20
Hypoglycemia	60	16	56
Symptomatic	20	10	—
Hypocalcemia	25	15	18 (<7 mg/100 ml)
Polycythemia	40	30	34
Hyperbilirubinemia	50	25	35
Heart failure	10 17‡	?	—
Renal vein thrombosis	?	?	2.4
Transient hematuria	8	8	—
Congenital anomalies	10	3	8

SOURCE: Refs. 6 and 11.

* Infants of insulin-dependent diabetic mothers.

† Infants of gestational diabetic mothers.

‡ Ref. 12.

These infants formerly were thought to be edematous at birth; however, pitting is not noted until after the first day of life. The data now indicate that the excessive body weight is a result of increased body fat, rather than fluid (13–15). When starved and deprived of water during the initial days after delivery, they lose more weight over a longer period than do normal infants (16). In the first 48 hr, urine volumes are larger than those from more mature infants of nondiabetic mothers. Renal sodium excretion is also higher when compared with infants of similar weight (17); however, when compared with infants of comparable gestation, this difference is insignificiant (18). Early feeding minimizes the weight loss and abolishes the difference when compared with nondiabetic controls (16).

VENTILATION AND ACID-BASE BALANCE

Prod'hom and associates (19) reported the adjustment of ventilation and acid-base balance in 20 asymptomatic white infants of diabetic mothers (classes B to F, as defined in Table III) and of 35 to 39 weeks' gestational age, delivered by elective cesarean section under spinal anesthesia. Apgar scores were greater than 4 at 1 min and above 8 at 5 min. Sixteen infants had normal x-rays of the chest; in four, there were varying degrees of hyperinflation and minimal infiltrates, and, in one, diffuse nodularity occurred at 1 hr but subsided by 24 hr. Adjustment of ventilation was found to be complete within 4 hr after delivery. A right-to-left shunt of 20 to 25% persisted throughout the first day of life. Although a slight respiratory acidosis was present for 1 to 4 hr, acid-base control was similar to that in infants of nondiabetic mothers. A low arterial pCO_2 was noted at 24 hr both in infants of diabetic mothers and in control infants. A respiratory rate above 60 was observed in 6 of 17 infants at 4 hr of age, all of whom had small tidal volumes, high physiologic dead space-to-tidal volume ratios, and relatively little increase in minute volume. These infants did not have other evidence of respiratory distress and

Table III.   Modified White Classification of Diabetes and Pregnancy

Class A—High fetal survival, no insulin, minimal dietary regulation.
    1. Gestational diabetes—abnormal glucose tolerance test during pregnancy which reverts to normal within a few weeks after delivery.
    2. Prediabetes—normal glucose tolerance test, but family history of diabetes, previous large infants or unexplained stillbirths.

Class B—Onset of diabetes in adult life after age 20 years, duration less than 10 years, no vascular disease.

Class C—Diabetes of long duration (10 to 19 years) with onset during adolescence (over 10 years) with minimal vascular disease.

Class D—Diabetes of 20 years of more duration, onset before age 10 years, evidence of vascular disease (i.e., retinitis, albuminuria, hypertension).

Class F—Patients with D plus nephritis and retinitis proliferans.

SOURCE: Refs. 4 and 10.

were otherwise well. These authors concluded that asymptomatic infants of diabetic mothers have as good ventilatory and acid-base control as normal infants.

RESPIRATORY DISTRESS

One of the most serious neonatal complications is respiratory distress.* Robert and associates (21) have surveyed 815 diabetic pregnancies from the Joslin Clinic population and confirmed the increased risk of these newborns for respiratory distress syndrome. Although RDS was previously considered to be due to such factors as the increased frequency of prematurity and delivery by cesarean section, this study demonstrated an increased risk of RDS in infants of insulin-dependent mothers irrespective of the gestational age or mode of delivery. Respiratory distress may be due to pulmonary edema, transient tachypnea, or hyaline membrane disease; or it may be related to intracranial anomalies or hemorrhage, cardiac failure, or aspiration. Pneumothorax or diaphragmatic hernia must also be considered. In addition to careful physical examination, roentgen studies are necessary to clarify the diagnosis. The presence of a fine, diffuse bilateral reticulogranular appearance in the x-ray of the chest is consistent with the diagnosis of respiratory distress syndrome associated with hyaline membrane disease.

The clinical criteria for diagnosis of hyaline membrane disease initially include an expiratory grunt, followed shortly by a pattern of difficult inspiratory breathing with retraction of the sternum and intercostal spaces while the abdomen is protruded. Later, flaring of the alae nasi and cyanosis may be present. The infant is irritable, with a "complaining cry" and hoarseness. The inspiratory effort is brief, and expiration is prolonged. Fine crackling rales may be heard. In infants whose course is unfavorable, an ashen color is associated with a fall in body temperature, declining respiratory rate, and apneic episodes. Both a respiratory and metabolic acidosis—(increased lactic acid

* This subject has been treated extensively by Avery and Fletcher in *The Lung and Its Disorders in the Newborn Infant* (23). The reader is referred to this source for a discussion of pulmonary physiology, diagnosis, and management.

and carbon dioxide tension, reduced buffer base, and decreased pH—are usually observed in the severe respiratory distress syndrome. Electrolyte abnormalities, including azotemia, hyperkalemia, and hyperphosphatemia, may occasionally be noted in these infants if the prenatal course has been difficult. These may be similar to the findings in "distressed" infants noted earlier by McCance and Widdowson (22).

Smith et al. (24) have studied lecithin synthesis and cellular growth in monolayer cell cultures from rabbit fetal lungs in late gestation. They found that cortisol enhances lecithin synthesis and reduces cellular growth. The addition of insulin abolishes the stimulatory effect of cortisol on lecithin synthesis but does not affect its growth-inhibiting activity. These observations may provide an important basis for understanding the pathogenesis of the increased frequency of respiratory distress syndrome observed in infants of diabetic mothers.

CARBOHYDRATE METABOLISM

Following delivery, glucose concentrations in offspring of diabetic mothers decline rapidly to values below those observed in normals. Approximately 60% of babies from insulin-dependent mothers (IDMs) have glucose concentrations below 30 mg/100 ml in the first 6 hr of life (25,26), as compared with a frequency of approximately 15% in infants of gestational diabetic mothers (IGDMs see Table II).

Observations by McCann et al. (27,28) and Chen et al. (29) have indicated that infants of diabetic mothers may be subdivided into those from mothers with gestational diabetes and those born of mothers with insulin-dependent diabetes. The infants from mothers with gestational diabetes had, on the average, lower blood sugars and free fatty acids (FFA) at 2 hr of age than did normal infants; however, the values were higher than those found in infants of insulin-dependent mothers. The rate of fall in blood sugar immediately after delivery was slowest in the normal infants, intermediate in the infants of mothers with gestational diabetes, and most rapid in those of insulin-dependent diabetics (Fig. 2).

The initial rate of fall in glucose concentration varied directly with the concentration in maternal blood at the time of delivery, with very high levels resulting in an initial precipitous decline. Light et al. (30) showed in a study of 18 infants of diabetic mothers that the cord blood glucose level was related to the rate of glucose infusion to the mother during delivery, to the route of delivery, and to the severity of the maternal diabetes. They found that the higher the cord blood glucose level, the more rapid the disappearance of glucose, the lower the level to which the glucose concentration falls, and the greater the prevalence of hypoglycemia during the first hours of life. In many infants, blood sugar rises spontaneously after 4 to 6 hr to values not unlike those found in infants of nondiabetics.

The course of changes in the blood sugar level in the hypoglycemic infants usually follows one of three patterns. The majority have a transient, asymptomatic phase soon after birth that lasts between 1 and 4 hr; then a spontaneous rise occurs. Some infants have a prolonged intial phase of hypoglycemia, often severe, below 15 mg/100 ml, which may persist for several hours and be associated with symptoms. Others, after an apparently benign initial phase, develop symptomatic hypoglycemia after 12 to 24 hr or as late as 5 days of age. Pennoyer and Hartmann (25) found that among 38 babies with blood sugar values under 30 mg/100 ml, only 16 had symptoms. Of these, only 5 did

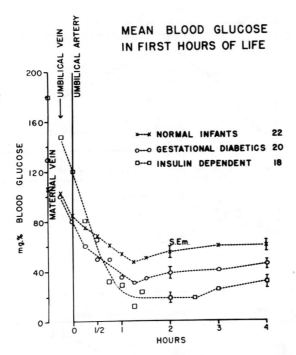

Figure 2. Serial changes in the concentration of glucose in the blood of infants immediately following delivery. The group from mothers with gestational diabetes had abnormal intravenous glucose tolerance tests during pregnancy but received no insulin therapy. [Adapted from McCann et al. *N. Engl. J. Med.* 275:1, 1966.]

not have associated problems that could have contributed to the clinical manifestations. Symptoms such as apnea, tachypnea, cyanosis, limpness, failure to suck, absence of the Moro reflex, listlessness, convulsions, and coma may be related to hypoglycemia alone or may be secondary to other pathologic conditions.

TREATMENT

When symptoms and hypoglycemia coexist at any age, therapy directed at elevating the concentration of glucose in the blood should be initiated. A prompt response to therapy is evidence that hypoglycemia was indeed the cause of the symptoms. However, if the hypoglycemia has been of long duration or if the symptoms are due to other causes, either a partial or delayed response to therapy may occur. During the first hours of life, glucagon in high dosage—300 μg/kg IV or IM to a maximum of 1 mg total dose—can elevate the blood sugar level for 2 to 3 hr in most infants (26) (Fig. 3). Wu et al. (31) have minimized the fall in blood glucose in IDMs by the intravenous administration of 30 μg/kg glucagon within 15 min after delivery. However, if the infant is severely ill, glucose administered intravenously is the treatment of choice. Unless blood sugar levels can be measured at 2- to 6-hr intervals, neither form of therapy may be adequate to keep the blood sugar at a proper level.

As noted above, meticulous control of maternal glucose during labor and delivery

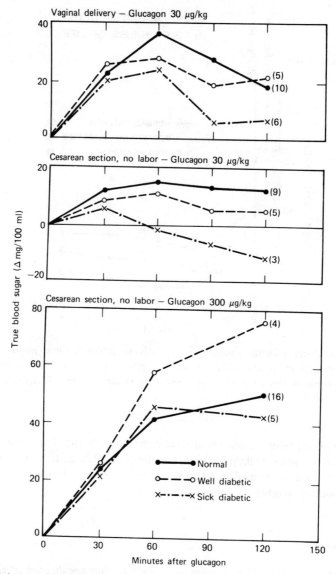

Figure 3. Relation of labor in the mother and condition of the infant to the concentration of blood sugar following small and large doses of glucagon. All infants were two hours of age or younger. [From Cornblath et a. *Pediatrics* 28:592, 1961.]

minimizes the frequency of hypoglycemia in the neonate. Various regimens for controlling blood glucose have been recommended (28), but none has been proved to have an advantage over intravenous glucose. Haworth et al. (32) found that a bolus injection of glucose produced marked variation in glucose levels from hyper- to hypoglycemia. Furthermore, epinephrine therapy was of no advantage and even produced serious lactic acidosis. McCann et al. (28) have administered a combination of glucose and fructose or fructose alone as a single injection soon after delivery to well infants of mothers with gestational diabetes, producing an elevated level of glucose for 2 or 3 hr. Infants treated with a combination of glucose and fructose were observed by Bergman et al. (33) to have higher blood glucose values at 24 hr of age compared with controls. Since fructose therapy has not been critically evaluated and may be dangerous to the undiagnosed infant with hereditary fructose intolerance, other treatment is preferable.

The significance of hypoglycemia without symptoms remains unknown. No specific recommendations for therapy for these asymptomatic infants seem justified. However, in those infants with excessively low blood sugar values—under 20 mg/100 ml—that persist for more than 1 hr, conservative management consists of supporting the blood glucose level.

CALCIUM METABOLISM

In addition to the electrolyte and acid-base derangement associated with the respiratory distress syndrome, occasional sick infants have other alterations related to calcium metabolism. Hypocalcemia with tetany is now recognized as a significant complication in the infant of the diabetic mother (33–38). Chvostek sign, carpopedal spasm, and Trousseau sign are unreliable indicators of tetany in any newborn infant. Neuromuscular and behavioral alterations have been described, but many of the symptoms and signs are nonspecific and similar to those described for hypoglycemia and hypoxia. Hyperexcitability seems to be a common observation.

Gittleman et al. (36) observed that 6 of 22 infants of diabetic mothers had serum calcium levels below 8.0 mg/100 ml, which was considered abnormal on the first day of life. In another group of infants of prediabetic mothers, who had either gestational or noninsulin-dependent diabetes, 7 of 36 infants had similarly low levels. Since most of these infants were delivered preterm, their calcium levels should be compared with those of infants of like gestation and mode of delivery. Previously, Gittleman et al. (39) had shown that many low birthweight infants may have low serum calcium values without symptoms. In infants delivered by elective cesarean section for cephalopelvic disproportion or for repeat cesarean section, hypocalcemia was noted in 13.7%. A similar incidence, 11.8%, was found for infants delivered by elective cesarean section in well-controlled diabetics. Tsang et al. (37) prospectively studied 28 infants of diabetic mothers with a comparable matched control group. The incidence of hypocalcemia was significantly increased in the infants of diabetic mothers, even when gestational age and perinatal complication were taken into consideration. It is of some interest that the low levels of calcium may persist, as in the two infants of diabetic mothers who were found to have idiopathic hypoparathyroidism (40).

The mechanism of the hypocalcemia in these infants is unknown. A decrease in serum protein concentrations and calcium binding does not explain the findings. Renal studies demonstrated no differences in excretion of calcium, magnesium, and phosphorus in infants of diabetic mothers compared with normal controls (37). The response of the kidney to exogenous parathormone was normal, as shown by a decrease in calcium and an increase in phosphate excretion. Since serum calcium was higher in the diabetic mothers, Tsang (37,38) speculated that relative maternal hyperparathyroidism leads to fetal hypoparathyroidism with resultant neonatal hypocalcemia. Serum parathyroid levels during the first 48 hr of life were compatible with this hypothesis but not conclusive (38). Although Bergman (33) verified the previously reported incidence of hypocalcemia in infants of diabetic mothers, he noted a significant decrease in ultrafilterable calcium. He also measured plasma parathyroid hormone values in four infants (IDMs); only one had an elevated level, and the others had low values. Calcitonin values in cord blood were in the same range as those of the adult; however, a significant rise occurred by 24 hr after birth in controls as well. In the IDMs there was a negative correlation between total calcium and calcitonin. Bergman suggested that hypoglycemia may be related to secretion of glucagon, which in turn stimulates calcitonin release. The latter would then inhibit mobilization of calcium from bone, thereby causing hypocalcemia. Unfortunately, this attractive hypothesis is not supported by the preliminary studies of Bloom and Johnston (41), who report diminished rather than increased glucagon levels in infants of diabetic mothers.

TREATMENT

Diagnosis of symptomatic hypocalcemia depends on obtaining a serum calcium determination and must be differentiated from manifestations of central nervous system disease, hypoglycemia, hypoxia, and other metabolic abnormalities. An electrocardiogram may be helpful in recognizing the infant with hypocalcemia, since prolongation of the QT interval may be present. Once the diagnosis of hypocalcemic tetany is suspected and blood obtained, intravenous calcium gluconate—5 to 10 ml as a 10% solution— should be given slowly and immediately, with EKG monitoring to avoid heart block. Thereafter, either calcium lactate or gluconate, in a total dosage of 1 to 2 g of calcium daily, may be given orally. Therapy may be continued by mouth for 1 week, with repeated determinations of serum calcium concentrations. Therapy should also include feedings of a low-solute milk with added calcium to provide a Ca : P ratio of 2 to 4 : 1 (g/g).

BILIRUBIN METABOLISM

Hyperbilirubinemia occurs more commonly in infants of diabetic mothers than in controls of comparable weight or gestation (42–44). Taylor et al. (44) reported that the serum bilirubin values in umbilical cord blood from infants of diabetic mothers were similar to values from controls, but significant differences in bilirubin concentrations between the groups were apparent at 48 hr of age. The 48-hr value for serum bilirubin did not correlate with the value for umbilical cord blood, with the degree of hepatomegaly or splenomegaly, or with the presence of edema. Although the number of nucleated red blood cells was high initially, a sharp drop was found on the second and third day of life. Hematologic studies did not suggest an explanation of the mechanism of the phenomenon. In particular, there was no evidence for increased hemolysis. Olsen et al. (43) drew similar conclusions from 94 surviving infants. Vaginal delivery was associated with a higher incidence of serum bilirubin, above 20 mg/100 ml, than was cesarean section. It was known that complicated vaginal delivery predisposes to hyperbilirubinemia. The observations of Zetterström et al. (42), who first emphasized the problem of hyperbilirubinemia in the infant of the diabetic mother, have not been confirmed with respect to the high incidence of ABO isoimmunization. It is noteworthy that kernicterus apparently is a rare complication of hyperbilirubinemia in these infants, even though hypoglycemia, asphyxia, and anoxia are often present and considered predisposing factors.

Effects of Early Feeding

Hubbell et al. (45) investigated the effects of early and late feeding of infants of diabetic mothers in the management of the respiratory distress syndrome. These authors found that infants fed as early as 4 hr after delivery had lower serum bilirubin levels at 72 hr of age than did the paired infants who had been fasted for 48 hr. Of 48 pairs of infants, 5 of the early-fed group versus 16 in the fasted group had serum bilirubin values above 20 mg/100 ml. The mechanism for this difference is unknown, although a relationship to glucose metabolism and glucuronide conjugation has been suggested. Volume changes with weight loss alone cannot account for these differences.

OTHER CLINICAL COMPLICATIONS

The sick infant of the diabetic mother may have a variety of other clinical problems, including intracranial, adrenal, or renal hemorrhage, congenital anomalies, renal vein thrombosis, or congestive heart failure. Roentgen examination often reveals a large heart in asymptomatic infants; this finding alone is not an indication for digitalization. In the presence of a rapidly enlarging liver, tachypnea, and tachycardia, however, such therapy is suggested. Seratto et al. (12) studied 42 consecutive infants of diabetic mothers; 20 of these were born to mothers with gestational diabetes. Multiple clinical problems were observed, including cardiorespiratory complications. Of 19 patients with tachypnea, 7 were found to have "wet lung" syndrome by x-ray, 7 were in congestive failure, 2 had infiltrates or aspiration pneumonia, and 4 had no abnormal x-ray changes. Abnormal electrocardiograms were observed in 15 patients. Of the 7 infants with congestive heart failure, 1 died, 6 had associated hypoglycemia, and 2 were hypocalcemic.

Renal Vein Thrombosis

Maternal diabetes was first recognized as a predisposing factor to renal vein thrombosis in the infant reported by Avery, Oppenheimer, and Gordon in 1957 (46). Since then Takeuchi and Benirschke (47) have reported a series of 16 cases, 5 from mothers with diabetes, 7 from prediabetics (presumptive), and 4 from women with unproved diabetic status. The incidence in infants born to diabetic mothers is unknown, although Francois et al. (5) found 4 of 168 with this complication. The presence of a mass in the flank or abdomen associated with proteinuria and hematuria suggests the diagnosis. Unilateral thrombosis may be treated conservatively and by nephrectomy (48). The pathogenesis of this complication is speculative at best; most authors have suggested it arises from polycythemia and local stasis of blood in renal veins, which could be secondary to an osmotic diuresis brought about by hyperglycemia. However this hypothesis is inadequate to explain the occurrence of thrombosis in infants born to mothers with prediabetes. The mechanism remains obscure. Transient hematuria of unknown origin has also been noted in both IDMs and IGDMs (11).

Polycythemia

The pathogenic basis for the increased hematopoiesis observed in the liver, the erythrocytosis (polycythemia), and the renal vein thrombosis (see above) remains ill-defined. Schwartz and associates (49) have speculated that these complications might be secondary to fetal hypoxia. Further, they have suggested a potential limitation in maternofetal oxygen transfer in pregnant diabetic women. Hemoglobin A_{Ic} (HbA_{Ic}), a normal minor variant of HbA, has glucose linked to the terminal valine of the beta chain. This glycohemoglobin, which does not interact well with 2,3-diphosphoglycerate (DPG), has a relatively high affinity for oxygen. The deoxyconformation of hemoglobin A, in contrast, facilitates DPG binding to the beta chains, stabilizing this conformation and lessening oxygen affinity. Schwartz et al. (49) have observed a significant increase in HbA_{Ic} as a percentage of total hemoglobin during the third trimester of pregnancy in women with gestational diabetes or insulin-dependent diabetes. Recent data suggest that these changes are acquired and are related to hyperglycemia. Widness and associates (49a) have related HbA_{Ic} in third trimester maternal blood to infant's birth weight as well as to degree of maternal glucose control (49b). Bleicher and Pang (50) noted an increase in erythrocyte 2,3-DPG of 30 to 35% during pregnancy. This increase was not modified by gestational or insulin-dependent diabetes. They note that there is conflicting data on maternal $P_{50}O_2$ during pregnancy. Future studies of organic phosphate intermediates and of oxygen transport between maternal and fetal blood in diabetic pregnancies should clarify this problem.

Neonatal Small Left Colon Syndrome

Davis and Campbell (51) have noted an unusually high incidence of obstruction in the lower part of the colon in infants of insulin-dependent mothers. Barium enema frequently reveals a colon uniformly narrowed from the splenic flexure to the anus; this disorder was observed in 8 of 20 symptomatic infants of insulin-dependent mothers. In a prospective analysis, the same authors observed similar roentgenographic features in 6 of 12 asymptomatic IDMs. The pathogenesis of this left-colonic lesion is obscure. No surgical intervention is required.

Congenital Anomalies

The infants of diabetic mothers have an increased incidence of congenital malformation (52–54). Recently, Pedersen et al. (55) reported an incidence of congenital anomalies of 6.4% in offspring of diabetic mothers as compared with 2.1% in a control group. They suggested that the incidence was correlated with the severity of vascular complications in the mother. Insulin reactions and hypoglycemia did not appear to affect the incidence of congenital malformations. Farquhar (56) reviewed 329 diabetic pregnancies with 251 survivors at late follow-up. He observed an 8.9% incidence of all types of malformations in those offspring from mothers treated with insulin and a 10.3% incidence in those treated by diet alone. Kucera (57) analyzed the world literature of 7101 fetuses from nine geographic and ethnic areas. Offspring of diabetic mothers had 4.79% incidence of anomalies compared with 0.65% for World Health Organization controls. There have been suggestions of higher frequency of skeletal malformations, including sacral agenesis. Soler et al. (58) have analyzed data for 701 infants born to diabetic women between 1950 and 1974 in Birmingham, England. The incidence of malformations in this series was 8.1% (three to four times the rate for the normal population); 3.8% of the infants had fatal malformations, Rowland and associates (59) reviewed 470 infants of diabetic mothers from the Joslin Clinic. Proved heart disease, with a 4% incidence, was five times that expected in the general population. Although the types of heart anomalies were highly variable, transposition of the great arteries, ventricular septal defect, and coarctation of the aorta together accounted for over one-half of the 19 cases reported. These authors observed no relationship between gestational factors and the incidence of heart defects. In recent years, the improvement in the management of the diabetic mother and her infant has been responsible for increasing the number of survivors. Thus the importance of diagnosing and treating correctable anomalies in these infants is apparent. Planned pregnancies with meticulous control prior to and during conception and organogenesis may be necessary in addition to prevention of long-term complications.

PATHOLOGY

The placenta of the diabetic mother is not remarkable. The fine structure of the chorionic villi is normal, and the capillary and epithelial basement membranes are not increased in width. Arteriolar narrowing of the placental bed is not a feature of this condition unless preeclamptic toxemia is present. However, Okudaira et al. (60), using electron microscopy in 13 placentas from patients with maternal diabetes, found that the most significant and constant alteration was an increase in basement membrane material in terminal chorionic villi, involving both the epithelial and capillary basement membrane and the stroma. Often there is excess amniotic fluid (61), the explanation of which is not apparent.

Gabbe et al. (62) have compared glycogen metabolism in placentas from full-term normal pregnancies with those from diabetic pregnancies. Vaginal and cesarean section had no effect on the values obtained in normal women. Glycogen concentrations were elevated in placentas from diabetic patients, although synthetase I levels were decreased. Both phosphorylase a and total phosphorylase were increased in diabetic placentas. Placental weights were decreased in patients with retinitis proliferans. These investigators suggested that insulin may be a controlling factor in placental glycogen metabolism and that hyperglycemia with increased glycogen may be responsible for the enzyme changes.

The infant of the diabetic mother shows characteristic pathologic alterations that explain, in part, his clinical condition. First, the large size observed at term is the result of increased body fat, rather than edema. Total body water is decreased (13), and fat determined by direct whole body tissue analysis is increased (15). The composition of adipose tissue fat with respect to long-chain fatty acids does not differ from that in normal infants (63). In infants delivered before term, gigantism and splanchnomegaly are less evident. The striking pathologic feature is the hypertrophy and hyperplasia of the beta cells in the islets of Langerhans (64–66). Van Assche (67) has found that the islets from babies whose mothers had reduced carbohydrate tolerance contain an increased proportion of β cells and silver-staining (Ag+) cells and those from babies with erythroblastosis or α-thalassemia do not. The latter, however, do show an increase in number and size of the islets of Langerhans. In addition, the pancreas has an unusual infiltrate of eosinophils. A similar eosinophilic infiltration has been observed in guinea pigs following the injection of large amounts of antibody to guinea pig insulin.

In these infants the liver has not always been found to be enlarged and glycogen-laden, but increased hematopoiesis has been a consistent observation. The heart is often overweight and enlarged. The brain is small for both body weight and gestation. The lungs frequently have features of hyaline membrane disease and hemorrhage (23). The kidneys show varying degrees of immaturity, as evidenced by fetal glomeruli, and this observation supports the concept that the infants are immature relative to their size. Hemorrhages have been reported in the adrenal gland and kidneys. Renal vein thrombosis also seems to occur more frequently in these infants. The pituitary and adrenal gland often do not have any demonstrable abnormalities.

PATHOPHYSIOLOGY

No single hypothesis has been proposed that satisfactorily accounts for the diverse metabolic abnormalities of the infant of the diabetic or prediabetic mother. Attention has been focused primarily on beta cell hyperplasia and glucose homeostasis. Although such infants have a rapid fall in the concentration of blood sugar in the period following delivery (25,68,69), the mechanism for this has only recently been demonstrated to differ from that observed in normal infants (see Fig. 2) (27). The administration of intravenous glucose, as in a tolerance test, results in a prompt, rapid disposal of glucose from the blood when compared with similar observations in infants of nondiabetic mothers (70) (Fig. 4). Understanding of the relationship between carbohydrate and fat metabolism has been extended with the elucidation of the role of free fatty acids (FFA) in blood plasma; this is a fraction of long-chain C_{12}-C_{18} fatty acids that exist in low concentrations bound to albumin in the plasma. FFA have a very rapid turnover and are an important source of energy for a variety of tissues (71). Previously, FFA have been shown to be elevated during starvation, in diabetes, and following the administration of epinephrine, growth hormone, or corticosteroid. Conversely, plasma FFA levels have been depressed by administration of glucose, glucagon, or insulin. Glucose uptake by adipose tissue inhibits FFA release, and glucose deprivation or unavailability stimulates FFA release. This concept has been extended to include a glucose–fatty acid cycle existing among adipose tissue, plasma, and muscle FFA in which the control of these factors by insulin is critical (72).

Melichar, Novak, Hahn, and Koldovsky (73) have reported low values of plasma FFA and glucose in infants of diabetic mothers. Chen and associates (29) have studied levels of glucose and FFA in plasma from infants of normal mothers, of gestational diabetics, and of insulin-dependent diabetics (Figs. 5 and 6). At delivery, maternal plasma FFA levels of diabetics were higher than those of control women, whether or not they were given glucose intravenously during labor and delivery. Plasma levels of FFA, both from the umbilical artery and vein, were low in all infants. In the infants of diabetic mothers, plasma free fatty acids rose to low normal levels by 120 min after birth, whereas values in control infants were significantly higher (Fig. 7). Persson et al. (74) confirmed the low plasma FFA concentrations in infants of diabetic mothers but showed that this reduction was accompanied by a rise in plasma glycerol. They suggested an increased rate of reesterification of FFA in adipose tissue to explain this dissociation. Another possible explanation is that FFA may have been used for energy, while glycerol

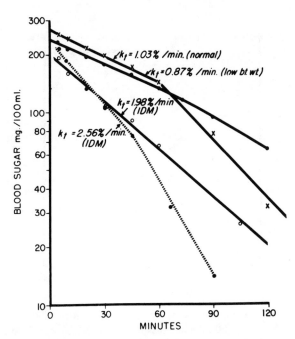

Figure 4. A semilogarithmic graph of blood glucose following intravenous injection of 1 g of glucose per kilogram of body weight. The rates of glucose disappearance (k_t) for normal (103) and low birth weight (104) infants are given for comparison. The two infants of diabetic mothers with fast k_t's were studied by Dr. Beverly F. Likly and provided data similar to those obtained by Baird and Farquhar (70).

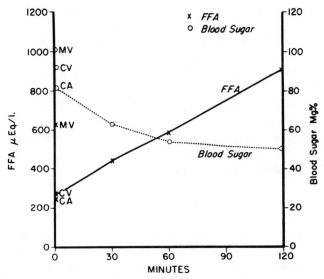

Figure 5. Data obtained from a vaginally delivered infant whose mother received glucose intravenously during labor. MV, CV and CA refer to maternal vein, umbilical cord vein, and cord artery. Observe the rapid rise in free fatty acid (FFA) in the normal infant at two hours of age. [From Cornblath, M., and Schwartz, R. *Disorders of Carbohydrate Metabolism in Infancy,* 2nd ed. W. B. Saunders Co., 1976.]

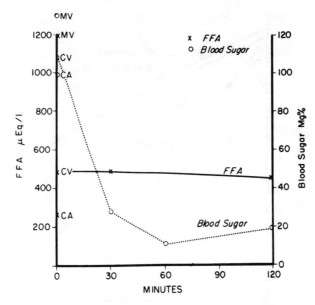

Figure 6. Data obtained in a vaginally delivered infant of a diabetic mother. In this patient, glucose fell to values below 30 mg/100 ml while plasma free fatty acids remained suppressed. These data suggest physiologic hyperinsulinism in the infant of the diabetic mother. [From Cornblath, M., and Schwartz, R. *Disorders of Carbohydrate Metabolism in Infancy*, 2nd ed. W. B. Saunders Co., 1976.]

accumulated because of a block in gluconeogenesis or decreased phosphorylation. Persson et al. (74) also determined β-hydroxybutyrate at birth in IDMs, IGDMs, and control infants. Maternal vein and umbilical vein values of β-hydroxybutyrate were directly correlated in all groups; IGDMs were found to have the highest levels. All groups of infants showed a significant fall in β-hydroxybutyrate levels during the first 30 to 60 min after birth; thereafter, the concentrations remained low and were essentially unchanged. Plasma total lipids in venous blood from the umbilical cord are low in infants from both diabetic and nondiabetic mothers (75,76). However, plasma cholesterol and phospholipid values tend to be slightly higher in the infant of diabetic mothers, even though maternal plasma contains much higher concentrations of the lipid fractions at delivery.

These physiologic observations of levels of glucose and free fatty acids suggest a state of functional hyperinsulinism in the infant of the diabetic mother. Baird and Farquhar (70) measured insulinlike activity in plasma using the rat diaphragm technique. Fasting values in six infants of diabetic mothers were similar to values in normal infants; however, following intravenous glucose, a greater rise in insulinlike activity was found in the former group. Hyperinsulinemia using radioimmunoassay techniques has now been reported in umbilical cord plasma from infants of mothers with gestational diabetes (77,78). There is a broad overlap with some normal values observed, suggesting that this represents a heterogeneous population. In most instances the elevated insulin level is appropriate for the degree of hyperglucosemia; however, in some cases there are disproportionately elevated insulin levels (Fig. 8).

Because of the transfer of maternal antibody to the fetus, radioimmunoassay of plasma from infants of insulin-treated mothers is unreliable unless maternal antibody is low. This technique has been obviated by the recent observation of Block et al. (79), who found elevated levels of C peptide, the connecting segment of the proinsulin molecule, in umbilical plasma from infants of diabetic mothers. Kalhan et al. (80) have shown that human insulin labeled with iodine-I^{125} does not cross the placenta to the fetus in either term normal women or diabetic women.

Studies performed on infants of gestationally diabetic mothers immediately after delivery have produced varied results as to insulin release. Acute glucose tolerance tests first performed by Isles and Farquhar (81,82) demonstrated a sharp early peak with a late delayed rise similar to that seen in normal adults but unlike that of normal infants; in normal infants the initial peak was minimal (Fig. 9). Pildes et al. (83) found in the IGDM an early rise in tolerance to oral glucose administered on the first day of life, as

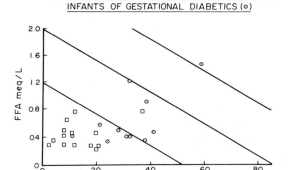

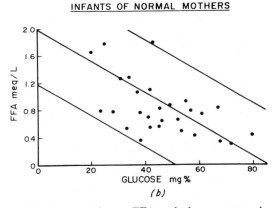

Figure 7. The relationship between plasma FFA and glucose at two hours of age in normal infants (●) and infants of diabetic mothers. Note that infants from insulin-dependent mothers (□) had both hypoglucosemia and suppressed free fatty acids while those from gestational diabetic mothers (O) overlapped the normal population. The lines represent the correlation (m plus 2 s.d.) for normal infants. [From observations of Schwartz, R., and associates. Modified from Chen, C.H., et al. *Pediatrics* 36:843, 1965]

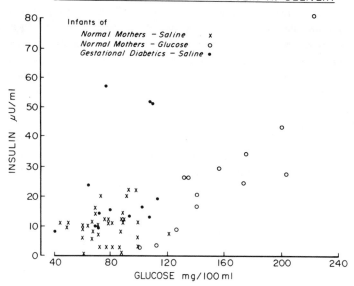

Figure 8. The effects of continued glucose infusion to normal mothers and gestationally diabetic mothers during labor upon umbilical plasma glucose and insulin levels at delivery. Note the overlap in insulin values for the infants of gestational diabetic mothers. [Personal observations of Schwartz, R., and associates. From Camerini-Davalos. R. A., and Cole. H. S. (eds.). *Early Diabetes in Early Life*. New York, Academic Press, Inc., 1975, p. 131. Modified from original observations of Obenshain et al. *N. Engl. J. Med.* 283:566, 1970.]

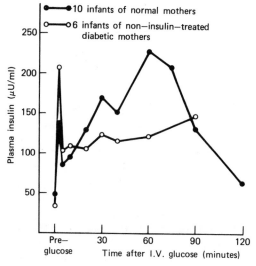

Figure 9. Mean plasma insulin levels following intravenous glucose 0.5 g/kg body weight). [From Isles, Dickson, and Farquhar. *Pediat. Res.* 2:198, 1968.]

626

compared with values for controls (Fig. 10). King et al. (84) could not distinguish between groups by the response to continuous infusion of glucose at high rates—12 to 24 mg/kg/min—at 2 hr of age. In the IGDM, intravenous arginine resulted in a slightly higher insulin response than in the normal infant; however, conversion to glucose, as judged from a rise in plasma glucose, was increased (85). Kalhan et al. (86) have determined glucose turnover by the prime-constant infusion technique of Steele, using glucose-l^{13}C. They have found turnover of glucose to be low in two IDMs— 2.8 and 3.2 mg/kg/min—compared with four normals—4.42 ± 0.39 mg/kg/min—studied at 2 hr of age. They suggest that variable intrauterine hyperglycemia and hyperinsulinemia in the IDM inhibited hepatic production of glucose immediately after birth.

These observations support the hypothesis of Pedersen (68) that maternal hyperglycemia may be an important factor in the metabolic abnormalities of such infants. According to this hypothesis, fetal hyperglycemia stimulates release of insulin by fetal islet cells, giving rise to persistent hyperinsulinism in the fetus. The insulin promotes glucose uptake in a variety of organs and tissues, including adipose tissue. The surfeit of glucose in the presence of excess insulin produces the characteristic obesity. This attractive theory is consistent with the observations in manifest diabetes. However, there is no evidence that latent or prediabetes is associated with fluctuations in the level of blood glucose in the pregnant woman; yet some infants from these women have the same embryopathy as infants of overtly diabetic mothers.

Other explanations of pathogenesis have even less evidence to support them. A genetic influence was suggested from the observations of Jackson (87) that infants of diabetic fathers have features similar to those of infants whose mothers are diabetic.

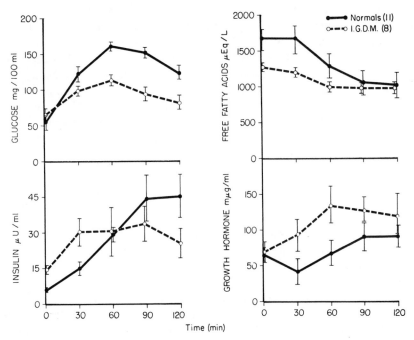

Figure 10. Blood glucose, plasma insulin, free fatty acids, and growth hormone values (mean ± S.E.) at fasting and during oral glucose tolerance tests in normal newborns and IGDM. [From Pildes, Hart, Warrner, and Cornblath. *Pediatrics* 44:76, 1969.]

This report has remained controversial. The adrenocortical theory suggested that hyperadrenocorticism was a major factor in diabetic embryopathy (88). However, the levels of plasma 17-hydroxycorticosteroids are similar in diabetic and control mothers at delivery, and the values in cord plasma are low (89). Hypercorticism prior to delivery remains unproved. It is true that urinary excretion of adrenal corticoids appears to be increased during the first days of life (90), but these data are inadequately controlled for the mode of delivery, and their significance has yet to be determined. Similarly, the pituitary growth hormone hypothesis is based on the large size and excessive growth of these infants. The data of Kalkhoff et al. (91) indicate that levels of growth hormone–like substances in cord plasma are elevated, but less so in infants of diabetic mothers than in controls. Joassin et al. (78) found growth hormone levels determined by radioimmunoassay to be similar to those of normal infants. Stern et al. (92) and Light and associates (93) have found diminished urinary catecholamines in some infants of diabetic mothers with low blood glucose values. Bloom and Johnston (41) have noted low plasma glucagon values persisting in the first hours of life in a comparable group of infants. Similarly, Luyckx et al. (94) reported a fall in glucagon after intravenous glucose in the IDM as contrasted to a rise in controls. Williams and associates (95) observed less increase in plasma glucagon in the first hour of life in infants of insulin-treated mothers than in normal infants or in those whose mothers were treated with diet alone. In contrast to control infants, IDMs given an intravenous bolus of alanine—150 mg/kg—at 1 hr of age did not show a rise in either blood glucose or glucagon. These observations require verification but raise questions concerning the role of counterregulatory factors in glucose homeostasis.

The final analysis of this complex problem will require techniques for study of the fetus in utero. The influence of the maternal environment is evident in overt diabetes. Maintenance of normoglycemia in the pregnant diabetic prevents excessive fetal growth. On the other hand, pathologic manifestations are present in some instances that suggest that factors intrinsic to the fetus may also be important. Peel (96) has reported an example of biovular twins, one of whom weighed 9 lb 2 oz at 37 weeks and was a typical "cushingoid" infant, and the other was 4 lb 12 oz and appeared normal. The placentas weighed 2 lb 10 oz and 14 oz, respectively. No data on blood sugars were available for these infants. Insulin may be an important fetal growth factor.

MANAGEMENT

Meticulous, ongoing, and cooperative management of the mother's diabetes and prenatal care are critical for the optimal outcome of the specific pregnancy. Therefore, the preparation for this event should be initiated at an appropriate age once the diagnosis of insulin-dependent diabetes mellitus has been established in the female child. This must be individualized but should be considered in the education of the preadolescent age group.

It is clear that the best way to attain optimal survival rates is by a collaborative effort on the part of the pediatrician, the obstetrician, and the internist. The pregnant diabetic requires careful supervision throughout pregnancy (97). Control of diet, activity, and insulin are necessary to achieve a stable maternal environment for the fetus (98). Prolonged and early hospitalization may be an economic way to achieve this. At delivery, meticulous attention to glucose and insulin administration is necessary to control maternal blood glucose within the normoglycemic range. Ketosis must be avoided throughout pregnancy and delivery. Delivery for the permanent diabetic is best individualized and may vary from 35 weeks to term, depending on the results of fetal and maternal monitoring. The gestational diabetic or prediabetic should be permitted to go to term unless monitoring suggests compromise of the fetoplacental unit.

Following delivery at a regional perinatal center, the initial management of the infant should be the responsibility of a pediatrician who is knowledgeable in the total care of the high-risk newborn. Apgar scores at 1 and 5 min after delivery are important and of prognostic value. After respirations are established, gastric emptying to obtain the volume of the stomach contents is indicated as a diagnostic measure for intestinal obstruction; the relationship of gastric aspiration to the subsequent development of the respiratory distress syndrome is still not established. Ideally, the precise state of control of the mother's diabetes at delivery will be known to the pediatrician. Blood sugar values should be obtained for maternal and cord veins at delivery. Thereafter, serial blood sugar determinations from peripheral sites for 1, 2, 4, and 6 hr will define the degree of hypoglycemia. Regardless of their size and maturity these infants should be cared for in an intensive-care nursery. Temperature, humidity, and oxygen should be monitored carefully and regulated according to the infant's response. Routine utilization of high oxygen and humidity is not indicated. Early—before 4 to 6 hr—oral feedings with glucose or water are recommended unless complications are present. Antibiotics are given only for known or suspected infections and not prophylactically.

A large proportion—40 to 60% of IDMs and 80% of IGDMs—of infants will have a relatively uneventful course and require nothing more than careful observation with determinations of base line electrolytes, glucose, bilirubin, and hematocrit values and a routine urinalysis before discharge. Even these infants, however, may be poor feeders, regain weight slowly, and require longer hospitalization than infants of nondiabetic mothers.

The following management procedures are recommended for the complications that occur in these infants (see Table II).

Therapy for the respiratory distress syndrome requires an intensive-care nursery with specialized personnel, equipment, and laboratory support. Attention must be given to body temperature, airway patency, oxygenation, and acid-base status. This requires arterial blood analyses, measurements for hypovolemia and anemia, chest roentgenograms, as well as determinations of fluid and electrolyte balance, all of which are critical. Adequate oxygenation may be achieved by increasing ambient oxygen concentration through continuous mechanical ventilation. Details of therapy may be found in the recommendations of Avery and Fletcher (23) and Tooley (99).

The transient asymptomatic hypoglycemia—glucose levels less than 20 mg/100 ml—during the first hours of life may be prevented (81) and will respond to intravenous glucagon—300 μg/kg body weight to a maximum total dose of 1 mg—(see Fig. 3). In addition to the glucagon, sick infants with hypoglycemia should be given intravenous glucose. In our experience, an initial single intravenous injection of 0.5 to 1.0 gm glucose per kilogram body weight as 25% glucose should be given; this initial dose must be followed by a continuous infusion of glucose in water at a rate of 4 to 8 mg/kg/min. The concentration of glucose depends on the total water requirement. (For example, at 6 mg/kg/min with a daily requirement of 60 ml/kg, 14 to 15% glucose would be needed.) This procedure usually maintains the blood glucose level within normal limits. If, on repeated assay, the concentration of glucose remains low—less than 30 mg/100 ml—the rate of infusion should be increased to 10 to 12 or even to 14 to 18 mg/kg/min. If hypoglucosemia persists, steroids or ACTH may be necessary. Careful and frequent observation of the infant is essential to avoid overhydration, heart failure, and pulmonary edema.

After blood sugar has remained stable for 12 hr, oral feedings should be initiated, and the rate of administration of glucose should be gradually reduced. This reduction in the glucose infusion rate should be accomplished stepwise in decrements of 4 to 6 mg/kg/min spaced at intervals of 4 to 6 hr. Thus the rate might be lowered from 14 to 10 to 6 to 2 mg/kg/min over a period of 12 to 18 hr. Decrements of the required size can be achieved by using 10 and then 5% glucose solutions. Blood glucose should be monitored throughout the period. These precautions are necessary in order to avoid reactive hypoglycemia.

Hypocalcemic tetany may be treated with 5 to 10 ml of 10% calcium gluconate, slowly administered intravenously with constant monitoring of the heart rate. Therapy should be continued for several days with oral calcium salts and a low solute formula.

The relationship among kernicterus, serum levels of bilirubin, marked hypoglycemia, and severe derangements in acid-base balance and oxygen saturation in the respiratory distress syndrome requires clarification before definite recommendations for the management of any specific bilirubin level are justified. Early feedings have been shown to be effective in preventing the rise in bilirubin (45), as have fluorescent lights.

A high index of suspicion for both hypoglycemia and hypocalcemia will result in appropriate diagnosis and early therapy and may prevent late sequelae.

PROGNOSIS

Only preliminary or retrospective data of the most general type are available to predict the outcome of infants of diabetic mothers. In an early study of 185 children in 1950 by White et al. (100), 9% of children of either diabetic mothers or diabetic fathers had "overt" diabetes. In contrast, in a prospective analysis Farquhar (56) followed up 329 diabetic pregnancies from 1948 to 1966 in Edinburgh. In his survivors (251), weights and heights were distributed over a normal range; however, an excess of both boys and girls, 9 and 13%, respectively, fell below the third percentile for height, and a comparable number fell above the ninety-seventh and below the third percentiles for weight. Only two—less than 1%—of his children developed manifest diabetes. It should be noted that diabetes in the father has no influence on perinatal outcome although genetic liability is present.

Subsequently, Francois et al. (5) evaluated 97 offspring of diabetic mothers between 2 and 16 years of age. Only one child (1%) developed manifest diabetes, and 6 of 49 (12%) had abnormal glucose tolerance tests. Of the latter 6, 2 showed delayed insulin secretion and 4 had hyperinsulinism. Height and weight were normal in all but 8 cases, who were above 2 S.D. in either parameter. Psychomotor development was normal in all but 5 children. It is noteworthy that in 2 children the cause of the encephalopathy was attributed to asymptomatic hypoglycemia—blood glucose values of less than 10 mg/100 ml—that persisted several days.

The collaborative study of cerebral palsy was not designed to determine the various metabolic abnormalities in diabetic pregnancies and their influence on infant outcome. For example, blood sugar and serum ketone measurements were not done systematically in either mothers or infants. Therefore, the report by Churchill et al. (101) that suggested, on the basis of data from this survey, that acetonemia has adverse effects on intrauterine brain development requires validation in a properly controlled prospective study.

Yssing (102) has advantageously used the unique pregnant diabetic population carefully studied by Pedersen and his associates over the past three decades. For example, she evaluated outcome relative to maternal estriol excretion in 154 pregnancies that resulted in 159 surviving children. At followup between 1 year 8 months and 10 years 1 month, major congenital abnormalities and cerebral damage were significantly more frequent in infants from mothers with subnormal estriol excretion.

Detailed prospective controlled studies considering multiple variables are necessary before definitive conclusions are justified.

SUMMARY (105,106)

Diabetes during pregnancy not only affects maternal metabolism but also has diverse effects on the fetus and newborn. Congenital anomalies of the fetus are more common. Anatomic alterations may include increased body fat, increased islet cells with beta cell hyperplasia, organomegaly, and increased hemopoiesis. Hyperinsulinism and hypoglycemia occur but do not often produce serious symptomatic effects. Respiratory distress is one of the more serious complications. The infant of the insulin-dependent or gestational diabetic mother, whether delivered early—37 weeks' gestation—or at term, is a high-risk infant who requires intensive nursing care as compared with the normal infant of similar weight or gestation. The mother should be delivered in an environment where optimal care for the infant can be provided. Prognosis for these infants continues to improve as knowledge accumulates concerning the pathophysiologic alterations in mother, fetus, and neonate.

REFERENCES

1. Farquhar, J. W.: The child of the diabetic woman. *Arch. Dis. Child.* 34:76, 1959.
2. Pedersen, J., Molsted-Pedersen, L., and Anderson, B.: Perinatal foetal mortality in 1245 diabetic pregnancies. *Acta Chir. Scand. Suppl.* 433:191, 1973.
3. O'Sullivan, J. B., Charles, D., Mahan, C. M., and Dandrow, R. V.: Gestational diabetes and perinatal mortality rate. *Am. J. Obstet. Gynecol.* 116:901, 1973.
4. White, P.: Diabetes mellitus in pregnancy. *Clin. Perinatol.* 1:331, 1974.
5. Francois, R., Picaud, J. J., Ruitton-Ugliengo, A., David, L., Cartal, M. Y., and Bauer, D.: The newborn of diabetic mothers. *Biol. Neonate* 24:1, 1974, and International Congress of Pediatrics, Buenos Aires, Argentina, October, 1974.
6. Eshai, R., and Gutberlet, R. L.: The infant of the diabetic mother. *Pediatr. Ann.* 4:12, 1975.
7. Kyle, G. C.: Diabetes and pregnancy. *Ann. Inter. Med.* 59(1), pt. 2 (suppl. 3), 1963.
8. White, P., Koshy, P., and Duckers, J.: The management of pregnancy complicating diabetes and of children of diabetic mothers. *Med. Clin. North Am.* 37:1481, 1953.
9. O'Sullivan, J. B., Mahan, C. M., Charles D., and Dandrow, R. V.: Medical treatment of the gestational diabetic. *Obstet. Gynecol.* 43:817, 1974.
10. Pedersen, J., Molsted-Pedersen, L., and Andersen, B.: Assessors of fetal perinatal mortality in diabetic pregnancy. *Diabetes* 23:302, 1974.

11. Warrner, R. A., and Cornblath, M.: Infants of gestational diabetic mothers. *Am. J. Dis. Child.* 117:678, 1969.

12. Serratto, M., Cantez, T., Harris, V., Yeh, T., and Pildes, R.: Cardiac, pulmonary and metabolic findings in infants of diabetic mothers. Presented to International Pediatric Conference, Buenos Aires, Argentina, 1974.

13. Garn, S. M.: Fat, body size and growth in the newborn. *Hum. Biol.* 30:265, 1958.

14. Osler, M., and Pedersen, J.: The body composition of newborn infants of diabetic mothers, Pediatrics 26:985, 1960.

15. Fee, B. A., and Weil, W. B., Jr.: Body composition of infants of diabetic mothers by direct analysis. *Ann. N.Y. Acad. Sci.* 110:869, 1963.

16. Farquhar, J. W., and Sklaroff, S. A.: The post-natal weight loss of babies born to diabetic and non-diabetic women. *Arch. Dis. Child.* 33:323, 1958.

17. Cook, C. D., O'Brien, D., Hansen, J. D. L., Beem, M., and Smith, C. A.: Water and electrolyte economy in newborn infants of diabetic mothers. *Acta Paediatr.* 49:121, 1960.

18. Osler, M.: Renal function in newborn infants of diabetic mothers. *Acta Endocrinol.* 34:287, 1960.

19. Prod'hom, L. S., Levinson, H., Cherry, R. B., Drorbaugh, J. E., Hubbell, J. P., Jr., and Smith, C. A.: Adjustment of ventilation, intrapulmonary gas exchange, and acid-base balance during the first day of life: Normal values in well infants of diabetic mothers. *Pediatrics* 33:682, 1964.

20. White, P.: Symposium on diabetes mellitus; pregnancy complicating diabetes. *Am. J. Med.* 7:609, 1949.

21. Robert, M. F., Neff, R. K., Hubbell, J. P., Taeusch, H. W., and Avery, M. E.: The association between maternal diabetes and the respiratory distress syndrome. *New Eng. J. Med.* 294:357, 1976.

22. McCance, R. A., and Widdowson, E. M.: Metabolism and renal function in the first two days of life. *Cold Spring Harbor Symp. Quant. Biol.* 19:161, 1954.

23. Avery, M., and Fletcher, B.: *The Lung and Its Disorders in the Newborn Infant,* 3rd ed. Philadelphia, W. B. Saunders Company, 1974. *Major Problems in Clinical Pediatrics,* vol. I.

24. Smith, B. T., Giroud, C. J. P., Robert, M. F., and Avery, M. E.: Insulin antagonism of cortisol action on lecithin synthesis by cultured fetal lung cells. *J. Pediatr.* 87:953, 1975.

25. Pennoyer, M. M., and Hartmann, A. F., Sr.: Management of infants born of diabetic mothers. *Postgrad. Med.* 18:199, 1955.

26. Cornblath, M., Nicolopoulos, D., Ganzon, A. F., Levin, E. Y., Gordon, M. H., and Gordon, H. H.: Studies of carbohydrate metabolism in the newborn infant: IV. The effect of glucagon on the capillary blood sugar in infants of diabetic mothers. *Pediatrics* 28:592, 1961.

27. McCann, M. L., Chen, C. H., Katigbak, E. B., Kotchen, J., Likly, B. F., and Schwartz, R.: The effects of fructose on hypoglucosemia in infants of diabetic mothers. *New Engl. J. Med.* 275:1, 1966.

28. McCann, M. L., Adam, P. A. J., Likly, B. V., and Schwartz, R.: The prevention of hypoglucosemia by fructose in infants of diabetic mothers. *New Engl. J. Med.* 275:8, 1966.

29. Chen, C. H., Adam, P. A. J., Laskowski, D. E., McCann, M. L., and Schwartz, R.: The plasma free fatty acid composition and blood glucose of normal and diabetic pregnant women and of their newborns. *Pediatrics* 36:843, 1965.

30. Light, I. J., Keenan, W. J., and Sutherland, J. M.: Maternal intravenous glucose administration as a cause of hypoglycemia in the infant of the diabetic mother. *Am. J. Obstet. Gynecol.* 113:345, 1972.

31. Wu, P. Y. K., Modanlov, H., and Karelitz, M.: Effect of glucagon on blood glucose homeostasis in infants of diabetic mothers. *Acta Paediatr. Scand.* 64:441, 1975.

32. Haworth, J. C., Dilling, L. A., and Vidyasagar, D.: Hypoglycemia in infants of diabetic mothers: Effect of epinephrine therapy. *J. Pediatr.* 82:94, 1973.

33. Bergman, L.: Studies on early neonatal hypocalcemia. *Acta Paediatr. Scand.* (suppl.) 248:5, 1974.

34. Zetterstrom, R., and Arnhold, R. G.: Impaired calcium-phosphate homeostasis in newborn infants of diabetic mothers. *Acta Paediatr.* 47:107, 1958.

35. Craig, W. S.: Clinical signs of neonatal tetany: With especial reference to their occurrence in newborn babies of diabetic mothers. *Pediatrics* 22:297, 1958.

36. Gittleman, I. F., Pincus, J. B., Schmerzler, E., and Annecchiarico, F.: Diabetes mellitus or the prediabetic state in the mother and the neonate. *Am. J. Dis. Child.* 98:342, 1959.

37. Tsang, R. C., Kleinman, L. I., Sutherland, J. M., and Light, I. J.: Hypocalcemia in infants of diabetic mothers. *J. Pediatr.* 80:384, 1972.

38. Tsang, R. C., Chen, I. W., Friedman, M. A., Gigger, M., Steichen, J., Koffler, H., Fenton, L., Brown, D., Pramanik, A., Keenan, W., Strub, R., and Joyce, T.: Parathyroid function in infants of diabetic mothers. *J. Pediatr.* 86:399, 1975.

39. Gittleman, I. F., Pincus, J. B., Schmerzler, E., and Saito, M.: Hypocalcemia occurring on the first day of life in mature and premature infants. *Pediatrics* 18:721, 1956.

40. Kunstadter, R. H., Oh, W., Tanman, F., and Cornblath, M.: Idiopathic hypoparathyroidism in the newborn. *Am. J. Dis. Child.* 105:499, 1963.

41. Bloom, S. I., and Johnston, D. I.: Failure of glucagon release in infants of gestational diabetic mothers. *Br. Med. J.* 4:453, 1972;

42. Zetterstrom, R., Strindberg, B., and Arnhold, R. G.: Hyperbilirubinemia and ABO hemolytic disease in newborn infants of diabetic mothers. *Acta Paediatr.* 47:238, 1958.

43. Olsen, B. R., Osler, M., and Pedersen, J.: Neonatal jaundice in infants born to diabetic mothers. *Dan. Med. Bull.* 10:1, 1963.

44. Taylor, P. M., Wolfson, J. H., Bright, N. H., Birchard, E. L., Derinoz, M. N., and Watson, D. W.: Hyperbilirubinemia in infants of diabetic mothers. *Biol. Neonate* 5:289, 1963.

45. Hubbell, J. P., Drorbaugh, J. E., Rudolph, A. J., Auld, P. A., Cherry, R. B., and Smith, C. A.: "Early" versus "late" feeding of infants of diabetic mothers. *New Engl. J. Med.* 265:835, 1961.

46. Avery, M. E., Oppenheimer, E. H., and Gordon, H. H.: Renal-vein thrombosis in newborn infants of diabetic mothers. *New Engl. J. Med.* 265:1134, 1957.

47. Takeuchi, A., and Benirschke, K.: Renal venous thrombosis of the newborn and its relation to maternal diabetes. *Biol. Neonate* 3:237, 1961.

48. Tevteras, E., and Rudstrom, P.: Renal thrombosis of the newborn: Report of a primary case successfully treated by surgery. *Acta Paediatr.* 45:545, 1956.

49. Schwartz, H. C., King, K. C., Schwartz, A. L., Edmunds, D., and Schwartz, R.: Effects of pregnancy on hemoglobin A_{1c} in normal, gestationally diabetic and diabetic women. *Diabetes.* 25:1118, 1976.

49a. Widness, J. A., Schwartz, H. C., Thompson, D., King, K. C., Kahn, C. B., Oh, W., and Schwartz, R.: Glycohemoglobin (HbA$_{1c}$): A predictor of birth weight in infants of diabetic mothers. *J. Pediatr.* 92:8, 1978.

49b. Widness, J. A., Schwartz, H. C., Thompson, D., Kahn, C. B., Oh, W. and Schwartz, R.: Hemoglobin A$_{1c}$ (Glycohaemoglobin) in diabetic pregnancy: An indicator of glucose control and fetal size. *Br. J. Obs. and Gyn.* 85:812, 1978.

50. Bleicher, S. J., and Pang, S. J.: Oxygen transport and the role of the erythrocyte 2,3 diphosphoglycerate, in Camerini-Davalos, R. A., and Cole, H. S. (eds.): *Early Diabetes in Early Life.* New York, Academic Press, Inc., 1975, p. 243.

51. Davis, W. S., and Campbell, J. B.: Neonatal small left colon syndrome. *Am. J. Dis. Child.* 129:1024, 1975.

52. Gellis, S. S., and Hsia, D. Y.-Y.: The infant of the diabetic mother. *Am. J. Dis. Child.* 97:1, 1959.

53. Dekaban, A., and Baird, R.: The outcome of pregnancy in diabetic women: I. Fetal wastage, mortality, and morbidity in the offspring of diabetic and normal control mothers. *J. Pediatr.* 55:563, 1959.

54. Hagbard, L.: Diabetes and prediabetes. *Mod. Probl. Pediatr.* 8:221, 1953 (Bibliotheca Paediatrica, fasc. 81).

55. Pedersen, L. M., Tygstrup, I., and Pedersen, J.: Congenital malformations in newborn infants of diabetic women. Correlation with maternal diabetic vascular complications. *Lancet* 1:1124, 1964.

56. Farquhar, J. W.: Prognosis for babies born to diabetic mothers in Edinburgh. *Arch. Dis. Child.* 44:36, 1969.

57. Kucera, J.: Rate and type of congenital anomalies among offspring of diabetic women. *J. Reprod. Med.* 7:61, 1971.

58. Soler, N. G., Walsh, C. H., and Malins, J. M.: Congenital malformations in infants of diabetic mothers. *Quarterly J. Med.* XLV 178:303, 1976.

59. Rowland, T. W., Hubbell, J. P., Jr., and Nadas, A. S.: Congenital heart disease in infants of diabetic mothers. *J. Pediatr.* 83:815, 1973.

60. Okudaira, Y., Hirota, K., Cohen, S., and Strauss, L.: Ultrastructure of the human placenta in maternal diabetes mellitus. *Lab. Invest.* 15:910, 1966.

61. Hagbard, L.: *Pregnancy and Diabetes Mellitus.* Springfield, Ill., Charles C Thomas, 1961. American Lecture Series No. 449 (Chapter 5).

62. Gabbe, S. G., Deniers, L. M., Greep, R. O., and Villee, C. A.: Placental glycogen metabolism in diabetes mellitus. *Diabetes* 21:1185, 1972.

63. King, K. C., Adam, P. A. J., Laskowski, D. E., and Schwartz, R.: Sources of fatty acids in the newborn. *Pediatrics* 47:192, 1971.

64. Cardell, B. S.: Hypertrophy and hyperplasia of the pancreatic islets in newborn infants. *J. Pathol.* 66:335, 1953.

65. Potter, E. L.: *Pathology of the Fetus and the Newborn,* 2nd ed. Chicago, Year Book Medical Publishers, Inc., 1961, p. 335.

66. McKay, D. G., Benirschke, K., and Curtis, G. W.: Infants of diabetic mothers: Histologic and histochemical observations of the pancreas. *Obstet. Gynecol.* 2:133, 1953.

67. VanAssche, F. A.: *The Fetal Endocrine Pancreas: A Quantitative Morphological Approach.* Proefschrift ingediend by de faculteit Geneeskunde der Katholieke Universiteit Leven, Belgium, 1970.

68. Pedersen, J., Bojsen-Moller, B., and Poulsen, H.: Blood sugar in newborn infants of diabetic mothers. *Acta Endocrinol.* 15:33, 1954.

69. Farquhar, J. W.: Hypoglycemia in newborn infants of normal and diabetic mothers, *S. Afr. Med. J.* 42:237, 1968.

70. Baird, J. D., and Farquhar, J. W.: Insulin-secreting capacity in newborn infants of normal and diabetic women. *Lancet* 1:71, 1962.

71. Dole, V. P.: The significance of nonesterified fatty acids in plasma. *Arch. Intern. Med.* 101:1005, 1958.

72. Randle, P. J., Garland, P. B., Hales, C. N., and Newsholme, E. A.: The glucose fatty acid cycle, its role in insulin sensitivity and the metabolic disturbances of diabetes mellitus. *Lancet* 1:785, 1963.

73. Melichar, V., Novak, M., Hahn, P., and Koldovsky, O.: Free fatty acids and glucose in the blood of various groups of newborns: Preliminary report. *Acta Paediatr.* 53:343, 1964.

74. Persson, B., Gentz, J., and Kellum, M.: Metabolic observations in infants of strictly controlled diabetic mothers. *Acta Paediatr. Scand.* 62:465, 1973.

75. Pantelakis, S. N., Cameron, A. H., Davidson, S., Dunn, P. M., Fosbrooke, A. S., Lloyd, J. K., Malins, J. M., and Wolff, O. H.: The diabetic pregnancy: A study of serum lipids in maternal and umbilical cord blood and of the uterine placental vasculature. *Arch. Dis. Child.* 39:334, 1964.

76. Mortimer, J. G.: Cord blood lipids of normal infants and infants of diabetic mothers. *Arch. Dis. Child.* 39:342, 1964.

77. Jorgensen, K. R., Deckert, T., Molsted-Pedersen, L., and Pedersen, J.: Insulin, insulin antibody and glucose in plasma of newborn infants of diabetic women. *Acta Endocrinol.* 52:154, 1966.

78. Joassin, G., Parker, M. L., Pildes, R. S., and Cornblath, M.: Infants of diabetic mothers. *Diabetes* 16:306, 1967.

79. Block, M. B., Pildes, R. S., Mossabhov, N. A., Steiner, D. F., and Rubenstein, A. H.: C-peptide immunoreactivity (CPR): A new method for studying infants of insulin-treated diabetic mothers. *Pediatrics* 53:923, 1974.

80. Kalhan, S. C., Schwartz, R., and Adam, P. A. J.: Placental barrier to human insulin I^{125} in insulin dependent diabetic mothers. *J. Clin. Endocrinol. Metab.* 40:139, 1975.

81. Isles, T. E., and Farquhar, J. W.: The effect of endogenous antibody on insulin-assay in the newborn infants of diabetic mothers. *Pediatr. Res.* 1:110, 1976.

82. Isles, P. E., Dickson, M., and Farquhar, J. W.: Glucose intolerance and plasma insulin in newborn infants of normal and diabetic mothers. *Pediatr. Res.* 2:198, 1968.

83. Pildes, R. S., Hart, R. J., Warrner, R. and Cornblath, M.: Plasma insulin response during oral glucose tolerance tests in newborns of normal and gestational diabetic mothers. *Pediatrics* 44:76, 1969.

84. King, K. C., Adam, P. A. J., Clemente, G. A., and Schwartz, R.: Infants of diabetic mothers: Attenuated glucose uptake without hyperinsulinemia during continuous glucose infusion. *Pediatrics* 44:381, 1969.

85. King, K. C., Adam, P. A. J., Yamaguchi, K., and Schwartz, R.: Insulin response to arginine in normal newborn infants and infants of diabetic mothers. *Diabetes.* 23:816, 1974.

86. Kalhan, S., Savin, S., Uga, N., and Adam, P. A. J.: Quantification of glucose turnover with glucose-1-^{13}C tracer: Attenuated glucose production in newborn infants of diabetic mothers. (Abstract, *Pediatr. Res.,* 10, 441, No. 660, 1976.)

87. Jackson, W. P. U.: Prediabetes: A survey. *S. Afr. J. Lab. Clin. Med.* 6:127, 1960.

88. Farquhar, J. W.: The possible influence of hyperadrenocorticism on the foetus of the diabetic woman. *Arch. Dis. Child.* 31:483, 1956.

89. Migeon, C. J., Nicolopoulos, D., and Cornblath, M.: Concentrations of 17-hydroxycorticosteroids in the blood of diabetic mothers and in blood from umbilical cords of their offspring at the time of delivery. *Pediatrics* 25:605, 1960.

90. Smith, E. K., Reardon, H. S., and Field, S. H.: Urinary constituents of infants of diabetic and non-diabetic mothers: I. 17-hydroxycorticosteroid excretion in premature infants. *J. Pediatr.* 64:652, 1964.

91. Kalkhoff, R., Schalch, D. S., Walker, J. L., Beck, P., Kipnis, D. M., and Daughaday, W. H.: Diabetogenic factors associated with pregnancy. *Tr. A. Am. Physicians* 77:270, 1964.

92. Stern, L., Ramos, A., and Leduc, J.: Urinary catecholamine excretion in infants of diabetic mothers. *Pediatrics* 42:598, 1968.

93. Light, I. J., Sutherland, J. M., Loggie, J. M., and Gaffney, T. E.: Impaired epinephrine release in hypoglycemic infants of diabetic mothers. *N. Engl. J. Med.* 277:394, 1967.

94. Luyckx, A. S., Massi-Benedetti, F., Falori, A., and Lefebvre, P. J.: Presence of pancreatic glucagon in the portal plasma of human neonates: Differences in the insulin and glucagon responses to glucose between normal infants and infants from diabetic mothers. *Diabetologica* 8:296, 1972.

95. Williams, P. R., Sperling, M. A., and Racasa, Z.: Blunting of spontaneous and amino acid stimulated glucagon secretion in infants of diabetic mothers. *Diabetes* 24(suppl. 2):411, 1975 (abstract).

96. Peel, Sr., J.: Diabetes in pregnancy, *Proc. R. Soc. Med.* 56:1009, 1963.

97. Gordon, H. H.: The infants of diabetic mothers. *Am. J. Med. Sc.* 244:129, 1962.

98. Persson, B., and Lunell, N. O.: Metabolic control in diabetic pregnancy. *Am. J. Obstet. Gynecol.* 122:737, 1975.

99. Tooley, W. H.: Idiopathic respiratory distress syndrome, in Gellis, S. S., and Kagan, B. M.: *Current Pediatric Therapy—7,* 7th ed. Philadelphia, W. B. Saunders Company, 1976, pp. 729–731.

100. White, P., Koshy, P., and Duckers, J.: Management of pregnancy complicating diabetes and the children of diabetic mothers. *Med. Clin. North Am.* 37:1481, 1953.

101. Churchill, J. A., Berendes, H. W., and Nemore, J.: Neuropsychological deficits in children of diabetic mothers. *Am. J. Obst. Gynecol.* 105:257, 1969.

102. Yssing, M.: Oestriol excretion in pregnant diabetics related to long-term prognosis of surviving children. *Acta Endocrinol.* (suppl. 185) 75:95, 1974.

103. Bowie, M. D., Mulligan, P. B., and Schwartz, R.: Intravenous glucose tolerance in the normal newborn infant: The effects of a double dose of glucose and insulin. *Pediatrics* 31:590, 1963.

104. Cornblath, M., Wybregt, S. H., and Baens, G. S.: Studies of carbohydrate metabolism in the newborn infant: VII. Tests of carbohydrate tolerance in premature infants. *Pediatrics* 32:1007, 1963.

105. Third International Symposium on Early Diabetes, December, 1974. Camerini-Davalos, R. A., and Cole, H. S.: *Early Diabetes in Early Life.* New York, Academic Press, Inc., 1975, pp. 1–615. (This volume serves as a detailed source for several of the areas covered in this chapter.)

106. Report of the National Commission on Diabetes to the Congress of the United States, Volumes I–IV, 1975, U.S. Government Printing Office. (May be purchased from the Superintendent of Documents. Publication Nos. DHEW-NIH-76-1018, 1019, 1020, 1021, 1022, 1023, 1024, 1031, 1032 and 1033. Nos. 1022 and 1023 are especially relevant to this chapter.) The report includes the details of two workshops that supplement the material presented: (1) Perinatal Problems, Pathophysiology and Treatment and (2) Workshop on Pregnancy of the Committee on SCOPE.

26

Nutrition of the Low Birthweight Infant

Philip Sunshine, M.D.

One of the major difficulties encountered in the care of the low birthweight infant is that of supplying nutrition in order for the infant to grow and develop adequately. The full-term infant is able to tolerate various types of milks and other nutriments with minimal, if any, difficulties. Such is not the case with the infant of low birthweight, who not only has an "immature" digestive system but also may have other major difficulties such as respiratory distress, cardiovascular abnormalities, hemorrhagic diathesis, and a relatively immature renal system. Although it is paramount to ensure that the infant is given adequate caloric intake, the ability of the infant to digest, absorb, and metabolize foodstuffs is limited. In this chapter, I concentrate primarily on the nutrition of the very low birthweight infant, that is, the infant who weighs less than 1500 g at birth and is usually less than 33 weeks' gestation.

HISTORICAL PERSPECTIVE

At the turn of the century, physicians caring for small premature infants were well aware of the inability of the infant to be fed by the usual feeding techniques and advocated early introduction of feedings, especially with human milk, in an attempt to supply adequate caloric intake for these babies. Studies by Levine and Gordon and coworkers beginning in the 1930s to the 1940s demonstrated that many preterm infants would not gain weight so rapidly if fed human milk as they would if they were fed milk with a protein content of 4 to 6%. Thus high-protein milks such as Alacta and Olac were designed for such small infants. Although there was no uniform agreement as to the amount of protein that should be fed to these small infants, most centers caring for premature infants used formulas in order to provide 6 to 9 g protein/(kg)(day).

In the late 1940s and early 1950s, it was also demonstrated that small infants could not excrete a "a water load" properly and often would take up to 48 hr or more to excrete the fluid ingested. Since many of these infants were edematous, had respiratory distress of one form or other, or had frequent episodes or apnea or cyanosis, it was recommended that early feedings were not needed, and often these infants were deprived of fluid intake for 48 and even 72 hr after birth. It was a common practice to place these tiny babies in incubators, to give them no feedings for 2 or 3 days, and if they were still alive after that time, to initiate feedings.

Several events occurred within a very short time in the late 1950s that altered the concepts of fluid and caloric requirements of the small preterm infants. A major breakthrough occurred when Reardon and her coworkers demonstrated that infants of diabetic mothers had a much greater rate of survival when given glucose plus saline than did those infants who received nothing by mouth or had very little fluid intake. Soon thereafter, Usher demonstrated that many infants with hyaline membrane disease would have an enhanced rate of survival if glucose in water and sodium bicarbonate were infused intravenously early in the course of their illness. This form of therapy became highly controversial. Many investigators attempting to duplicate Usher's results would be unable to do so because they would often wait until the infants had severe acidosis and hypercarbia before beginning the infusion of glucose and sodium bicarbonate. In such situations, sodium bicarbonate often would be detrimental rather than beneficial.

The studies by Silverman and coworkers and Day and coworkers also were significant in noting that careful regulation of thermal environment was beneficial in enhancing the survival of low birthweight infants. Other studies verified that the caloric expenditure and rate of catabolism were decreased markedly if the infants were maintained in a neutral thermal environment.

The use of early intravenous feedings of low birthweight infants was clarified by a very important observation by Cornblath and coworkers; they demonstrated a marked improvement in the survival of very small premature infants when intravenous dextrose was given immediately after birth and continued until the infants could take feedings orally. Thus, it became a routine in most nurseries throughout the country to begin the infusion of dextrose in water immediately after birth in order to decrease catabolism, prevent hypoglycemia, and avoid early caloric deprivation.

In the mid- to late 1960s, data in laboratory animals were being accumulated that showed that prenatal and early neonatal caloric deprivation would result in severe and often permanent growth retardation, especially of the central nervous system. Thus, the pendulum began to swing in the opposite direction, as many of those caring for neonates became very concerned about the effect of nutritional deprivation in low birthweight infants, and various techniques were introduced in an attempt to have these babies grow at the same rate as they would had they remained in utero. Peripheral alimentation, total parenteral nutrition via a central catheter, transpyloric feedings, or combinations of these techniques were initiated often with hazardous rather than beneficial results. Intravenous infusions of hypertonic glucose, amino acids, emulsified fat, and even ethanol were given, and complications of hyperglycemia, hyperosmolality, hyperammonemia, acidosis, fluid overload, and ethanol intoxication were recognized. Gastrointestinal perforation, an increased incidence of neonatal necrotizing enterocolitis, and other gastrointestinal catastrophes were encountered more frequently as overzealous attempts to feed these low birthweight infants were used.

Presently, we are beginning to recognize the need for early feedings and yet at the same time attempting to prevent complications that can ensue readily. Although intravenous nutrition has been known to be an important adjunct in the care of the low birthweight infant, oral feedings are paramount to ensure that adequate growth does take place. Often this is extremely difficult because of other problems that the infant may have that tend to limit both intravenous and oral supplementation of nutriments. To understand better some of the difficulties encountered in trying to provide adequate nutrition, it is important to understand certain aspects of the gastrointestinal tract during development, and how these relate to the nutrition of the infant.

DEVELOPMENT OF THE GASTROINTESTINAL TRACT

Morphological Development

The gastrointestinal tract develops from entoderm and a mesoblastic mesenchymal layer, which together are called the splanchnopleure, on about the fourteenth day of intrauterine life. By 3.5 weeks of gestation, the foregut and hindgut as well as the liver buds are discernible, and by the fourth week of gestation, the intestine has assumed a tubular shape. At the same time pancreatic buds, liver cords and ducts, and a gallbladder begin to form. Over the next 1 to 2 weeks, the intestine elongates very rapidly and forms a loop that protrudes along the yolk stalk into the umbilical cord.

Between the sixth and tenth weeks, the small intestine continues to grow rapidly, rotating and coiling inside the cord; it reenters the abdominal cavity, with the jejunum leading the way and filling the left part of the abdominal cavity. The ileum fills the right half of the abdominal cavity, and then the colon reenters, after which time, the cecum becomes fixed close to the right ileac crest, and the ascending and transverse colon come to lie in their respective positions. Abnormalities of this type of rotation and reentry lead to various types of nonrotation or malrotation, the most severe type being an omphalocele.

The intestine continues to grow rapidly, so that from the fifth to fortieth week of intrauterine life, the intestine increases approximately 1000-fold. At term, the length of the small intestine is approximately three to four times the crown-rump length, or about 250 cm in length.

By the seventh week of intrauterine life, villi begin to form in the duodenum and proximal jejunum. By the tenth to twelfth week, primitive crypts of Lieberkühn begin to form. The development of the intestine proceeds craniocaudally, so that by 19 weeks of intrauterine life, well-developed villi and crypts are found throughout the small intestine, including the ileum.

The enterocytes develop microvilli by 8 to 10 weeks of intrauterine life. By 12 weeks of intrauterine life, the microvilli have well-developed microfilaments present. The crypt cells have less defined microvilli and tend to lag behind the development of the cells in the villi, but they mature as they progress up the villus.

Although there are many data regarding cellular proliferation in laboratory animals, very few data are available in humans. A few studies that have been done in man suggest that the time for the cells of the crypt to migrate to the tip of the villi is approximately 48 to 72 hr.

The same data have been described in other adult mammals, but studies of the suckling animal, especially in the rat and mouse, where intense investigation has been carried out, show that the rate of migration may be two to three times longer than that of the adult. Whether this very slow rate of migration occurs also in the human newborn is not known, but these findings might well explain the clinical impression that there is a great delay in healing after severe insult to the intestine of the infant as compared with the adult.

Enzymatic Development

The activity of alkaline phosphatase, ATPase, and amino peptidase are all present in the intestine of the 7- to 8-week-old fetus. From about the fourteenth week onward, the enzymes are active in the ileum. Beginning about the twelfth or fourteenth week disaccharidases are detectable in very low activity, but they increase rapidly, so that by the twenty-fourth week of gestation the enzymes have reached significant levels of activity. The activity of lactase tends to lag behind the development of other disaccharidases and often is not well developed until the thirty-second to thirty-fourth week of gestation. Many preterm babies are found to have very low activity of lactase, but lactose intolerance is encountered infrequently.

The peptidases have been found to be present and active beginning in the eleventh to twelfth week of gestation, and the activities of these enzymes increase slowly during gestation.

The enzymes of the exocrine pancreas can usually be detected between the sixteenth and eighteenth weeks of intrauterine life. The activity of lipase is still low at term but markedly increases after birth and continues to do so during the first 9 months of life. There appears to be high enough activity of lipase present even in the very small preterm infant to hydrolyze most triglycerides adequately. Amylase activity, which is detected by 22 weeks of gestation, remains low even after birth and may be decreased until 4 to 6 months of age. Tryptic activity is detected at approximately 16 weeks of age and increases rapidly after 28 weeks of intrauterine life. If enterokinase is added to the assay, marked activity of trypsin can be detected even at 24 weeks' gestation. The other proteolytic enzymes parallel the activity of trypsin. Enterokinase does not become active until late gestation and even at term is only 20% as active as it is in older children.

Functional Development of the Intestine

The fetus of 24 to 26 weeks' gestation is capable of absorbing and digesting protein appropriately in most situations. The activities of the proteolytic enzymes of the pancreas appear active enough to hydrolyze the protein found in milk. Also the pancreas can respond well to stimulation by secretin and pancreozymin. The intestinal peptidases are adequate for complete digestion and absorption of substrate, so that, except for the very immature infant, the ability to digest and absorb protein is essentially intact.

Although lipid can be absorbed by pinocytosis in the twelve-week human fetus, the preterm infant has incomplete digestion of fat until approximately 34 to 36 weeks' gestation. The activity of pancreatic lipase appears to be adequate for lipolysis, but the concentration and the pool of bile acids are decreased in preterm infants. The concentration of bile acids increases rapidly over the first several months of extrauterine life, and fat absorption is enhanced. It is well recognized that the preterm infant often has a reduced capacity to absorb fat, especially if the milk contains large quantities of saturated fats.

By the twenty-fourth week of intrauterine life, the activities of the disaccharidases are probably adequate for digestion, even though the activity of lactase lags behind the development of the other sugar-splitting enzymes. However, except for lactase, the rate limiting step in carbohydrate absorption is the ability to transport glucose. Although the fetuses can transport glucose both aerobically and anaerobically by the tenth week of gestation, they soon loose the ability to transport the monosaccharides anaerobically and can do so only under aerobic conditions. Even up to approximately 12 months of age, the infant can transport increased concentrations of glucose only about one-third to one-fourth as well as the adult. Despite the decreased activities of lactase and pancreatic amylase and decreased glucose transport, carbohydrate malabsorption is rarely encountered even in the very immature infant. Obviously, if the feedings contain great quantities of carbohydrate, especially lactose or starch, the infant's capabilities to digest such a load could be taxed. Also, if the infant has suffered from asphyxia or hypoxia, the transport of monosaccharides is impaired; monosaccharide malabsorption is not uncommon in such infants.

Development of Motility

As with the development of the intestine, the factors involved in its motility develop in a cranial-caudal fashion. By 9 weeks of intrauterine life, Auerbach's plexus is detected, and by 13 weeks Meissner's plexus is noted. The muscle layers, both the longitudinal and circular, appear by 12 weeks of gestation. By 24 weeks of gestation, the muscularis mucosae and the smooth muscle layers of the intestine are fairly well developed. Ganglion cells have reached the rectum but are rather immature in appearance. They continue to mature throughout the first 5 years of life. Swallowing is detected in the human fetus by 16 to 17 weeks of intrauterine life; however, the coordination of sucking and swallowing is usually not well developed prior to 33 to 34 weeks' gestation. Esophageal motility is poorly developed in the preterm infant, and there is poor coordination in response to swallowing as well. The lower esophageal sphincter pressure is decreased, and reflux is common. Gastric emptying time appears to be delayed, but factors such as the amount of hydrochloric acid the infant can produce or pepsin secretion rates do not appear to be correlated with delayed gastric emptying time. After delivery, the rate of gastric emptying time is greatly influenced by the position in which the infant is placed.

The relatively immature muscle layers, the poor coordination of peristaltic waves, the increased number of antiperistaltic waves, and possible decreased hormonal secretions all tend to lead to prolonged transit time, which is frequently encountered in the preterm infant. Many of the infants act as if they have a functional intestinal obstruction with stasis and distention. The stasis can, in time, lead to bacterial overgrowth and intestinal infection.

Development of Immunological Function

In the fifteenth week, fetal lymphopoiesis is present, and the Peyers patches are recognized by 20 weeks of intrauterine life. These increase in size and number until the child is 10 years of age. Although immunoglobulins can be found in the intestinal mucosa of the 13- to 14-week fetus, secretory IgA appears to be absent from the lumen of the intestine of preterm as well as some term infants. The ability of even the term infant to respond immunologically to foreign protein is severely hampered.

Although the intestinal tract is capable of adapting readily to the extrauterine environment by the time the fetus has reached 36 to 38 weeks' gestation, the ability of the small preterm infant's intestinal tract to adjust is markedly limited. The gastrointestinal tract is immature in that there is poor coordination of motility, incomplete digestive and absorptive processes, and probably decreased rate of cellular turnover. The ability to respond by immunological mechanisms is also delayed. These and perhaps other factors predispose the immature infant to develop gastrointestinal malfunction and make the process of providing adequate nutrition more difficult.

NUTRITIONAL NEEDS OF THE PRETERM INFANT

Having discussed development of the gastrointestinal tract, and having outlined the difficulties that the preterm infant can encounter, we can now focus on the food requirements of the low birthweight infant.

Fluid Requirements

The quantity of fluid required by the low birthweight infant has been the subject of much controversy over the years. The total body water decreases from about 80 to 85% when the infant is at 28 weeks' gestation to 70 to 72% when the infant is at term. Most of these changes occur in the extracellular fluid, which decreases from about 55 to 58% to approximately 42 to 45% over the same period. The large amount of extracellular fluid, the large surface area of the infant in relationship to weight, the decreased capability of the kidney to conserve fluid, and the increased permeability of the skin, all enhance fluid loss and make the problems of fluid management more difficult. Although the term infant can readily adjust to wide fluctuations of fluid intake, certainly between 90 and 200 ml/(kg)(day), the low birthweight infant cannot. Although the infant requires at least 90 ml/(kg)(day) to remain in positive fluid balance, attempts to provide the infant with increasing amounts of fluid can often lead to edema, congestive heart failure, and other abnormalities associated with fluid overload. This is especially true in the infant who has hyaline membrane disease, is receiving ventilatory support, or has a complication of a patent ductus arteriosus. Although it is paramount to provide the infant with adequate fluid intake, often, slight increases of fluid infusion may lead to congestive heart failure.

If the infant is cared for in a conventional incubator, especially if covered with a heat shield, the amount of insensible fluid loss can be kept to a minimum of about 1 to 1.3 ml/(kg)(hr). Factors that increase the insensible fluid loss include the use of radiant warmers, which can triple the insensible water loss, and phototherapy, which can double the insensible water loss especially if the infant is not on servocontrol. Increased amounts of fluid can be given inadvertently when the infant is cared for on a mechanical ventilator in which warm and humidified gases are being delivered. Also supersaturating a head hood with warm mist can increase fluid uptake by the infant (Table I).

In most situations, the infants cared for in a conventional incubator with a heat shield have decreased insensible water loss, and fluid requirements can readily be achieved with an infusion of 100 to 115 ml/(kg)(day). If the infant has to be cared for under a radiant warmer, it is important to recognize that the insensible water loss may be tripled unless appropriate care is instituted. This becomes an extremely difficult problem to manage because some of the infants weighing less than 1000 g may require a great deal of fluid, which is usually supplied as 5% dextrose in water. This in turn may lead to hyperglycemia and hyperosmolality. We have found that if the infants are covered with a transparent blanket made from plastic packing material, fluid loss can be

Table I. Factors Influencing Fluid Loss in Preterm Infants

Use of radiant warmer (especially infrared warmer)	↑↑↑
Phototherapy (loss decreased if patient servocontrolled)	↑
Ambient temperature above neutral thermal zone	↑↑
Elevated body temperature	↑↑
Respiratory distress	↑
Increased activity of infant	↑
Use of heat shield	↓↓
Use of "thermal blanket"	↓↓
High relative humidity (>40%)	↓
Use of warm humidified air via endotracheal tube	↓

SOURCE: Modified from Oh, W., in *Neonatology*, ed. G. B. Avery. J. B. Lippencott Co., Philadelphia, 1975.

decreased markedly. The insensible water loss can be decreased by over 70% if such "thermoblankets" are used.

The initial fluid infusion for the small low birthweight infant is usually 40 to 60 ml/(kg)(day) but may vary, depending on the infant's condition. Over the first week, the fluid intake is usually increased so that the infant is receiving between 110 and 150 ml/(kg)(day). Obviously, there is wide fluctuation in requirements, especially if the infant is being supported with ventilatory systems. The infant's urine output and specific gravity must be monitored carefully, and it is best to maintain the infant's urine specific gravity between 1.005 and 1.012. If possible, the infant should be weighed at least twice a day and have careful and frequent examinations in order to detect edema and congestive heart failure.

After the infant has recovered from such initial problems as hyaline membrane disease or apnea, the fluid intake may be increased appropriately; at that time the infant may tolerate up to 160 to 170 ml/(kg)(day).

Caloric Requirements

The caloric requirements of the low birthweight infant vary markedly, depending on the infant's condition and the associated illnesses that may also be present. Generally speaking, after the first or second week of life the infant requires approximately 120 cal/(kg)(day). This includes 40 to 50 cal/(kg)(day) for basal requirements, 15 cal/(kg)(day) for activity, up to 10 cal/(kg)(day) for cold stress, 10 to 15 cal/(kg)(day) for fecal losses, and 25 to 30 cal/(kg)(day) for growth (Table II). Some infants fail to gain appropriately on 120 cal/(kg)(day), especially if they are in a stage of catchup growth after being calorically deprived.

Protein

There has been great controversy over what constitutes the ideal protein intake in premature infants. For many years, it was felt that the infant would grow best if provided with 6 g of protein/(kg)(day). In an elegant study, Davidson and coworkers demonstrated that there was rapid growth of low birthweight infants when they were fed 3 to 6 g of protein/(kg)(day). When the infant was fed 2 g/(kg)(day), the rate of

Table II.   Caloric Requirements of the Preterm Infant (Cal/kg/day)

Basal requirements	40–50
Activity	5–15
Cold stress	0–10
Fecal losses	10–15
Specific dynamic action	8–10
Growth	20–30
	83–130

growth was decreased, and those fed over 6 g/(kg)(day) developed significant azotemia (Fig. 1). Obviously too little protein is associated with increasing amounts of edema and poor weight gain, and too much protein is associated with azotemia, tyrosinemia, and an increasing incidence of late metabolic acidosis as well as hyperammonemia. Goldman and coworkers also demonstrated that excessive protein intake in the very low birthweight infants appeared to be injurious to the developing central nervous system; they found an increased number of low birthweight infants with mental subnormality among a group fed 6 g of protein/(kg)(day) as compared with those who were fed 3 g/(kg)(day).

In recent studies in Finland, Raiha, Gaull, and coworkers have demonstrated that small preterm infants gained weight appropriately when fed pooled human milk.

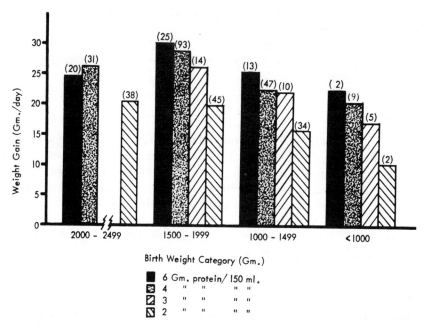

Figure 1. Effect of protein intake on weight gain. Infants were fed 2, 3, 4, or 6 g of protein/(kg)(day). From Davidson, M., Levine, S. F., Bauer, C. H., and Dann, M. Feeding studies in low birth weight infants. *J. Pediat.* 70:695–713, 1967. Reproduced with permission of senior author and the C. V. Mosby Co.

Although the fluid intake of these was 170 ml/(kg)(day) and the infants did have a greater initial weight loss than those infants fed proprietary formulas, they gained weight at the same rate as those who were fed a higher protein-containing formula. These investigators pointed out that certain amino acids such as cystine and taurine are present in greater concentration in human milk than in cow's milk formulas. Although these are not essential amino acids in adults, they may be essential in the preterm infant. Thus, human milk, despite its low protein content, may actually provide "high value" protein intake and be adequate for growth of these infants.

Fat Requirements

The fat requirement in the preterm infant is usually in the range of 3 to 5 g/(kg)(day). It is imperative that linoleic acid and arachidonic acid be included, as they are essential fatty acids for the preterm as well as the term baby. It is recognized that unsaturated fats are absorbed much more readily than saturated fats, and this may be due to the presence of a binding protein in the intestine that facilitates the absorption of unsaturated fats. Thus, an infant fed a diet containing an increased amount of unsaturated fat has a greater absorption of these nutriments.

As previously mentioned, the preterm infant has decreased concentrations of the bile acids needed to facilitate fat absorption. The concentration of bile acids present in the duodenum correlates very well with the amount of fat that is absorbed. The lower the concentration of bile acids, the lower the fat absorption. However, data of Signer and coworkers have demonstrated that, although bile acids are decreased in the lumen of the premature infant's intestine, the fat in human milk is absorbed well regardless of the concentration of bile acids.

Carbohydrates

Carbohydrate, which in most milks is lactose, provides 35 to 50% of the daily calories. Despite the fact that the activity of lactase may be very low in the small preterm infant, lactose intolerance is rarely manifest except in in unusual circumstances. Lactase activity also appears to be decreased when the infant is exposed to phototherapy. If the infant remains hypoxic or hypercarbic, carbohydrate intolerance, especially monosaccharide malabsorption, is manifested by increased amounts of reducing substances in the stool and increased water loss.

Vitamins

Even in the very low birthweight infant, vitamin deficiency is encountered infrequently, especially since most preterm infants are given supplemental vitamins A, C, and D. Because of decreased activity of hepatic tyrosine transaminase, the ability of the preterm infant to metabolize tyrosine and phenylalanine adequately is limited. Vitamin C is a necessary cofactor that allows the infant to metabolize these amino acids normally. An adequate intake of the B vitamin is enhanced by the supplementation of the B vitamins in most formulas; also these vitamins are present in adequate amounts in human milk. Deficiency of vitamin K is rare in the term and preterm infant, as routine injections of this vitamin are given soon after the infant's delivery in the amount of 0.25 to 1.0 mg. Infants who receive antimicrobial agents may be predisposed to develop vitamin K deficiency and hemorrhagic tendencies. Administration of supplemental vitamin K every other or every third day while the infant is on antimicrobial agents tends to obviate the difficulties that the infants might encounter. Excessive vitamin K given to infants may lead to hyperbilirubinemia and cause hemolytic anemia. Vitamin E is poorly transmitted from the mother to the infant through the placenta, and the infant is born with low stores of this particular vitamin. If the infant has steatorrhea, vitamin E absorption may be markedly impaired. The preterm infant is predisposed to vitamin E deficiency because vitamin E is an antioxidant that may be exhausted if the infant is placed in high concentrations of oxygen for cardiorespiratory difficulties. The absorption of vitamin E appears to be decreased when increased amounts of iron are present in the diet. Also, if increased amounts of polyunsaturated fats are ingested, the requirements of vitamin E are increased. The absorption of vitamin E is unpredictable in most premature infants, and if the infant has vitamin E deficiency with hemolytic anemia, edema, hypoproteinemia, or a skin rash, an injectable form of vitamin E, which is at present a non-FDA approved drug, may have to be given.

Mineral and Trace Elements

The infant requires approximately 4 to 6 mEq of calcium/(kg)(day) and 2 to 4 mEq of phosphorus/(kg)(day). Ideally, maximum absorption of both is present when the calcium to phosphorus ratio is 2:1, a ratio found in human milk (Table III). In most modified milk formulas, although calcium concentration is much greater, the phosphorus content is also greater, and phosphorus tends to be absorbed more readily than calcium. Term infants fed cow's milk preparations may develop hypocalcemia, but such is not the case in infants fed human milk.

It has long been recognized that the preterm infant needs additional iron in order to

Table III. Estimated Mineral and Vitamin Requirements for Low Birthweight Infants

Mineral	mEq/kg/day	Vitamin	Amount/day
Sodium	2–3	A	500 IU
Potassium	2–3	Thiamine	0.2–0.4 mg
Chloride	2–3	Riboflavin	0.4–0.5 mg
Calcium	4–6	Pyridoxine	200–400 ug
Phosphorus	2–4	B$_{12}$	0.5–1.0 ug
Magnesium	1	C	25–50 ug
Iron	6–10 mg/day	D	400 IU
Zinc	2–3 mg/day	E	5–30 IU
		K	5–15 ug
		Folic acid	50 ug
		Niacin	5 mg

SOURCE: Modified from Ziegler, G. G. E., and Fomon, S. J., *Infant Nutrition*, ed. by S. J. Fomon, 2nd ed, W. B. Saunders, Philadelphia, 1974; Anderson, T. A., and Fomon, S. J., *ibid.*; and Fanaroff, A. A., and Klaus, M. H., in *Care of the High Risk Neonate*, ed. by M. H. Klaus and A. A. Fanaroff, W. B. Saunders, Co., Philadelphia, 1973.

avoid the complications of iron deficiency anemia. Modified cow's milk formulas with supplemental iron are currently available for preterm infants. However, in the low birthweight infant, an increasing amount of iron in formula has led to the development of deficiency of vitamin E. Also, the iron contained in human milk appears to be readily absorbed, even though the concentration of the iron is much less than in the iron-fortified formulas. Normal full-term infants fed exclusively on human milk for a period of 1 year, during which time they more than tripled their birthweight, had normal concentrations of hemoglobin and demonstrated no evidence of iron deficiency anemia. Whether this same type of absorptive facility occurs in the preterm infant remains to be investigated. It should be pointed out that indiscriminate supplementation of iron is to be avoided and at the same time appropriate amounts of iron may have to be added either to formulas or to human milk in order to enhance the absorption.

The deficiency of zinc in preterm infants is not readily recognized, but since there are marginal concentrations of zinc in both human and preparatory formulas, it is possible that zinc deficiency may be more common than generally recognized. Zinc deficiency is certainly a problem in infants who have malabsorption or who receive parenteral nutrition. It has also recently been demonstrated that patients with acrodermatitis enteropathica have decreased ability to absorb zinc. Although very few data are currently available regarding zinc requirements in infancy, it appears that the zinc content of human milk is adequate to prevent any complications of zinc deficiency.

Parenteral Nutrition

Total parenteral nutrition has been shown to be a very effective technique in the management of children as well as adults with severe gastrointestinal disorders, especially those which are complicated by extensive resection of the small intestine. This armamentarium has been of immense help to pediatricians caring for neonates with gastrointestinal catastrophes or various types of intractable diarrhea. It became obvious that the use of total parenteral nutrition might be of some benefit to small preterm infants in an attempt to supplement them with additional calories intravenously. Although the initial reports of the use of total parenteral nutrition in preterm infants were promising, as more and more experience was gathered, it became obvious that not all the small preterm infants could tolerate even 10% dextrose plus amino acids, let alone 15 to 20% dextrose.

Difficulties with hyperglycemia, hyperosmolality, acidosis, hyperammonemia, hyperaminoacidemia, and azotemia were encountered as well as those complications which are associated with the use of indwelling catheter. In order to avoid the complications of the indwelling catheter, peripheral veins were used to provide supplemental nutrition. The small preterm infants seemed to tolerate infusion of hypertonic solutions into peripheral veins much better than older infants and children.

Using peripheral alimentation, it was shown in a few preterm infants that the infusion of 12.5% dextrose and 2.5% crystalline amino acids providing 60 cal/(kg)(day) would result in weight gain and the maintenance of these infants in positive nitrogen balance. Although such is not the case in all infants, it is obvious that in some small preterm infants, if their metabolic activity is minimal, temperature control is exact, and they have no added complications, as little as 60 cal/(kg)(day) may be adequate to maintain minimal weight gain.

Fat Emulsion

Although a great deal of experience has been gained in Europe and Canada with the use of intravenous fat emulsions, it was not until recently that the drug Intralipid was approved for use by the FDA. Intralipid is a 10% emulsion of soybean oil that is stabilized with 1.2% egg phospholipid and made isotonic with 2.5% glycerol. It is rich in polyunsaturated fats, yields 1.1 cal/ml, and has a metabolic fate that is similar to that of naturally occurring chylomicrons. As with the use of glucose and amino acid infusions, the infusion of Intralipid has been a great asset in the care of infants and children with gastrointestinal difficulties. Its use in preterm infants has not been so extensive, but several factors have been observed. Intralipid clearance rates in newborn infants are similar to those of adults. Decreased tolerance has been noted in preterm infants of less than 32 weeks' gestation. Similarly, those infants who were small for gestational age have decreased utilization of Intralipid, which often is much more severe than that found even in the small preterm infant.

Concentrations of triglycerides and free fatty acids following the infusion of Intralipid in infants who are small for gestational age are often two to three times higher than that noted in term and preterm infants who are appropriate for gestational age. It has also been demonstrated in laboratory animals that Intralipid is not well metabolized when the animal is hypoxic, and it has therefore been suggested that if hypoxia is present, Intralipid should not be used.

In normal adults, it has been found that pulmonary diffusing capacity has been decreased following the infusion of Intralipid, and deposition of pigmented materials in alveolar macrophages has been observed at necropsy in patients who have received intravenous infusions of Intralipid.

Although Intralipid does not displace bilirubin from albumin, at least in in vitro studies, as the Intralipid is metabolized to release free fatty acids, these in turn might possibly displace bilirubin from albumin. Therefore, the judicious use of Intralipid in jaundiced infants is indicated. Increased concentrations of Intralipid in plasma have also been shown to interfere with the assay of bilirubin and have led to spuriously high readings of bilirubin in serum by certain spectophotometric methods. Hyponatremia has also been reported to occur when Intralipid is infused, especially if the emulsion is not cleared rapidly. This is due to the space-occupying effect of fat and results in a spuriously low level of sodium in serum.

Despite these precautions, a great deal of experience has been gathered in preterm infants with the use of Intralipid, which may supply as much as 40% of the caloric intake. Thus, a combination of Intralipid with glucose and amino acids can be infused in order to supply as much as 90 to 100 cal/(kg)(day). This infusion contains approximately 50% of the calories in the form of glucose, 40% in the form of Intralipid, and 10% in the form of protein.

Alcohol

Infusions of alcohol have also been recommended in conjunction with peripheral nutrition, and a solution containing intravenous fat, glucose, amino acid, and 0.5 to 1% alcohol has been used. Although many term infants and some preterm infants can tolerate intravenous alcohol, there have been reports of markedly elevated levels of alcohol in the blood of these infants despite the fact that only 0.5 to 1% ethanol was infused. Interestingly, many of these infants have no signs of ethanol intoxication, and only when very high concentrations of alcohol are found in serum are they correlated with evidence of apnea or lassitude. It has been our recommendation that intravenous ethanol not be used in preterm infants, because the activity of alcohol dehydrogenase in liver is markedly reduced in the term infant and might even be more greatly reduced in the liver of preterm infants. Thus, with the use of Intralipid, glucose, and amino acids, the need for an additional caloric intake with the use of intravenous alcohol is obviated.

APPROACH TO THE NUTRITION
OF THE LOW BIRTH WEIGHT INFANT

It is obvious that the digestive capacity of the preterm infant is developmentally impaired, and judicious use of oral feedings is indicated. It is also obvious that early infusions of fluid and glucose are indicated in almost all low birthweight infants, especially those weighing less than 1500 g and of less than 32 to 33 weeks' gestation. Oral feedings are begun when the infant's condition is stable and gradually increased as the infant is able to absorb and digest the nutriments adequately. As the oral intake is increased, the intravenous supplementation is appropriately decreased. Thus, the small preterm infant should be given intravenous infusions of approximately 40 to 60 ml/(kg)(day) for the first 24 to 48 hr, and the amount of fluid should be increased until the infant is taking approximately 120 to 150 ml/(kg)(day) by the end of the second week. If the infant has difficulties with oral intake, supplemental calories can be provided intravenously beginning with 5 to 10% dextrose and then gradually adding amino acids and Intralipid. The concentration of dextrose can be increased slowly to 10 and even 15%, concomitantly with the gradual addition of 0.5 to 1.5% of amino acids and 10% of Intralipid. By the end of the tenth day of life, 40% of the calories can be given in the form of fat, 50% from glucose, and approximately 10% from protein. Careful monitoring of the infant receiving intravenous alimentation is necessary in order to detect hyperglycemia, hyperosmolality, azotemia, and hyperlipidemia. Obviously, a multivitamin preparation must be used that supplies adequate concentrations of A, B, C, D, E, and K. The electrolytes and minerals are also added to the infusion as necessary. It is extremely difficult to provide adequate concentrations of calcium; as infants maintained on total parenteral nutrition for a period of time develop osteopenia.

Oral feedings should be introduced early, but, with use of intravenous supplementation, this can be done gradually. In some of the very low birthweight infants, total caloric intake by mouth may not be achieved until the infant is 30 to 40 days of age. It has been our practice to use human milk to feed low birthweight infants, especially those who weight less than 1250 g. We continue the human milk until the infant has regained his birthweight and often until the infant weighs 1500 g or more.

Realizing that pooled human milk often has a protein concentration of less than 0.8% and a caloric concentration of less than 17 or 18 cal/oz (0.5 to 0.55 cal/ml), we have increased the amount of intake of these infants so that they may have to consume 170 ml/(kg)(day) in order to receive adequate calories by mouth. Supplementation of human milk with cornstarch solids (polycose) and medium-chain triglycerides has been advocated in the small preterm infant, but their efficacy has not been carefully evaluated.

We have attempted to avoid the 24 cal/oz formulas as well as elemental formulas that have much higher osmolar concentrations.

We feel that human milk has a definite advantage in the feeding of the low birth-weight infant in that the quality of protein is "better" than that of casein and that various amino acids are present in increased amounts as compared with those found in casein. These include cystine and taurine, which may be essential amino acids for the small preterm infant. The calcium/phosphorus ratio of 2:1 of human milk enhances the absorption of both; the absorption of iron is enhanced in human milk, and the fat is extremely well absorbed even in the presence of low concentrations of bile acid. The various host-resistant factors in human milk, including secretory IgA, lysozymes, lactoferrin, and growth factors for lactobacilli, make this a very attractive method for feeding the "immunologically deficient" preterm infant. If fresh human milk is available directly from the mother, additional benefits from lymphocytes and macrophages can decrease the colonization of the gut with *E. coli* and probably *klebsiella*. Obviously, if the milk is frozen, the leukocytes are destroyed; and if the milk is pasteurized, much of the immunoglobulins is also destroyed.

We have encouraged mothers of preterm infants to collect their milk either by manual expression or preferably with an electric breast pump for use in their own infant. The parents tend to be fastidious in their hand-washing and milk-collecting techniques, and bacterial contamination has not been a problem. We have given this milk directly to the preterm infant. Not only do we feel that the milk is more readily digestible by the infant and has various forms of protective effects, but we find that the mothers are more intimately involved with the care of their preterm infant and have a greater sense of attachment to their baby.

It appears that we have come full circle in our thinking regarding the nutrition of small preterm infants since the days of Goodhart and Hess. Early feedings, the use of human milk in the feeding of preterm infants, and the careful monitoring of these babies has given us a greater facility in providing adequate nutrition without jeopardizing the infants in attempting to get them to grow normally. Attempts to "overfeed" the infant in order to get him to grow along the rate that the infant would have grown if he remained in utero probably are not feasible in most preterm infants. However, the ability to provide adequate calories for growth is certainly within the present realm of our knowledge and capabilities.

REFERENCES

1. Agate, F., and Silverman, W. A.: The control of body temperature in the small newborn infant by low energy infra-red radiation. *Pediatrics* 31:725, 1963.

2. Ames, R. B.: Urinary water excretion and neurohypophyseal function in full term and premature infants shortly after birth. *Pediatrics* 12:272, 1953.

3. Anderson, T. A., and Foman, S. J.: Vitamins in Infant Nutrition, 2nd ed., ed. by S. J. Foman. W. B. Saunders Co., Philadelphia, 1974.

4. Andrew, G., Chan, G., and Schiff, D.: Lipid metabolism in the neonate: I. The effects of intralipid infusion on plasma triglyceride and free fatty acid concentrations in the neonate. *J. Pediat.* 88:273, 1976.

5. Bakken, A. F.: Temporary intestinal lactase deficiency in light-treated jaundiced infants. *Acta Paed. Scand.* 66:91, 1977.

6. Cashore, W. J., Sedaghatian, M. R., and Usher, R. H.: Nutritional supplements with intravenously administered lipid, protein hydrolysate and glucose in small preterm infants. *Pediatrics* 56:8, 1975.

7. Cornblath, M., Forbes, A. E., Pildes, R. S., et al.: A controlled study of early fluid administration on survival of low birth weight infants. *Pediatrics* 38:547, 1966.

8. Davidson, M., Levine, S. Z., Bauer, C. H., and Dann, M.: Feeding studies in low birth-weight infants: I. Relationship of dietary protein, fat, and electrolyte to rates of weight gain, clinical courses, and serum chemical concentrations. *J. Pediat.* 70:695, 1967.

9. Day, R. L., Caliguiri, L., Kamenski, C., et al.: Body temperature and survival of premature infants. *Pediatrics* 34:171, 1964.

10. Fanaroff, A. A., and Klaus, M. H.: Feeding the low birth weight infant, in *Care of the High Risk Infant,* ed. M. H. Klaus and A. A. Fanaroff. W. B. Saunders Co., Philadelphia, 1973.

11. Goldman, H. I., Freudenthal, R., Holland, B., and Karelitz, S.: Clinical effects of two different levels of protein intake on low birth weight infants. *J. Pediat.* 74:881, 1969.

12. Goldman, H. I., Goldman, J. S., Kaufman, I., et al.: Late effects of early dietary protein intake on low birth weight infants. *J. Pediat.* 85:764, 1974.

13. Goodhart, J. F. *The Diseases of Children,* 9th ed. Blakestones & Co., Philadelphia, 1910, pp. 47–91.

14. Gordon, H., and Levin, S. Z.: The metabolic basis for the individualized feeding of infants, premature and full-term. *J. Pediat.* 25:464, 1944.

15. Grand, R. J., Watkins, J. B., and Torti, F. M.: Development of the human gastrointestinal tract: A Review. *Gastroenterology* 70:790, 1976.

16. Hansen, J. D. L., and Smith, C. A.: Effects of withholding fluid in the immediate postnatal period. *Pediatrics* 12:99, 1953.

17. Hess, J. H.: Premature and congenitally diseased infants. Lea and Febiger, Philadelphia, 1922, pp. 171–204.

18. Kagan, B. M., et al.: Body composition of premature infants: Relation to nutrition. *Am. J. Clin. Nutr.* 25:1153, 1972.

19. Katz, L., and Hamilton, J. R.: Fat absorption in infants of birth weight less than 1300 grams. *J. Pediat.* 85:608, 1974.

20. McMillan, J. A., Landaw, S. A., and Oski, F. A.: Iron sufficiency in breast-fed infants and the availability of iron from human milk. *Pediatrics* 58:686, 1976.

21. Oh, W.: Fluid and electrolyte management in neonatology, ed. G. B. Avery. J. B. Lippincott Co., Philadelphia, 1975.

22. Peden, V. H., Sammon, T. J. and Downey, D. A.: Intravenously induced infantile intoxication with ethanol. *J. Pediat.* 83:490, 1973.

23. Räihä, N. C. R., Heinonen, K., Rassin, D. K., and Gaull, G. E.: Milk protein quantity and quality in low birthweight infants: I. Metabolic responses and effect on growth. *Pediatrics* 57:659, 1976.

24. Reardon, H. S., et al.: Treatment of acute respiratory distress in newborn infants of diabetic and "prediabetic" mothers. *Am. J. Dis. Child.* 94:558, 1957. (Abs.).

25. Signer, E., Murphy, G. M., Edkins, S., and Anderson, C. M.: Role of bile salts in fat malabsorption of premature infants. *Arch. Dis. Child.* 49:174, 1974.

26. Smith, C. A.: Reasons for delaying the feeding of premature infants. *Ann. Paediat. Fenniae* 3:261, 1977.

27. Usher, R.: Reduction of mortality from respiratory distress syndrome of prematurity with early administration of intravenous glucose and sodium bicarbonate. *Pediatrics* 32:966, 1963.

28. Watkins, J. B., Ingall, D., Szczepanik, P., et al.: Bile-salt metabolism in the newborn. *New Engl. J. Med.* 288:431, 1973.

29. Winick, M., Brasel, J., and Rosso, P.: Nutrition and cell growth, in *Nutrition and Development,* ed. M. Winick. John Wiley & Sons, New York, 1972.

30. Wu, P. Y. K., and Hodgman, J. E.: Insensible water loss in preterm infants: Changes with postnatal development and non-ionizing radiant energy. *Pediatrics* 54:704, 1974.

31. Ziegler, E. E., and Fomon, S. J.: Major minerals, in *Infant Nutrition,* ed. S. J. Fomon. W. B. Saunders Co., Philadelphia, 1974.

27

The Low Birthweight Infant: General Considerations and Bilirubin Metabolism

John D. Johnson, M.D.

Infants weighing 2500 g or less at birth are generally considered to be of low birthweight. Until the 1960s this weight designation was also widely used to define premature birth. However, the work of Gruenwald (1966), Battaglia and Lubchenco (1967), and Yerushalmy (1967) in the 1960s has totally reshaped our thinking regarding infants of low birthweight (LBW). These workers have pointed out the necessity for classifying newborn infants both by birthweight *and* gestational age in order to understand morbidity and mortality risks more clearly. The Colorado classification of newborns uses birthweight, gestational age, and the pattern of intrauterine growth. Thus, infants of low birthweight (≤2500 g) may be born prematurely and be large, appropriate, or small for gestational age, or they may be born at term or postterm and be small for gestational age.

For the purposes of this chapter, we subdivide the low birthweight infant into two major groups, the preterm infant of less than 38 weeks' gestation, recognizing that such infants may have deviations from normal intrauterine growth, and the infant who is small for gestational age (SGA) with a birthweight below the tenth percentile on the Colorado growth scale, recognizing that such infants have wide variations in gestational age.

In the United States between 7 and 8% of all deliveries result in low birthweight infants, and approximately one-third of all low birth birthweight infants are SGA (Gruenwald, 1964). Thus, the incidence of preterm births in the United States is between 5 and 6%. In the United States, the incidence of low birthweight is considerably higher for nonwhites than for whites. There are also marked worldwide differences in the incidence of LBW infants, varying from less than 5% in Norway to almost 12% in Hungary and presumably even higher in many developing countries that do not have adequate birth recording. It has been estimated that about half the difference in infant mortality rates between the United States and certain Western European countries such as Sweden and the Netherlands can be accounted for by the higher incidence of LBW in the United States. The high mortality of LBW infants makes even small increases in the proportion of LBW infants assume major significance (Chase and Byrnes, 1972).

There is a striking relationship between LBW and neonatal mortality. The neonatal mortality risk for LBW infants is 25 to 30 times greater than for infants with birthweight greater than 2500 g and increases sharply as birthweight decreases. In the LBW category, mortality risks are markedly influenced by gestational age. A study from the University of Colorado demonstrated that infants with birthweights between 1000 and 1500 g who were preterm and of appropriate size for gestational age had a 50% mortality; infants of similar birthweight but with gestational ages of greater than 34 weeks (SGA) had a 13% mortality (Battaglia, 1970). Thus, for infants with comparable birthweights, the greater the gestational age, the lower the mortality. However, at any given gestational age, the lower the birthweight, the greater the neonatal mortality. Neonatal morbidity risks follow a very similar pattern to mortality risks when considering both birthweight and gestational age.

THE PRETERM INFANT

The pathogenesis of preterm delivery is incompletely understood. Epidemiologic studies have identified many associations with preterm delivery, but it is often difficult to establish independence of a particular factor from many others. Also, one should not confuse correlations or associations with true causality. The settings in which preterm delivery are most likely to occur are listed in Table I. The prevention of prematurity should be the major goal of perinatal medicine; yet our current inadequate knowledge of its pathogenesis allows us very few points of attack. One cause that is totally preventable is elective cesarean section prior to term. Advances being made in understanding the

Table I. Etiology of Preterm Delivery

Epidemiologic associations
   Lower socioeconomic status
   Primiparas and grand multiparas
   Both young (<20 years) and older women
   Women in developing countries
   Female infants
   Multiple births
   History of previous premature infant(s)
Maternal illnesses or conditions
   Uterine malformations
   Blood-group incompatibilities with sensitization
   Acute systemic infection
   Urinary tract infection
   Premature rupture of membranes with amnionitis
   Preeclampsia
   Incompetent cervical os
   Placenta abruptio, placenta previa
   Anemia
   Inadequate nutrition (?)
   Elective cesarean section prior to term

Table II. Physiologic Handicaps of the Preterm Infant

Handicap	Potential Pathologic Result
Pulmonary immaturity	Respiratory distress syndrome Wilson-Mikity syndrome Chronic pulmonary insufficiency of prematurity
Cardiovascular immaturity	Suboptimal perfusion Systemic hypotension Patent ductus arteriosus Congestive heart failure Persistent pulmonary hypertension
Inadequate thermoregulation	Hypothermia Hyperthermia
Central nervous system immaturity	Birth asphyxia Apnea Poorly coordinated suck and swallow: aspiration
Gastrointestinal immaturity	Diminished tolerance to oral feedings: malnutrition Fat malabsorption Necrotizing enterocolitis
Hematologic difficulties	Hemorrhage Anemia
Immunologic immaturity	Severe infections
Incomplete hepatic development	Jaundice Hypoglycemia
Renal immaturity	Acidosis Fluid overload Antibiotic toxicity

maintenance of pregnancy and the initiation of labor will provide the physiologic base line from which a more systematic analysis of deviations can be launched.

The physiologic handicaps under which the preterm infant must labor were lucidly presented by Levine and Gordon in 1942, and very little has been added since that time. Immaturity of pulmonary, cardiovascular, gastrointestinal, renal, nervous, hematologic, and immunologic systems contributes to the high morbidity and mortality of the preterm infant (Table II). A complete discussion of the physiologic handicaps is beyond the scope of this chapter. Several other chapters in this volume address specific difficulties encountered by the preterm infant in considerable detail. We consider one specific area later in the chapter, namely, bilirubin metabolism and jaundice.

THE INFANT WHO IS SGA

There are several known and many unknown causes of intrauterine growth retardation resulting in low birthweight infants who are SGA (Table III). The cause may reside in the fetus, itself, e.g., chromosomal abnormalities or congenital infections. However, growth retardation in most fetuses is presumably the result of an adverse maternal or placental environment. Low socioeconomic status, low or high maternal age, high altitude, and possibly poor maternal nutrition are factors that correlate with fetal growth retardation. Maternal smoking and drug use—heroin, alcohol—result in smaller-than-normal infants for gestational age. Rarely, specific placental disorders—infection, infarction, tumors—are found in association with SGA infants. Although placental size is generally reduced with intrauterine growth retardation, attempts to relate placental pathology to fetal growth have generally been unsuccessful. The smaller of discordant twins may be severely growth-retarded. One of the most important maternal conditions in which fetal growth retardation is seen is hypertensive cardiovascular disease. This is true both for severe, prolonged preeclampsia, and also for essential hypertension, renal hypertension, and the vascular disease of advanced diabetes.

Despite all these recognized associations of maternal diseases and conditions and SGA infants, many infants who are SGA are not suspected to be so prior to delivery, and in many instances the cause of fetal growth retardation is not obvious. In one recent series, only 33% of 105 SGA newborns were diagnosed antenatally. During this period 25% of all perinatal deaths were related to intrauterine growth retardation. Two-thirds of these deaths were stillbirths in undiagnosed SGA fetuses at or after 37 weeks' gestation (Tejani et al., 1976). Ultrasonic cephalometry, especially when performed serially, can improve the detection rate of SGA fetuses but still misses many and has a high inci-

Table III. Etiology of the Infant Who Is SGA

Inherent reduction in fetal growth
    Congenital malformations
    Chromosomal anomalies
    Congenital infections
    Twins
Maternal conditions
    Low socioeconomic status
    Low or advanced maternal age
    Poor nutrition
    Smoking
    Maternal addiction—heroin, alcohol
    Hypertensive cardiovascular disease
    Previous history of infant who was SGA
    Hemoglobinopathy (SS)
Environmental conditions
    High altitude
    Irradiation
    Teratogens
Placental conditions
    Infarction
    Hemangiomas
    Premature placental separation
    Single umbilical artery

Table IV. Physiologic Handicaps of the Fetus or Infant Who Is SGA

Handicap	Potential Pathologic Result
Inadequate placental "reserve" during labor and delivery	Fetal distress Stillbirth Asphyxia neonatorum Meconium aspiration syndrome Pulmonary hemorrhage
Disorders of carbohydrate homeostasis	Hypoglycemia (common) Hyperglycemia (rare)
Hypoxia in utero with increased erythropoetin production	Polycythemia, hyperviscosity: seizures, heart failure, respiratory distress
Decreased subcutaneous fat leading to poor thermoregulation	Hypothermia
Hypermetabolic state	Poor growth if not supplied with adequate calories
Impaired immunocompetence	Increased incidence of infection (?)

dence of false positives (Queenan et al., 1976). Campbell (1974) has suggested that the head/abdominal circumference ratio, determined by ultrasound, may be a valuable technique for assessing fetal growth in late gestation. This ratio is greater than 1 in the second trimester, about 1 at 36 weeks, and less than 1 in the last 4 weeks of gestation. In most SGA fetuses, reversal of the ratio late in gestation does not occur. Refinements in ultrasound measurements and the development of other diagnostic techniques for the accurate detection of the SGA fetus, thus facilitating fetal therapy or more optimal timing of delivery, represent major challenges for perinatologists.

The neonatal morbidity of the infant who is SGA has a different pattern than that seen in the preterm infant whose size is appropriate for gestational age (Table IV). There is a high incidence of fetal distress with resultant neonatal asphyxia and meconium aspiration syndrome in SGA infants. They are also quite prone to hypoglycemia and occasionally develop transient neonatal diabetes. Hyperviscosity secondary to polycythemia also occurs with increased frequency in SGA infants.

THE NEWBORN INTENSIVE CARE NURSERY

The present-day neonatal intensive care nursery can be thought of as an arena in which second-level preventive medicine as well as the more dramatic life support is being practiced. Although preterm delivery or intrauterine growth retardation may not have been prevented, many causes of morbidity in these low birthweight infants are recognized and fairly well understood. Morbidity can thus be anticipated and in many instances avoided. This approach has resulted in significantly reduced neonatal mortality and morbidity for the low birthweight infant over the past decade. Data from the province of Quebec show that neonatal mortality in both low birthweight infants and in those of greater than 2500-g birthweight is lowest for hospitals with intramural neonatal intensive care units (NICUs), only slightly higher for hospitals that have no NICU of their own but regularly refer sick and low birthweight infants to extramural NICUs, and significantly higher in hospitals that have no NICU and do not regularly refer sick and low birthweight infants to extramural NICUs (Usher, 1975).

Survival of infants with birthweights of 501 to 1000 g has increased to 30% or more in some units, and for those with birthweights of 1001 to 1500 g survival may be 75% or more. Overall survival for infants with the respiratory distress syndrome is 80 to 90% in many NICUs.

PROGNOSIS OF THE LOW BIRTHWEIGHT INFANT

Fortunately, follow-up of low birthweight survivors of NICUs indicates an improving long-range prognosis. Stewart and Reynolds (1974) have reported that 90% of infants with birthweight less than or equal to 1500 g treated at University College Hospital, London, between 1966 and 1970, are without detectable handicaps at a mean age of 5 years. Several follow-up studies of children surviving with the aid of mechanical ventilation as neonates have reported more than 80% to be free of significant intellectual and neurologic impairment.

Despite these encouraging statistics, mortality and morbidity rates can and should be reduced further. The Committee on Perinatal Welfare of the Massachusetts Medical Society (1971) analyzed perinatal deaths for that state for 1967 and 1968 and concluded that fully one-third of the deaths were preventable. Although the overall long-term prognosis for infants of very low birthweight is good, Fitzhardinge et al. (1976) recently reported that 48% of infants with birthweight less than or equal to 1500 g surviving with the aid of mechanical ventilation had significant handicaps on follow-up. Continued refinements in perinatal and neonatal care for the LBW infant will be necessary to improve these mortality and morbidity statistics further.

Many follow-up studies of the low birthweight infant have failed to differentiate between the true preterm infant and the infant who is SGA. Lubchenco and coworkers (1972) have reported that gestational age and birthweight are equally important in determining outcome. For a group of preterm infants, in any gestational age category, the incidence of handicaps increased with decreasing birthweight; infants with the shortest gestational ages had the highest incidence of handicaps.

On the other hand, term infants who are SGA have a low incidence of neurological handicaps such as spastic diplegia and an average IQ but high incidences of minimal cerebral dysfunction and of school failure (Fitzhardinge and Steven, 1972). Follow-up studies of SGA infants born in the era of NICUs should tell us whether aggressive treatment of asphyxia, hypoglycemia, polycythemia, and other disorders results in improved prognosis for this group.

Bilirubin Metabolism and Jaundice in Low Birthweight Infants

Hyperbilirubinemia occurs almost invariably in low birthweight infants, particularly those who are preterm. Its magnitude is greater than that seen in full-term infants, and its peak occurs later—at 4 to 6 days—than in term infants (3 days). Furthermore, a high incidence of kernicterus has been observed at autopsy in very low birthweight infants dying between 3 and 6 days of age, despite peak concentrations of bilirubin between 9 and 15 mg/dl, concentrations much lower than normally considered dangerous in term infants.

There are many pathological causes of exaggerated hyperbilirubinemia that may occur in preterm as well as term infants, e.g., red blood cell isosensitization and congenital infections. These conditions are well known to pediatricians. What is discussed here is our current understanding of bilirubin metabolism in the newborn and the factors that influence it.

BILIRUBIN PRODUCTION

Most bilirubin is derived from the catabolism of the heme moiety of the hemoglobin from senescent erythrocytes. In adults, this source accounts for 75% of total bilirubin formation. Accurate quantitation of the percentage contribution of this source to total bilirubin formation in newborns is not available. A priori one would expect greater bilirubin production, relative to body weight, in the newborn compared with the adult because of the increased red cell mass of the newborn and the known shortened red cell life span. Preterm infants have an even shorter red cell life span than do full-term newborns (Pearson, 1967). In fact, total bilirubin formation in the full-term human newborn has been estimated from endogenous carbon monoxide production or pulmonary excretion and found to be two to three times greater than in adults when expressed per kilogram of body weight (Wranne, 1967; Fallstrom, 1968; Maisels et al., 1971; Ostrander et al., 1976).

From simple calculations, it seems unlikely that the shortened red cell life span of the newborn can account totally for this increased rate of bilirubin production, so that one must consider other potential sources of bilirubin formation as contributing to the overall elevation of the rate of production. When an isotopic precursor of bilirubin such as ^{15}N-glycine is administered to an animal or man, a significant amount of isotopically labeled bilirubin is formed over the first 2 to 3 days following administration and is known as the "early-labeled peak" (ELP) of bilirubin formation. This peak accounts for about 25% of total bilirubin formation in the human adult (Berk et al., 1976).

The contribution of ELP bilirubin formation to overall production in the human newborn has not been clearly delineated. Although Vest (1967) found a greater percentage of the total isotopically labeled bilirubin in the ELP in newborns than others had found in adults—greater still in preterm newborns—the isotopic precursor of bilirubin in these studies was administered several days after birth, a time at which erythropoiesis is suppressed. Thus, the "late peak" of bilirubin production, that derived from red cell hemoglobin breakdown, may have been lower than that existing in early postnatal life from red cells formed in utero. Expressing ELP as a percentage of the total in these studies may be misleading. Nevertheless, by inference, ELP bilirubin production may be significantly elevated in the newborn period.

At least two sources of ELP have been identified. One is of erythropoietic origin, arising from ineffective erythropoiesis, hemolysis of "stress reticulocytes," and, presumably, breakdown of hemoglobin bound to the nucleus of erythroid precursor cells during the process of nuclear extrusion. It has been suggested that a subpopulation of red cells of the newborn behave like stress reticulocytes (Zipursky, 1965); the rapid destruction of these cells could contribute to elevated ELP bilirubin formation in the neonatal period.

A second source of the ELP is hepatic in origin and appears to result from the rapid turnover of heme, which serves as the prosthetic group for several hepatic proteins, such as cytochrome P-450, and which may also exist as a "free" or unassigned heme pool. The rate-limiting enzyme for the conversion of heme to bilirubin, microsomal heme oxygenase, has much higher activity in hepatocytes from newborn rodents than in adult animals, suggesting increased conversion of heme to bilirubin in the suckling period (Thaler et al., 1972). Furthermore, the activity of this enzyme system in liver increases in response to fasting, hypoglycemia, and glucagon or epinephrine administration (Bakken et al., 1972). Whether bilirubin production by the liver changes in response to these dietary, physiologic, and hormonal stimuli in the human newborn is not known.

From this discussion, it is plausible that several factors may contribute to the increased rate of production of bilirubin in the human newborn. Few studies comparing rates of production of bilirubin in low birthweight infants *versus* full-term infants have been reported. Total bilirubin production can be quantitated by determining carbon monoxide production or excretion, since CO and bilirubin are produced in equimolar quantitites during heme catabolism, CO is not significantly metabolized before excretion, and no other significant sources of endogenous CO are thought to exist. Qualitative estimates of bilirubin production can be obtained by determining blood carboxyhemoglobin concentration, and most studies on bilirubin production in the newborn have used this measurement. There is one study showing that blood carboxyhemoglobin levels are much higher in "severely jaundiced" preterm infants than in a group of normal full-term infants (Necheles et al., 1976). Landaw et al. (1973) have found higher corrected carboxyhemoglobin concentrations in a small group of preterm infants than in full-term controls. Gross and coworkers (1977) have recently reported that even healthy preterm infants have markedly elevated blood carboxyhemoglobin concentrations compared with full-term infants on day 4 of life, with the concentration in term infants being significantly higher than in normal adults. However, in preliminary studies, we have found only a slight difference in endogenous carbon monoxide excretion in healthy preterm infants during the first week of life when compared with a group of healthy term infants (Bartoletti et al., 1977). On the other hand, we have seen elevated bilirubin production in a small group of preterm infants of diabetic mothers. Gartner et al. (1977) did not find the endogenous load of bilirubin presented to the liver to be increased in premature monkeys compared with term monkeys; however, production is only one component of the endogenous load, the other being enteric reabsorption of bilirubin (see below). Further studies of the rate of bilirubin production under various physiologic and environmental conditions are warranted to define more clearly the role of production in contributing to neonatal hyperbilirubinemia.

BILIRUBIN TRANSPORT

Bilirubin is transported from its sites of formation to the liver firmly bound to serum albumin. The association constant for bilirubin binding to human albumin is approximately 10^8 at the primary binding site, and the binding capacity at this site is 8.5 mg bilirubin/g albumin. There are probably weaker binding sites with association constants of 10^6 to 10^7. Experimentally, once the primary binding site is almost saturated, bilirubin begins to appear in increasing amounts "free" in plasma and is deposited in cell membranes. It is at this point that toxic effects of bilirubin are observed, resulting in kernicterus or bilirubin encephalopathy.

It is now known that various exogenous and endogenous anions compete with bilirubin for access to the binding sites on albumin. Exogenously administered substances that are well known to be competitive in this binding are sulfasoxizole and salicylate. More recently, other effective competitors have been reported. These include the benzoate anion, used, for example, as a preservative for the intravenous preparation of diazepam; the parabens, used as preservatives in many pharmaceutical preparations; and several diuretics, including furosemide, ethycrynic acid and the chlorothiazides (Rasmussen et al., 1976; Loria et al., 1976; Shankaran and Poland, 1977; Wenneberg et al., 1977). It should be obvious by this time that any drugs introduced into the armamentarium of the neonatologist should be tested for this effect before clinical usage. Endogenous anions that may compete with bilirubin for binding to albumin include bile acids; hematin, which is increased in the presence of Rh-hemolytic disease; and high concentrations of free fatty acids, which are elevated in the presence of cold stress, starvation, hypoglycemia, and during intravenous administration of fat emulsions.

Although elevated hydrogen-ion concentration (acidosis) has been reported to reduce bilirubin binding to albumin, this effect has not been found using all binding assays (Jacobsen and Brodersen, 1976). Nevertheless, acidosis and anoxia predispose animals to bilirubin deposition in the central nervous system. The mechanism for these effects may be increased susceptibility of brain cells to bilirubin toxicity.

From this brief discussion of the pathogenesis of bilirubin encephalopathy, it should not be surprising that sick preterm infants frequently have pathological evidence of kernicterus at autopsy despite total serum bilirubin levels that are not considered dangerous in healthy term infants (Stern and Denton, 1965; Gartner et al., 1970). In addition to their low serum albumin concentrations (decreased binding capacity), such infants are frequently acidotic, hypoxic, starved, and subjected to cold stress—all factors that potentially increase the risk of bilirubin encephalopathy.

HEPATIC UPTAKE OF BILIRUBIN

Bilirubin is rapidly and selectively transported from plasma to hepatic parenchymal cells. The mechanism involved is not well understood. One view holds that there are specific receptors on the cell membrane of the hepatocyte that account for the uptake process. An alternative theory is that ligandin or Y protein, an abundant cytoplasmic protein found in liver, as well as kidney and small intestine, which binds a number of organic anions including bilirubin, is a major determinant of the net flux of bilirubin from plasma into the liver cell (Levi et al., 1968). The latter hypothesis is attractive, since this protein is capable of regulation because of a short half-life and induction or stabilization by various drugs and chemicals.

From the point of view of neonatal jaundice, hepatic ligandin is absent during the initial half of fetal life in several species and present at only 5 to 20% of the adult concentration at birth; its concentration in the liver of the newborn mammal then increases to adult levels in the first few days following parturition. It can be induced with phenobarital and its rate of synthesis decreased by starvation. If further investigation shows a definite role for ligandin in the hepatic uptake of bilirubin, these latter characteristics of the protein would suggest impaired uptake in the neonatal period and the capacity to alter uptake with various physiologic and pharmacologic manipulations.

Altered hepatic blood flow following birth, with a change from perfusion by an arterial blood supply to perfusion predominantly by portal venous blood, could alter hepatic function and bilirubin uptake. Patency of the ductus venous, brought about, for example, by hypoxemia associated with the respiratory distress syndrome, would impair uptake of bilirubin by diverting blood flow away from the sinusoidal circulation. All these areas deserve further study.

BILIRUBIN CONJUGATION

The major metabolic pathway for the hepatic biotransformation of bilirubin is its conjugation with 2 moles of glucuronic acid by bilirubin glucuronyl transferase to form bilirubin diglucuronide. The in vitro activity of this enzyme system was shown to be very low in the liver of fetal and newborn rodents (Brown and Zuelzer, 1958; Lathe and Walker, 1958). Subsequent studies have generally supported these early findings and have been extended to include the nonhuman primate. Gartner et al. (1977) have reported limited hepatic uptake and excretion of bilirubin in the newborn rhesus monkey, but hepatic conjugation of bilirubin was the rate-limiting step in bilirubin disposition, existing at only 5% of adult capacity in this species that does exhibit "physiologic" jaundice. The prematurely born rhesus monkey had even lower activity of hepatic bilirubin glucuronyl transferase, but only two such animals were studied.

In addition to this age-related limitation of bilirubin conjugation, other factors can influence conjugation capacity. Serum from pregnant women has inhibitory activity toward glucuronyl tranferase activity measured in vitro. Occasionally this inhibitory activity is very potent and results in transient familial neonatal hyperbilirubinemia (Arias et al., 1965). The inhibitory substance has not been identified, and its level does not always correlate with the degree of neonatal hyperbilirubinemia (Cole and Hargreaves, 1972).

The milk of 0.5 to 1% of breast-feeding mothers contains potent inhibitory activity toward bilirubin glucuronyl transferase and results in the syndrome known as "breast milk jaundice." The identification of this inhibitor as pregnane-$3\alpha,20\beta$-diol (Arias et al., 1964) has been questioned by a subsequent study showing that this steroid does not inhibit bilirubin glucuronyl transferase in human liver slices (Adlard and Lathe, 1970). Hargreaves (1973) has shown that unsaturated fatty acids of chain length 18 to 20 carbon atoms are potent inhibitors of the glucuronyl transferase activity of rat liver. Human milk contains lipase activity which allows hydrolysis of triglycerides in milk to occur and which probably accounts for the increasing inhibitory activity of stored milk. Luzeau et al. (1975) found that milk from mothers of infants with breast milk jaundice had higher lipoprotein lipase activity than did milk from controls. However, it is difficult to extrapolate these in vitro findings to the in vivo situation, especially since it is thought that fatty acids released during digestion are resynthesized into triglycerides in the intestinal mucosa. Continued investigation into the pathogenesis of breast milk jaundice will be necessary to further our understanding of this interesting condition.

Novobiocin is a known inhibitor of glucuronyl transferase. Starvation of newborn rats and experimentally induced hemolysis retard the age-related increase in enzyme activity, and phenobarbital increases the activity.

BILIRUBIN EXCRETION

Conjugated bilirubin is excreted from the liver cell into the biliary canaliculi against a concentration gradient and subsequently, in the adult, is reduced to urobilinogen by gut bacteria. Conjugated bilirubin cannot be reabsorbed across the intestinal mucosa, but the lipid-soluble unconjugated molecule can be. Although there is minimal enterohepatic circulation of bilirubin in the human adult (Lester and Schmid, 1963), the potential for significant intestinal reabsorption of bilirubin exists in the newborn period. The bacterial flora necessary for reducing bilirubin to urobilinogen are not present, and conjugated bilirubin can be deconjugated by the enzyme β-glucuronidase, which is present in intestinal mucosal cells. In fact, unconjugated bilirubin has been found in the feces of human newborns (Brodersen and Hermann, 1963). As mentioned, unconjugated bilirubin can be absorbed from the intestinal lumen. If it is not cleared from the portal circulation in one pass through the liver, it will gain access to the systemic circulation and contribute to the serum bilirubin level.

Although this potential exists, there is no easy or safe way to quantitate its contribution to the total hepatic bilirubin load and to neonatal hyperbilirubinemia in the human. Poland and Odell (1971) have fed agar, a substance that binds bilirubin in the intestine and prevents reabsorption, to a group of human newborns and demonstrated lower serum bilirubin and increased fecal excretion of bilirubin when compared with a control group. They have interpreted these findings as indicating interruption of the enterohepatic circulation of bilirubin in the agar-fed group, thus implying that normally this mechanism contributes significantly to "physiologic" jaundice. An alternative explanation for the effect of agar would be that it "traps" bilirubin diffusing from the intestinal microcirculation across the intestinal wall. Other investigators have found no evidence of decreased serum bilirubin following administration of agar.

However, certain clinical observations suggest that enterohepatic circulation of bilirubin in the newborn exists and is significant. Unconjugated hyperbilirubinemia is commonly seen in association with obstruction of the small bowel in the newborn. Stasis of excreted bile with deconjugation and reabsorption of bilirubin could explain this observation. Early feeding of newborns, even with sterile water, results in levels of serum bilirubin that are lower than those seen in infants who are fasted. Increased intestinal motility induced by feeding could reduce the time available for deconjugation and reabsorption of bilirubin. Further studies of the enterohepatic circulation of bilirubin should be conducted to clarify its role in producing neonatal jaundice.

SUMMARY

Despite numerous advances in the prevention and treatment of neonatal jaundice and a better understanding of its pathogenesis, we continue to be plagued by the occurrence of bilirubin encephalopathy in the sick low birthweight infant. More subtle neurological damage may be occurring in all birthweight categories, even with serum bilirubin values of 10 to 14 mg/dl (Scheidt et al., 1977).

Our current understanding of bilirubin metabolism in the newborn period suggests that several factors contribute to neonatal hyperbilirubinemia. An increased bilirubin load presented to the liver, probably secondary to both elevated bilirubin production and an enterohepatic circulation, and restricted hepatic conjugation capacity are important factors in the genesis of neonatal jaundice. Impaired hepatic uptake may also play a role. Further research in this area should be directed at quantitating the contribution of these factors under various circumstances and elucidating conditions that influence these steps in bilirubin metabolism. Perfecting bilirubin-albumin binding assays and correlating binding parameters with long-term outcome deserve continued attention. Only by a more thorough understanding of normal bilirubin metabolism will we be able to devise more effective approaches to the prevention and therapy of neonatal hyperbilirubinemia. A detailed discussion of the current status of therapy for neonatal jaundice—phototherapy, phenobarbital, exchange transfusion—is beyond the scope of this chapter but has been extensively reviewed by Maisels (1972). In the low birthweight infant, phototherapy and exchange transfusions are used at lower concentrations of serum bilirubin than in term infants because of the greater susceptibility to kernicterus.

BIBLIOGRAPHY

Arias, I. M., Gartner, L. M., Seifter, S., and Furman, M.: Prolonged neonatal unconjugated hyperbilirubinemia associated with breast feeding and a steroid, pregnane-3(alpha),20(beta)-diol, in maternal milk that inhibits glucuronide formation in vitro. *J. Clin. Invest.* 43:2037, 1964.

Arias, I. M., Wolfson, S., Lucey, F. J., and McKay, R. J., Jr.: Transient familial neonatal hyperbilirubinemia. *J. Clin. Invest.* 44:1442, 1965.

Bakken, A. F., Thaler, M. M., and Schmid, R.: Metabolic regulation of heme catabolism and bilirubin production: I. Hormonal control of hepatic heme oxygenase activity. *J. Clin. Invest.* 51:530, 1972.

Bartoletti, A. L., Ostrander, C. R., and Johnson, J. D.: Carbon monoxide excretion as an index of bilirubin production in newborn infants. *Pediat. Res.* 11:531, 1977 (abst.)

Battaglia, F. C.: Intrauterine growth retardation. *Am. J. Obstet. Gynecol.* 106:1103, 1970.

Battaglia, F. C., and Lubchenco, L. O.: A practical classification of newborn infants by birthweight and gestational age. *J. Pediat.* 71:159, 1967.

Berk, P. D., Blaschke, T. F., Scharschmidt, B. F., Waggoner, J. G., and Berlin, N. I.: A new approach to quantitation of the various sources of bilirubin in man. *J. Lab. Clin. Med.* 87:767, 1976.

Brodersen, R., and Hermann, L. S.: Intestinal reabsorption of unconjugated bilirubin: A possible contributing factor in neonatal jaundice. *Lancet* 1:1242, 1963.

Brown, A. K., and Zuelzer, W. W.: Studies on the neonatal development of the glucuronide conjugating systems. *J. Clin. Invest.* 37:332, 1958.

Campbell, S.: The assessement of fetal development by diagnostic ultrasound. *Clin. Perinatol.* 1:507, 1974.

Chase, H. C., and Byrnes, M. E.: *Trends in "Prematurity" United States: 1950–67.* U.S. National Center for Health Statistics. Vital and Health Statistics Series 3, No. 15, 1972.

Cole, A. P., and Hargreaves, T.: Conjugation inhibitors and early neonatal hyperbilirubinemia. *Arch. Dis. Child.* 47:415, 1972.

Committee on Perinatal Welfare of the Massachusetts Medical Society: Report on perinatal and infant mortality in Massachusetts, 1967 and 1968, December, 1971.

Fallstrom, S. P.: Endogenous formation of carbon monoxide in newborn infants: IV. On the relation between the blood carboxyhaemoglobin concentration and the pulmonary elimination of carbon monoxide. *Acta Paediat. Scand.* 57:321, 1968.

Fitzhardinge, P. M., Pape, K., Arstikaitis, M., Boyle, M., Ashby, S., Rowley, C., Netley, C., and Swyer, P. R.: Mechanical ventilation of infants of less than 1,501 g birthweight: Health, growth, and neurologic sequelae. *J. Pediat.* 88:531, 1976.

Fitzhardinge, P. M., and Steven, E. M.: The small-for-date infant: II. Neurological and intellectual sequelae. *Pediatrics* 50:50, 1972.

Gartner, L. M., Snyder, R. N., Chabon, R. S., and Bernstein, J.: Kernicterus: High incidence in premature infants with low serum bilirubin concentrations. *Pediatrics* 45:906, 1970.

Gartner, L. M., Lee, K., Vaisman, S., Lane, D., and Zarafu, I.: Development of bilirubin transport and metabolism in the newborn rhesus monkey. *J. Pediat.* 90:513, 1977.

Gross, S. J., Landaw, S. A., and Oski, F. A.: Vitamin E and neonatal hemolysis. *Pediatrics* 59:995, 1977.

Gruenwald, P.: Infants of low birth weight among 5,000 deliveries. *Pediatrics* 34:157, 1964.

Gruenwald, P.: Growth of the human fetus: I. Normal growth and its variation. *Am. J. Obstet. Gynecol.* 94:1112, 1966.

Hargreaves, T.: Effect of fatty acids on bilirubin conjugation. *Arch. Dis. Child.* 48:446, 1973.

Jacobsen, J., and Brodersen, R.: The effect of pH on albumin-bilirubin binding affinity, in Bergsma, D., and Blondheim, S. H. (eds.): *Bilirubin Metabolism in the Newborn II.* Amsterdam, Excerpta Medica, 1976, p. 175.

Landaw, S. A., Kandall, S. R., and Thaler, M. M.: Corrected carboxyhemoglobin (COHB) as an index of hemolysis in "non-hemolytic" neonatal hyperbilirubinemia. *Clin. Res.* 21:321, 1973 (abst.).

Lathe, G. H., and Walker, M.: The synthesis of bilirubin glucuronide in animal and human liver. *Biochem. J.* 70:705, 1958.

Lester, R., and Schmid, R.: Intestinal absorption of bile pigment: II. Bilirubin absorption in man. *N. Engl. J. Med.* 269:178, 1963.

Levi, A. J., Gatmaitan, Z., and Arias, I. M.: Two cytoplasmic proteins from rat liver and their role in hepatic uptake of sulfobromophthalein (BSP) and bilirubin. *J. Clin. Invest.* 47:61, 1968.

Levine, S. Z., and Gordon, H. H.: Physiologic handicaps of the premature infant. *Am. J. Dis. Child.* 64:274, 1942.

Loria, C. J., Echeverria, P., and Smith, A. L.: Effect of antibiotic formulations in serum protein: bilirubin interaction of newborn infants. *J. Pediat.* 89:479, 1976.

Lubchenco, L. O., Delivoria-Papadopoulos, M., and Searls, D.: Long-term follow-up studies of prematurely born infants: II. Influence of birthweight and gestational age on sequelae. *J. Pediat.* 80:509, 1972.

Luzeau, R., Odievre, M., Levillain, P., and Lemonnier, A.: Activité de la lipoproteine lipase dans les laits de femme inhibiteurs in vitro de la conjugaison de la bilirubine. *Clin. Chim. Acta* 59:133, 1975.

Maisels, M. J.: Bilirubin: On understanding and influencing its metabolism in the newborn infant. *Pediat. Clin. No. Amer.* 19:447, 1972.

Maisels, M. J., Pathak, A., Nelson, N. M., Nathan, D. G., and Smith, C. A.: Endogenous production of carbon monoxide in normal and erythroblastotic newborn infants. *J. Clin. Invest.* 50:1, 1971.

Necheles, T. F., Rai, U. S., and Valaes, T.: The role of haemolysis in neonatal hyperbilirubinaemia as reflected in carboxyhaemoglobin levels. *Acta Paediat. Scand.* 65:361, 1976.

Ostrander, C. R., Johnson, J. D., and Bartoletti, A. L.: Determining the pulmonary excretion rate of carbon monoxide in newborn infants. *J. Appl. Physiol.* 40:844, 1976.

Pearson, H. A.: Life-span of the fetal red blood cell. *J. Pediat.* 70:166, 1967.

Poland, R. D., and Odell, G. B.: Physiologic jaundice: The enterohepatic circulation of bilirubin. *N. Engl. J. Med.* 284:1, 1971.

Queenan, J. T., Kubarych, S. F., Cook, L. N., Anderson, G. D., and Griffin, L. P.: Diagnostic ultrasound for detection of intrauterine growth retardation. *Am. J. Obstet. Gynecol.* 124:865, 1976.

Rasmussen, L. F., Ahlfors, C. E., and Wennberg, R. P.: The effect of paraben preservatives on albumin binding of bilirubin. *J. Pediat.* 89:475, 1976.

Scheidt, P. C., Mellits, E. D., Hardy, J. B., Drage, J. S., and Boggs, T. R.: Toxicity to bilirubin in neonates: Infant development during first year in relation to maximum neonatal serum bilirubin concentration. *J. Pediat.* 91:292, 1977.

Shankaran, S., and Poland, R. L.: The displacement of bilirubin from albumin by furosemide. *J. Pediat.* 90:642, 1977.

Stern, L., and Denton, R. L.: Kernicterus in small premature infants. *Pediatrics* 35:483, 1965.

Stewart, A. L., and Reynolds, E. O. R.: Improved prognosis for infants of very low birthweight, *Pediatrics* 54:724, 1974.

Tejani, N., Mann, L. I., and Weiss, R. R.: Antenatal diagnosis and management of the small-for-gestational-age fetus. *Obstet. Gynecol.* 47:31, 1976.

Thaler, M. M., Gemes, D. L., and Bakken, A. F.: Enzymatic conversion of heme to bilirubin in normal and starved fetuses and newborn rats. *Pediat. Res.* 6:197, 1972.

Usher, R. H.: The special problems of the premature infant, in Avery, G. (ed.): *Neonatology.* Philadelphia, J. B. Lippincott, Co., 1975, p. 157.

Vest, M. F.: Studies on hemoglobin breakdown and incorporation of (^{15}N) glycine into haem and bile pigment in the newborn, in Boucher, A. D., and Billing, B. H. (eds.): Bilirubin Metabolism. Oxford, Blackwell Scientific Publications Ltd., 1967, p. 47.

Wennberg, R. P., Rasmussen, L. F., and Ahlfors, C. E.: Displacement of bilirubin from human albumin by three diuretics. *J. Pediat.* 90:647, 1977.

Wranne, L.: Studies on erythro-kinetics in infancy: VII. Quantitative estimation of the haemoglobin catabolism by carbon monoxide technique in young infants. *Acta Paediat. Scand.* 56:381, 1967.

Yerushalmy, J.: The classification of newborn infants by birthweight and gestational age. *J. Pediat.* 71:164, 1967.

Zipursky, A.: The erythrocytes of the newborn infant. *Semin. Hematol.* 2:167, 1965.

Index